Acute Medicine

D1323444

Acute Medicine

A symptom-based approach

Edited by

Stephen Haydock
Consultant Physician, Taunton and Somerset NHS Foundation Trust, UK

Duncan Whitehead
Consultant Nephrologist and Physician, Taunton and Somerset NHS Foundation Trust, UK

Zoë Fritz
Consultant Acute Physician, Cambridge University Hospitals NHS Foundation Trust and Wellcome Trust Research Fellow in Bioethics at the Universities of Warwick and Cambridge, UK

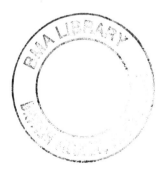

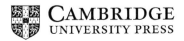

CAMBRIDGE
UNIVERSITY PRESS

University Printing House, Cambridge CB2 8BS, United Kingdom

Cambridge University Press is part of the University of Cambridge.

It furthers the University's mission by disseminating knowledge in the pursuit of
education, learning and research at the highest international levels of excellence.

www.cambridge.org
Information on this title: www.cambridge.org/9781107633575

© Cambridge University Press 2015

First published 2015
Reprinted 2015

Printed in the United Kingdom by Clays, St Ives plc

A catalogue record for this publication is available from the British Library

Library of Congress Cataloguing in Publication data
Acute medicine (Haydock)
Acute medicine : a symptom-based approach / [edited by] Stephen Haydock,
Duncan Whitehead, Zoë Fritz.
    p. ; cm.
Includes bibliographical references and index.
ISBN 978-1-107-63357-5 (hardback)
I. Haydock, Stephen, 1960– , editor.   II. Whitehead, Duncan (Nephrologist), editor.
III. Fritz, Zoë, editor.   IV. Title.
[DNLM: 1. Emergency Service, Hospital–Great Britain–Case Reports.   2. Acute
Disease–Great Britain–Case Reports.   3. Diagnosis, Differential–Great Britain–Case
Reports.   4. Emergency Treatment–methods–Great Britain–Case Reports. WX 215]
RA971
362.110941–dc23
2014032220

ISBN 978-1-107-63357-5 Paperback

Contents

Contributors

Iftikhar Ahmed MD MRCP
Specialist Registrar in Gastroenterology, North Bristol
NHS Trust

Chris Allen MA MD FRCP
Consultant Neurologist, Addenbrooke's Hospital,
Cambridge

Sani H. Aliyu MB BS FRCP FRCPath
Consultant in Microbiology and Infectious Diseases,
Department of Infectious diseases, Addenbrooke's
Hospital, Cambridge

Pawel Bogucki MB BS MRCP
Specialist Registrar in Dermatology, Royal Devon and
Exeter Hospital

Darshan H. Brahmbhatt MA MRCS MRCP
Specialist Registrar, Addenbrooke's Hospital,
Cambridge

Ewen Cameron MD MA MB BChir FRCP
Consultant Gastroenterologist, Addenbrooke's
Hospital, Cambridge

Peter M. F. Campbell FRCP
Consultant Physician and Geriatrician, Musgrove
Park Hospital, Taunton

Jane Chalmers MRCP
Specialist Registrar in Gastroenterology, Weston
General Hospital, Somerset

Wendy Chamberlain RGN BPhil MSc
Nurse Consultant Critical Care, Musgrove Park
Hospital, Taunton

Tony Coll PhD FRCP
University Lecturer/Honorary Consultant
Physician, Wolfson Diabetes and Endocrine Clinic,
Addenbrooke's Hospital, Cambridge

Gareth Corbett MB BS MRCP(UK) MRCP(Gastro)
Specialist Registrar in Gastroenterology,
Addenbrooke's Hospital, Cambridge

Julia Czuprynska MRCP FRCPath
Consultant Haematologist, King's College Hospital,
London

Carla Davies BM BS DTM & H
Core Medical Trainee, Musgrove Park Hospital,
Taunton

Mark Dayer PhD FRCP
Consultant Cardiologist, Musgrove Park Hospital,
Taunton

Edward Fathers MA FRCP
Consultant Neurologist, Musgrove Park Hospital,
Taunton

Mark Fish MD MRCP
Consultant Neurologist, Musgrove Park Hospital,
Taunton

Zoë Fritz MA MRCP
Consultant in Acute and General Medicine,
Addenbrooke's Hospital, Cambridge

Jonathan Fuld PhD FRCP
Consultant in Respiratory and General Medicine,
Addenbrooke's Hospital, Cambridge

Luke Gompels MRCP PhD
Consultant Rheumatologist, Musgrove Park Hospital,
Taunton

**Daniel E. Greaves BSc (Hons) MB BChir
MPhil MRCP**
Specialist Registrar in Microbiology and Infectious
Diseases, Clinical Microbiology and Public Health
Laboratory, Addenbrooke's Hospital, Cambridge

Emma Greig PGCertNutMed PhD FRCP
Consultant Gastroenterologist, Musgrove Park Hospital, Taunton

Stephen Haydock MA PhD FRCP
Consultant Physician, Musgrove Park Hospital, Taunton

Matthew R. Hayman PhD MRCP
Consultant in Acute and Geriatric Medicine, Musgrove Park Hospital, Taunton

Jonathan Hills BM BS
Department of Anaesthetics, Colchester General Hospital, Colchester

John Kalk FRCP
Consultant in Diabetes and Endocrinology, Musgrove Park Hospital, Taunton

Catherine Laversuch FRCP
Consultant Physician and Rheumatologist, Musgrove Park Hospital, Taunton

Cliff Mann FCEM FRCP
Consultant in Emergency Medicine, Musgrove Park Hospital, Taunton

Deepak Mannari FRCPath PhD
Consultant in Haematology, Musgrove Park Hospital, Taunton

Rudi Matull MD FRCP
Consultant in Gastroenterology, Musgrove Park Hospital, Taunton

Marko Nikolić MA MB BChir MRCP
Wellcome Trust PhD Programme for Clinicians Fellow, Cambridge Stem Cell Institute, University of Cambridge and Honorary Specialty Registrar in Respiratory Medicine, Addenbrooke's Hospital, Cambridge

Marguerite Paffard MRCPsych
Consultant Psychiatrist, Wellsprings Hospital Site, Taunton

Kate R. Petheram BSc MB ChB MRCP
Consultant Neurologist, Sunderland Royal Hospital, Sunderland

Lucy Pollock MB BChir FRCP
Consultant in Medicine for the Elderly, Musgrove Park Hospital, Taunton

Kobus Preller MB ChB MRCP EDIC DICM FFICM
Consultant Physician in Acute Medicine and Critical Care, Addenbrooke's Hospital, Cambridge

Christopher J. S. Price BSc MB BS PhD MRCP
Neurologist, Musgrove Park Hospital, Taunton

Peter J. Pugh MD FRCP FESC
Consultant Cardiologist, Addenbrooke's Hospital, Cambridge

Charlotte Rutter BSc(Hons) MB ChB MRCP PGCert TLHP FHEA
Specialist Registrar in Gastroenterology and General Internal Medicine, Gloucestershire Royal Hospital

Gillian Sims Dip Couns MBACP (Accred)
Alcohol Liaison Worker, Somerset Drug and Alcohol Service, Musgrove Park Hospital, Taunton

Robert A. Stone MB BS BSc PhD FRCP
Consultant in Respiratory Medicine, Musgrove Park Hospital, Taunton

David Tate MRCP
Specialist Registrar in Gastroenterology, Gloucestershire Hospitals NHS Foundation Trust

Paul D. Thomas MD FRCP
Consultant Gastroenterologist, Musgrove Park Hospital, Taunton

Satish Thomas William MD(STD) MRCP Dip. GUM Dip. HIV
Consultant in Genitourinary Medicine and HIV, Musgrove Park Hospital, Taunton

Andrew Thompson MRCP
Consultant Physician, Musgrove Park Hospital, Taunton

Marianne Tinkler MB BCh MRCP Dip Pal Med
Specialist Registrar in Respiratory Medicine, North Bristol NHS Trust

Gareth Walker MRCP
Specialist Registrar in Gastroenterology, Musgrove Park Hospital, Taunton

Stuart Walker MD FRCP
Consultant Cardiologist, Musgrove Park Hospital, Taunton

Nic Wenninke MRCP
Consultant Physician, Musgrove Park Hospital, Taunton

Christopher Westall MB BS BmedSci MRCP
Specialist Registrar in Acute Medicine & Intensive Care, Addenbrooke's Hospital, Cambridge

Duncan Whitehead MRCP AHEA
Consultant Physician and Nephrologist, Musgrove Park Hospital, Taunton

Rob Whiting MRCP
Consultant in Stroke Medicine, Musgrove Park Hospital, Taunton

Penny Williams MRCP
Specialist Registrar in Dermatology, Royal Devon and Exeter Hospital

Cally Williamson BSc (Hons) MCSP
Senior Physiotherapist, Musgrove Park Hospital, Taunton

Mohamed Yousuf MRCP
Consultant Acute Physician, Musgrove Park Hospital, Taunton

Preface

The assessment and management of patients presenting on the 'acute medical take' remains a fundamental skill for all physicians in training, whether they eventually intend to practise in acute medicine or in a medical specialty. With this in mind, the Royal College of Physicians in the UK have identified a core of around 20 common and 40 other medical presentations, which trainees should be able to competently assess and manage. These presentations, with minor differences, are common to several training schemes, namely Acute Core Common Stem (ACCS), Core Medical Training (CMT), General Internal Medicine (GIM) and Acute Internal Medicine (AIM), spanning the period from early medical training to the award of a Certificate of Completion of Training. The original idea for this book sprang from discussions with Cambridge University Press back in 2009. It was felt that a single volume that covered the approach to these common presentations would be a useful resource for physicians in training.

During development of the book, the lists of common presentations have undergone some changes with promotion and demotion of some conditions. For the sake of completeness, we have prepared chapters on presentations that are currently or were previously listed in the 60 important presentations. Each chapter by one or two authors covers a single presentation. A short scenario is included to put the problem into a clinical context and the reader is talked through the approach to such a patient by experienced clinicians dealing with such problems on a daily basis. Authors have been requested to consider common pitfalls and questions they are frequently asked by juniors when dealing with such problems. Initially aimed at registrars training in acute medicine, it is relevant to all physicians in training. The book should also be of value to medical students and foundation year doctors as they gain experience on the acute medical take.

Acknowledgements

In preparation of the text I was able to call on the help of some 50 trusted current and former colleagues from both teaching and district general hospitals. The fact that they (almost!) all made the required submission deadlines made a difficult editorial task much less onerous than it might have been. I am deeply indebted to all the contributing authors. I was also very fortunate in having the assistance of Duncan Whitehead in Taunton and Zoë Fritz in Cambridge. As the book progressed, it became clear that their help should be formally recognized, and I was pleased that they agreed to share the editorial responsibility for the final work. In addition, other clinicians at various stages of training from FY1 to consultant reviewed and commented on the draft chapters. I would particularly like to thank the following junior and senior colleagues for their helpful comments: Andrew Greenhalgh, Andrew Savva, Ben Grimshaw, Ed Saxby, Francesca Neuberger, Jemmima Scott, Joalice Stark, Jonathan Witherick, Paul Lambert, Susan Robinson and Sam Khanna. I am also much obliged to Nisha Doshi and Jane Seakins of the editorial team at Cambridge University Press who have been patient, supporting and above all tolerant! I thank them for all their help and advice.

Finally I must acknowledge and thank my wife Kate and sons Christopher and David for their support, putting up with my complaints and the many weekends I was sat in front of the laptop, drinking gallons of tea and answering their questions with grunts at worst and monosyllables at best.

Stephen Haydock, Williton, Somerset

Abbreviations

A&E	Accident and Emergency		BPH	benign prostatic hypertrophy
AAA	abdominal aortic aneurysm		bpm	beats per minute
ABC	airway, breathing, circulation		CAD	coronary artery disease
ABCDE	airway, breathing, circulation, disability, exposure/examination		CBT	cognitive behaviour therapy
			CD	Crohn's disease
ACE	angiotensin-converting enzyme		CI	confidence interval
ACS	acute coronary syndrome		CIWA	Clinical Institute Withdrawal Assessment
ADPCKD	autosomal dominant polycystic kidney disease		CJD	Creutzfeldt–Jakob disease
AF	atrial fibrillation		CK	creatine kinase
AIDP	acute inflammatory demyelinating polyneuropathy (Guillain–Barré syndrome)		CKD	chronic kidney disease
			CLL	chronic lymphocytic leukaemia
			CML	chronic myeloid leukaemia
AKI	acute kidney injury		CMV	cytomegalovirus
ALF	acute liver failure		CNS	central nervous system
ALP	alkaline phosphatase		COPD	chronic obstructive pulmonary disease
ALS	advanced life support		CPAP	continuous positive airways pressure
ALT	alanine aminotransferase		CPR	cardiopulmonary resuscitation
ANA	anti-nuclear antibody		CRP	C-reactive protein
ANCA	anti-neutrophilic cytoplasmic antibodies		CSF	cerebrospinal fluid
			CT	computed tomography
AP	alkaline phosphatase; anteroposterior		CTEPH	chronic thromboembolic pulmonary hypertension
APTT	activated partial thromboplastin time			
5-ASA	5-aminosalicylic acid		CTKUB	CT of kidney, ureter and bladder
ASD	atrial septal defect		CTPA	CT pulmonary angiography
AST	aspartate aminotransferase		CVE	cerebrovascular event
ATN	acute tubular necrosis		CVP	central venous pressure
ATP	adenosine triphosphate		CXR	chest X-ray
AV	atrioventricular		D2	dopamine D2 receptors
AVNRT	atrioventricular nodal re-entry tachycardia		DEXA	dual energy X-ray absorptiometry
			DI	diabetes insipidus
AVRT	atrioventricular re-entry tachycardia		DIC	disseminated intravascular coagulation
bd	twice daily		DIP	distal interphalangeal
BiPAP	bi-level positive airways pressure		DM	diabetes mellitus
BJP	Bence Jones protein		DNACPR	do not attempt cardiopulmonary resuscitation
BLS	basic life support			
BMI	body mass index		DVT	deep vein thrombosis
BNF	*British National Formulary*		EBV	Epstein–Barr virus
BNP	brain natriuretic peptide		ECF	extracellular fluid
BP	blood pressure		ECG	electrocardiogram

ED	emergency department	IM	intramuscular
EEG	electroencephalogram	INR	international normalized ratio
eGFR	estimated glomerular filtration rate	ITU	intensive therapy unit
ENT	ear, nose and throat	IV	intravenous
EPS	electrophysiological testing	K	potassium
ESBL	extended spectrum beta-lactamase	KUB	kidney, ureter and bladder
ESR	erythrocyte sedimentation rate	LAHB/LPHB	left anterior hemiblock/left posterior hemiblock
ESRF	end-stage renal failure	LBBB	left bundle branch block
ET	essential tremor	LFT	liver function tests
ETOH	ethyl alcohol	LMWH	low molecular weight heparin
FAST	focused assessment with sonography for trauma	LOS	lower oesophageal sphincter
FBC	full blood count	LP	lumbar puncture
FEV_1	forced expiratory volume in 1 second	LUTI	lower urinary tract infection
FFP	fresh frozen plasma	LVEF	left ventricular ejection fraction
FNA	fine needle aspiration	LVF	left ventricular function
FVC	forced vital capacity	LVH	left ventricular hypertrophy
GABA	gamma-aminobutyric acid	MAHA	microangiopathic haemolytic anaemia
GBM	glomerular basement membrane		
GCS	Glasgow Coma Scale	MAP	mean arterial pressure
GFR	glomerular filtration rate	MAU	medical assessment unit
GHB	gamma-hydroxybutyrate	MCA	Mental Capacity Act
GI	gastrointestinal	MC&S	microscopy, culture and sensitivity
GORD	gastro-oesophageal reflux disease	MCV	mean corpuscular volume
GRACE	Global Registry of Acute Coronary Events	MDT	multidisciplinary team
GTN	glyceryl trinitrate	MHA	Mental Health Act
GUD	genital ulcer disease	MI	myocardial infarction
HAS	human albumin solution	MMSE	Mini-Mental State Examination
Hb	haemoglobin	MRI	magnetic resonance imaging
HbA_{1c}	glycosylated haemoglobin	MRSA	meticillin-resistant *Staphylococcus aureus*
HCG	human chorionic gonadotrophin		
HCM	hypertrophic cardiomyopathy	MSM	men who have sex with men
HDU	high dependency unit	MSU	mid-stream urine
HELLP	haemolysis, elevated liver enzymes and low platelets	MTP	metatarsophalangeal
		MUS	medically unexplained symptoms
HOCM	hypertrophic obstructive cardiomyopathy	MUST	Malnutrition Universal Screening Tool
HR	heart rate		
HRT	hormone replacement therapy	NEAD	non-epileptic attack disorder
HSV	herpes simplex virus	NG	nasogastric
5-HT	5-hydroxytryptamine (serotonin)	NGU	non-gonococcal urethritis
HUS	haemolytic uraemic syndrome	NICE	National Institute for Health and Care Excellence
IBD	inflammatory bowel disease		
IBS	irritable bowel syndrome	NIHSS	National Institutes of Health Stroke Scale
ICF	intracellular fluid		
ICH	intracranial haemorrhage	NILS	non-invasive liver screen
ICP	intracranial pressure	NMDA	N-methyl-D-aspartate
ICU	intensive care unit	NSAID	non-steroidal anti-inflammatory drug
IHD	ischaemic heart disease		
IIH	idiopathic intracranial hypertension	NSTEMI	non-ST-elevation myocardial infarction
IL	interleukin		

NYHA	New York Heart Association
OCP	oral contraceptive pill
od	once daily
25OHD	25-hydroxy vitamin D
OTC	over the counter
PCR	polymerase chain reaction
PD	Parkinson's disease
PE	pulmonary embolism
PEFV	peak expiratory flow volume
PEG	percutaneous endoscopic gastrostomy
PFO	patent foramen ovale
PID	pelvic inflammatory disease
PIP	proximal interphalangeal
PMR	polymyalgia rheumatica
PMT	pacemaker-driven tachycardia
PO	by mouth
POTS	postural orthostatic tachycardia syndrome
PPI	proton pump inhibitor
PR	per rectum
prn	as required
PSA	prostate specific antigen
PT	prothrombin time
PTH	parathyroid hormone
PVD	peripheral vascular disease
qds	four times a day
RA	rheumatoid arthritis
RBBB	right bundle branch block
RBC	red blood cell
RF	rheumatoid factor
ROSC	return of spontaneous circulation
RRT	renal replacement therapy
RUQ	right upper quadrant
RV	right ventricle
SAAG	serum-ascites-albumin gradient
SALT	speech and language therapy/therapist
SaO$_2$	oxygen saturation in arterial blood
SBP	spontaneous bacterial peritonitis; systolic blood pressure
SC	subcutaneous

SIADH	syndrome of inappropriate ADH secretion
SLE	systemic lupus erythematosus
SNARI	serotonin noradrenergic reuptake inhibitor
SOB	shortness of breath
SOL	space-occupying lesion
SPECT	single photon emission computed tomography
SSRI	selective serotonin reuptake inhibitor
STEMI	ST-elevation myocardial infarction
STI	sexually transmitted infection
SvcO$_2$	central venous oxygen saturation
SVR	systemic vascular resistance
SVT	supraventricular tachycardia
TB	tuberculosis
tds	three times a day
TFT	thyroid function test
TIA	transient ischaemic attack
TLoC	transient loss of consciousness
TNF	tumour necrosis factor
TNM	tumour node metastasis
TSH	thyroid stimulating hormone
TTP	thrombotic thrombocytopenic purpura
U&E	urea and electrolytes
UC	ulcerative colitis
USS	ultrasound scan
UTI	urinary tract infection
V/Q	ventilation/perfusion
VaD	vascular dementia
VF	ventricular fibrillation
VIP	vasoactive intestinal peptide
VT	ventricular tachycardia
VTE	venous thromboembolism
VZV	varicella zoster virus
WBC	white blood cell
WCC	white cell count
WPW	Wolff–Parkinson–White
ZN	Ziehl–Neelsen

Introduction: presentations to acute medicine

This book has been written to serve several functions. We have noted many highly competent SHOs in medicine turn away from the medical career path due to fear of having the medical registrar on-call responsibility. There still remains a certain mystique and thankfully a respect for the 'med. reg.' on-call, the person in the hospital overnight who will know what to do, no matter what the situation; they remain *the lynchpin of the hospital at night*. Certainly the med. reg. should be experienced and knowledgeable, but a pragmatic rational approach applying fundamental medical principles to unusual or complex circumstances is often the asset that most sets them apart.

The conditions within this textbook and the scenarios described are situations that you will encounter, or may have already encountered, while on-call on the medical take.

To illustrate the diversity and relative frequency of presentations seen on the medical take we include the following table of 500 real unselected acute medical patients presenting to a busy district general hospital in Somerset. The conditions are listed in order of frequency within this group of patients, and it should be remembered that these are primary diagnoses. For example, the patient presenting with 'cough' due to

pneumonia, with an associated acute kidney injury and atrial fibrillation with a fast ventricular response, would be listed under pneumonia. The patient with a syncopal episode may be included under either 'syncope' or 'blackout' as there is an overlap in these two areas of the curricula!

The fear of medical SHOs (meaning all training grades between FY1 and ST3) to take the next step up the physician's career ladder is often misplaced and we believe the best way to achieve the required confidence as a recently appointed medical registrar is through knowledge. Included within these pages are many words of wisdom from a broad range of physicians and allied healthcare professionals whom the editors hold in high regard. There is advice that would enable appropriate assessment and management of each of these 500 acute medical patients included within the chapters of this book. This should augment your already significant knowledge base (*most medics are excessively modest about their knowledge*).

We the editors have learnt and applied many of the lessons held within this book during the editing process, and we are confident they will help you in your practice as a medical registrar and beyond as a consultant physician.

Table 1 Summary of 500 admissions to a busy District General Hospital in Somerset. To reflect seasonal variation, this was separated into 250 consecutive patients presenting during the summer and 250 during the winter of 2012. The primary diagnosis was identified from the discharge summary and categorized according to the Royal College of Physicians acute and general internal medicine curricula. Data collection and analysis by Dr Carla Davies BM BS DTM & H, CT1 in Medicine, Taunton and Somerset NHS Trust

Curriculum topic	Total (per 500 admissions)	Summer		Winter	
Chest pain	71	NSTEMI	11	NSTEMI	7
		Angina	10	Angina	4
		Non-cardiac chest pain	8	Non-cardiac chest pain	7
		Musculoskeletal chest pain	8	Musculoskeletal chest pain	10
		ST-elevation myocardial infarction	3	ST-elevation myocardial infarction	2
		Pericarditis	1		

Table 1 (*cont.*)

Curriculum topic	Total (per 500 admissions)	Summer		Winter	
Breathlessness	59	Congestive cardiac failure	8	Congestive cardiac failure	12
		Exacerbation of COPD	10	Exacerbation of COPD	14
		Exacerbation of asthma	1	Exacerbation of asthma	1
		Pleural effusion	1	Pleural effusion	4
		Anaemia	3	Anaemia	3
		Pneumothorax	1		
		Haemothorax	1		
Cough	53	Lower respiratory tract infection	12	Lower respiratory tract infection	12
		Community-acquired pneumonia	11	Community-acquired pneumonia	9
		Hospital-acquired pneumonia	3	Hospital-acquired pneumonia	1
		Aspiration pneumonia	3	Aspiration pneumonia	2
Leg swelling	24	Cellulitis	7	Cellulitis	7
		DVT	2	DVT	3
		DVT excluded	2	DVT excluded	3
Weakness/paralysis (stroke)	23	TIA	7	TIA	3
		Ischaemic stroke	9	Ischaemic stroke	1
		Haemorrhagic stroke	2	Haemorrhagic stroke	1
Palpitations	22	Atrial fibrillation	5	Atrial fibrillation	6
		Atrial flutter	2	Atrial flutter	5
		Supraventricular tachycardia	1	Atrial tachycardia	1
				Symptomatic ectopic beats	2
Dysuria	19	Urinary tract infection	10	Urinary tract infection	9
Sepsis	19	Neutropenic sepsis	1	Sepsis of unknown origin	2
		Urosepsis	6	Urosepsis	3
				Line sepsis	2
				Groin abscess	1
				Neutropenic sepsis	3
				Intraperitoneal sepsis	1
Poisoning	19	Mixed overdose	4	Mixed overdose	7
		Paracetamol overdose	1	Paracetamol overdose	2
		Opioid overdose	1	Opiate overdose	2
		MDMA overdose	1	Lorazepam overdose	1
Palliative care	18	Pain control	9	Pain control	9
Syncope and presyncope	17	Postural hypotension secondary to medications	2	Syncope	6
		Aortic stenosis	2	Cardiac induced syncope	3
		2:1 Block	1	Bradycardia second to medications	1
		Bradycardia	1		
		Anorexia causing bradycardia	1		

Table 1 (*cont.*)

Curriculum topic	Total (per 500 admissions)	Summer		Winter	
Falls	12	Multifactorial fall	4	Multifactorial fall	3
		Mechanical fall	3	Mechanical fall	1
				Medication-related fall	1
Haematemesis and melaena	12	Upper GI bleed	4	Upper GI bleed	8
Headaches	12	Hypertensive headache	2	Hypertensive headache	1
		Viral meningitis	2	IIH	1
		Chronic headache	2	Migraine	2
		Migraine	1		
		Idiopathic intracranial hypertension	1		
Dyspepsia	11	GORD	4	GORD	7
Acute kidney injury and chronic kidney disease	9	Acute kidney injury	4	Acute kidney injury	5
Fever	9	Viral illness	2	Viral illness	4
		Infective endocarditis	1	EBV	2
Diarrhoea	8	Diarrhoea and vomiting	3	Gastroenteritis	4
		Clostridium difficile	1		
Haemoptysis	8	Haemoptysis secondary to lower respiratory tract infection	1	PE	2
		Haemoptysis secondary to malignancy	2		
		Pulmonary embolus	3		
Confusion	7	Dementia	2	Confusion, unclear cause	2
		Acute on chronic confusion	1	Non-organic confusion	1
		Delirium secondary to steroids	1		
Weight loss	6	New diagnosis of malignancy	4	New diagnosis of malignancy	2
Blackouts	6	Complete heart block	1	Complete heart block	1
		Trifascicular block	1	Long QT syndrome	1
		GTN-induced collapse	1	HOCM	1
Rash	5	Exanthematous pustulosis	1	Viral rash	1
		Vasculitis	1	Viral papilloma	1
				Exfoliative dermatitis	1
Abdominal pain	4	Diverticular colitis	1	Abdominal pain	2
		Diverticulitis	1		
Incidental findings	4	Anorexia causing hypokalaemia	1	Anorexia-induced hypokalaemia	1
				Hyperkalaemia secondary to spironolactone	1
				Ventricle thrombus	1
Jaundice	4	Decompensated liver cirrhosis	1	Decompensated cirrhosis	1
		Deranged LFTs secondary to antibiotics	1		
		Chronic pancreatitis	1		

Table 1 (*cont.*)

Curriculum topic	Total (per 500 admissions)	Summer		Winter	
Anaphylaxis	3	Allergic reaction	2		
		Hereditary angio-oedema	1		
Fits and seizures	3	Seizure? cause	1	Epilepsy	2
Polydipsia	3	Diabetic ketoacidosis	1	Diabetic ketoacidosis	1
		Addison's crisis	1		
Polyuria	3	Poor diabetic control, high capillary blood glucose	2	Diabetes secondary to steroids	1
Pruritus	3	Gallstones	2	Gallstones	1
Visual disturbance	3	Hypertensive retinopathy	1	Central retinal vein occlusion	1
		Opsoclonus	1		
Weakness/paralysis (excluding stroke)	3	Viral neuropathy	1	Hyponatraemia	1
		Chronic idiopathic demyelinating polyneuropathy exacerbation	1		
Abdominal swelling and constipation	2			Constipation	2
Memory loss	2	Global amnesia	1	Global amnesia	1
Rectal bleeding	2	Inflammatory colitis	1	Crohn's colitis	1
Swallowing difficulties	2			Dysphagia	2
Unconscious patient	2	Hypoglycaemia	1	Addison's crisis	1
Unsteadiness, balance disturbance	2	Labyrinthitis	1	Labyrinthitis	1
Alcohol and substance dependence	1	Alcohol withdrawal	1		
Bruising and spontaneous bleeding	1	High INR	1		
Haematuria	1			Vasculitis	1
Head injury	1			Head injury	1
Immobility	1			Pain control, bony metastases	1
Involuntary movement disorders	1			Myoclonic jerks	1
Loin pain	1	Pyelonephritis	1		
Medical problems following surgery	1			Sepsis post transrectal ultrasound guided biopsy	1
Shocked patient	1			Spontaneous bacterial peritonitis	1
Vomiting and nausea	1			Unwell following chemotherapy	1

Four patients had two separate presentations.

Chapter

1

Abdominal mass/hepatosplenomegaly

David Tate

Introduction

The identification of an abdominal mass can be a stressful time for the patient. It is imperative to carefully formulate a differential diagnosis based upon the abdominal findings and the clinical context: *patients rarely present with just an abdominal mass*. A prompt diagnosis may enable the patient to quickly be reassured of a benign cause or rapidly provided with access to appropriate specialist care and treatment.

No table can be entirely inclusive on this topic; we are confident you could recall additional causes under each aetiological heading listed in Table 1.1.

> **Scenario 1.1**
>
> *A 75-year-old woman presents on a Saturday to the emergency department; struggling to cope at home, she reports a 4-week history of progressive abdominal swelling. During this time she has not been eating well and has lost a significant amount of weight. On examination she is cachectic and jaundiced; she has ascites and an epigastric mass which is 5 cm in diameter, craggy in nature and tethered to the underlying structures.*

This patient has been deteriorating for some time and unfortunately (*but not uncommonly*) presented out of hours. She probably has advanced cancer, and this should be recognized by the admitting doctor from the outset; the differential diagnosis at this early stage is wide and so this diagnosis should not be given to the patient without further confirmation.

History

A careful and comprehensive history is required. In particular:

Systemic enquiry ('red flags' for malignancy)

- Fever and night sweats
- Weight loss (unintentional ≥ 3 kg)
- Dysphagia
- Change in bowel habit
- Blood per rectum
- Visible haematuria
- Intermenstrual bleeding
- Anorexia

Family history

- Malignancy
- Polycystic kidney disease

Drug history

- Prescribed
- Over the counter

Social history

- Alcohol consumption (binges?)
- Travel history, including areas visited (rural or urban), activities engaged in (safaris, water sports, etc.); did they take malaria prophylaxis and have the recommended vaccinations?
- Sexual history (protected, high risk partners?)
- Intravenous drug use (clean needles or shared?)
- Occupation (e.g. sheep farming, associated with hydatid disease)

Past medical history

- Tuberculosis
- Diverticular disease
- Inflammatory bowel disease
- Solid tumours or haematological malignancy

The presence of 'red flags' requires the exclusion of malignancy as a priority when planning investigations, bearing in mind that they can clearly be compatible

Acute Medicine, ed. Stephen Haydock, Duncan Whitehead and Zoë Fritz. Published by Cambridge University Press. © Cambridge University Press 2015.

Table 1.1 Common and important causes of an abdominal mass by aetiology

Aetiology	Diagnosis
Neoplastic	*Malignant*
	Primary malignancy
	• Pancreatic
	• Colorectal
	• Hepatocellular carcinoma
	• Gastric
	• Renal
	• Ovarian
	• Endometrial
	Secondary/metastatic disease
	• Hepatic metastasis
	• Lymphadenopathy (testicular spread to para-aortic nodes)
	• Splenomegaly (CML)
	• Peritoneal spread
	Benign
	• Uterine fibroids
	• Lipoma (anterior abdominal wall)
Infective	*Abscess*
	• Diverticular
	• Appendix
	• Empyema of the gallbladder (may progress from cholecystitis)
	• Crohn's disease
	• Liver abscess (most commonly caused by ascending pathogens from biliary tract)
	Hepatomegaly
	• Malaria
	• Leptospirosis
	• Viral hepatitis
	Splenomegaly
	• Immune hyperplasia (bacterial endocarditis, EBV, etc.)
Vascular	*Abdominal aortic aneurysm*
	Hepatomegaly
	• Congestion (right heart failure/tricuspid regurgitation, may be pulsatile)
	• Budd–Chiari syndrome (hepatic vein occlusion, normally by thrombus)
	Splenomegaly
	• Portal hypertension (liver cirrhosis)
Inherited	*Renal*
	• Autosomal dominant polycystic kidney disease (ADPCKD)
	Hepatomegaly
	• Riedel's lobe (normal variant)
	• ADPCKD with hepatic cysts (♀>♂)
Mechanical obstructive	*Intestinal distension*
	• Obstruction
	• Constipation
	Renal enlargement
	• Hydronephrosis (severe)
	Bladder
	• Urinary retention
Degenerative	*Hernia*
	• Umbilical
	• Paraumbilical
	• Spigelian
Inflammatory	*Pancreatic pseudocyst*
	Hepatomegaly
	• Sarcoidosis
	• Early cirrhosis with portal hypertension (with splenomegaly)
	• Non-alcoholic steatohepatitis
	Splenomegaly
	• Sarcoidosis
	• Systemic lupus erythematosus
Metabolic	*Hepatomegaly*
	• Amyloidosis
Iatrogenic	*Renal transplant* (right or left iliac fossa mass with scar overlying)
	Implants
	• Buscopan pump (used in multiple sclerosis)
	• Gastric pacemaker
	Embedded peritoneal dialysis catheter (inserted ready for externalizing when dialysis is required)
	Incisional hernia
Idiopathic	*Splenomegaly*
	• Idiopathic thrombocytopenic purpura
Physiological	*Pregnancy*

with other aetiologies: a patient with a liver abscess will develop anorexia and lose weight, so initially it is important to keep an open mind and equally open differential diagnosis. Try not to increase the patient's anxieties at this early stage.

Examination

Perform a full examination of the patient, including: respiratory, cardiovascular and neurological examinations alongside the abdominal examination. Many pathologies resulting in an abdominal mass or organomegaly will have manifestations in other systems as well. There are often some subtle clues to the aetiology which may be present, so take care to examine for *anaemia, splinter haemorrhages and lymphadenopathy*.

Once organomegaly or a mass has been identified, examine it carefully and clearly document:

- site (consider which organ it may be, or is associated with)
- size
- shape
- nature (smooth or craggy, soft or firm)
- mobility
- reducibility (if it could represent a hernia)
- appearance of the overlying skin (scar, stretch marks).

In addition a *digital rectal examination and urinalysis are essential elements of the clinical examination which must not be forgotten*.

After completing the examination you may have findings that require you to go back and revisit the history. Patients rarely mind a few additional questions asked after or during the examination; it shows their physician is interested and considering their case carefully.

Investigation

Blood tests

- FBC
- U&E
- LFT
- CRP
- Calcium
- Clotting screen
- Tumour markers (use selectively, with caution)
- Blood film (if haematological malignancy is suspected)
- If infective symptoms
  - Blood cultures
  - Urine cultures
  - Stool culture (if diarrhoea)
  - According to history; malaria screening, HIV, hepatitis serology, CMV, EBV

These can be helpful in narrowing the differential diagnosis and identifying the unwell from the clinically stable patient.

- Anaemia is *never normal* and always has a cause or causes; it should prompt haematinics (B_{12}, folate, iron studies) to be checked and acted upon.

- Raised inflammatory markers suggest infection, but are significantly raised in IBD and frequently elevated with neoplasia.
- Low albumin, raised platelet count and anaemia all suggest neoplasia, but are compatible with significant inflammation of other causes.
- Tumour markers *should be used with caution in assisting initial diagnosis* as none are specific for a given malignant disease; they are more useful for monitoring response to treatment:
  - CA19-9, pancreatic cancer
  - CA125, ovarian cancer
  - CEA, colorectal cancer.

Radiological imaging

Always give careful consideration to deciding the most appropriate initial imaging modality (Table 1.2). The aim is to gain *accurate diagnostic information in the shortest time frame with the minimum of risk to the patient*. The modality selected will depend upon the differential diagnosis formed, which guides *the question you are asking of the imaging*:

- Has this well 45-year-old woman with nodular hepatomegaly whose grandfather died of renal failure got ADPCKD with multiple liver cysts?
- *Ultrasound scanning will rapidly answer this question with virtually no risk to the patient.*
- In the 53-year-old male smoker who drinks 50 units of alcohol a week, who has lost 6 kg of weight over 2 months and examination revealed craggy hepatomegaly and anaemia, the question needing an answer is 'has he got cancer?' and if so 'what is the primary and has it metastasized?'
- *CT chest, abdomen and pelvis with contrast is the first-line imaging modality of choice, giving diagnostic and prognostic information, also clarifying potential biopsy sites for histological confirmation.*

It is not the case that USS is more sensitive for liver lesions than CT, but it does avoid exposing the patient to the risks of ionizing radiation and iodinated contrast.

Surgical exploration

Despite modern imaging modalities, in certain circumstances surgical exploration by laparotomy or more frequently laparoscopy into the cause of an abdominal mass is still warranted. This needs careful

Table 1.2 Comparison of different abdominal imaging modalities

Modality	Advantages	Disadvantages
Ultrasound	Excellent in experienced hands Modality of choice for RUQ pain, acute jaundice and pelvic masses	Limited by body habitus Limited by operator experience Limited information on metastatic spread or tissue invasion Images not standardized and more difficult to interpret for someone who has not performed the scan
CT	Quick to perform Readily available Wealth of experience in interpretation Can detect metastatic spread, and tissue invasion Easily reviewed by multidisciplinary team (MDT)	High dose of ionizing radiation Limited resolution compared to MRI Iodinated contrast exposure (see Chapter 39)
Abdominal X-ray	Good acute investigation to exclude obstruction and toxic bowel dilatation	If normal may need further imaging Will often require CT imaging if abnormal
MRI	Excellent diagnostic detail	Not readily available Difficult to interpret (limited expertise) Slow image acquisition Claustrophobic patients often struggle with the examination

Adapted from the American College of Radiology, 2010 [1].

consideration and discussion between the physician, surgeon and patient.

Strengths

- Direct visualization
- Potential to biopsy abnormal tissues if seen
- Can proceed to definitive operation (if included in the consent process)

Weaknesses

- Risk of general anaesthesia and paralysis
- Operative risk (infections, bleeding, pain, etc.)
- Expensive
- Emotional trauma and anxiety provoking

Although laparoscopy can be an excellent tool in the evaluation of the abdominal mass, it is rarely required.

Endoscopy

Endoscopy (*gastroscopy and colonoscopy*) is usually performed in response to imaging showing a suspected lesion of gastric or colonic origin. It is the only investigation to provide direct visualization of the gastrointestinal mucosa. *Gastroscopy* is the first-line investigation for patients presenting with dysphagia or an epigastric mass, alongside CT imaging of the abdomen. Endoscopic ultrasound can provide excellent definition of mucosal and deeper infiltration of cancers. It is often the modality of choice for determining operability of cancers, particularly oesophageal.

Acute management of 'suspected cancer'

> **Scenario 1.1 continued**
>
> *A CT chest, abdomen and pelvis is requested. The CT imaging reveals a tumour at the head of the pancreas (Figure 1.1), which was invading local structures. Metastases are evident in the liver and a large amount of ascites is present. Following the CT scan the patient and her son were keen to know what it showed. It was explained that a pancreatic mass was seen and this might represent cancer; however, it was made clear to them that at this point the diagnosis was not confirmed, but further results would soon be available and diagnostic certainty was needed before any specific treatments could be planned. Abdominal paracentesis was performed and ascitic fluid sent for urgent cytological examination. The next day the cytology from her ascitic fluid had been processed and showed adenocarcinoma cells.*

It is clear from the previous imaging discussion that a contrast-enhanced CT of chest, abdomen and pelvis was the most appropriate first-line imaging. This was likely to reveal the nature of the primary tumour with information about distant spread. When cancer is suspected, cytology or histology should always be obtained if possible to confirm the diagnosis and classify the type of cancer. *Beware the many cancer mimics which have caused physicians to mistakenly diagnose cancer from CT scans!*

For this patient urgent sampling of the ascitic fluid for cytology was the easiest and safest way to try to confirm the diagnosis.

Ensuring the diagnosis is followed up – the MDT approach

NICE recommends that every patient with a new diagnosis of cancer is reviewed by an MDT (multidisciplinary team) meeting. Such meetings (e.g. upper GI, lower GI, gynaecological) commonly involve the relevant physician, surgeon, radiologist, pathologist, oncologist and oncology specialist nurse. The patient's current performance status and co-morbidities are considered alongside the CT imaging, cytology and pathology results. The tumour is staged according to the TNM classification (Box 1.1). Initial treatment is decided: surgery, chemotherapy, radiotherapy or symptom control and palliative care.

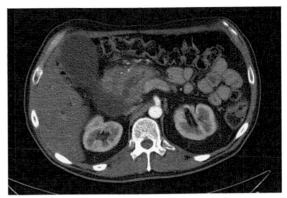

Figure 1.1

Box 1.1 TNM staging of cancer
Tumour – T1–T4 describes different levels of local invasion specific to the type of tumour
Nodes – N0–N3
Metastases – M0/M1 indicates presence or absence of metastases

---

Within the NHS, quality targets exist for the investigation of symptoms suggestive of a cancer diagnosis and subsequent treatment [2–4].

- All patients referred with suspected cancer from a GP have a maximum wait of 2 weeks from referral to see a specialist.
- All cancer patients should wait no more than one month (31 days) from diagnosis to first definitive treatment.
- A maximum 2-month (62-day) wait from urgent GP referral for suspected cancer to first definitive treatment for all cancers.

If a patient is referred to the acute medical take with suspected cancer, the admitting team should always consider whether outpatient investigation would be more appropriate. Systems are in place to ensure the rapid outpatient investigation of patients with suspected malignancy. Admission may be required for associated problems:

- symptom control, e.g. pain, breathlessness
- inability to cope in their current state and home circumstances
- emergency complication, e.g. acute cord compression.

If they are to be discharged, *robust arrangements for appropriate investigations and follow-up should be in place at discharge*; this should not impede early discharge.

Communicating bad news

It is frequently the responsibility of the medical team looking after the patient on the ward to communicate the prognosis and treatment plan to the patient. It is devastating for most patients and relatives when a diagnosis of cancer is given and this must be given with the utmost sensitivity. Once the diagnosis has been confirmed, it should be communicated in as timely a manner as possible. In this setting some patients are fully aware of the likely cause of their recent ill health, others are either in denial or blissfully ignorant of the true situation.

Communication of a cancer diagnosis requires a thoughtful and empathic approach. In some situations the hospital palliative care team and oncology nurse specialists can be called upon to help support these conversations. They can offer continuity, accessibility and time to patients and their families unrivalled by physicians; their role should never be underestimated and they should be involved as early as possible in such cases.

The principles of breaking bad news

- Choose an appropriate location; quiet and unlikely to be disturbed.
- Allow time to perform this vital role properly without rushing the patient or their relatives.
- Ensure that you know who you are speaking to and have the patient's consent.
- Check prior knowledge.
- Send a 'warning shot'.
- Explain in clear and easy to understand language the diagnosis and the likely outcome.
- Do not shy away from words like 'cancer'; all too often 'tumour' or other medical terminology is used, which clouds the situation.
- Ensure that the family and patient have a follow-up plan and have a point of contact (often the specialist cancer nurse).

Communication should be honest and upfront at all times. There is often heightened emotion which can be represented as anger towards medical and nursing staff in this situation; this should be handled sensitively and not taken personally.

Imagining yourself in the patient's or the relative's shoes is a distressing and uncomfortable exercise, but it clearly helps empathy with the patient and better appreciation of their reactions. The need for simple clear unambiguous language in delivering this news can never be overstated. Repetition of the message can also be valuable as it can be 'blocked out' initially by patients or their relatives.

Enlargement of liver and/or spleen

Hepatosplenomegaly

The commonest cause of hepatosplenomegaly in the UK is liver cirrhosis with portal hypertension (Table 1.3). This can present acutely and is often seen by acute physicians and intensivists.

The acute complications seen in these patients are generally related to the portal hypertension:

- Ascites with associated risk of spontaneous bacterial peritonitis (see Chapter 3)
- Oesophageal and gastric varices, which can bleed torrentially (see Chapter 26)
- Hepatic encephalopathy, certainly under-recognized at admission (see Chapter 36)
- Hepatorenal failure, less common at presentation but also indicates a poor prognosis; bear in mind

that hypovolaemia is the commonest precipitator of acute kidney injury in this patient group.

In addition, significant hepatosplenomegaly is commonly encountered in the context of both myeloproliferative and lymphoproliferative disorders. Outside the UK, the following causes predominate:

- malaria
- tuberculosis
- schistosomiasis
- kala-azar.

Isolated hepatomegaly

Hepatomegaly commonly results from cirrhosis (usually alcoholic in origin), malignancy and congestion due to cardiac failure (Table 1.4). It can be misdiagnosed in patients with hyperinflation due to COPD, due to downward displacement of the liver by the diaphragm. It may arise acutely, when it is frequently painful and/or tender as in viral or alcoholic hepatitis, or chronically, and more commonly painless as in fatty liver or amyloidosis. The presence of hepatomegaly should be confirmed by ultrasound imagining, which will provide information regarding the liver architecture.

The size of the liver is not an indicator of the severity of disease as demonstrated in ADPCKD where occasionally massive hepatomegaly occurs with minimal impairment of liver function.

Isolated splenomegaly

The spleen is the largest lymphoid organ at 7–10 cm in length, and only has efferent lymphatic vessels. It is generally only palpable when twice normal size. For this reason splenomegaly is often diagnosed on imaging rather than examination. The functions of the spleen should be recalled when managing the patient with splenomegaly.

Splenic functions include:

- reservoir of erythrocytes and thrombocytes, in case of significant haemorrhage
- destruction and recycling of old erythrocytes, life span ≈120 days
- immune function destroying many bacteria and viruses that enter the circulation, especially important for encapsulated bacteria: *Pneumococcus*, *Meningococcus*, *Haemophilus influenzae* type b (Hib), *Klebsiella*, salmonella and group B streptococcus
- haematopoiesis during gestation.

Table 1.3 Common causes of significant hepatosplenomegaly that may present on the acute medical take

Aetiology	Comments
Portal hypertension	
• Liver cirrhosis	Stigmata of chronic liver disease
• Budd–Chiari syndrome	Rapid development of ascites with pain
Myeloproliferative disorders	
• Chronic myeloid leukaemia	
• Myelofibrosis	
Lymphoproliferative disorders	
• Lymphoma	Associated lymphadenopathy
• Chronic lymphatic leukaemia	
Infectious	
• Viral hepatitis	Stigmata of intravenous drug use
• EBV, CMV, toxoplasmosis	Glandular fever like illnesses
• Brucellosis	Farmers
• Leptospirosis	Environmental exposure to pathogen, jaundiced
• Malaria, schistosomiasis, kala-azar, tuberculosis	Patient travel history, outside of UK (although TB increasingly present in some UK communities)
Metabolic	
• Amyloidosis	May have evidence of primary cause
• Gaucher's disease (glucocerebrosidase deficiency)	May be massive splenomegaly in patient with known diagnosis
Blood dyscrasias	
• Sickle cell disease	Characteristic features in patient with known diagnosis
• Thalassaemia major	

Thankfully for the asplenic patient it is not the seat of 'one's emotions or passions', as our predecessors thought!

The cause of enlargement may be pathology requiring upregulation of these functions:

- *Increased turnover of red blood cells* as in inherited spherocytosis.
- *Increased immune activity* due to infection, most commonly in the UK due to glandular fever (Epstein–Barr virus), but the infective causes are numerous and include several tropical diseases:
  - malaria*
  - leishmaniasis*
  - trypanosomiasis
  - ehrlichiosis
  - brucellosis
  - typhoid fever.
- Abnormal immunoregulation in some patients with autoimmune conditions such as SLE and rheumatoid arthritis can also result in splenomegaly.
- *Haematopoiesis* and splenic enlargement can occur in adult life if the bone marrow is failing, as in myelofibrosis*.

Other mechanisms (and examples) for development of splenomegaly include:

- *Infiltrative*: amyloid, sarcoidosis, metastases or in Gaucher's disease*
- *Neoplastic*: lymphomas, chronic lymphocytic leukaemia (CLL) and chronic myeloid leukaemia* (CML)
- *Congestive*: increased pressure within the venous system such as portal hypertension or more rarely splenic vein thrombosis.

(*May cause 'massive' splenomegaly >20 cm in length.)

Acute complications of splenomegaly

Left upper quadrant pain: this can be the presenting feature of patients with splenomegaly, most likely occurring as with most organ pain from rapid expansion or inflammation.

Hypersplenism is an abnormally high rate and premature destruction of circulating blood cells; this may result due to the underlying cause of the splenomegaly such as in chronic malaria or TB. The complications include:

Table 1.4 Common causes of significant isolated hepatomegaly that may present on the acute medical take

Aetiology	Comments
Cancer	
• Hepatocellular carcinoma	Hepatoma may occur in context of cirrhosis
• Secondary deposits	Malignancy often causes tender nodular hepatomegaly
Toxic	
• Alcoholic hepatitis	Stigmata of alcoholic liver disease
• Alcoholic cirrhosis	Acute alcoholic hepatitis is frequently painful
Lymphoproliferative disorders	
• Lymphoma	Associated lymphadenopathy
• CLL	
Infectious	
• Viral infections, e.g. hepatitis, EBV	History of intravenous drug use or recent glandular fever like illness
• Leptospirosis	Environmental exposure to pathogen, jaundiced
• Hydatid disease	Sheep farmers, especially in Wales
• Amoebic abscess	Tropical exposure
Liver congestion	
• Cardiac failure	Other features of right heart failure
• Budd–Chiari syndrome	Rapid development of ascites with pain
• Tricuspid regurgitation	Pulsatile liver
Metabolic/granulomatous	
• Haemochromatosis	Slate grey skin pigmentation, hypogonadism, diabetes mellitus, arthritis, cardiomyopathy
• Amyloidosis	May be evidence of primary cause
• Sarcoidosis	Lupus pernio, erythema nodosum, hilar lymphadenopathy, hypercalcaemia
Miscellaneous	
• Riedel's lobe	Tongue-like enlargement of right lobe of liver. Benign anatomical variant
• COPD	Spurious apparent enlargement due to downward displacement of diaphragm

- thrombocytopenia and potentially spontaneous bruising
- anaemia
- leucopenia and potentially serious secondary sepsis.

Splenic rupture: any patient with an enlarged spleen should be cautioned to avoid contact sports or heavy lifting activities which may increase the risk of splenic rupture. This will often cause a large intra-abdominal bleed and hypovolaemic shock, requiring urgent surgical assessment. This is a recognized cause of death in patients with EBV infection.

References

1. American College of Radiology. Appropriateness Criteria, 2010.

2. NICE. Referral guidelines for suspected cancer CG27. Clinical Guideline, 2005. Available to download at www.nice.org.uk/cg027.

3. HM Government. Cancer Reform Strategy, 2007. Available to download at www.nhs.uk/NHSEngland/NSF/Documents/Cancer%20Reform%20Strategy.pdf.

4. Department of Health. National Cancer Strategy, 2011. Available to download at www.gov.uk/government/publications/the-national-cancer-strategy.

Abdominal pain

Stephen Haydock and Gareth Walker

Introduction

Establishing the cause of abdominal pain can be diagnostically challenging in certain patient groups such as the elderly, women (especially if pregnant) and immunosuppressed. A successful approach should be based upon:

- understanding of the mechanisms of how pain is generated and/or perceived in relation to abdominal structures
- recognizing that patterns of presentation exist based upon the localization of the pain, its quality and radiation
- recognizing 'red flags' suggestive of significant and potentially life-threatening pathology
- recognizing that chronic abdominal pain is often functional in origin.

Abdominal pain is commonly described in terms of parietal, visceral or referred pain.

Parietal pain: afferent nerves originate in the parietal peritoneum and enter the ipsilateral dorsal root ganglion at the corresponding superficial dermatomal level. The pain receptors respond to irritation from infection, chemical or other inflammatory processes. It is usually perceived as a sharp, well-localized pain and results in localized tenderness and guarding that can progress to generalized peritonitis with abdominal rigidity and rebound tenderness.

Visceral pain: afferent nerves originate in the walls of hollow organs (responding to ischaemia, distension and inflammation) and capsules of solid organs (responding to capsular stretching). They enter the ipsilateral and contralateral cord at multiple levels. The pain is therefore poorly characterized (dull, cramping, aching) and poorly localized (being felt generally around the midline). It is interpreted at the cortical level as originating

from the approximate spinal cord level determined by the embryological origin of the organ:

- *Epigastric pain* due to organs of *foregut* origin (stomach, duodenum, biliary system)
- *Periumbilical pain* due to organs of *midgut* origin (small bowel, appendix, caecum)
- *Hypogastric/suprapubic pain* due to *hindgut* organs (colon, intraperitoneal parts of genitourinary system).

Referred pain is perceived as arising distant from its source and results from convergence of nerve fibres at the spinal cord. It also reflects embryological origins. Examples include:

- scapular pain due to biliary colic
- groin pain due to renal colic
- shoulder pain due to blood or infection causing diaphragmatic irritation
- ureteric obstruction causing ipsilateral testicular pain.

Acute abdominal pain

Scenario 2.1

You are asked to review a 75-year-old woman on the care of the elderly ward in the early hours of the morning. She has been awoken from sleep with a generalized abdominal pain. On examination she looks unwell, has a tachycardia of 130 beats per minute, irregularly irregular, with blood pressure of 100/70 having been 140/95 prior to the pain. She has mild generalized abdominal tenderness but no guarding or rebound tenderness. Her bowel sounds are increased. Her medication includes digoxin and warfarin for atrial fibrillation, prednisolone 30 mg for a recent diagnosis of polymyalgia rheumatica and regular tramadol.

Acute Medicine, ed. Stephen Haydock, Duncan Whitehead and Zoë Fritz. Published by Cambridge University Press. © Cambridge University Press 2015.

This patient is unwell and requires urgent resuscitation and surgical referral. The suspicion, given the atrial fibrillation, generalized pain and increased bowel sounds, is of gut ischaemia. The absence of severe pain, tenderness, guarding and rebound is still consistent with this, especially in a patient on regular high dose steroids and analgesia. The presentation of an acute abdominal problem in the elderly is often less clear than in a younger individual and often results in significant delays in diagnosis and appropriate life-saving intervention.

Clinical assessment of acute abdominal pain

Some patients with acute abdominal pain may be very unwell and require urgent resuscitation; as always this is the priority.

History

- When did the pain start?
- Did it come on suddenly or gradually?
  - Sudden onset suggests vascular occlusion (ischaemic gut, torsion), small tubular obstruction (biliary or ureteric colic).
  - Gradual onset suggests inflammatory disorder or bowel obstruction.
- Can you describe the quality of the pain? Dull or sharp, constant or waxing/waning, colicky?
  - Burning pain of dyspepsia
  - Tearing pain of dissection
  - Colicky pain of biliary or ureteric colic
  - Sharp localized pain of peritoneal inflammation.
- Where in abdomen do you feel it? Localized or generalized?
- Does it radiate anywhere? Shoulder, groin, back?
- Does anything make it better or make it worse?
  - Relation to meals (peptic ulcer better, biliary colic worse)
  - Relation to position and movement (agitation of renal colic, curled up, still patient with peritoneal inflammation).
- Has it changed in quality or location since onset?
  - Generalized visceral pain becomes localized as overlying peritoneum is inflamed.
  - Progression of renal stones down ureter.
  - Progression of a vascular dissection.

- Other associated symptoms:
  - cardiorespiratory (may present as upper abdominal pain)
  - vomiting
  - diarrhoea
  - rectal bleeding
  - dysuria, frequency
  - scrotal swelling, penile discharge
  - vaginal discharge
  - fever
  - weight loss
  - vaginal bleeding and discharge.
- Take a detailed medical, drug and social history. In particular note:
  - previous abdominal disease and surgery
  - recent sexual contact for females; was protection used?
  - alcohol intake
  - smoking history
  - previous surgery or recent instrumental procedures
  - immunosuppression due to HIV or drugs
  - vascular disease including hypertension, atrial fibrillation
  - other major co-morbidities that would influence surgical risk.

The location of the pain and its radiation can help narrow the differential diagnosis.

But remember the possible pitfalls:

- Poor localization of visceral pain
- Localization of pain in relation to embryological origins
- Anatomical variants, e.g. retrocaecal appendix
- Change in the nature of pain over time, e.g. poorly localized pain of appendicitis becoming localized with onset of peritonitis.

Examination

A full examination of all major systems is required as abdominal pain may result from other systems (cardiovascular, respiratory, musculoskeletal) but in particular:

- Is the patient unwell, do they look pale, are they sick and in pain?
- Review the observations; are they tachycardic, tachypnoeic, hypotensive, pyrexial (elderly patients with infection may be hypothermic)?
- Remember restlessness of renal colic and the still, curled up patient with peritonitis.

- Inspect for abdominal scars and other stigmata of chronic disease; examine skin for bruising (Cullen's sign, Grey Turner's sign) and rash of herpes zoster.
- Palpate all areas of the abdomen, elicit localized tenderness, rebound tenderness, organomegaly (liver, kidneys and spleen) and palpate the abdominal aorta.
- Remember that signs of peritonitis may be diminished in the elderly.
- Auscultate carefully for bowel sounds (usually 2–12 of medium pitch per minute is normal).
- Perform a rectal examination.
- Perform a testicular examination in men.
- Perform a pelvic examination in women or request a gynaecological opinion if indicated and you are no longer familiar/confident with pelvic examination.

Investigations

Blood and urinalysis

- FBC
- CRP
- Glucose
- U&E
- LFTs
- Amylase
- Lactate
- Beta-HCG in woman of childbearing age
- Urinalysis and urine culture
- Blood culture if indicated

ECG for ischaemia; abrial fibrillation

Plain radiology

- *Plain abdominal and erect chest radiographs* are quick, cheap and require minimal radiation exposure. However, they are only diagnostically useful in specific conditions. It is often difficult to position patients who are unwell; an erect chest radiograph (CXR) requires a patient to be sat upright for 5–10 minutes. The sensitivity of an erect chest film is poor and it cannot be used to rule out a perforated viscus. Plain abdominal and erect chest radiographs may indicate:
  - obstruction and ileus
  - caecal and sigmoid volvulus

  - bowel perforation (*absence of free air does not exclude perforation*)
  - radiopaque foreign bodies
  - constipation
  - pulmonary pathology presenting as abdominal pain.

Ultrasound scanning of the abdomen

Ultrasound is a rapid non-invasive imaging modality [1] that can be performed at the bedside and is the accepted imaging modality of choice in pregnancy. Focused assessment with sonography for trauma (FAST) is routinely performed in the emergency department as a screening investigation for haemopericardium and haemoperitoneum in patients admitted following trauma. Emergency department scanning in the context of acute abdominal pain is also useful to exclude abdominal pain due to an abdominal aortic aneurysm. The ability to detect other pathologies is highly dependent on the expertise of the sonographer as well as patient factors such as obesity. Ultrasound imaging of the abdomen performed by an experienced sonographer may be useful in the confirmation of:

- abdominal aortic aneurysm
- gallbladder disease
- pancreatitis
- hydronephrosis/renal calculi
- ectopic/intrauterine pregnancy
- ovarian pathology
- testicular pathology
- appendicitis (*especially in children*).

Studies suggest that initial ultrasound scanning in patients presenting with acute abdominal pain increases the sensitivity for urgent diagnosis and reduces radiation exposure. The increasing focus on the acquisition of ultrasound skills in acute and emergency medicine may lead to the increasing use of ultrasound imaging prior to CT scanning in the acute setting.

Computed tomography

CT imaging of the abdomen and pelvis remains the modality of choice in the investigation of abdominal pain. It has a high diagnostic yield and is particularly useful in the elderly, where the diagnosis is often obscure. It has a high sensitivity and specificity, as well as being readily available, non-operator dependent and able to identify a wide range of disease processes, including appendicitis and diverticulitis. However, it requires a significant radiation exposure and potential risk of IV contrast reactions. Unlike bedside ultrasound, the patient must be clinically stable to undergo imaging.

Oral contrast-enhanced scans

- Offer better resolution than unenhanced scans in bowel obstruction and ileus.
- Probably better differentiation in acute appendicitis.
- Oral (iodinated) barium sulphate is a thicker liquid with lower risk of aspiration but contraindicated in suspected intestinal perforation.
- Oral water-soluble Gastrografin has a higher aspiration risk but is safer in suspected perforation.

Intravenous contrast-enhanced scans

- Improves the visualization of inflammatory, infectious and neoplastic lesions.
- Improved discrimination of focal pathology of solid organs.
- Necessary for CT angiography to visualize mesenteric vasculature in ischaemic bowel.
- Risk of adverse reactions is lower with modern non-ionic iodinated contrast agents (0.7% adverse events with only 2% of these events rated as severe).

Unenhanced scans

- The development of modern spiral/helical multi-detector CT scanners has enabled rapid data acquisition with minimal movement artefact, thinner image slices and improved contrast detection. These technological advancements have increased the diagnostic yield of non-contrast-enhanced scans in the acute setting.

Magnetic resonance imaging

- Indicated in pregnant woman where ultrasound has not been helpful and CT imaging is best avoided due to the risks of radiation exposure.

Management

The specific management will depend on the underlying condition but the following general principles apply.

Resuscitation

- According to standard ABC guidelines in accordance with the degree of intravascular fluid deficit.
- Establish IV access and administer crystalloid.
- Consider urinary catheterization to assist with fluid resuscitation.

Analgesia

- One of the first concerns should be the relief of pain. There has been a traditional belief that the administration of analgesia should be deferred until a diagnosis has been secured, as the analgesia may mask the symptoms and interfere with the diagnostic evaluation.
- Two separate Cochrane reviews of the published literature in this area, most recently in 2011 [2], have challenged this belief. It is now established that opioid analgesia *does not* increase the risk of diagnostic error or error in decision making regarding the management of acute abdominal pain.
- Therefore, reduce pain to manageable levels by administration of IV morphine 2–5 mg at 15-minute intervals; consider co-administration of an antiemetic.
- Pain that persists despite adequate doses of opioid analgesia is suggestive of a *severe underlying condition*.
- Remember that opioid dependent patients will require increased analgesic dosages.

Nasogastric tube

- Ensure patient is nil by mouth.
- Place wide-bore nasogastric tube in patients with copious vomiting, bowel obstruction or ileus.

Surgical acute abdomen

An urgent surgical opinion should be sought if clinical assessment suggests a 'surgical acute abdomen', that is an underlying condition causing acute abdominal pain with a rapidly worsening prognosis in the absence of surgical intervention.

Such a situation is suggested by:

History

- Severe abdominal pain of sudden onset that persists for greater than 6 hours and is refractory to opioid analgesia

- Severe *generalized* abdominal pain (mesenteric ischaemia/infarction can cause profound pain and distress without obvious peritonism)
- High risk individual: elderly, immunosuppressed, pregnant

Examination

- Persistent, localized abdominal tenderness with guarding and rebound suggestive of localized peritoneal inflammation (including on rectal or pelvic examination)
- Bruising of abdominal wall (Cullen's and Grey Turner's sign)
- Features of intestinal obstruction or ileus (vomiting with increased or absent bowel sounds)
- Palpable mass, e.g. intussusception, incarcerated hernia, appendix abscess and diverticular abscess

Investigation

- Markedly elevated serum amylase/lipase in pancreatitis
- Markedly elevated lactate suggestive in bowel infarction
- Free air under diaphragm in perforated abdominal viscus
- Dilated small or large bowel loops

Abdominal pain in the elderly

The diagnosis and management of acute abdominal pain in the elderly poses particular challenges [3]. Studies show that patients over 65 years are much more likely to be misdiagnosed and have significantly increased mortality due to:

- decreased immune function with age
- multiple co-morbidities, e.g. diabetes mellitus, chronic renal disease, cardiovascular disease
- increased prevalence of life-threatening abdominal pathology, e.g. aortic aneurysm and ischaemic gut
- chronic analgesic and anti-inflammatory usage (steroids and NSAIDs) that mask symptoms of serious pathology
- delay in seeking medical help
- vague and atypical presentations of serious pathology
- inability to communicate severity and nature of pain and other symptomatology.

Chronic abdominal pain

Scenario 2.2

You have been referred a 40-year-old woman by the emergency department. She has been brought to the ED after taking an overdose of tramadol and morphine. She is drowsy but reveals that she took the medication to 'get rid of the stomach pains that are ruining her life'. Old notes show that she has presented on numerous occasions over the past 2 years with abdominal pain to the surgical department, where she has had extensive radiological and endoscopic investigation. The last discharge summary states that 'if this patient presents again she should not be referred to surgery as there is no surgical condition to treat'. Each admission has been associated with an escalation in her opioid analgesia.

Chronic abdominal pain is an extremely common and troublesome condition in which patients describe persistent or intermittent abdominal pain, with or without other symptoms of several months duration. *Most patients will have a functional disorder* without serious underlying pathology. The Rome diagnostic criteria [4] are the most widely accepted diagnostic classification for functional gastrointestinal disorders and describe:

Functional dyspepsia (see Chapter 20)
Functional abdominal pain with at least 6 months of pain, poor relation to gut function and with some loss of daily activities

- Functional abdominal pain syndrome
- Non-specific functional abdominal pain

Functional bowel disorders characterized by characteristic symptoms for at least 12 weeks in the preceding 12 months in the absence of a structural or biochemical explanation

- Irritable bowel syndrome
- Functional abdominal bloating
- Functional constipation
- Functional diarrhoea
- Unspecified functional bowel disorder

It is important to understand that although 'functional', these conditions are a cause of *considerable distress and suffering to those affected*. In addition they are associated with a high financial burden due to the cost of medical expenses and loss of income due to absenteeism from work.

Investigation of chronic abdominal pain

Most patients who present to secondary care with a worsening of chronic abdominal pain will do so because of inadequate symptom control. They will usually have already had extensive investigation in primary and often secondary care. It is therefore important *to find out what has already been done to investigate the condition and when it was done,* using patient notes and discussion with the patient's general practitioner. For the occasional patient who has not been investigated, the following (NICE guideline 2008 [5]) are suggestive of a significant underlying problem:

- unintentional or unexplained weight loss
- rectal bleeding
- family history of bowel or ovarian cancer
- altered bowel habit with looser and/or more frequent stools for >6 weeks if over 60 years
- abdominal or rectal masses
- any features of ovarian malignancy.

In addition the following findings on initial screening merit further investigation:

- anaemia
- raised inflammatory markers (ESR or CRP)
- hyperglycaemia
- elevated serum amylase
- abnormal liver function
- raised antibody titre of endomysial antibodies or tissue transglutaminase.

Great caution is needed in making a diagnosis of a functional illness in a patient presenting after 50 years of age due to the high risk of malignancy.

Irritable bowel syndrome (IBS)

IBS is the most commonly recognized cause of functional abdominal pain. It is more common in women and is found in 15–20% of adolescents and adults in Western societies. It follows a chronic relapsing and remitting course and shows overlaps with other functional gastrointestinal disorders. IBS should be considered in patients with a six month history of abdominal pain that is either relieved by defecation or associated with altered bowel frequency (constipation or diarrhoea predominant IBS) or stool form [5]. In addition at least two of the following should be present:

- altered stool passage (straining, urgency or incomplete evacuation)
- abdominal bloating (especially in women), distension, tension and hardness
- symptoms worsened by eating.

Lethargy, nausea, backache and bladder symptoms are also commonly described. The aetiology is not well understood but it is generally thought that there is abnormal gut motility associated with visceral hypersensitivity.

Management

- General advice on lifestyle, physical activity and diet.
- Dietary fibre intake can be decreased or increased according to predominant symptoms. Insoluble fibre, contained within foods such as wholegrain bread, bran, cereals, nuts and seeds (except golden linseeds), can worsen symptoms in diarrhoea predominant IBS. Soluble fibre, contained within food such as oats, barley, rye, fruit, root vegetables and golden linseeds, can help in patients with constipation predominant symptoms.
- New evidence for using a diet low in FODMAPs (fermentable oligosaccharides, disaccharides, monosaccharides and polyols) that aims to reduce dietary intake of fermentable sugars to reduce malabsorptive symptoms such as disabling diarrhoea, wind and bloating. This type of diet improves symptoms by almost 80% when introduced by a specialist dietitian.
- Antispasmodic agents.
- Probiotics, such as *Bifidobacterium infantis*, may be of use.
- Laxatives or antimotility agents according to symptoms (aiming for Bristol stool scale type 4 stool).
- Use of tricyclic antidepressants (TCAs) for analgesic effect starting at low dose (5–10 mg amitriptyline nocte) with careful dose escalation (up to 30 mg). TCAs are good in patients with diarrhoea as they tend to be slightly constipating. Selective serotonin reuptake inhibitors (SSRIs) are better used for patients with constipation.
- Cognitive therapy, hypnotherapy or other psychological interventions are recommended by NICE in refractory IBS (ongoing symptoms after 12 months of pharmacological treatment).

Functional abdominal pain

Functional abdominal pain is less common than IBS and probably affects about 2% of the adult population.

It is defined as pain that persists for greater than 6 months without evidence of an underlying physiological/pathological disorder that is not related to eating, defecation or menstruation and interferes with daily functioning. It is poorly understood but appears to be related to hyperalgesia resulting in altered pain perception in the context of psychosocial factors (see Chapter 48). A similar approach to excluding an organic cause is indicated as above for suspected IBS.

Management

- Confident and supportive explanation of the condition and how the pain is generated and perceived, psychosocial support (e.g. cognitive therapy) aiming at minimizing the adverse impact of the pain, e.g. absence from work.
- Analgesic agents, e.g. NSAIDs, H2-blockers and TCAs.
- Avoiding opiates as these can rapidly lead to dependence and in the long term may even worsen pain due to opioid-induced hyperalgesia.
- Consider psychiatric referral if there is coexisting depression or other psychological problems.

References

1. McGahan JP, Richards J, Gillen M (2002) The focused abdominal sonography for trauma scan: pearls and pitfalls. *Journal of Ultrasound in Medicine* 21(7): 789–800. Available to download at www.jultrasoundmed.org/content/21/7/789.full.

2. Manterola C, Vial M, Moraga J, Astudillo P (Editorial Group: Cochrane Colorectal Cancer Group). Analgesia in patients with acute abdominal pain. Published online 19 January 2011. Available online at http://onlinelibrary.wiley.com/doi/10.1002/14651858.CD005660.pub3/pdf.

3. Laurell H, Hansson LE, Gunnarsson U. (2006) Acute abdominal pain among elderly patients. *Gerontology* 52(6): 339–344.

4. Drossman DA (2006) The functional gastrointestinal disorders and the Rome III process. *Gastroenterology* 130: 1377–90. Available to download at http://romecriteria.org/rome_III_gastro/.

5. NICE (2008) Clinical Guideline 61: Irritable bowel syndrome in adults: Diagnosis and management of irritable bowel in primary care. Available to download at http://publications.nice.org.uk/irritable-bowel-syndrome-in-adults-cg61.

Abdominal swelling and constipation

Charlotte Rutter

Introduction

Abdominal distension may be caused by medical, surgical and gynaecological problems and you should keep in mind the traditional 5 F's – *fat, flatus, faeces, fluid or fetus*.

The patient may present with an acute problem requiring urgent intervention:

- ascites with decompensated chronic liver disease
- acute intestinal obstruction

or have a more chronic problem:

- constipation
- pseudo-obstruction.

As always, a structured and focused history and examination is required to guide appropriate management.

Clinical assessment of abdominal distension (all causes)

History

Presenting complaint

- Onset of abdominal distension: acute or chronic, and duration
- Associated pain: site, character, duration and radiation
- Change in bowel habit
  - Diarrhoea: frequency, stool type, steatorrhoea, overflow, urgency, incontinence, nocturnal (suggests pathological cause)
  - Constipation: frequency, stool type, excess straining, sensation of incomplete stool evacuation, digitation
  - Passage of blood or melaena per rectum
  - Flatus and wind

- Jaundice, bruising, confusion, peripheral oedema, shortness of breath
- Nausea and vomiting
- Dyspepsia
- Dysphagia
- Weight loss
- *Past medical history* focusing on:
- GI disease
- Liver disease
- Cardiac disease – right-sided failure
- Causes of bowel obstruction – abdominal surgery (adhesions), malignancy, radiotherapy
- Gynaecological history
- Causes of wind and bloating
  - Diabetes mellitus – gastroparesis
  - Scleroderma – small bowel bacterial overgrowth
  - Coeliac disease
  - Thyroid disorders
  - Air swallowing and chewing gum
  - Nissen fundoplication surgery
- *Psychiatric history*: consider anorexia nervosa, bulimia, depression, anxiety, physical or sexual abuse in patients who have a non-organic cause
- *Drug history* in relation to:
  - liver patients (diuretics, opiates, laxatives, NSAIDs, ACE inhibitors, angiotensin-II antagonists)
  - volvulus (history of chronic constipation and laxative abuse is common)
  - pseudo-obstruction/ileus (opiates, tricyclics, anticholinergics, calcium channel blockers)
  - constipation (laxatives, opiates, antispasmodics, tricyclics, antipsychotics, antiparkinsonian drugs, anticonvulsants,

Acute Medicine, ed. Stephen Haydock, Duncan Whitehead and Zoë Fritz. Published by Cambridge University Press. © Cambridge University Press 2015.

calcium channel blockers, iron, calcium, barium)
- over the counter medicines and herbal remedies
- *Family history*: malignancy (particularly gastrointestinal)
- *Dietary history*: fluids, fibre, vegetarian, carbohydrates, exclusions (dairy, gluten, lactose)
- *Social history*: accommodation, mobility, family, work, alcohol, smoking, recent travel, intravenous or any other drug use, sexual history

Examination

- *Basic nursing observations* (temperature, blood pressure, heart rate, oxygen saturations, respiratory rate)
- *General observations*
  - Abdominal distension, scars, masses
  - Jaundice, encephalopathy, spider naevi, caput medusa, bruising, gynaecomastia
  - Hepatic flap
- *Palpation*: tenderness, guarding (document location), peritonism
- *Masses*: hepatosplenomegaly, renal, abdominal (malignancy, stools, abscess)
- *Percussion*: resonant suggestive of air or flatus (obstruction, pseudo-obstruction, ileus) or dull (fluid or faeces)
- *Elicit shifting dullness* (ascites):
  - Percuss from umbilicus to iliac fossa
  - At dull point keep your hand there and ask the patient to roll over (left iliac fossa patient turns on right side, right iliac fossa patient turns on left side)
  - Percuss again and assess whether the fluid has shifted
- *Bowel sounds*: absent (strangulation, ischaemia or ileus), tinkling (fluid obstruction)
- *Hernial orifices*: reducible or strangulated
- *Rectal examination*: tone, masses, blood, melaena, impaction
- *Signs of underlying cause*: e.g. cardiac failure (cardiomegaly, raised JVP, peripheral oedema)

Investigations

Blood tests

- Full blood count

- Clotting
- Serum urea and electrolytes
- Liver function tests
- C-reactive protein
- Non-invasive liver screen if suspicion of chronic liver disease (urgent USS indicated)
- Group and save or cross match if evidence of upper gastrointestinal haemorrhage
- Consider coeliac screen if anaemic or predominant symptoms are of diarrhoea, bloating, nausea or weight loss
- Consider thyroid function test if diarrhoea, constipation or weight loss
- Consider haematinics if anaemia or weight loss (malignancy, coeliac disease, alcohol excess, B_{12} or folate deficiency)
- Consider calcium if symptoms of confusion or constipation which may be due to hypercalcaemia with underlying malignancy (add on parathyroid hormone if patient is hypercalcaemic)
- Consider calcium, magnesium and phosphate if patient is dehydrated or had profuse diarrhoea

Other investigations

- *Urinalysis*: pregnancy test, microscopy, culture and sensitivities, protein to look for nephropathy
- *Stool sample*: microscopy, culture and sensitivities, *Clostridium difficile* toxin if gastroenteritis suspected, also oocytes, cysts and parasites
- *Electrocardiogram*: atrial fibrillation, which may cause bowel ischaemia
- *Arterial blood gas*: acidosis or raised lactate suggestive of AKI, sepsis or surgical cause

Imaging

- Chest X-ray: possible infection, pleural effusion, cardiomegaly, pneumoperitoneum
- Abdominal X-ray (perforated viscus, faecal loading, dilated bowel loops, volvulus)
- Urgent abdominal ultrasound with hepatoportal vein Doppler to rule out portal vein thrombosis (Budd–Chiari) or hepatocellular carcinoma
- CT abdomen and pelvis (mechanical bowel obstruction)

Abdominal distension due to ascites

> **Scenario 3.1**
>
> *A 46-year-old man is referred to the medical assessment unit from the emergency department with a swollen abdomen, confusion and jaundice. He has a history of alcohol excess but denies drinking in recent months and has never been admitted to hospital. He has no other significant past medical history. He is married with two children and works as a solicitor.*

This is a relatively common referral to the medical team and may represent an acute hepatological emergency which requires input from gastroenterology, and potentially the intensive care team or regional liver unit. See Chapter 36 for the investigation and management of decompensated liver failure.

All patients with ascites in the context of decompensated liver disease must have an urgent ascitic tap to rule out spontaneous bacterial peritonitis.

Ascitic tap procedure (Table 3.1)

A high INR or low platelet count is not a contraindication to an ascitic tap as patients are likely to be coagulopathic and thrombocytopenic. FFP or platelet cover is not required for an ascitic tap [1].

Pathophysiology of ascites

- Ascites refers to fluid within the abdominal cavity and is the most common complication of cirrhosis; about 60% of patients with compensated cirrhosis develop ascites within 10 years [2].
- Its pathogenesis in liver disease is due to two main factors:
  - *Portal (sinusoidal) hypertension*: structural changes due to cirrhosis result in increased splanchnic blood flow. It exerts a local hydrostatic pressure resulting in increased production of lymph and transudation of fluid into the peritoneal cavity. Ascites only develops once the wedge hepatic portal venous gradient is >12 mmHg.
  - *Water and sodium retention*: systemic vasodilatation causes a decrease in effective circulating blood volume and a hyperdynamic circulation. This activates the sympathetic nervous system and renin–angiotensin system, promoting water and salt retention.

- (Low serum albumin is *no longer thought to be causative* in pathogenesis.)
- It indicates a poor prognosis, with mortality approximately 40% at 1 year and 50% at 2 years [2].
- In 25% of patients, ascites is caused by malignancy, cardiac failure, tuberculosis, pancreatic disease or other miscellaneous causes.

Interpretation of ascitic tap results

- Calculate serum-ascites-albumin gradient (SAAG), which is:
- *serum (albumin) – ascites (albumin).*
- SAAG is more accurate in identifying the cause of ascites (portal hypertension or not) than using Light's criteria.
- *SAAG >11 g/L (or 1.1 g/dL) suggests ascites due to portal hypertension*:
  - cirrhosis
  - right heart failure
  - Budd–Chiari (portal vein thrombosis)
  - spontaneous bacterial peritonitis, TB, malignancy (in portal hypertensive patient).
- *SAAG <11 g/L (or 1.1 g/dL) suggests ascites not due to portal hypertension*:
  - nephrotic syndrome
  - malnutrition
  - protein-losing enteropathy
  - hypothyroidism
  - malignancy
  - TB
  - pancreatitis
  - spontaneous bacterial peritonitis (in hypoalbuminaemic patient).
- Neutrophils >250/μL or WCC >500/μL is diagnostic of spontaneous bacterial peritonitis.

Management

All patients

- ABCDE + glucose approach
- Two large-bore cannulae and fluid resuscitation if evidence of upper gastrointestinal haemorrhage or hypovolaemia
- Correction of coagulopathy if evidence of active bleeding or disseminated intravascular coagulation (DIC) due to sepsis (FFP, platelets, vitamin K and cryoprecipitate)
- Correction of hypoglycaemia

Table 3.1 How to perform an ascitic tap

Informed consent	• Quote a complication rate of 1% due to formation of abdominal haematomas (rarely serious or life-threatening). More serious complications such as haemoperitoneum or bowel perforation are rare (0.1% of procedures). • If patient unable to give informed consent then discuss with family and proceed acting in the patient's best interests
Equipment needed	• Dressing pack, sterile gloves, sterile gauze, chlorhexidine • Orange needle and 2 green needles • 5 mL and 20 mL syringe (50 mL if sending for cytology) • 5 mL 1% or 2% lidocaine • 2 white top specimen bottles (3 if sending for cytology) • Aerobic and anaerobic blood culture bottles (yield is increased from 40% to 72–90% compared to specimen bottles) • Plaster and tape
Aseptic technique	• Elicit shifting dullness and identify site for aspiration (commonly left or right lower quadrants) • Clean skin • Draw up lidocaine into 5 mL syringe • Make a skin bleb with an orange needle and then change for a green needle • Insert needle perpendicularly into the skin, aspirating before infiltrating lidocaine. Advance the needle repeating this until you enter the peritoneal cavity and aspirate ascites. Withdraw the needle. • Allow time for local anaesthetic to take effect whilst changing to a 20 mL syringe (50 mL if sending for cytology) • Advance the needle through the same tract, through the peritoneum and into the peritoneal cavity. Aspirate 20–50 mL of ascitic fluid
Send specimens	• Divide the fluid into the specimen pots and blood culture bottles (send at least 20 mL to cytology) • Send specimens for: WCC and MC&S (contact on-call microbiology technician if out of hours) Albumin (to calculate SAAG – see p. 18) Cytology Lactate dehydrogenase (identifies secondary SBP) Amylase (if pancreatitis suspected) Mycobacteria (if TB suspected)
Documentation	• Document procedure in medical notes, including appearance of ascites (straw coloured, cloudy, bloody, chylous) and investigations requested

- Analgesia for pain
- Antibiotics if evidence of sepsis (chest, urine, SBP, diverticulitis, perforation, abscess)

Decompensated liver disease with ascites

- *Pabrinex* two pairs, three times a day intravenously for nine doses. Continue with oral thiamine and vitamin B compound-strong once Pabrinex completed.
- *Fluid resuscitation* ideally with 4% human albumin solution if readily available but alternatively Hartmann's or normal saline. *Never give dextrose until one dose of Pabrinex is given as the sugar load can precipitate Wernicke's encephalopathy.* Patients who are intravascularly depleted will die of hypovolaemia before salt overload and fluid is likely to go into the abdomen, but this can be drained. *Correction of intravascular volume depletion is the priority.*
- Fluid replacement should correct renal impairment in most patients with acute kidney injury. If this is not the case after 24 hours, they may have hepatorenal syndrome and should be discussed with the gastroenterology team to consider vasopressor (terlipressin) and albumin therapy. The patient may need haemofiltration in the intensive care setting.
- Stop all *drugs* that may contribute to confusion, acute kidney injury or electrolyte disturbance.
- *Lactulose* to ensure three soft stools a day.

- Urgent *dietitian review* and consider *early NG tube insertion* for facilitation of drugs and enteral nutrition.
  - Clinical trials comparing enteral nutrition with corticosteroids showed no difference in 28-day mortality.
  - Evidence shows that patients with alcoholic hepatitis who are enterally fed (high protein, high calorie diet) have an improved survival.
  - Concerns over precipitating variceal haemorrhage with nasogastric tubes have not been confirmed in clinical trials [2,3].
- *No added salt* diet (80–120 mmol sodium a day) [2].
- *Treat infection* with appropriate antibiotics.
- *Tense ascites +/– respiratory compromise should be drained*:
  - <5 L fluid drained: prescribe 500 mL normal saline for fluid replacement.
  - >5 L drained: prescribe 100 mL 20% HAS for every third litre drained (i.e. 5th, 6th, 9th, 12th, etc.) to prevent circulatory compromise.
  - The drain should *never* be clamped; the aim is to drain to dryness as quickly as possible.
  - The drain should be removed after a *maximum of 6 hours* to reduce the risk of introducing infection.
  - Malignant ascites does not require HAS cover.
- *Non-tense ascites does not require drainage.*
- *Diuretics*
  - Spironolactone (side effects include gynaecomastia, acute kidney injury).
  - Start at 50–100 mg once daily and monitor daily weights; aim for 0.5 kg weight loss a day.
  - If this is not achieved by day 3, double the dose of spironolactone and titrate up to a maximum of 400 mg a day.
  - If the patient does not respond to spironolactone or becomes hyperkalaemic, add in furosemide 40 mg once daily and titrate up in 40 mg doses to a maximum of 160 mg a day.
  - If sodium drops below 125 mmol/L stop diuretics (cirrhotic patients are hyponatraemic due to their disease and this is an independent prognostic factor).
  - Malignant ascites is often refractory to diuretics.
- Fluid restriction should only be applied if the patient is clinically euvolaemic with normal renal function and not taking diuretics.

- Patients who do not respond to initial resuscitative therapy should be discussed with the high dependency/intensive care teams as they should be managed in a level 2 or above setting.

In addition

- Oesophagogastroduodenoscopy once patient stabilized if evidence of upper gastrointestinal haemorrhage. This should also be done electively in cirrhotic patients for variceal surveillance.
- Refer to liver specialist nurse who can provide further information and support. In addition they can review patients in clinic and arrange outpatient ascitic drainage.
- Refer to the alcohol liaison team.
- If cytology or SAAG is suggestive of metastatic ascites, arrange appropriate investigations to find primary neoplasm, refer to multidisciplinary team and palliative care if required.

Spontaneous bacterial peritonitis (SBP)

- SBP is present in 1.5–3.5% of outpatients with cirrhosis and ascites; this rises to 10% in hospitalized patients. Mortality has been reduced from 90% to 20% due to early diagnosis and treatment [2].
- Those who recover from SBP have a cumulative recurrence rate of 70% at 1 year. Survival at 1 year is 30–50% and falls to 25–30% at 2 years. Therefore, these patients should be considered for liver transplantation [2].
- If clinical suspicion of SBP is high (tender abdomen or peritonitis, decompensation) broad spectrum antibiotics should be commenced early and continued even if ascitic fluid cultures are negative.
- Antibiotic choice is driven by local microbiology protocol and sensitivities (commonest cause is Gram-negative rods such as *E. coli*).
- Prescribe 20% HAS 1.5 g/kg intravenously on day 1 of diagnosis and 1 g/kg on day 3. Hepatorenal syndrome (HRS) occurs in approximately 30% of patients with SBP treated with antibiotics alone and is associated with a poor survival. Albumin decreases the frequency of HRS and improves survival [2].
- Patients who have had one episode of SBP should be prescribed long-term antibiotic prophylaxis

(ciprofloxacin 500 mg od or norfloxacin 400 mg od) [1,2].

Other important causes of abdominal distension

1. Constipation

- Pathological causes should be ruled out (colonic/rectal/anal malignancy or stricture).
- If associated with abdominal bloating and distension in a young person it is more suggestive of a functional cause.
- Due to normal transit, slow transit or incoordination of the rectum, anus or pelvic floor. Remember constipation with overflow diarrhoea.
- Further investigations
  - Flexible sigmoidoscopy and colorectal biopsies (left-sided stenosis, melanosis coli, Hirschsprung's disease, obstructing rectal/anal malignancy)
  - Abdominal X-ray (faecal loading, megarectum)
  - Colonic transit studies (normal or slow transit)
  - Anorectal physiology (absent recto-anal inhibitory reflex is diagnostic of Hirschsprung's disease)
  - Defecating proctogram (rectocele, prolapsed, intussusception)
  - Endoanal US (sphincter function).
- *General advice*
  - *Drugs review*: avoid those that reduce gut motility
  - *Dietary review*: increase fluids, increase soluble fibre, wholegrains, oats and golden linseeds. Give patient the NICE IBS diet sheet if appropriate [4].
- *Glycerin suppositories* before enema to soften the stools. May need general anaesthetic and manual evacuation if impacted (and flexible sigmoidoscopy to rule out underlying carcinoma).
- *Hypercalcaemia* – rehydrate and check PTH; investigate for underlying malignancy.
- *Behavioural therapy*
  - Toilet habit training
  - Biofeedback (teaches patient to normalize pelvic floor function whilst watching real-time feedback about sphincter function)

- Psychological support, cognitive behavioural therapy, hypnotherapy.
- ***Laxatives***
- Drugs used to hasten gut transit time and encourage defecation
- Patients are advised to avoid chronic laxative use if possible as it does not provide sustained relief. BSG guidelines [5] recommend bulk-forming laxatives (isphagula) as first-line therapy
- *Bulk forming*
  - Bran, methylcellulose and isphagula husk
  - Increases the volume of non-absorbable solid residue in the gut, distending the colon and stimulating peristalsis
  - Best for constipation with small, hard stools and patient must increase fluid intake. Clinical effects may take several days to develop
  - *Side effects*: Flatulence, abdominal distension and obstruction. Impaction can occur above strictures.
- ***Stimulant***
  - Senna, bisacodyl, sodium picosulfate
  - Stimulate the enteric nerves resulting in gastrointestinal peristalsis and increased water and electrolyte secretion by the mucosa
  - Contraindicated in bowel obstruction
  - *Side effects*: Cramps. Chronic use can cause hypokalaemia, and nerve damage resulting in an atonic colon. Should be used for short periods only.
- *Osmotic*
  - Lactulose, macrogols (Movicol and Laxido) and saline purgatives (magnesium hydroxide or sodium salts)
  - Increases water in the bowel by retaining the fluid it was administered with or by drawing it out from the body
  - Lactulose should only be prescribed for liver patients (it produces osmotic diarrhoea of low faecal pH and discourages the proliferation of ammonia-producing organisms. It is therefore useful in the treatment of hepatic encephalopathy)
  - *Side effects*: flatulence, cramps and abdominal discomfort; avoid magnesium hydroxide in renal failure due to magnesium toxicity.
- *Stool softeners*
  - Sodium docusate and liquid paraffin

- Soften or lubricate faeces to aid passage through gastrointestinal tract
- Best for constipation, faecal impaction, haemorrhoids and anal fissures
- *Side effects*: Should not be used long term.

- *5-HT₄ agonists* (prucalopride)
  - A selective serotonin receptor agonist that predominantly stimulates colonic motility.
  - Recommended by NICE as treatment for women with constipation that has not responded to at least two laxatives from different classes, at the highest tolerated doses for at least 6 months. It should be trialled for 4 weeks and stopped if not effective [6].
  - *Side effects*: headache, abdominal pain, nausea and diarrhoea.

2. Small bowel obstruction

- Commonest causes are adhesions and irreducible external hernias (inguinal, femoral or umbilical).
- Less common causes are:
  - Crohn's disease (stricturing with, or without, active disease)
  - caecal carcinoma causing obstruction of the ileocaecal valve
  - ischaemic stricture secondary to radiation enteritis or mesenteric ischaemia
  - intussusception, gallstone ileus, small bowel volvulus.
- Commonest symptom is colicky abdominal pain:
  - distal obstruction (progressive abdominal distension and dehydration)
  - mid small bowel obstruction (severe colic)
  - high small bowel obstruction (can be pain free, vomiting and rapid dehydration).
- Distended, fluid-filled small bowel loops on plain abdominal X-ray.
- Management of small bowel obstruction:
  - surgical review: urgent surgery only if suspicion of strangulation
  - 'drip and suck' – nil by mouth and nasogastric tube
  - intravenous fluid resuscitation and correct electrolyte imbalances
  - if suggestion of active Crohn's disease, involve gastroenterology team to optimize medical

therapy (may require antibiotics and/or steroids).

3. Large bowel obstruction

- The obstructed colon slowly distends as small bowel contents pass through the ileocaecal valve; colonic peristalsis tries to overcome the obstruction, causing colicky abdominal pain. The risk of perforation of the thin-walled caecum is greatly increased with ongoing dilatation.
- Commonest cause is colorectal cancer (40 000 new cases each year in the UK – NICE colorectal cancer guideline [7]).
- Less common causes include:
  - sigmoid or caecal volvulus
  - pseudo-obstruction
  - chronic constipation and faecal impaction
  - diverticular stricture or acute diverticulitis.

4. Ileus

- Paralytic ileus presents with symptoms of bowel obstruction but there is no mechanical cause.
- It is due to intestinal hypomotility and is multifactorial in origin. It results in a lack of coordinated peristalsis resulting in the accumulation of bowel gas and fluids.
- *Causes include*:
  - surgery
  - electrolyte disturbance: hyponatraemia, hypokalaemia, hypo- or hypermagnesaemia
  - drugs
  - intra-abdominal inflammation: diverticulitis, appendicitis, perforated duodenal ulcer
  - retroperitoneal inflammation: pancreatitis, pyelonephritis
  - intestinal ischaemia: arterial embolus or thrombosis, mesenteric venous thrombosis
  - systemic sepsis.
- Ileus is common postoperatively – small bowel motility usually returns after 24 hours, followed by gastric motility in 2 days and colonic motility in 3–5 days.
- *Management includes*:
  - surgical review but management is conservative
  - limit oral intake, correct intravascular volume, correct electrolyte imbalances

- nasogastric tube if distension or vomiting
- if lasts for more than 5 days, look for another cause.

5. Pseudo-obstruction

- Mimic of a true mechanical bowel obstruction.
- *Caused by abnormal gut motility due to*:
  - disorders of smooth muscle (primary due to rare visceral myopathies, secondary due to amyloid, radiation, SLE, muscular dystrophy or systemic sclerosis)
  - disorders of myenteric plexus
  - neurological diseases (Parkinson's, autonomic dysfunction)
  - small bowel diverticulosis
  - drugs.
- Initial investigations include plain abdominal radiograph showing dilated fluid loops with air/fluid levels. Computed tomography (CT) or barium follow-through showing a diffusely distended small bowel with no transition point suggests chronic intestinal pseudo-obstruction and may obviate the need for laparotomy. Scintigraphy may be used to assess gastric, small bowel, colonic or whole gut transit.
- *Management includes*:
  - initial correction of electrolyte imbalances (potassium, calcium and magnesium) and intravenous fluids
  - prokinetics rarely work, erythromycin (motilin agonist) or octreotide may be of benefit
  - low residue, low fat and low lactose diet
  - occasionally massive caecal distension may occur requiring decompression by colonoscopy or caecostomy
  - in rare cases patients may become malnourished or dehydrated and require long-term home parenteral nutrition.

References

1. Moore KP, Aithal GP (2006). Guidelines on the management of ascites in cirrhosis. *Gut* 2006; 55: 1–2. Doi:10.1136/gut.2006.099580.

2. European Association for the Study of the Liver (2010). EASL clinical practice guidelines on the management of ascites, spontaneous bacterial peritonitis and hepatorenal syndrome in cirrhosis. *Journal of Hepatology* 53: 397–417.

3. Stickel F, Hoehn B, Schuppan D, Seitz HK (2003). Review article: nutritional therapy in alcoholic liver disease. *Alimentary Pharmacology and Therapeutics* 18: 357–373.

4. National Institute for Health and Care Excellence (2008). NICE Irritable Bowel Syndrome and diet. Available at www.nhs.uk/conditions/incontinence-bowel/documents/nice%20guidelines%20ibs.pdf (accessed 2 July 2014).

5. R Spiller, Q Aziz, F Creed, et al. Guidelines on the irritable bowel syndrome: mechanisms and practical management. *Gut* 2007; 56: 1770–1798. doi: 10.1136/gut.2007.119446.

6. National Institute for Health and Care Excellence (2010). Prucalopride for the treatment of chronic constipation in women. Available at http://guidance.nice.org.uk/TA211/Guidance/pdf/English (accessed 9 May 2013).

7. National Institute for Health and Care Excellence (2011). Colorectal cancer: the diagnosis and management of colorectal cancer. CG131. Available at http://guidance.nice.org.uk/CG131/NICEGuidance/pdf/English (accessed 12 June 2013).

Further reading

NHS Choices – Liver transplant – Who can use it? www.nhs.uk/Conditions/Liver-transplant/Pages/Who-can-use-it.aspx (accessed 9 June 2013).

Paine P, McLaughlin J, Lal S (2013). Review article: the assessment and management of chronic severe gastrointestinal dysmotility in adults. *Alimentary Pharmacology and Therapeutics* 38: 1209–1229.

Chapter

4

Abnormal sensation

Edward Fathers

Introduction

This is a practical guide on how to assess patients with disturbance of sensation in the emergency setting. You will be relieved to know that you require very little knowledge of neuroanatomy. It is worth appreciating that there are very few patients who present with pure sensory disturbance. There are usually other accompanying symptoms such as clumsiness, weakness, unsteadiness or disturbance of sphincter function.

Scenario 4.1

A 30-year-old woman is referred urgently by her GP. She gives a 2-week history of back pain associated with a progressive paraesthesia of the legs and gradually worsening leg weakness. She has been a frequent attender at her GP practice with various somatic symptoms related to underlying anxiety and depression and her symptoms were initially viewed in a similar light. However, today she is unable to stand and pass urine. On examination you find her to have significant lower limb weakness with increased tone and hyperreflexia. There is profound sensory loss with a clear sensory level at T10. She is in acute retention of urine.

Clinical assessment

The majority of the clinical assessment is asking the right questions; there is surprisingly little extra information gained after performing a neurological examination.

What is the character of the sensory disturbance?

Patients often struggle to find the right vocabulary to describe their altered sensation. In practice all you need to know is has the sensation:

- disappeared altogether

- become reduced
- become heightened.

What anatomical site is affected?

Try and get an accurate description of the area affected by sensory disturbance and find out if the area has enlarged or changed over time and if so how quickly this took place.

Are the sensory symptoms continuous or intermittent?

If they are continuous do they fluctuate over time but never actually disappear.

Some general rules

1. Sensory symptoms that come and go are rarely significant. Patients use the terms tingling and 'pins and needles' interchangeably; they both mean the same thing. Tingling is a symptom that everyone gets, it is a part of normal physiology. In isolation, the symptom of tingling is usually not significant. Tingling in the fingertips that is worse at night and disturbs sleep is usually due to carpal tunnel syndrome. Tingling that moves around different parts of the body at different times is not usually due to an underlying neurological disease process.

2. A region of altered sensation that has been present continuously for more than 48 hours in the same place is usually pathological and requires investigation.

3. Altered sensation accompanied by pain in the same area usually indicates a problem in the peripheral nervous system (a peripheral nerve root or a peripheral nerve lesion).

4. Remember to think anatomically, where would a lesion have to be to give rise to this pattern of sensory disturbance? Is it located in the brain,

---

Acute Medicine, ed. Stephen Haydock, Duncan Whitehead and Zoë Fritz. Published by Cambridge University Press. © Cambridge University Press 2015.

brainstem, spinal cord, nerve root, plexus or peripheral nerve?

Clinical entities commonly encountered in the emergency situation

1. Spinal cord lesions

- Any disease process affecting the spinal cord will usually produce a 'sensory level', that is a horizontal line usually across the abdomen or thorax below which everything feels different and above which everything feels normal.
- There is sometimes a band-like area a few centimetres in size where there is a transition of altered sensation.
- Usually a spinal cord lesion will cause a sensory level affecting both sides of the body, but if just one side of the cord is damaged this will cause a contralateral sensory level.
- In theory, a sensory level could be anywhere from the knees up to the neck but in practice it is usually somewhere on the trunk, most frequently at around a level of the umbilicus to the mid-thorax.
- *A note of caution*: a peripheral neuropathy can produce a stocking distribution of sensory loss which could extend up to the mid-thigh. A lower spinal cord lesion can give rise to the same pattern of sensory loss. In this uncommon situation it can therefore be difficult to differentiate between a lesion in the spinal cord and peripheral nerves.
- Most patients can tell you exactly where the sensory level is on the trunk. It is unusual for the neurological examination to demonstrate that the level is in a different location.
- It is important to ask the right questions when testing for a sensory level. Remember that the majority of patients do not lose sensation altogether; they do, however, have altered or reduced sensation. So, for example, when testing pin prick sensation do not ask the question 'Can you feel it?' as the answer is probably yes; the correct question to ask is: '*Does it feel sharp or perhaps does it feel different?*' *and get the patient to tell you when the sensation changes to normal.* You may need to show them first how sharp the pin feels by lightly pressing it on the upper body first.

- Neurological examination should of course also include an assessment of the tone and power in the limbs as well as coordination and walking. It is worth noting that spinal cord pathology usually evolves over time and therefore the physical signs often change, sometimes quite rapidly. Be aware that with an acute spinal cord injury the lower limb reflexes can diminish or become absent; after a period of several days they will then become brisk. This is due to the phenomenon of spinal shock. There will often be an extensor plantar response but this is not always present.
- Imaging of the spinal cord needs to be performed urgently; if there is an external compressive lesion then outcome and prognosis is improved with rapid diagnosis and treatment.
- A common mistake is to request an MRI scan of the wrong region. Often patients who have a sensory level below the umbilicus have a lumbar spine MRI scan requested. This is the incorrect test. There are two important points to remember. Firstly, the spinal cord only extends down as far as the L1 vertebra, therefore to image the spinal cord you need to request a cervical and thoracic MRI scan. Secondly, a sensory level tells you the lowest possible extent of the lesion. It can be anywhere above that. Patients with a sensory level at the umbilicus will often have problems within the cervical spinal cord not in the lower thoracic cord.
- If MRI imaging indicates external compression of the spinal cord then an urgent surgical referral is required. If the spinal cord appears inflamed (usually identified by high signal changes within the cord), this is referred to as transverse myelitis and needs appropriate investigation. Inflammation of the cord can sometimes be subtle and doesn't always show abnormalities on an MRI scan. The causes of suspected transverse myelitis are shown in Table 4.1.

2. Peripheral neuropathy

- A mild length-dependent sensorimotor peripheral neuropathy is common in the general population. It is particularly prevalent in patients over the age of 70 years and is present in the majority of patients who have had diabetes for more than 10 years. You will therefore find evidence of a peripheral neuropathy in many patients that you examine.

Table 4.1 Causes of transverse myelitis

Aetiology	Examples
Idiopathic	Often a specific cause is not identified
Autoimmune	Multiple sclerosis
	Devic's disease (neuromyelitis optica)
Systemic inflammatory	SLE
	Sjögren's syndrome
	Sarcoidosis
Infections	*Bacterial:*
	Tuberculosis
	Syphilis
	Lyme disease
	Viral:
	Herpes simplex
	EBV
	Influenza
	HIV

- Usually the evidence for this is the absence of ankle reflexes combined with distal sensory loss. There is often reduced or absent sensation for a vibrating tuning fork at the feet combined with reduced awareness of sharp pin prick sensation in a stocking distribution usually somewhere on the foot extending up to the mid-calf level. Less commonly you may find evidence of distal weakness in the form of mild bilateral foot drop.
- For the purposes of this chapter I am concentrating on the *causes of peripheral neuropathy which present acutely*. Most peripheral nerve problems evolve slowly over months or years.
- There are peripheral nerve disorders that can evolve rapidly over a few days or weeks. The conditions that you need to know about are:
  - Guillain–Barré syndrome
  - mononeuritis multiplex due to vasculitis
  - neuropathy due to acute infection (HIV seroconversion, Lyme disease)
  - peripheral nerve toxicity, e.g. due to chemotherapy agents (vincristine).

These conditions will all present with a *combination of sensory symptoms and motor weakness*.

Guillain–Barré syndrome

- An autoimmune condition triggered by prior exposure to foreign antigens (viral infections, e.g. CMV, influenza, and bacteria, e.g. *Campylobacter jejuni*) resulting in antibody production that cross-react with human Schwann cell antigens causing acute demyelination of peripheral sensory and motor nerves.
- Patients may give a history of antecedent viral or enteric infection.
- Frequently causes tingling to appear simultaneously in the toes and the fingers; the tingling is usually continuous and often accompanied by some subtle loss of sensation.
- There is often a progression of symptoms which occurs rapidly over 2 or 3 days. The tingling and numbness rises up the legs and hands, and at the same time the patients start to become aware of weakness.
- Unlike other peripheral nerve disorders the pattern of weakness in Guillain–Barré syndrome is *predominantly proximal* in many patients in the first few days of the illness.
- It is often painful, due to localized demyelination in the nerve roots; it frequently causes back pain, or nerve root type pain radiating down the limbs.
- Most patients with acute Guillain–Barré syndrome will have many sensory symptoms but when you examine them neurologically there are usually very few sensory signs. Tests of pin prick sensation, light touch, temperature and vibration sensation are often normal. However, patients are usually quite weak.
- The weakness in Guillain–Barré syndrome evolves rapidly and usually peaks at around day 10 to 14 though occasionally it can take up to 4 weeks to reach its maximum severity.
- Patients develop areflexia but this can take a few days to appear, so on initial assessment in the emergency room deep tendon reflexes may still be present.
- Principal concern in the acute phase is respiratory muscle paralysis. Patients require careful monitoring of vital capacity. You should have a *low threshold for involving HDU* where the patient can have close monitoring and urgent intubation by skilled staff if this becomes necessary. In a person of average size, a vital capacity of less than 2 litres should raise concern; if the vital capacity is between 1.0 and 1.5 litres then there is an urgent need for discussion with HDU or ITU.
- Management is largely supportive and most patients will make a good recovery. However,

the mortality is 2–3% and 5% will recover with significant disability. Treatment is with IV immunoglobulins or plasmapheresis [1]. Each are equivalent in effectiveness. Combination treatment is no better than either alone. Immunoglobulins are easier to administer. Corticosteroids are ineffective. Treatment is recommended for patients with significant weakness (unable to walk unaided). The treatment is effective if given within the first 2 weeks of the onset of weakness. *It does not need to be given urgently in the middle of the night.*

Mononeuritis multiplex

- Multiple individual peripheral nerves are being damaged, usually due to interruption of the blood supply to each nerve, most commonly due to vasculitis.
- Patients will present with a rapidly evolving pattern of asymmetric peripheral nerve damage with corresponding sensory deficits and motor weakness appropriate for whichever peripheral nerve has been affected. It is often painful.
- There may be important clues from the blood tests, including a raised eosinophil count, ESR, C-reactive protein or a positive ANCA.

Infective

- Infective causes are rare.
- If there is bilateral facial weakness (this may be quite subtle) then consider Lyme disease.
- Infection with HIV can affect any part of the nervous system. Peripheral nerve complications include a presentation similar to Guillain–Barré syndrome, mononeuritis multiplex and a distal symmetrical polyneuropathy.

Drug-induced neuropathies

- There are only a small number of drugs that cause an acute rapidly evolving peripheral neuropathy; these are mostly chemotherapy agents. The list includes vincristine, paclitaxel, cisplatin, suramin and thalidomide.

3. Sensory disturbance due to multiple sclerosis

- Multiple sclerosis is an inflammatory disorder of the central nervous system; it commonly presents with a relapsing and remitting clinical course. Localized areas of inflammation within the brain or spinal cord can cause demyelination, which disturbs normal axonal signalling giving rise to symptoms that correspond to the pathways involved.
- Non-neurologists often find it difficult to determine if new sensory symptoms could be a manifestation of multiple sclerosis. The difficulty arises because multiple sclerosis lesions can appear anywhere in the central nervous system and therefore any anatomical site could be affected. However, there are usually certain patterns to the sensory symptoms that make them relatively easy to identify. The most common sites are:
  - optic nerve (optic neuritis)
  - spinal cord (giving rise to partial transverse myelitis)
  - brainstem
  - cerebral hemispheres.
- The typical features of an MS relapse are as follows:
  - *Duration.* The symptoms must be present for greater than 24 hours continuously; usually they are present for 2–8 weeks in total.
  - *Anatomical site.* This is usually quite large. For example, a whole limb or distal limb is usually affected, sometimes a whole region or quadrant of the body. Patches of numbness only a few centimetres in size anywhere on the body are usually not due to multiple sclerosis relapses.
  - *Time course.* The sensory disturbance usually evolves over hours to days. There may be an initial small area of sensory disturbance which rapidly enlarges over this time course.
- The sensory symptoms are often associated with other motor problems. For example, the sensory loss in a limb frequently causes interference with proprioception which in turn leads to clumsiness and reduced function.
- If a patient with a previous established diagnosis of multiple sclerosis presents with new sensory symptoms that fit the pattern described above, then the diagnosis of a sensory relapse is usually fairly straightforward. The diagnosis is usually a clinical one and does not usually require MRI.
- The natural history of an MS relapse is that the majority of symptoms will recover spontaneously within 6–8 weeks. The speed of recovery can be hastened slightly by offering the patient high dose corticosteroids; however, the eventual recovery that takes place is not influenced by the use of

corticosteroids. There is therefore no long-term benefit of administering these drugs.

- Neurologists would usually recommend only offering high dose corticosteroids *if the symptoms were severe and disabling.* A typical regimen of treatment would be methylprednisolone orally 500 mg once per day for 5 consecutive days.

4. Altered facial sensation

- This is a clinical problem often seen in neurology outpatient clinics. It presents less often to emergency physicians.
- Intermittent tingling in the face is a common symptom which does not require investigation.
- Patients with a persistent (greater than 24 hours) area of altered sensation on the face usually do require investigating.
- If the area of sensory disturbance increases in size over time and spreads to the inside of the mouth or the tongue, then the probability of finding a cause is high.
- In this group of patients an MRI brain scan is required. The common causes of persistent altered facial sensation include:
  - demyelination
  - intrinsic brain tumours
  - extrinsic benign tumour causing brainstem compression (vestibular schwannoma).
- Rarer causes of facial sensory loss that would not be identified on an MRI brain scan include trigeminal sensory neuropathy due to Sjögren's syndrome.

5. Nerve entrapment

The 'trapped nerve' diagnosis is overused. The peripheral nerves are vulnerable to compression at a small number of specific areas:

- *Nerve root* as it passes laterally through the vertebrae:
  - foraminal stenosis
  - disc herniation.
- *Peripheral nerve* entrapment:
  - median nerve at the wrist causing *carpal tunnel syndrome*
  - ulnar nerve at the elbow causing *cubital tunnel syndrome*
  - ulnar nerve at the wrist causing *Guyon's canal syndrome*

- common peroneal nerve at the fibular head causing *peroneal nerve compression syndrome.*

Some more general rules

1. Nerve root compression is painful. So if there is no history of significant pain it is very unlikely that you're dealing with sensory symptoms due to a nerve root compression. Root pain is usually not well localized; it often has a deep aching quality.
2. Nerve root lesions can give rise to reflex loss at the corresponding level.
   C5/6 Biceps
   C7/8 Triceps
   L3/4 Knee
   S1 Ankle
3. Peripheral nerve entrapment often has both motor and sensory loss. Carpal tunnel syndrome is a slight exception as patients often have diffuse tingling and pain throughout the hand, not just in the median nerve distribution. Symptoms are often worse at night and disturb sleep. Neurological examination often reveals normal sensory testing and normal motor function.
4. Radial nerve lesions are rare. There is usually very little sensory loss, though it can produce a patch of numbness on the dorsum of the hand.

Scenario 4.1 continued

This young woman has a spinal cord lesion somewhere above T10. MRI of the cervical and thoracic cord confirmed an extensive thoracic transverse myelitis. MRI of the brain and nerve conduction studies were both normal.

Reference

1. Hughes RA, Raphael JC, Swan AV, van Doorn PA. Intravenous immunoglobulin for Guillain–Barré syndrome. *Cochrane Database Syst Rev* CD002063, 2006.

Further reading

Patten J. *Neurological Differential Diagnosis*, 2nd edn. Springer; 1998.

Acute back pain

Luke Gompels

Introduction

Acute back pain is one of the commonest problems seen in primary care, affecting up to one-third of the UK population each year of whom 20% will consult their GP. Many such patients have 'non-specific low back pain' due to precipitating musculo-ligamentous injury or skeletal degenerative change and will have significant resolution of their pain within 6 weeks. Providing the history is uncomplicated, further investigations are not required. Radiological imaging of such patients often adds little to diagnosis and short-term use of analgesia, continued encouragement to keep mobile and physiotherapy are all helpful.

There is, however, a broad differential diagnosis for a patient presenting with acute back pain that includes:

- significant neurological compromise
- infection
- malignancy
- abdominal pathology
- other systemic diseases including ankylosing spondylitis and other inflammatory disorders.

When confronted with an acute hospital admission for back pain such significant pathologies need consideration and exclusion.

> ### Scenario 5.1
> *A 57-year-old man presents with severe low back pain radiating to the left buttock and left knee. The pain is severe with progressive increases in his analgesic prescriptions. His medical history includes a recent diagnosis of rheumatoid arthritis with commencement on methotrexate and previous systemic and local treatment for prostatic carcinoma.*

History

1. Does the patient have a history to suggest neurological compromise?

- Ensure that there is no history to suggest major or progressive motor or sensory deficit, new onset bladder or bowel incontinence or urinary retention.
- Bladder or bowel dysfunction may suggest compression of the *cauda equina*. This is the serious clinical complex of:
  - low back pain
  - lower limb motor weakness
  - saddle anaesthesia
  - bowel and/or bladder disturbance (usually urinary retention but occasionally overflow incontinence).
- This is a medical emergency and is most commonly caused by malignancy but can be caused by massive disc herniation.
- Patients may give a history of *sciatica* – a sharp or burning sensation radiating down the back of the leg to the knee or ankle.

2. Consider the following 'red flag' findings

- Exclude any trauma related to age:
  - injury related to a fall
  - minor fall or heavy lifting in a patient with osteoporosis or suspected osteoporosis (increased risk of fragility fracture: risk factors include female gender, prior history of fractures, positive family history, steroid use, inflammatory joint disease, drug or alcohol abuse, low BMI, smoking)

Acute Medicine, ed. Stephen Haydock, Duncan Whitehead and Zoë Fritz. Published by Cambridge University Press. © Cambridge University Press 2015.

- History of malignancy
- Fever/night sweats
- Age of onset <20 and >50
- Unexplained weight loss, severe fatigue or malaise
- Thoracic pain
- Duration of pain >1 month or not at all responsive to analgesia
- Pain not relieved by lying down
- Other symptoms suggestive of inflammatory disease:
    - early morning spinal stiffness
    - response to NSAIDs
    - improvement with activity
    - positive family history
    - sacroiliac pain (can be unilateral or bilateral)
    - extra-articular features.

3. Is there evidence of alternative pathology with pain referred to the back?

Two per cent of low back pain is due to visceral disease; some possibilities to consider are included below.

Thoracic pain

- Cardiac or pericardial disease
- Thoracic dissection
- Pulmonary or pleural disease

Lumbar pain

- Peptic ulcer disease
- Pancreatitis
- Cholecystitis
- Abdominal aortic aneurysm
- Diverticulitis

Lumbar sacral

- Renal disease (nephrolithiasis, pyelonephritis, perinephric abscess)
- Disease of pelvic organs (prostatitis, endometriosis, chronic pelvic inflammatory disease, tubal pregnancy)

4. Does the patient have musculoskeletal back pain due to non-specific causes?

Non-specific low back pain is tension, soreness and/or stiffness in the lower back region for which it is not possible to identify a specific cause of the pain.

Several structures in the back, including the joints, discs and connective tissues, may contribute to symptoms. If history and examination are supportive and other factors as listed above have been considered or excluded then diagnostic imaging and further investigation may not be required. These patients will often be managed in the community without the need for hospital admission.

Physical examination

Inspection

Assess posture ideally with patient standing and note:

- loss of cervical or lumbar lordosis
- kyphosis or scoliosis.

Palpation

- Check for point tenderness suggesting an underlying pathological cause, e.g. osteoporotic or pathological vertebral collapse or discitis.
- Superficial tenderness and multiple trigger points for pain in surrounding areas – may suggest more 'yellow flag' features and further psychosocial history taking will be required (described later).
- Tenderness within a dermatomal distribution should be followed up with further neurological assessment as below.

Range of motion

- Check degree of forward flexion, extension, lateral flexion and rotation:
  Thoracolumbar flexion: patient bends forward at the waist with the knees fully extended, attempting to touch the toes with the fingertips. Normal lumbar flexion involves progressive reversal of lumbar curvature from lumbar lordosis in the standing position to flattening of the lordosis in mid-flexion and even slight kyphosis at full flexion.
  Lumbosacral extension: patient bends backward while supporting the low back and shoulders (normal range 15–25 degrees).
  Lumbar lateral flexion: patient bends to the left and right with the knee extended.
  Thoracolumbar rotation: patient places the hands on opposite shoulders and rotates the spine to the left and right while fixing the pelvis (normal range 50–70 degrees). This can be performed with the patient seated if required. Movement of the lumbar spine includes 40–60 degrees forward

Table 5.1 Summary guide for identifying common cervical and lumbar nerve root lesions

Nerve	Sensory loss	Motor weakness	Reflex
C5	Lateral arm	Deltoid, biceps	Biceps
C6	Lateral forearm, thumb, index finger	Wrist extensors, biceps	Supinator
C7	Middle finger	Wrist flexors, finger extensors, triceps	Triceps
C8	Medial forearm, ring finger, little finger	Finger flexors, thumb extensors	None
T1 (rare)	Medial arm	Finger abductors	None
L3	Anterior/medial thigh	Hip flexion	Patella
L4	Anterior leg, medial foot	Tibialis anterior (ankle dorsiflexion)	Patella
L5	Lateral leg, web of big toe	Extensor hallucis longus (big toe extension)	None
S1	Posterior leg, lateral foot	Peroneus muscles (foot eversion)	Achilles

flexion, 20–35 degrees extension, 15–20 degrees lateral flexion and 10–20 rotation.

Thoracic spinal movements are closely integrated with the lumbar spine and can be hard to assess independently. Thoracic spine movements are limited to:

Flexion	20–40°
Extension	20–45°
Lateral flexion	35–50°
Rotation	35–50°

Schober's test assesses the amount of lumbar flexion, may be considered if inflammatory back pain is suspected. A mark is made at the level of the iliac crests (dimples of Venus if present) on the vertebral column – this is about at the level of L5. One mark is made 5 cm below this and another at about 10 cm above. The patient is then instructed to touch their toes. If the increase in distance is less than 5 cm then this is indicative of a limitation of lumbar flexion.

Neurological assessment

This is directed by both history and especially whether there are any neurological symptoms. Screening techniques can be used:

- Walk on their heels
- Walk on their toes
- Single leg dip.

Straight leg raise

Tests for evidence of nerve root tension or radiculopathy.

With the patient supine, the leg is raised while fully extended with the ankle dorsiflexed; the test is positive if there is pain between 10–60 degrees of movement. The most common lesion that will produce a positive test is either an L5 or S1 disc lesion (see sensory testing below):

- L5 motor nerve root testing evaluates strength of ankle and great toe dorsiflexion. L5 sensory nerve root damage would result in numbness in the medial foot and the web space between the first and second toe.
- The S1 nerve root is tested by evaluating ankle reflexes and sensation at the posterior calf and lateral foot. S1 radiculopathy may cause weakness of plantar flexion, but is difficult to detect. It can also be worth checking foot eversion.

A complete neurological examination assessing tone, power reflexes, plantar responses and sensation may also be required depending on history and symptoms (see Table 5.1).

General evaluation

With particular attention to assessing for any clinical evidence of malignancy:

- Breast examination
- Prostate examination
- Check for lymphadenopathy (see Chapter 45).

Scenario 5.1 continued

Key considerations would include a thorough assessment for neurological signs in the lower limbs. The history of carcinoma merits particular assessment for cauda equina syndrome. A cord compression would be less common for prostatic carcinoma progression, but require stronger consideration for breast, lung, renal and bowel cancer. Recent urological instrumentation, surgery or dental work is sometimes a potential risk factor for bacteraemia leading to discitis. Rheumatoid arthritis may at a late stage involve the spine but this tends to affect the atlanto-axial joint leading to subluxation – is there any evidence of upper motor neurone signs? Seronegative arthritides such as ankylosing spondylitis are the group most likely to present with mid or low back stiffness. Has immune suppression increased risk of infection or has the patient had longer-term steroid exposure contributing to an osteoporotic crush fracture? Are there other risk factors for osteoporosis?

Investigations

Laboratory requests

- *Urinalysis*: a screen for UTI so often missing from clerking notes, so repeat if uncertainty.
- *FBC*: anaemia of chronic disease.
- *ESR, CRP*: evidence of acute infection/ inflammation. In patients with back pain and a high CRP where there is no other explanation or where there is an explanation but acute back pain is ongoing and there is spinal tenderness, discitis requires exclusion.
- *U&E, LFTs, bone profile*: remember that elevated alkaline phosphatase can be an acute phase response.
- *Amylase*: patients with central back pain.
- *PSA*.

Note: the specificity of a positive HLA B27 antigen for diagnosing ankylosing spondylitis is low and it should not be used as a screening test for this disorder.

Imaging

Chest radiograph

- Should be considered in all patients requiring admission.
- Useful as a screen for any other sources of infection.
- Ensure no evidence of TB, neoplastic lesions.

Spinal radiographs

- This can be helpful to exclude any evidence of vertebral collapse or fracture, particularly in elderly patients with suspected osteoporosis.
- Lytic lesions can also be detected although not all are radiolucent.

- Often *not helpful* in younger patients, and *unnecessary radiation exposure* should be avoided.
- Is not a reliable test in the acute setting to diagnose sacroiliitis or other early inflammatory changes.

MRI

Should be considered when needed to exclude the following:

- cauda equina and other concerns regarding acute neurological compromise
- spinal malignancy
- infection
- fracture
- ankylosing spondylitis or other inflammatory disorders.

CT spine

- Considered when MRI is contraindicated or patients are unable to tolerate scanner environment.
- Can be helpful for delineating bony anatomy and whether there is evidence of fracture but is not helpful in determining whether there is evidence of neurological compromise.

Radionucleotide imaging (technetium bone scans)

- These can be helpful where there is concern regarding diffuse pathology and plain X-rays have not found a cause and there are too many areas to examine with MRI.

Other imaging may be indicated when there is evidence of visceral disease, e.g. abdominal CT for suspected abdominal aortic aneurysm.

Other tests

- *Nerve conduction studies*: helpful to determine whether there is evidence of radiculopathy if there are acute symptoms.
- *Electromyelography*: evidence of myelopathy/ myositis (proximal muscle weakness, elevated CK).

Scenario 5.1 continued

Screening blood tests were normal. A plain X-ray excluded osteoporotic collapse. In this case with a number of differing considerations in the history an MRI was requested. This demonstrated a canal stenosis at L2/3 with a large

> osteophyte compressing the L3 nerve root. This was amenable to surgical intervention and the patient had a good outcome following surgery.

Management

Analgesic treatments

Pharmacological

Paracetamol (1 g qds) given regularly can be an effective initial treatment and prevent unnecessary use of NSAIDs and excess opioid use.

NSAIDs (ibuprofen 400 mg tds or preferably naproxen 500 mg bd) are particularly effective in patients with inflammatory back pain. Significant side effects (GI bleeding and renal dysfunction), especially in elderly patients and those with evidence of kidney disease. Use with caution in patients who are septic. Co-prescribe a PPI in patients over 45.

Opioids: give consideration to risk of opioid dependence; examples include codeine and dihydrocodeine and tramadol. All can cause confusion, particularly in elderly patients, and should be used with caution. Consider referral to pain team if dose requirement is increasing.

Low dose benzodiazepines for a short course if patients are having particular difficulty mobilizing, but caution should be given regarding dependence issues and yellow flag features regarding back pain as detailed below.

Non-pharmacological treatments for acute back pain

Patient education: advise to stay as active as possible and return to normal activities as soon as possible (avoiding lifting). Referral to a back pain service with a patient education programme is the most helpful if it is locally available.

Physiotherapy: patients should be referred for acute physiotherapy.

Treatments that are not supported by strong evidence:

- Systemic steroids are not helpful.
- Acupuncture has no clear evidence base.
- Spinal manipulation and chiropractic techniques are commonly used by patients, especially for chronic pain. There is low quality evidence to demonstrate that spinal manipulation may have short-term benefits for pain reduction, but is not effective in treating disability. Chiropractic techniques are considered safe if performed by a well-trained practitioner but have no clear evidence base.

- Bed rest is *not* recommended and can worsen outcome, including joint stiffness, muscle wasting, loss of bone density and pressure ulcers, and is a risk for developing VTE.

Notes on specific conditions

Spinal infection

History

Often moderately severe pain with spinal tenderness, with generalized evidence of sepsis. Onset can be insidious with a particular pattern of non-mechanical, constant pain and not relieved by rest.

Risk factors for developing spinal infections include:

- advanced age
- IV drug use
- HIV infection
- long-term steroid use
- diabetes.

Examination

- Pyrexia.
- Local tenderness to palpation should direct imaging to that area.
- Ensure there is no evidence of urinary retention and check for signs of a psoas abscess (e.g. flank pain and limitation of pain on hip movement).
- Fully assess lower limb neurology.

Investigations

- Elevated inflammatory response in almost all cases (elevated ESR, CRP, WCC).
- Alkaline phosphatase may be raised as part of an acute phase response.
- Blood cultures are required, and should be repeated during temperature spikes. Antibiotics should be delayed if at all possible until confirmation of septic source – this is usually with MRI.
- Consider local biopsy.

Vertebral osteomyelitis is the most common form of spinal infection and can develop from infections in surrounding areas and from bacteraemic spread following surgery.

Intervertebral disc space infections involve the space between adjacent vertebrae.

Spinal canal infections (least common) include:

- spinal epidural abscess (often significant neurological signs combined with evidence of sepsis)
- adjacent soft tissue infections including cervical and thoracic paraspinal lesions and lumbar psoas muscle abscess.

Pathophysiology

- Infection usually starts in the anterior portion of the vertebral body (rich arterial supply), spreading to the rest of the vertebral body through the medullary space.
- The lumbar region is most often affected (50% of cases), followed by the thoracic spine (35% of cases) and the cervical spine rarely.
- *Staphylococcus aureus* causes over 50% of cases. Other causes include *Streptococcus* (groups B and G especially in patients with diabetes), *Pneumococcus, Enterococcus, Escherichia coli, Salmonella* (particularly after urinary tract instrumentation), *Pseudomonas* and *Candida* (particularly in IV drug users) and *Klebsiella*.
- Tuberculosis accounts for approximately 2% of infections overall. The thoracolumbar region is most commonly affected. Multifocal involvement is rare, can be difficult to detect and almost never occurs in immunocompetent hosts or those with normal pulmonary findings.
- Tuberculous spondylitis (Pott disease) generally begins with inflammation of the anterior intervertebral joints, typically spreading via the anterior ligament to the adjacent vertebrae, and once two vertebrae are involved can enter the intervertebral disc space (leading to the appearance of disc sparing, see below). The avascular disc tissue can then necrose leading to vertebral collapse, subsequent deformity and kyphosis, which can result in neurological compromise.
- Spinal tuberculosis most commonly involves the thoracic spine. MRI can be helpful here; typical features include evidence of a well-defined paraspinal high signal region, with evidence of abscess and subligamentous spread to three or more vertebral levels with involvement of the entire vertebral body.
- With two vertebral levels involved in a destructive process it can be hard to tell the difference between neoplastic and infectious causes of disc destruction. A destructive bone lesion associated with well-preserved endplates is more likely to be secondary to an underlying neoplastic lesion.

Investigation

- Avoid unnecessary X-ray imaging of lumbar/pelvic region in younger patients and proceed to MRI.
- MRI may demonstrate typical findings such as vertebral endplate destruction, bone marrow and disc abnormalities and paravertebral or epidural abscesses.
- Radionucleotide imaging can be considered if the patient is unable to tolerate MRI.
- Biopsy is usually done under CT guidance.
- The possibility of concurrent infective endocarditis should be considered in patients with underlying cardiac defects and in this case echocardiography should be considered.

Management

- Often require long-term antibiotics, hence requirement for accurate microbiological diagnosis.
- Surgery may be required if significant bone involvement, neurological deficit, failure of needle biopsy and evidence of spinal instability.
- CRP will be expected to normalize more rapidly than ESR in response to correct antibiotics. Maintenance of CRP within the normal range is a helpful way of ensuring that antibiotics have been given for a sufficient duration.

Osteoporotic vertebral compression fractures

History

- Commonly lower thoracic and lumbar vertebrae.
- Spontaneous acute severe pain, with anterior radiation and flank pain being common; leg radiation is rare.
- Abdominal and chest pain can occur.
- The severe pain usually persists for several weeks, with moderate discomfort for several months.
- A history of risk factors for osteoporosis should be sought, particularly in patients with kyphosis and

those with a prior history of low trauma fractures (wrist and hip).

Examination

- It is rare that patients present with the cauda equina syndrome or other manifestations of neurological compromise (but always consider and exclude on the basis of robust history and examination).

Investigation

- Plain X-rays may identify fractures, but may not help to decide if there is an acute change.
- MRI to age fracture and identify alternative cause of pain.
- Bone scanning is helpful if multiple compression fractures are suspected.
- The radiological features include:
  - end-plate deformity with a reduction in the mid-vertebral height (biconcavity)
  - decrease in the anterior vertebral height (wedging)
  - reduction in the anterior and posterior vertebral height (compression).
- Serum investigations should include full blood count, ESR and CRP, biochemical profile (urea, electrolytes, albumin, total protein and liver function tests), bone profile, (serum calcium, phosphate and alkaline phosphatase) and thyroid function tests.
  - Hypercalcaemia suggests primary hyperparathyroidism, myeloma or skeletal metastases.
  - Hypocalcaemia, hypophosphataemia and raised alkaline phosphatase suggests osteomalacia.
- Serum and urine electrophoresis should also be performed if the ESR or CRP is elevated, or there are concerns regarding myeloma.
- In younger patients with unexplained osteoporosis, anti-endomysial antibodies can be considered to exclude coeliac disease, particularly if there is suspicion of malabsorption.
- In men measure serum testosterone, sex hormone binding globulin and gonadotrophins and PSA if there are symptoms of prostatism or sclerosis on spine X-rays.

- 25OHD and PTH measurements may be useful in excluding vitamin D deficiency and secondary hyperparathyroidism in patients with limited sunlight exposure, previous gastric resection, malabsorption or anticonvulsant treatment.
- Bone density measurements are assessed using a dual energy X-ray absorptiometry (DEXA) test. This compares bone density to a control population level at peak bone density (this occurs in the mid 20s); this is the T-score. In younger patients the Z-score can be used; this is an age-matched control. Osteoporosis is diagnosed with a T-score of −2.5 or lower with evidence of prior fracture with osteopenia defined as a T-score of −1.5 to −2.5.

Management

Evidence supports use of the following in *acute* pain:

- IV bisphosphonates (pamidronate and zoledronate) for acute pain control.
- intranasal salmon calcitonin

Invasive techniques to stabilize *acute* fractures and reduce pain levels include:

- *Vertebroplasty* where cement is injected in the fracture site.
- *Kyphoplasty* where a balloon is inflated in the bone matrix to restore vertebral height.

Spondyloarthritis

Spondyloarthritis refers to a family of diseases that share several clinical features including:

- inflammation of axial joints (especially sacroiliac joints)
- asymmetric oligoarthritis (especially lower extremities, knees and ankles)
- dactylitis (sausage digits)
- enthesitis (inflammation at sites of ligamentous or tendon attachment to bone, especially Achilles tendon).

Additional features are:

- genital and skin lesions
- eye and bowel inflammation
- association with preceding/ongoing infection.

Back pain is the most common symptom (70%) of patients at presentation. Clinical features of inflammatory spinal disease include:

- onset before the age of 40 years
- insidious onset

- improvement with exercise
- no improvement with rest
- nocturnal pain
- good response to NSAIDs.

Spondylosis

Spondylosis describes arthritis of the spine seen radiographically as disc space narrowing with arthritic changes in the facet joint.

Spondylolisthesis

Spondylolisthesis is the anterior or posterior displacement of one vertebra on the one beneath it.

- Low-grade spondylolisthesis (<50%) may not be symptomatic or require treatment.
- While this may occur due to spondylosis in the younger patient as above, degenerative spondylolisthesis is a disease of the older adult that develops as a result of facet joint arthritis and remodelling.
- Slips can be asymptomatic but can worsen the symptoms of neurogenic claudication when associated with lumbar spinal stenosis.

Radiculopathy

Radiculopathy describes impairment of specific nerve roots.

- May cause radicular pain, weakness or altered sensation in the distribution of the nerve.
- *Sciatica* (lumbosacral radiculopathy) is a set of symptoms including:
  - pain that may be caused by general compression or irritation of one of five spinal nerve roots of the sciatic nerve
  - lower back pain, buttock pain, numbness or weakness in the leg and foot
  - neurological compromise with pins and needles or tingling and difficulty in moving/ controlling the leg
  - compressed, inflamed or ischaemic nerves.

Myelopathy

Myelopathy refers to pathology of the spinal cord.

- Clinical manifestations depend on which spinal level and which part of the cord is affected (anterior, posterior or lateral).

- Features may include:
  - upper motor neurone signs (weakness, spasticity, increased tone, hyperreflexia)
  - upgoing plantars
  - sensory deficit
  - bladder/bowel dysfunction.

Socioeconomic impact of chronic low back pain

Acute low back pain due to non-specific causes is usually self-limiting (recovery rate 90% within 6 weeks) but 2–7% of people develop chronic pain. Recurrent and chronic pain account for up to 75% of work-related sick leave.

Risk factors for developing acute and chronic back pain are poorly understood; they include:

- heavy physical work
- repetitive bending, twisting, lifting, pulling and pushing
- working in a long-term fixed position
- exposure to vibration.

Psychosocial risk factors include:

- stress, distress, anxiety, depression
- cognitive dysfunction
- pain behaviour
- job dissatisfaction
- work-related stress.

Psychosocial 'yellow flags' are factors that increase the risk of developing, or perpetuating, chronic pain and long-term disability (including) work-loss associated with low back pain. Examples include:

1. Attitudes and beliefs about back pain – that it is harmful or severely disabling, or have high expectation of passive treatments rather than a belief that active participation will help.
2. Behaviour – belief that pain may be inappropriate (fear-avoidance and consequent reduced activity levels).
3. Compensation issues and employment-related problems.
4. Depression – depression, anxiety, stress, tendency to low mood and withdrawal from social interaction represent a high risk.

Identification of 'yellow flags' should lead to appropriate cognitive and behavioural management. However, there is no evidence on the effectiveness of psychosocial assessment or intervention in acute low back pain.

Further reading

NICE Guidance Clinical Knowledge Summaries: Acute low back pain (up to 6 weeks) and chronic low back pain (more than 6 weeks). Available to download at http://cks.nice.org.uk/back-pain-low-without-radiculopathy (accessed 2 December 2013).

Patten JP. *Neurological Differential Diagnosis*, 2nd edn. Springer, 1998.

Acute kidney injury (AKI) and chronic kidney disease (CKD)

Duncan Whitehead

Acute kidney injury

The terms acute renal failure, dysfunction and impairment alongside the myriad of definitions that accompanied them are now obsolete. International consensus in terminology and definition was achieved by the 2007 publication of the AKI network criteria [1] defining AKI as any one of:

- increase in serum creatinine by ≥26.5 μmol/L within 48 hours
- increase in serum creatinine of 1.5 times baseline, known or presumed to have occurred within 7 days
- urine volume <0.5 mL/kg/h for 6 hours (oliguria).

AKI is associated with an increased length of hospital stay and in-hospital mortality, the risks are greater the more severe the AKI. Long term there is increased risk of death, CKD and hypertension in patients who have had AKI, even following a full or near full recovery of renal function.

Therefore physicians should aspire to prevent the occurrence or prevent the progression of AKI.

AKI is commonly predictable in hospital inpatients [2]. Common risk factors for developing AKI include:

- age over 65 years
- co-morbidities (DM, IHD, LVF, PVD, liver disease)
- medications (ACE inhibitors, angiotensin-II inhibitors, NSAIDs, diuretics)
- CKD (eGFR<60 mL/min)
- hypovolaemia
- sepsis
- poor nutritional status.

AKI always has at least one cause. Through accurate assessment and diagnosis and removal/treatment of risk factors the progression/development of AKI can often be prevented.

> ### Scenario 6.1
>
> *Mr ARF, an 86-year-old man, was found on the floor by his cleaner and referred by his GP to MAU. He had been on the floor for 26 hours. His past medical history includes ischaemic heart disease and left ventricular failure for which he takes ramipril 5 mg od and furosemide 40 mg od. On assessment his BP = 90/50, HR = 105 bpm, and he is clinically hypovolaemic with a reduced skin turgor, cold peripheries and a reduced central capillary refill time. He is confused and unable to give a clear history. Blood tests reveal a urea = 42.5 mmol/L, creatinine = 425 μmol/L, K= 4.1 mmol/L.*

This is a common presentation to the medical assessment unit. It is clear this man is hypovolaemic and his acute kidney injury is at least in part pre-renal and he may have started to develop acute tubular necrosis as a consequence of renal hypoperfusion. Initial treatment should include intravenous hydration with balanced crystalloid solution (*serum potassium being normal*), to rapidly restore euvolaemia and renal perfusion. Repeated fluid challenges are the safest approach to fluid resuscitation.

The more astute admitting doctor will proceed to give further consideration to other causes of this man's AKI, which should include checking a serum creatine kinase and reviewing his FBC. Examine for a palpable bladder; urine dipstick analysis and a septic screen should also be performed. Obtain previous creatinine results to gauge his baseline renal function, and any further past medical history or drug history is essential to be able to offer good quality care.

Management should proceed with close monitoring of urine output, regular clinical fluid assessments

---

Acute Medicine, ed. Stephen Haydock, Duncan Whitehead and Zoë Fritz. Published by Cambridge University Press.
© Cambridge University Press 2015.

and daily blood tests to gauge progress and inform on further intravenous fluid requirements. Furosemide and ramipril should be crossed off his drug chart, *not 'held' for a day or two*. An escalation plan should be made with the benefit of further background regarding his normal function and additional co-morbidities.

Common causes of AKI

Consider the cause by location of pathology.

Pre-renal

- Inadequate renal perfusion resulting in reduced capillary glomerular pressure (which drives the glomerular filtration rate (GFR)).
- Treatment consists of improving renal perfusion, often with intravenous fluid resuscitation and withdrawing antihypertensive medication.
- Fully and rapidly reversible.

Renal

Tubular interstitial

Acute tubular necrosis (ATN)

- Renal tubular cells are highly metabolically active, due to active membrane transporter proteins responsible for electrolyte and water reabsorption.
- Tubular cells have a correspondingly high oxygen requirement and are very vulnerable to hypoxia-induced necrosis.
- Hypoperfusion is the commonest cause of renal hypoxia; pre-renal AKI will progress to ATN if renal perfusion is not restored; the longer the delay, the more severe the ATN.
- Severe ATN often recovers, but not always or fully; with sustained adequate perfusion, this can take several weeks while requiring renal replacement therapy.
- Polyuria can occur during the recovery phase.
- ATN can result from direct tubular cell toxicity (gentamicin, contrast-induced nephropathy).

Acute interstitial nephritis

- Normally suspected on clinical grounds, confirmation requires renal histology which shows leucocytes, often eosinophils, infiltrating the renal parenchyma.
- Commonly caused by a local (renal) drug reaction – antibiotics, NSAIDs and proton pump inhibitors are the commonest causes:

- AKI often resolves on stopping the offending agent
  - steroids are used in more severe cases.
- Can occur secondary to infection.
- Rare causes include sarcoidosis and SLE.

Sepsis-induced AKI

- Severe sepsis is defined as organ dysfunction due to infection.
- Pathophysiology is multifactorial; biopsies commonly demonstrate ATN with or without interstitial nephritis.
- Treat sepsis with prompt antibiotics and optimal fluid management with organ support when indicated.
- Most patients will recover to independence from renal replacement therapy.

Rhabdomyolysis

- Muscle breakdown releases myoglobin into the circulation, which is broken down releasing haem pigment.
- AKI results from direct toxicity of haem to the tubular cells and cast formation within the tubules causing obstruction (unlikely if CK <5000 units/L).
- Forced diuresis (200–300 mL/h) with intravenous hydration, diluting the urine reduces both effects and can prevent or lessen the AKI – care is required as fluid overload might result if oliguric renal failure is developing.
- Urinary alkalization (pH >6.5) with IV sodium bicarbonate may be beneficial but is unproven.

Glomerular

Crescentic glomerulonephritis/rapidly progressing glomerulonephritis

- Histological diagnosis demonstrating aggressive disease which untreated will irreversibly destroy glomeruli, often resulting in ESRF.
- Rare: ≈2% of AKI admissions to an acute medical unit, so *easily missed*.
- *Urine dipstick;* if no *blood or protein* is present a glomerulonephritis is *unlikely*.
- Hypertension is common but not universal.
- High index of suspicion is required in those with no obvious cause of AKI.
- Associated haemoptysis suggests a *pulmonary-renal syndrome*, a potentially life-threatening situation.

- Causes include: ANCA-positive vasculitis, anti-GBM disease, lupus nephritis, post-streptococcus glomerulonephritis and IgA nephropathy.

Haemolytic uraemic syndrome (HUS)

- Subdivided into diarrhoea positive (D+) and the rarer inherited diarrhoea negative (D−) HUS.
- Shiga toxin producing organisms such as *E. coli* 0157:H7 are the causative pathogen in D+ HUS.
- HUS is a microangiopathic haemolytic anaemia (MAHA):
  - the clotting cascade is inappropriately activated within the renal capillary bed
  - fibrin strands form within the renal capillaries, erythrocytes are cleaved by the fibrin strands (haemolysis) resulting in *helmet cells/schistocytes on blood film*
  - thrombus formation occurs around the fibrin strands, platelet aggregation results, explaining the *low platelet count*
  - thrombus in the renal capillaries causes a reduced blood flow and GFR.
- Triad of anaemia, thrombocytopenia and AKI.
- Platelet infusions should be avoided if possible; they will rapidly aggregate with the thrombus and worsen the situation in the renal vascular bed.

Post-renal

- The pressure gradient between the blood in the glomerular capillary and ultrafiltrate in Bowman's capsule drives the filtrate across the glomerular basement membrane.
- In an obstructed system, pressure is conducted back via the urine to the renal tubules and Bowman's capsule.
- The fall in pressure gradient across the glomerular basement membrane results in a reduction in GFR.
- If unresolved CKD develops:
  - the pathophysiology of this irreversible damage is complex involving many cytokines and vasoactive factors
  - progressive tubular interstitial fibrosis results.
- Early drainage to decompress the renal parenchyma is the treatment of choice.
- The intervention required depends on the level of obstruction.

Myeloma kidney

Multiple myeloma causes AKI and CKD through several distinct mechanisms:

- Hypercalcaemia and the resulting hypovolaemia
- Renal calculi resulting from hypercalciuria due to hypercalcaemia
- Cast nephropathy occurs if Bence Jones protein (BJP) precipitates out within the tubules, most commonly when urinary concentration of BJP is high (e.g. hypovolaemia during septic episode)
- NSAID use for bone pains
- Renal amyloid deposition, causing progressive CKD with or without nephrotic syndrome.

Chronic kidney disease

The recognition of CKD improved when estimated glomerular filtration rate (eGFR) reporting became standard practice (Table 6.1). Reported eGFR is calculated using the modification of diet in renal disease equation (MDRD), which factors age, gender and creatinine. This gives a reasonable approximation for average sized individuals; it is less good at extremes of size, where the Cockcroft–Gault formula (calculator available at http://nephron.com/cgi-bin/CGSI.cgi) is more reliable as it includes weight. No eGFR formula is perfect and interpretation in the clinical context is essential.

Despite the terminology not all patients with CKD truly have a disease. From 40 years old everybody loses ≈1 mL/min/year of GFR so in the eighth decade of life an eGFR ≈50 mL/min is normal, without any disease process being present.

Common causes of CKD

Diabetic nephropathy

- Develops contemporaneously with retinopathy; the vessels affected are of similar size
  - microalbuminuria is the first sign
  - poor glycaemic control and high blood pressure result in more rapid progression.
- The cause of ESRF in ≈20–25% of UK dialysis population.

Hypertensive nephropathy/ischaemic nephropathy

- Hypertension is a risk factor for progression of all CKD; a target BP <130/80 mmHg is acceptable, or <125/75 mmHg if proteinuria ≥ lg/24hrs.

Table 6.1 Classification of CKD

CKD stage	eGFR (mL/min)	Description	Prevalence (%)
1	>90	Normal/increased eGFR, with evidence of kidney damage	3.3
2	60–89	Slight decrease in eGFR, with evidence of kidney damage	3.0
3A	45–59	Moderate decrease in eGFR, with or without other evidence of kidney damage	4.3
3B	30–44		
4	15–29	Severe decrease in eGFR, with or without other evidence of kidney damage	0.2
5	<15	Established or end-stage renal failure (ESRF)	0.2

Renal artery stenosis

- Commonly due to atherosclerotic disease, although in young patients the cause may be fibromuscular dysplasia.
- Stenting is controversial in atherosclerotic renal artery stenosis; generally believed beneficial in those with flash pulmonary oedema, rapidly deteriorating renal function or highly resistant hypertension.

Chronic glomerulonephritis

- Glomerulonephritides are histological diagnoses characterized by glomerular inflammation.
- Pathophysiology of each type is not fully understood although aberrant immunological responses are often implicated.
- All result in blood or protein on urine analysis.
- The rate of renal decline, quantity of proteinuria, hypertension and the renal interstitial appearance on biopsy guide the renal prognosis.

IgA nephropathy

- The most common glomerulonephritis.
- Varied prognosis from aggressive crescentic glomerulonephritis to benign chronic glomerulonephritis causing only invisible haematuria.

Membranous glomerulonephritis

- Commonest cause of nephrotic syndrome in adults.
- Treatment is challenging although ≈30% enter spontaneous remission.

Autosomal dominant polycystic kidney disease

- Commonest inherited cause of ESRF within the UK.

Chronic interstitial nephritis

- NSAIDs, analgesic nephropathy is the commonest cause.
- Commonly presents with hypertension or incidental abnormal blood test.

Post-obstructive nephropathy

- If delayed resolution of the obstruction, often due to limited symptoms.

Chronic reflux nephropathy

- Recurrent episodes of pyelonephritis cause renal scarring and loss of function.

Post AKI

- *Any cause of AKI* can result in permanent loss of functional glomeruli.

Nephrectomy

- Anticipate ≈50% drop in eGFR post nephrectomy.

Prescribing in CKD and AKI

Essential considerations when prescribing in this context are:

1. The drug's potential to worsen renal function or delay recovery; is it *essential* (≈20% of AKI is drug associated)?
2. Will the low GFR affect drug or metabolite clearance requiring dose reduction?
3. Dose increases may be needed as/if AKI recovers.

In patients with AKI the eGFR is meaningless; it is safest to assume a low GFR <20 mL/min when prescribing in any patient with AKI.

Commonly used medications requiring careful prescribing in this setting include analgesics and antibiotics.

Analgesia

No patient should be left in pain, but analgesia must be used safely, a practically applicable adaptation of the WHO pain ladder:

1. Paracetamol 1 g qds PO
   Avoid non-steroidal anti-inflammatory drugs (NSAIDs), *they INFLAME nephrologists*
2. Tramadol 50 mg tds ≈30% and 60% of metabolites renally excreted
   Buprenorphine patch <30% renal excretion
3. Oxycodone ≈10% renal excretion
   Fentanyl patch/patient-controlled analgesia <10% excreted in the urine

NSAID effects on the kidney: constriction of the afferent glomerular arterial results from a reduction of prostaglandin synthesis, reducing intraglomerular pressure, resulting in a fall in GFR. Downstream blood flow to the tubular cells is also reduced, increasing the risk of developing ATN. Interstitial nephritis can occur in susceptible individuals.

Antibiotics

Trimethoprim and co-trimoxazole (Septrin)

- Normally 15% of urinary creatinine is secreted by the tubules; in CKD this can be as high as 50%.
- Both drugs block tubular secretion of creatinine, causing a rise in serum creatinine without reducing GFR, most pronounced in CKD.
- Uncertainty about the significance of a creatinine rise follows; is it true AKI or a benign drug effect?
- Effect lasts ≈7–10 days after stopping the antibiotic.
- Prescribe with these words of caution in mind.

Nitrofurantoin

- Poor efficacy in CKD stage 3 or worse as often not excreted in high enough concentration to be bactericidal in the urine.

Gentamicin

- Directly toxic to tubular cells related to urinary concentration so more likely in hypovolaemia or if excessively high serum levels.
- Excreted unchanged by the kidney; prolonged half-life in CKD and AKI, so close monitoring of levels is essential.

Vancomycin

- AKI is a recognized rare side effect.
- Reduced renal clearance, so requires close serum monitoring.

Penicillins

- Beta-lactam neurotoxicity from accumulation is rare but serious; when prolonged high doses are indicated a dose reduction is required.
- Can cause interstitial nephritis.

The Renal Drug Handbook (see Further reading) provides comprehensive prescribing guidance for patients with AKI, CKD and those on renal replacement therapy.

Distinguishing AKI from first presentation of CKD

- Old creatinine results remain the best guide to acuity and every effort should be made to retrieve previous results.
- Ultrasound scanning can suggest CKD:
  - small kidneys, renal length <10 cm
  - reduced cortical thickness results from glomerular loss
  - simple cysts accumulate with damage
  - polycystic kidney disease and obstructive nephropathy can be diagnosed.
- Secondary complications of CKD may be present:
  - renal anaemia (normocytic)
  - secondary hyperparathyroidism.

These complications should be interpreted with caution as there are other causes which might be present in a patient with AKI.

- If uncertainty remains assume it is AKI, the safest approach.
- Renal histology can clarify chronicity, diagnosis and prognosis but should be used sparingly as it comes with a risk of haemorrhage.

Life-threatening complications of AKI

The life-threatening complications of AKI are the four main indications for dialysis alongside drug accumulation as a consequence of AKI:

1. Acidosis
2. Hyperkalaemia
3. Uraemia
4. Fluid overload

5. Drug toxicity.

The mainstay of treatment for all of these includes restoration of renal function as soon as is possible; sometimes this is inevitably slow or impossible to achieve.

If they result as part of the dying process then palliative management to alleviate suffering is the treatment of choice.

Acidosis

- Enzyme systems throughout the body are affected by acidosis; many consequences occur such as reduced cardiac contractility.
- *Sodium bicarbonate* is useful to treat the metabolic acidosis (bicarbonate <22 mmol/L) caused by AKI, orally 1 g tds.
- IV sodium bicarbonate 1.26% to 1.4% 500 mL given over 2 to 4 hours should be used if profound acidosis or coexisting hyperkalaemia is present. Caution in:
  - hypocalcaemia – calcium will fall
  - hypokalaemia – potassium will fall
  - fluid overload
  - anuria; if the urine output is not rapidly restored the patient needs more definitive treatment with renal replacement therapy
  - IV calcium administered through the same cannula will precipitate out as calcium carbonate!
- Hyperkalaemia will normally improve over several hours on correction of the acidosis; potassium moves into cells and urine.

A pH <7.1 due to renal failure is an indication for urgent RRT.

Hyperkalaemia

Hyperkalaemia is a common complication of AKI and CKD; it deserves prompt assessment and treatment as cardiac arrest due to arrhythmia can ensue.

Potassium >6 mmol/L is significant and requires assessment:

- Exclude pseudo-hyperkalaemia; causes include:
  - thrombocytosis (retest using a lithium heparin tube)
  - haemolysis, i.e. delay to processing sample.
- ECG; abnormalities vary including tented T waves, complete heart block, ventricular tachycardia and fibrillation.

Potassium >6.5 mmol/L, or >5.5 mmol/L with ECG changes, requires urgent treatment:

- IV calcium gluconate (10 mL of 10%) for any ECG abnormality.
- Insulin and glucose infusion (10 units Actrapid, 50 mL, 50% glucose over 30 minutes) causes intracellular movement of potassium lasting a few hours.
- Salbutamol nebulizers use the same channels as insulin and glucose to move potassium, and increase the risk of tachyarrhythmia, so are not recommended.
- Medication review; *stop contributing drugs* where possible: beta-blockers, ACE inhibitors, angiotensin-II inhibitors, spironolactone and LMWH.
- Sodium bicarbonate IV as in acidosis section.

In the setting of CKD additional strategies are beneficial:

- Low potassium diet
- Prevent constipation.

A persisting potassium >6.0 mmol/L without improvement in AKI or with persistent ECG changes is an indication for renal replacement therapy.

Uraemia

Uraemia is a description of symptoms not serum urea concentration. Neurological toxicity is caused by many unmeasured nitrogen-based substances which accumulate in patients with renal failure. Uraemic features include:

- anorexia
- nausea and vomiting
- myoclonic 'uraemic' jerks
- confusion
- reduced consciousness
- seizures
- pericardial effusion.

The presence of any of these is an indication for RRT, unless AKI is rapidly improved with initial treatments.

Fluid overload

- Pulmonary oedema can be life-threatening and is often iatrogenic through excessive intravenous fluid resuscitation in oliguric/anuric AKI.
- Exclude an obstructed urinary system.
- Initial treatment with high dose IV loop diuretic (furosemide 120 mg IV).

- Nitrate infusions can ameliorate the situation by causing vasodilation to offload the patient until RRT can be commenced.
- Fluid restrict ≤1 litre/24 hours.

Poor response to diuretics is an indication for RRT; if a diuresis is achieved then further IV furosemide can be given.

Drug accumulation

- Opiate toxicity from codeine or morphine is commonest due to accumulation of active metabolites.
- IV naloxone is the treatment of choice; it has a shorter half-life than the opiate metabolites, so an infusion is required to prevent a relapse of respiratory depression.
- See Chapter 49 for specific toxins requiring dialysis, e.g. lithium, ethylene glycol.

Assessing fluid status

Always assess and document the intravascular fluid status of a patient at risk of or who has AKI. Accurate clinical assessment of intravascular fluid status is a difficult skill; every clue should be considered to improve accuracy:

History

- Thirst
- Insensible losses:
  - diarrhoea and vomiting
  - fever
  - high stoma output
- Poor fluid intake

Examination

- JVP
- Capillary refill time
- Temperature of peripheries compared to chest
- Skin turgor
- Mucous membranes
- BP
- Postural BP
- HR
- Auscultation for a third heart sound
- Lung bases for crepitations
- Peripheral oedema

No clinical sign is fully reliable, all have limitations.

Investigations

- Raised serum lactate; anaerobic respiration due to hypoperfusion of tissues is the commonest cause – *shock*
- Disproportionally raised urea to creatinine
- CXR for fluid overload

Monitoring

- Fluid balance charts with hourly input and output recorded
- Daily weights *(1 litre of water = 1 kg of weight, the beauty of metric!)*
- Regular clinical assessment and documentation of fluid status

Prescribing fluids in AKI, oliguria and polyuria

Initial fluid prescription

- Balanced crystalloid solution is the fluid of choice, unless hyperkalaemia is present.
- Aim to rapidly restore euvolaemia and renal perfusion.
- If uncertain use fluid challenges of 250 mL boluses and assess physiological response and clinical fluid status; repeat until confident that the patient is euvolaemic.

Maintenance fluid prescription

Intravenous fluid requirement depends upon:

- insensible losses
- oral fluid intake
- urine output.

Oliguria

Three causes:

1. *Pre-renal*: inadequate renal perfusion; ensure the patient is euvolaemic and optimize cardiac output.
2. *Renal*: kidneys unable to produce more urine.
3. *Post-renal*: obstructed urinary system.

Polyuria

Defined as >3 litres/24 hours urine production; causes include:

- restoration of homeostasis in hypervolaemic patient with recovering AKI
- recovering ATN:

- regenerating tubular cells are unable to reabsorb electrolytes and water, so cannot concentrate the urine; typically resolves over a few days
- euvolaemia should be maintained and parenteral fluids are often required
- post relief of an obstructed urinary system, similar to recovering ATN
- iatrogenic:
  - over-judicious use of intravenous fluids
  - inappropriate diuretic use, *always review the prescription chart*
- osmotic diuresis (hyperglycaemia).

The causes of polyuria in resolving AKI can be difficult to differentiate; the well-meaning physician can drive polyuria with liberal IV fluids in a well-filled patient. The fluid prescription needs regular review; stopping intravenous fluids and close observation with a view to restarting if required is often appropriate.

AKI initial investigation

The initial investigations are to gauge severity and possible life-threatening consequences, the secondary questions are chronicity and aetiology of the renal failure.

Urine dipstick

This *must* be performed at the earliest opportunity; interpretation is covered in Chapter 27.

Blood tests

- Urea, creatinine and electrolytes
- Bicarbonate
- Liver function tests
- Corrected calcium
- Phosphate
- Glucose
- Full blood count (FBC)
- C-reactive protein (CRP)

Consider:

- immunoglobulins, electrophoresis, serum free light chains
- lactate
- HIV
- hepatitis B and C.

If haematuria or proteinuria is present on urine dipstick or the cause is uncertain consider investigation of haematuria with blood tests (see Chapter 27).

Imaging

- CXR – consolidation represents alveoli containing:
  - white cells
  - red cells
  - water
- Bladder scan:
  - a normally functioning bladder will hold 400–500 mL of urine, post-micturition volumes ≥100 mL confirm retention
- Ultrasound KUB:
  - within 24 hours if concern of obstruction or unexplained AKI

Nephrology referral for AKI

Specialist referral is required in a minority of patients with AKI; indications for referral include:

- indications for dialysis
- suspicion of acute glomerulonephritis
- unexplained AKI
- poor response to treatment
- severe AKI (creatinine ≥354 μmol/L, creatinine >3× baseline, anuria >12 hours)
- CKD stage 4 or 5
- renal transplant.

Always treat patients with AKI as unwell and give due consideration to the underlying causes. Prompt treatment of all reversible causes identified maximizes the chance of a good outcome.

References

1. Mehta RL, Kellum JA, Shah SV, et al. Acute Kidney Injury Network: report of an initiative to improve outcomes in acute kidney injury. *Crit Care* 2007;11(2): R31. Available to download at http://ccforum.com/content/pdf/cc5713.pdf.

2. NCEPOD. Adding Insult to Injury. A review of the care of patients who died in hospital with a primary diagnosis of acute kidney injury (acute renal failure). 2009.

Further reading

AKI – KDIGO guidelines. www.kdigo.org/clinical_practice_guidelines/pdf/KDIGO%20AKI%20Guideline.pdf.

Ashley C, Currie A. *The Renal Drug Handbook*, 3rd revised edn. Radcliffe Publishing, 2008.

Coresh J, Astor BC, Greene T, Eknoyan G, Levey AS. Prevalence of chronic kidney disease and decreased kidney function in the adult US population: third national health and nutrition examination study. *Am J Kidney Dis* 2003; 41(1): 1–12.

NICE. Acute kidney injury. National Institute for Health and Care Excellence Clinical Guideline 169 (2013). Available to download at http://guidance.nice.org.uk/CG169/Guidance/pdf/English.

NICE. Chronic kidney disease: early identification and management of chronic kidney disease in adults in primary and secondary care. National Institute for Health and Care Excellence Clinical Guideline 73 (2008). Available to download at http://guidance.nice.org.uk/CG73/Guidance/pdf/English.

RCPE UK Consensus Conference on 'Management of acute kidney injury: the role of fluids, e alerts and biomarkers', 16 and 17 November 2012, members of Consensus Panel: Feehally J (Co-Chair); Gilmore I (Co-Chair) et al. www.rcpe.ac.uk/clinical-standards/standards/uk-consensus-statement-on-management-of-acute-kidney-injury-nov-2012.pdf.

Renal Association (UK) guidelines. www.renal.org/Clinical/GuidelinesSection/Guidelines.aspx.

The ASTRAL Investigators. Revascularization versus medical therapy for renal-artery stenosis. *N Engl J Med* 2009; 361:1953–1962.

Aggressive/disturbed behaviour

Stephen Haydock

Introduction

The 2002/2003 British Crime Survey found that 5% of health and social services professionals had experienced violence and aggression at work. Those working in Mental Health and front line emergency medical services are most at risk. Violent and aggressive behaviour can take the form of verbal abuse or physical assault. Verbal abuse is the use of inappropriate words or behaviour causing distress and/or continuing harassment, including threats of physical assault that are not carried out. Physical assault is the intentional application of force to the person of another without lawful justification, resulting in physical injury or personal discomfort.

NHS staff should be competent to assess the risk of violence posed by an individual and understand how to manage that risk to ensure their personal safety. Staff should be aware of those factors associated with an increased risk of violent behaviour:

- Previous history of violent/aggressive behaviour
- Alcohol and substance abuse
- Acute delirium
- Dementia
- Acute psychoses.

The NHS has a 'zero tolerance' approach in respect of violence towards staff. All NHS Trusts should have in place policies that are designed to protect staff and patients. The 1974 Health and Safety at Work Act and the 1992 Management of Health and Safety at Work Act seek to ensure the safety of staff in the work environment by ensuring that potential risks are documented and appropriate advice and training to protect staff is provided.

NHS staff experience aggression and violence from individuals who:

- act aggressively in the context of a co-morbid organic or psychiatric illness which significantly impairs their judgement at the time of the incident
- act aggressively in the absence of such mitigating circumstances.

> **Scenario 7.1**
>
> *The nursing staff of MAU contact you regarding a 50-year-old woman who is a 'frequent flyer' and has been discharged following a further brief admission with 'non-cardiac chest pain'. Her husband has come to pick her up but is unhappy that there is no clear diagnosis. He is behaving **very** aggressively towards the nursing staff who have encountered him previously and seen him behave in a similar manner. He is refusing to leave and demanding to see a doctor.*

Such situations can generally, but not always, be dealt with by a sympathetic and understanding approach. When dealing with such an individual it may be appropriate to involve hospital security staff by having them available for support if needed; indeed the nursing staff will often have already done so if they feel threatened.

In approaching the patient you should be aware of *warning signs of incipient violent behaviour*. People may become aggressive and violent without warning. However, overtly aggressive and violent behaviour is usually preceded by a recognizable escalation:

- increasingly loud speech, shouting, swearing and verbal abuse
- standing too close, adopting an aggressive stance, pointing and jabbing with the finger
- stamping feet, kicking objects, walking away
- inability to concentrate and over-sensitivity
- sweating, shaking

Acute Medicine, ed. Stephen Haydock, Duncan Whitehead and Zoë Fritz. Published by Cambridge University Press. © Cambridge University Press 2015.

- clenching teeth and jaws, clenching fists
- muscle tension, restlessness and fidgeting
- rapid breathing/sharp drawing in of breath
- flushing or extreme facial pallor, staring eyes
- crying.

De-escalation

This is the recommended technique in a potential crisis situation that aims to prevent an individual causing harm to themselves or others. It may involve moving the individual to a less confrontational area.

First the golden *do nots* … (TACOS):
Never:

- Threaten the aggressor
- Argue or contradict the aggressor
- Challenge the aggressor
- Order or command the aggressor
- Shame or disrespect the aggressor.

De-escalation is based around three concepts:

Self-control

- Appear calm and self-assured.
- Speak in a low monotone.
- Show respect even when limit setting.
- Do not be defensive even when insulted.
- Understand what back-up resources are available and when to leave!
- When the person gets up, comes up to you, shouts, points or wags his finger: then it is time to leave!

Physical presence

- Ensure you have clear access to exit.
- Keep at same height and avoid direct eye contact as can appear challenging (stand if he stands/sit if he sits).
- Stand at an angle from patient and more than three feet away.
- Never turn your back.
- Avoid smiling as may interpret as mockery or anxiety.
- Do not touch the person.
- Keep hands in view.
- Do not point, shake finger or argue or try to convince the person.

Communication

- Do not yell or talk over, wait for gaps and then talk calmly.
- Answer information questions appropriately and truthfully.
- Try to understand the concerns (may have a genuine reason for anger).
- Do not respond at all to verbal abuse.
- Empathize with feelings and not behaviour.
- Give limits and rules in a firm tone, ideally with choices, e.g. talk calmly now or talk later when you are more relaxed.
- Calmly explain consequences of aggressive behaviour. e.g. stop shouting or I will not continue conversation.

Scenario 7.1 continued

Despite your best attempts the situation escalates and he becomes increasingly aggressive, overturning a table in the room, shouting verbal abuse and threatening violence.

In these circumstances you should remove yourself from danger and get help quickly if you have not already done so. All Trusts should have a policy in place that permits the summoning of assistance and *you should be aware of the process within the Trust where you are working*. There are generally two levels of escalation, often referred to as *priority one* and *priority two*.

Priority one (external assistance)

A direct call via the switchboard to request urgent police assistance. You should provide:

- the precise location (on the hospital site)
- exact nature of situation
- who and how many people are involved in the incident
- whether a weapon is involved.

Alternatively the ward can dial 999 directly to request assistance depending on the degree of urgency.

When to involve the police

It is appropriate to summon police assistance if there is an *immediate threat of physical harm*:

- direct threat of violence (verbal or physical threats)
- damage to property
- increasingly noisy and aggressive behaviour despite appropriate attempts to de-escalate the situation
- weapon involved.

If the police are called then:

- Back off from further negotiation.
- You do not need to inform the person that police have been called as this in itself can be a challenge causing further escalation.
- Do not prevent the police from attending if the person appears to calm down.
- Ensure the on-call hospital manager is aware that police have been called.

Priority two (internal assistance)

This is usually the route taken when:

- urgent medical review is required for a difficult patient
- urgent need for 'specialing' of a patient
- urgent need for internal security.

Following such an incident the Trust will have a reporting procedure that should be followed. This may result in action to protect staff from further behaviour by the individual and commonly involves a red and yellow carding system. 'Carding' is appropriate for patients and visitors, who are *aware of their violent behaviour and persistently behave in an unacceptable manner, regardless of attempts made to resolve the situation*.

Yellow card

This is a formal warning to a patient to explain to them that they will be refused treatment if they continue to behave in a manner that is unacceptable.

Red card

A red card excludes a patient from receiving *planned treatment* by the specific NHS Trust. Alternative arrangements for care must be made for the patient. This usually lasts for a defined period such as a year. Emergency treatment will be provided but internal security or police will be in attendance as required.

Scenario 7.2

You are called to the MAU to review a 65-year-old man who is becoming increasingly aggressive. He is under treatment for pneumonia and has a history of heavy alcohol consumption and mild cognitive impairment. He has already struck one of the nursing staff when she prevented him from leaving the ward. When you arrive, security staff have managed to get him into the relatives room and are watching him from the door of the room where he is walking up and down, swearing loudly to an imaginary companion and apparently 'waiting for the bus home'.

In this situation a clinical assessment of the physical and mental state of the patient is required. Patients frequently exhibit aggressive or violent behaviour in the context of an acute psychotic episode.

Acute psychosis

An acute disorder of thought and perception characterized by:

- hallucinations (especially auditory)
- delusions (unshakeable false beliefs that are inconsistent with educational, cultural and social background)
- sometimes negative symptoms of apathy and withdrawal
- lack of insight into their illness
- alterations in memory, self-awareness, social behaviour and emotion.

Causes

Psychiatric disorders

- Schizophrenia
- Bipolar affective disorder
- Severe depression including postnatal depression

Physical causes

- CNS tumours
- CNS inflammatory disorders
- Alzheimer's disease
- Multiple sclerosis

Drug related

Illicit drugs (intoxication or withdrawal)

- Alcohol
- Cocaine
- Amphetamine and metamphetamine
- Mephedrone
- MDMA (ecstasy)
- Cannabis
- LSD
- Psilocybins (magic mushrooms)
- Ketamine

Therapeutic medications

- Corticosteroids
- L-dopa

Table 7.1

	Organic	Non-organic
Age	>40 years old	<40 years old
Hallucinations	predominantly visual	predominantly auditory
Orientation	disorientated	orientated
Cognition and attention	fluctuating deficit	constant deficit
Psychomotor	retardation, tremor, ataxia	repetitive activity, rocking, posturing
Memory	recent impairment	remote impairment
Examination/investigation	abnormal	normal

Distinguishing between an organic and non-organic acute psychosis

When faced with a new presentation of psychosis, Table 7.1 may help decide if an underlying organic problem is responsible.

Legal framework

See Chapter 59 for a more detailed explanation of the application of the Mental Capacity and Mental Health Acts.

The 2005 Mental Capacity Act codifies the common law doctrine of '*necessity*'. This allows for the restraint and treatment of *mentally incapacitated* adults which is necessary and in their best interests, without exposing those treating the patient to incur liability for a charge of battery.

The 1983 Mental Health Act constitutes the basis for detaining and treating patients for a mental disorder (including physical consequences) without their consent and commonly referred to as '*sectioning*'.

The relevant articles of *the 1998 European Convention on Human Rights*

Article 2 Right to life

Article 3 Right to be free from torture or inhuman or degrading punishment or treatment

Article 5 Right to liberty and security of a person save in prescribed cases

Article 8 Right to respect for private and family life and principle of 'proportionality'

Guidelines for safe, rapid sedation

It is sometimes necessary to sedate patients who are assessed as lacking capacity. The use of such an approach may require the use of safe restraint techniques by appropriately trained staff and needs to be *proportional to the risk and threat posed* to both the patient and those around them. The following is based upon the *2005 NICE recommendations* [1]. In addition, *always consult local policy*:

1. Offer oral medication first.
2. Intramuscular is preferred parenteral route.
3. Prescribe oral and intramuscular route separately (never write O/IM on the drug chart).
4. First line for behavioural disturbance in absence of acute psychosis:
   a. oral lorazepam alone
   b. intramuscular lorazepam if required.
5. First line for behavioural disturbance in context of acute psychosis:
   a. oral haloperidol plus oral lorazepam
   b. intramuscular haloperidol plus oral lorazepam.
6. Intramuscular haloperidol carries risk of acute dystonic reactions and parenteral benzatropine or procyclidine should also be available.
7. Intravenous route used only in exceptional circumstances and with agreement of a senior clinician.

Following rapid sedation, patients will require close monitoring of basic vital signs, hydration status and pulse oximetry at a frequency determined by medical staff. More careful monitoring is required if:

- IV route used (patient should always be attended by a staff member with sufficient experience to recognize complications)
- consciousness is impaired
- BNF dose limit is exceeded
- relevant medical disorder
- the patient has taken alcohol and/or illicit drugs.

Addendum
Pharmacology and therapeutics of sedative drugs

Stephen Haydock

Benzodiazepines

Mechanism

- Enhance effect of the inhibitory transmitter GABA resulting in reduced arousal, sedation, muscle relaxation and amnesia.

Side effects

- Sedation
- Respiratory depression
- Insomnia
- Ataxia
- Dependence occurs readily and withdrawal is well recognized; this has led to a marked reduction in their use in recent years.

Antipsychotics

Mechanism

Classical agents block dopamine D2 receptors in the mesolimbic system, newer agents act on several different systems including the $5\text{-}HT_2$ receptor and may have specificity for the D2 receptors in the meso-limbic system compared to other parts of the brain.

Side effects

Side effects vary between agents and are less with newer atypical agents such as olanzapine and risperidone.

- Movement disorders (D2 blockade)
    - parkinsonian syndrome
    - dystonia
    - akathisia (motor and psychological restlessness)
    - tardive dyskinesia
- Postural hypotension (alpha-1 blockade)
- Hyperprolactinaemia causing galactorrhoea, gynaecomastia and menstrual disturbances due to dopamine blockade in posterior pituitary
- Sedation
- Neuroleptic malignant syndrome

Reference

1. NICE. The short term management of violent and aggressive behaviour in in-patient psychiatric settings and emergency departments (2005). NICE Clinical Guideline no. 25. Available as a download at www.nice.org.uk/nicemedia/pdf/cg025niceguideline.pdf.

Alcohol and substance dependence

Gillian Sims and Stephen Haydock

Introduction

In recent years the effects of excessive alcohol use on our society have been given far greater publicity; the costs in terms of health, unemployment, relationship breakdown and associated crime have been better appreciated. Over 24% of the population of England (2:1 male to female ratio) consumes alcohol at a level considered harmful or potentially harmful to health. Back in 2002 the World Health Organization's Global Burden of Disease Study [1] identified alcohol as the third most important risk factor for European ill health and premature death after smoking and raised blood pressure. They defined three levels of alcohol use:

- *Increasing/hazardous risk*: a pattern of alcohol consumption that increases someone's risk of harm, including psychological problems, alcohol-related accidents and physical illness.
- *Higher/harmful risk*: a pattern of alcohol consumption that *will cause actual harm*.
- *Dependent drinking*: alcohol consumption which leads to a difficulty in controlling alcohol use regardless of consequences. It affects 6% of men and 2% of women in England between the ages of 16 and 65.

In the UK alcohol consumption is described in units where 1 unit = 8 g (10 mL) of pure ethanol. The unit alcohol content of an alcoholic drink can be calculated:

$$[\text{Volume of drink (in mL)} \times \% \text{ alcohol by volume}] \div 1000$$

Thus an average 75 cL (750 mL) bottle of wine (12%) will contain 9 units, a 70 cL bottle of whisky (40%) will contain 28 units.

The UK Department of Health guidelines [2] identifies alcohol use as:

- *Lower risk*: no more than 3–4 units per day for a man or 2–3 units per day for a woman with two 24-hour alcohol-free periods during the week.
- *Increasing risk*: drinking over 3–4 units per day for a man or over 2–3 units per day for a woman.
- *High risk*: drinking over 8 units per day or over 50 units per week for a man and over 6 units per day or 35 units per week for a woman. The definition of the word 'risk' within these guidelines includes an array of different aspects including: health, social, employment, family and criminal risk. Alcohol consumption is associated with both acute and chronic toxicity.

Alcohol is not a stimulant but may produce stimulant effects by suppressing normal inhibitions. As a depressant compound it is associated with a characteristic syndrome of withdrawal:

- Socially consumed doses probably produce perceived benefits by acting on the brainstem reticular formation.
- Large amounts produce cortical depression, and general anaesthesia with loss of consciousness occurring at blood concentrations ≈300 mg/100 mL.
- Death from respiratory depression occurs typically with a blood concentration ≈400 mg/100 mL. The more common cause of death in acute alcohol poisoning is in fact hypoxia from the inhalation of vomit.

Alcohol in small quantities will cause:

- sensory impairment with reduced visual acuity, delayed recovery from visual dazzle and impairment of taste, smell and hearing
- reduced attention especially to the peripheral visual field

Acute Medicine, ed. Stephen Haydock, Duncan Whitehead and Zoë Fritz. Published by Cambridge University Press.
© Cambridge University Press 2015.

Table 8.1 Increased disease risk associated with chronic excess alcohol consumption

Condition	Relative risk
Liver cirrhosis	13
Mouth cancer	5.4
Larynx cancer	4.9
Oesophagus cancer	4.4
Hypertension	2.0–4.1
Liver cancer	3.6
Haemorrhagic stroke	3.3–3.6
Ischaemic stroke	2.7–3.0
Cardiac arrhythmias	2.2
Breast cancer (women)	1.6
Coronary heart disease (CHD) in middle age	1.3–1.7

- worse muscular coordination and steadiness, with delayed reaction times, nystagmus and vertigo
- increased confidence, reduced decision making skills, leading classically to overconfidence and an underestimation of errors (*observe UK men flirting in the pub on a Friday night*).

Chronic excess alcohol consumption is associated with an increased risk of many chronic diseases and premature death (Table 8.1, Box 8.1).

Box 8.1 Wernicke–Korsakoff syndrome

Chronic alcohol abuse can result in recognized neuropsychiatric manifestations due to impairment of the uptake and utilization of thiamine (vitamin B_1). Wernicke's encephalopathy describes the triad of mental confusion, ataxia and ophthalmoplegia whereas Korsakoff syndrome is a more advanced neuropsychiatric disorder characterized by loss of memory and confabulation.

The financial cost of alcohol in terms of health and crime is considerable. The Department of Health concluded in 2008 that alcohol misuse cost the NHS £2.7 billion per annum. Estimates for alcohol-related crime vary between £9 billion and £15 billion per annum [3].

- 6% of all hospital admissions relate to alcohol.
- Up to 35% of A&E attendances and ambulance costs are alcohol related.
- Up to 70% of A&E attendances at weekend peak times are alcohol related.
- 23–35% of deaths from falls are linked to alcohol.
- 30–38% of deaths from drowning are linked to alcohol.
- 38–45% of deaths from fire injuries are linked to alcohol.

An estimated *8.2% of adults used illegal drugs* in England and Wales in the financial year 2012/13, the lowest level since records began in 1996 [4]. According to the Department of Health Drug Misuse Statistics for England, in 2011 there were 6640 admissions to hospital with a primary diagnosis of drug-related mental health and behavioural disorder [5]. The UK spends 0.48% of GDP on its drugs policy, more than any other European country.

The Home Office classify all controlled drugs into three categories:

Class A: heroin, cocaine, crack, ecstasy, magic mushrooms, LSD, injected amphetamine

Class B: amphetamine, cannabis, methylphenidate (Ritalin), pholcodine, betamine

Class C: tranquillizers, some painkillers, gamma-hydroxybutyrate (GHB).

The decline in the use of illegal drugs corresponds to an increase in the use of chemicals often termed 'legal highs' that reproduce the depressant, hallucinogenic or stimulant effects of banned substances. These are substances of abuse that:

- are not controlled by the 1971 Misuse of Drugs Act
- are not licensed for legal use
- are not advertised or sold for human consumption and therefore not subject to medicines regulation
- mimic the effects of controlled drugs.

Such compounds are generally bought from high street 'head shops' or online. They are marketed as '*not for human consumption*' and as '*bulk research chemicals*' or bath salts, pond cleaner, room odorizers, incense, etc. They are either natural products or synthetic substances made by chemical synthesis from a natural precursor (semi-synthetic) or entirely synthetic. Commonly, the marketed 'herbal high' is inert organic material that has been soaked with synthetic cannabinoids.

There is often confusion, especially in the media, about the status of such compounds. For example, mephedrone (*meow meow*) is often referred to as a 'legal high' although it was in fact banned in the UK in 2010. To get round the confusion the term '*novel psychoactive substance*' is preferred (Table 8.2).

Table 8.2 Some commonly abused novel psychoactive substances

Active ingredient	Street names
Catathione	Khat
Cannabinoid agonists (e.g. AM2201)	Spice, K2, Majik, Black Mamba, Zulu, Doob
Mephedrone	Bubbles, meow meow
1-Benzofuran-6-ylpropan-2-amine (6-APB)	NRG3, benzofury
Desoxypipradol (2DPMP)	Ivory Wave, Whack

Table 8.3 Classification of common drugs of abuse by user experience

Depressants	Hallucinogens	Stimulants
Alcohol	Ecstasy	Cocaine
Heroin	Magic mushroom	Crack
Tranquillizers	LSD	Amphetamine
GHB	Ketamine	Ritalin
	Cannabis	

The rise of such drugs is not simply due to price; in fact many illegal drugs have become cheaper over the past 20 years. The rise in popularity can be attributed to:

- a fall in availability and purity of some traditionally popular illicit drugs
- ease of purchase through head shops and online
- increasing chemical production and marketing of many new 'legal' substances especially from China
- established usage in the dance club culture.

Like alcohol excess, drug abuse is associated with a considerable socioeconomic burden to the abuser, their family and society as a whole. It increases the break-up of relationships, domestic violence and criminal behaviour to fund the habit. There is a major financial burden to society through the costs of treating drug-related health problems and drug enforcement. This is in addition to the loss of productivity from unemployment, illness and premature death. *Intravenous drug abuse* is associated with well-documented risks of infection:

- *Viral pathogens*: HIV, hepatitis
- *Bacterial pathogens*: endocarditis, osteomyelitis, septic arthritis, abscess formation at injection site and distant sites, infection with gas-forming organisms.

Drug and alcohol misuse are associated with an increased prevalence of mental illness. The mental illness may have contributed to the development of abuse or developed as a consequence. Drug and/or alcohol abusers have an increased prevalence of co-morbid depression, anxiety, mania and acute psychosis. In particular the use of cannabinoids in the teenage years has been linked to an increased risk of schizophrenia in later life. The long-term use of ecstasy may result in permanent memory disturbance.

Drug and alcohol dependence and withdrawal

Drugs of abuse differ widely in chemical structure and cellular targets (Table 8.3). However, evidence is accumulating that the '*final common path*' of addictive drugs (including ethanol and nicotine) is the activation of dopaminergic neurones of the medial forebrain bundle. All drugs of addiction therefore ultimately act through this mechanism to modulate the brain reward system that physiologically functions to reinforce key pleasurable behaviours such as eating and sexual activity. This results in instant reward to the substance user and chronic changes in the reward system resulting in addiction.

Repeated use of the addictive drug can result in:

- *Psychological dependence* (all drugs of abuse) – cravings for the drug result in profound anxiety, sleep disturbance and dysphoria when the drug is withheld.
- *Physical dependence* (depressant drugs only) – later adaptive changes within body tissues result in tolerance; an increased amount of drug is required to obtain the desired effect, which occurs by alteration in the target receptors and downstream pathways of the drug together with an increased rate of metabolism.

When both psychological and physical dependence have developed, withholding the drug results in a characteristic withdrawal syndrome, with craving and dysphoria due to psychological dependence and rebound overactivity due to physical dependence. The physical withdrawal symptoms associated with depressant drugs may require management through a supervised detoxification programme.

Alcohol withdrawal

- Symptoms appear within 12 hours of stopping or significantly reducing consumption; characterized by tremors, insomnia, anxiety, GI disturbances and autonomic overactivity: tachycardia, tachypnoea, hyperthermia, sweating.

- Severe withdrawal develops within 48 hours; characterized by disorientation, agitation and hallucinations along with severe autonomic hyperactivity.
- Alcohol withdrawal seizures have a peak incidence 24 hours after stopping drinking and tend to be brief, generalized tonic-clonic seizures that respond to benzodiazepines. Status epilepticus is rare and should prompt a search for another problem such as a significant head injury.
- Delirium tremens develops within 48–72 hours, characterized by profound disorientation, agitation, hallucinosis (psychosis) and severe autonomic dysfunction.

Opioid withdrawal

- The speed of onset depends on the half-life of the opiate abused; heroin withdrawal symptoms peak at 36–72 hours and persist for 7–10 days.
- Patients describe a severe flu-like illness with rhinorrhoea, lacrimation, sneezing and leg cramps.
- Gastrointestinal symptoms are common; cramping, abdominal pain, nausea, vomiting and diarrhoea.
- Altered mentation (disorientation and hallucinations) *does not occur* with opioid withdrawal.

Scenario 8.1

A 55-year-old man was admitted via the emergency department following a witnessed tonic-clonic seizure. The next day he has recovered from the seizure but is extremely agitated and shaky. He admits drinking a bottle of vodka per day for the last 4 months following the break-up of his marriage; prior to this he had been drinking quite heavily but not to this extent.

Approach to alcohol misuse

Always remember that admission to hospital is an excellent *'teachable moment'* where alcohol and drug misuse can be addressed, especially when the presentation is linked to the substance misuse.

There are no simple tests that reliably identify patients who are abusing alcohol; clues include:

- macrocytosis
- deranged LFTs including elevated γ-GT (gamma-glutamyl transpeptidase)
- laboratory evidence of liver disease.

If suspected such patients should be routinely given nutritional support: high dose oral vitamin replacement plus parenteral supplements (Pabrinex) in particular to prevent the consequences of vitamin B_1 deficiency (Wernicke–Korsakoff syndrome).

There are many ways of raising the subject of alcohol consumption; some examples include:

- 'In this hospital we ask everyone about their alcohol use, do you mind if I ask you about your drinking?'
- 'Sometimes low mood/anxiety/weight can be affected by alcohol, do you mind if I ask you about your alcohol use?'
- 'Alcohol is often used as a way of coping; can I ask you how you're managing at the moment?'

A common fear about asking patients about alcohol use is that they may want to talk at length about past life events. This occasionally happens, but generally patients recognize that they will be asked questions about their lifestyle, whether that is smoking, weight, or substance use, and are willing to answer honestly provided the questioner appears non-judgemental.

Routinely asking *all patients* reduces the stigma for the doctor and the patients and reinforces the message that alcohol is a significant health issue. Alcohol use is not limited to young people; do not prejudge, routinely *ask all adults regardless of age*.

Alcohol use can be subjective; to give appropriate care an accurate documentation of the pattern of use is key:

- The term *social drinker* is often used but is ambiguous; this could mean 'meets friends in the pub after work each evening' or 'has one or two glasses of wine at Christmas and parties'.
- 'ETOH++' likewise does not document how much or how often; this could mean 'attended drunk due to low tolerance' or 'drinking high levels every day'.
- Few patients understand what one unit of alcohol is; changing the question from 'how many units do you drink each week' to *'how much do you buy and how often'* can give a more accurate idea of weekly consumption.

- There are numerous screening tools for identifying problematic alcohol use; all aim to clarify how much and how often the patient is drinking.
- The National Institute for Health and Care Excellence recommends the use of the Alcohol Use Disorders Identification Test (AUDIT).

Brief intervention for alcohol misuse

Evidence from numerous studies has shown Identification and Brief Advice (IBA) undertaken within the hospital setting can lead to reduced alcohol consumption. These benefits last for 2 years and perhaps up to 4 years.

The Scottish Intercollegiate Guidelines Network identified that ~8 people need to be provided with a brief intervention for one to reduce their alcohol intake to 'low-risk' levels. Adding to this the calculation, £5 saved for every £1 spent on treatment [6], brief interventions to address *increasing risk* and *high risk drinking* are one of the most cost-effective preventative measures:

- Brief intervention can last anywhere between 5 and 45 minutes but begins with simple *screening* and asking the patient about their alcohol intake.
- *Personalized feedback* alone is sometimes enough to reduce alcohol consumption.
- *Motivational interviewing* can promote positive changes; this encompasses: empathizing, avoiding confrontation or labelling while guiding patients to identify the difference between their current drinking habit and safe levels/patterns of drinking. Try to enable them to gain insight into the health risks of not altering their behaviour and give an appreciation for their ability to change.
- Brief interventions should be aimed at people who are drinking at increasing and high risk levels; there is no benefit for those who are alcohol dependent.
- Anyone drinking above 50 units per week or showing signs of dependence should be referred to the Hospital Alcohol Liaison service, to arrange an agreed treatment package before discharge.
- Alcohol withdrawal symptoms do not necessitate inpatient detoxification unless there are further medical problems or other specific issues. The Hospital Alcohol Liaison service will be able to

advise on how to link the patient into the relevant community or outpatient services.

Approach to opiate abuse

- One of the first things to establish is whether the patient is receiving medication and if so, how much and where they collect it. All opiate users will be able to say which pharmacy they collect from and there are a number of reasons to check this, including:
  1. Clarification of prescription (dose and drug)
  2. Check when the last prescription was issued
  3. If the script is not collected for three consecutive days the medication is stopped; the pharmacist needs to be informed if the patient is in hospital so the medication is continued on discharge.
- If no medication is currently being prescribed, follow the hospital protocol for substance misuse. This will help relax the patient and help with compliance if the possibility of opiate withdrawal symptoms is reduced.
- Two days prior to discharge, contact the local drug treatment service to arrange for treatment to continue in the community, if required.
- Remember drug and alcohol dependence often go hand in hand and such patients have:
  - severe dependence issues
  - higher levels of co-morbid psychiatric problems
  - higher risk of suicide
  - higher risk of accidental death from drug/alcohol interactions.

Treatment of alcohol dependence

In the UK, every local council has a Community Drug and Alcohol Action Team or Drug Partnerships which fund local services encompassing all substance misuse treatment. These services differ between areas, some offering treatment to both drug and alcohol users under one umbrella, while other areas separate services for alcohol and drug misuse.

Whatever the local arrangement, substance misusers will be offered a similar range of services including prescribed medication, detoxification and psychosocial treatment packages. Clients coming through community services for alcohol problems will generally be offered detoxification. This could take place in a number of ways:

1. GP prescribed chlordiazepoxide in a reducing regimen to self-administer

This is not generally perceived as best practice, as it leaves the patient to carry the responsibility for administering the medication. Risk of overdose and continued alcohol consumption whilst taking the medication are a significant concern. Accordingly GPs are generally not willing to prescribe for unsupported self-detoxifications.

2. Community detoxification supported by a specialist nurse

With this form of alcohol detoxification the patient is supported in the community [7], following an assessment by the doctor linked to the community service. The community detox nurse arranges with the patient to ensure they have robust support 24 hours per day from a friend or family member for the next 5–7 days.

Medication is prescribed by the service doctor and the nurse visits the home 2–3 times per day. On each visit blood pressure and pulse rate are checked, the patient is breathalysed and a CIWA completed indicating the amount of chlordiazepoxide to be taken. The night-time dosage is left for the supervising adult to issue, and they are advised about contacting the GP or calling an ambulance if the patient is struggling or has seizures. Typically the detox runs from Monday and the nurse continues to visit until Friday when, if still required, small amounts of chlordiazepoxide are left with the patient to complete the detox over the weekend.

3. Inpatient detoxification

Inpatient detoxifications tend to take place either in a specific detox unit or within a mental health unit. As with the community detox programme, this is planned as part of a treatment package and not spontaneous; there is often a longer wait for the patient as beds are limited. Alcohol detoxification still takes approximately one week, and no medication is provided on discharge.

Following alcohol detoxification, medication can be offered to assist patient abstinence in the form of:

- *Acamprosate*: reduces craving for alcohol, by reducing the effect of excitatory amino acids such as glutamate and GABA. If taken for a year,

it increases the number of alcohol-free days and frequency of complete abstinence. Benefit may persist for up to a year after stopping treatment.

- *Disulfiram (Antabuse)*: is an acetaldehyde dehydrogenase inhibitor so that even small amounts of alcohol exposure lead to rapid accumulation of acetaldehyde resulting in immediate unpleasant symptoms of vasodilation, breathlessness, headache, dizziness, nausea and vomiting. This requires the patient to review lifestyle and avoid buying anything that contains alcohol, e.g. deodorants, face creams, aftershave, cleaning fluids, etc.

Clinical Institute Withdrawal Assessment (CIWA) scoring

Most NHS Trusts in the UK now use a patient scoring system to guide prescribing of benzodiazepines (generally chlordiazepoxide) for alcohol withdrawal. Patients at risk of withdrawing from alcohol are assessed on 10 parameters on a 7-point scale (4-point scale for orientation and clouding of sensorium) in conjunction with measurement of vital signs:

- nausea and vomiting
- tremors
- anxiety
- agitation
- paroxysmal sweats
- orientation and clouding of sensorium
- tactile disturbances
- auditory disturbances
- visual disturbances
- headache.

The score guides benzodiazepine administration, with subsequent scoring of response and further administration if indicated until symptoms are controlled.

Treatment of opiate dependence

The two main prescribed drugs used are opioids:

1. Methadone (Physeptone)
2. Buprenorphine (Subutex).

- Both of these are *amber drugs* which need to be initially prescribed by a specialist substance misuse doctor. An initial assessment is completed and the patient is slowly titrated up to an optimum dose which then reduces the effects of any heroin used in addition.

- Once stabilized, the prescribing is generally passed to the GP to continue, with regular contact maintained with the drug treatment service. The majority of opiate users collect their medication on a daily supervised consumption basis from a local pharmacy.

With any substance misuse, a comprehensive treatment package should include a psychosocial component. This will be provided by the treatment service as part of the care planning agreed with the client.

References

1. WHO (2002) *World Health Report. Reducing Risks, Promoting Healthy Life*. WHO, Geneva.

2. Department of Health (2008) *Safe, Sensible, Social Consultation on Further Action*. http://webarchive. nationalarchives.gov.uk/+/www.dh.gov.uk/en/ Consultations/Liveconsultations/DH_086412.

3. Department of Health. *Reducing Alcohol Harm: health services in England for alcohol misuse*. Report by the Comptroller and Auditor General. HC 1049 Session 2007–2008; 29 October 2008. Available to download at www.nao.org.uk/wp-content/ uploads/2008/10/07081049.pdf.

4. Drug Misuse: Findings from the 2012–2013 Crime Survey for England and Wales July (2013) www.gov.uk/ government/publications/drug-misuse-findings-from-the-2012-to-2013-csew/drug-misuse-findings-from-the-2012-to-2013-crime-survey-for-england-and-wales.

5. The Information Centre (2011) *Statistics on Drug Misuse: England 2011*. www.hscic.gov.uk/catalogue/ PUB03024.

6. Raistrick D, Heather N, Godfrey C (2006) *Review of the Effectiveness of Treatment for Alcohol Problems*. National Treatment Agency for Substance Misuse, London. www.nta.nhs.uk/uploads/nta_review_of_the_ effectiveness_of_treatment_for_alcohol_problems_ fullreport_2006_alcohol2.pdf.

7. Scottish Intercollegiate Guidelines Network (2003) *The Management of Harmful Drinking and Alcohol Dependence in Primary Care*, Clinical Guideline 74. www.sign.ac.uk/pdf/sign74.pdf.

Further reading

Haydock SF (2012) Drug dependence. In: Bennet PN, Brown MJ and Sharma P (eds.) *Clinical Pharmacology*, 11th edn. Churchill Livingstone, Chapter 11.

NICE (2011) *Alcohol Dependence and Harmful Alcohol Use*, Clinical Guideline 115. Available to download at http:// guidance.nice.org.uk/CG115.

Anaphylaxis

Jonathan Hills

Introduction

Anaphylaxis is defined as a severe, life-threatening, generalized or systemic hypersensitivity reaction. It is estimated that 1 in 1,133 of the English population has experienced anaphylaxis at some point in their lives [1]. A total of 213 fatal reactions occurred in the UK between 1992 and 2001; half of these were iatrogenic, with a significant number occurring in hospitals (Table 9.1). Of the non-iatrogenic causes, half were related to venom (e.g. wasp sting) and the remainder were due to foods.

Pathophysiology

The final common pathway involves stimulation and degranulation of mast cells or basophils (either IgE mediated or other immunological mechanisms) resulting in the release of inflammatory mediators, namely histamine, leukotrienes, tryptases and prostaglandins. These substances increase in mucus production, bronchial smooth muscle tone and vascular permeability [3] resulting in:

- airway obstruction
- breathing difficulty
- circulatory compromise.

The term anaphylactic reaction is commonly used for hypersensitivity reactions that are IgE mediated; i.e. a previous exposure to a foreign protein (allergen) resulting in the formation of IgE antibodies, with a reaction occurring on re-exposure. The term anaphylactoid reaction implies that it is non-IgE mediated (as seen with contrast media). It is recommended that the term anaphylactoid is no longer used. Invalid assumptions of a non-IgE (anaphylactoid) cause have led to fatal re-exposure [4]. Clinically it is not possible to distinguish the two and, in both treatment and investigation are the same.

Table 9.1 Suspected triggers for fatal anaphylactic reactions in the UK, 1992–2001 [2]

Stings	47	29 wasp, 4 bee, 14 unknown
Nuts	32	10 peanut, 6 walnut, 2 almond, 2 brazil, 1 hazel, 11 mixed or unknown
Food	13	5 milk, 2 fish, 2 chickpea, 2 crustacean, 1 banana, 1 snail
Food, possible causes	17	5 during meal, 3 milk, 3 nut, 1 each – fish, yeast, sherbet, nectarine, grape, strawberry
Antibiotics	27	11 penicillin, 12 cephalosporin, 2 amphotericin, 1 ciprofloxacin, 1 vancomycin
Anaesthetic drugs	39	19 suxamethonium, 7 vecuronium, 6 atracurium, 7 at induction
Other drugs	24	6 NSAIDs, 3 ACE inhibitors, 5 gelatins, 2 protamine, 2 vitamin K, 1 each – etoposide, acetazolamide, pethidine, local anaesthetic, diamorphine, streptokinase
Contrast media	11	9 iodinated, 1 technetium, 1 fluorescein
Other	3	1 Latex, 1 hair dye, 1 hydatid

Reproduced with permission of the UK Resuscitation Council.

Acute Medicine, ed. Stephen Haydock, Duncan Whitehead and Zoë Fritz. Published by Cambridge University Press. © Cambridge University Press 2015.

You are fast bleeped to a 21-year-old brittle asthmatic. She is severely short of breath on the admissions unit. A junior doctor had seen the patient earlier that day and had diagnosed an asthma exacerbation secondary to a lower respiratory tract infection. The patient cannot speak due to breathlessness and within a few minutes starts to lose consciousness. Her nurse tells you she had been improving before she administered her IV antibiotics, 5 minutes ago. An urticarial rash is developing over her body with swelling around her lips.

Clinical features and diagnosis

Anaphylaxis presents with a wide range of symptoms and signs (Table 9.2), none of which are entirely specific to an anaphylactic reaction. The Resuscitation Council UK [2] has proposed a combination of criteria that makes the diagnosis more likely:

Anaphylaxis is more likely when all of the following three criteria are met:

- Sudden onset and rapid progression of symptoms
- Life-threatening airway and/or breathing and/or circulatory collapse
- Skin and/or mucosal changes (flushing, urticarial, angio-oedema)

The following support the diagnosis:

- Exposure to known allergen for the patient

Remember:

- Skin or mucosal changes alone are not a sign of an anaphylactic reaction
- Skin and mucosal changes can be gastrointestinal symptoms (e.g. vomiting, abdominal pain and incontinence)

Speed of onset:

Relates to the route of exposure:

- Intravenous routes typically within 5 minutes
- Stings within 15–30 minutes
- Foods around 30–35 minutes.

Rarely, reactions can take a slower time course but these are less likely to be fatal.

Differential diagnosis

Anaphylaxis has clinical features which are similar or identical to many conditions. Emergency treatment of

Table 9.2 The frequency of clinical manifestations of anaphylaxis*†‡ [5]

Signs and symptoms	Present
Cutaneous	
Urticaria and angio-oedema	85–90%
Flushing	45–55%
Pruritus without rash	2–5%
Respiratory	
Dyspnoea, wheeze	45–50%
Upper airway angio-oedema	50–60%
Rhinitis	15–20%
Dizziness, syncope, hypotension	30–35%
Abdominal	
Nausea, vomiting, diarrhoea, cramping pain	25–30%
Miscellaneous	
Headache	5–8%
Substernal pain	4–6%
Seizure	1–2%

*On the basis of a compilation of 1865 patients.

† Percentages are approximations.

‡ Children may have a lower frequency of cutaneous symptoms in anaphylaxis.

Reproduced with permission from Bernstein DI, Bernstein JA, Burks W, Feldweg AM, Fink JN, Greenberger PA, Golden DB, James, JM, Kemp SF, Ledford DK, Lieberman P, Sheffer AL. The diagnosis and management of anaphylaxis practice parameter: 2010 Update. *J Allergy Clin Immunol* 2010; 126 (3): 477–480e42.

'anaphylaxis' will not help many of these conditions and may make matters worse. Where time permits a meticulous history, with emphasis on exposure to potential triggers and events preceding the reaction, and sometimes but not always supported by a laboratory test such as an elevated mast cell tryptase, can differentiate most causes. In emergency situations or difficult cases, senior help should be called for early.

Angio-oedema causes symptoms related to pressure effects on neighbouring structures, particularly in the airway where life-threatening obstruction can occur. It results from increased vascular permeability with subsequent oedema affecting the subcutaneous and submucosal tissues. Airway compromise may require prompt intubation or even emergency tracheostomy. Unlike anaphylaxis, wheeze and urticaria do not occur (except in allergic angio-oedema).

Allergic angio-oedema results from mast cell degranulation and can present with either cutaneous signs or full blown anaphylaxis. Previous exposure is not always necessary (as in the non-IgE-mediated reactions). Treatment and investigations are similar to standard anaphylaxis.

ACE-inhibitor related angio-oedema results from bradykinin accumulation and occurs in 0.1–0.5% of patients treated with ACE inhibitors. Symptoms usually involve the lips and mouth and typically develop 2 weeks after starting treatment but reactions can occur sporadically. A lack of family history and normal C3 and C4 levels support the diagnosis. Treatment consists of drug cessation and future avoidance of ACE inhibitors. Subcutaneous and nebulized adrenaline should be administered in cases of airway compromise, alongside early anaesthetic review [6].

C1 esterase inhibitor deficiency leads to uncontrolled complement activation with subsequent localized, non-pitting, non-pruritic, non-erythematous, demarcated angio-oedema. The face, extremities and genitalia are the commonest sites to swell, but airway and bowel obstruction can occur. Misdiagnosis is common with some patients undergoing procedures for suspected surgical abdomens or even referred for psychiatric opinion. The condition can be either hereditary or acquired, which are clinically indistinguishable. Screening for this condition involves testing C3 and C4 levels together with C1 esterase inhibitor levels. Plasma or recombinant C1 esterase inhibitor concentrate infusion leads to rapid improvement of symptoms. Adrenaline, antihistamines and steroids are *not* considered to be effective.

Idiopathic angio-oedema causes acute or recurrent episodes without an obvious trigger and is a diagnosis of exclusion. Treatment consists of antihistamines and, in refractory cases, corticosteroids.

Scombroid fish poisoning is a self-limiting condition that can occur 30 minutes after the ingestion of spoiled fish, such as mackerel or tuna. It is characterized by flushing, headache, sweating, dizziness, burning of the mouth and throat, abdominal cramps, nausea, vomiting and diarrhoea. The mean duration of symptoms is 4 hours. Treatment is supportive and antihistamines may help alleviate symptoms.

Systemic mastocytosis and carcinoid syndrome can both cause episodes of flushing, urticaria, bronchospasm and hypotension, sometimes precipitated by alcohol. Stings and opioids can cause non-IgE-mediated anaphylaxis in patients with mastocytosis.

Monosodium glutamate (MSG) symptom complex causes flushing and bronchospasm. It can be differentiated from anaphylaxis by the absence of urticaria and angio-oedema and the presence of headache, chest pain, and burning or numbness in the upper trunk, face and neck. It is diagnosed when typical symptoms occur within 30 to 60 minutes of eating foods with high concentrations of MSG. The condition is also known as '*Chinese restaurant syndrome*' as MSG is a common ingredient in Chinese foods. The symptoms usually go away without treatment in about 2 to 3 hours.

The following may also sometimes be mistaken for anaphylaxis:

- *Munchausen/hysterical anaphylaxis* by patients who can feign stridor or by deliberate exposure to allergen in patients with known allergies
- *upper airway infection* (also have pyrexia, pain and trismus)
- *panic attacks* (including victims of previous anaphylaxis who think they have been re-exposed).

Management/resuscitation

The diagnosis may not be immediately clear but the management of any critically ill patient remains the same irrespective of the underlying cause [2].

Deal with life-threatening problems first and call for skilled help early. The patient in Scenario 9.1 should have a cardiac arrest call made immediately!

The Resuscitation Council UK algorithm is recommended (see Figure 9.1).

- Remove the trigger where possible (induced vomiting is not recommended in the cases of food-induced anaphylaxis).
- Apply high flow oxygen via an oxygen reservoir system in all cases.
- Fluids should be administered as soon as intravenous access is acquired. If intravenous access proves difficult, intra-osseous access can be considered. Colloid fluids have *not* been found to be superior to crystalloids for resuscitation purposes.
- Colloids should be changed to crystalloids if infused before the reaction occurred, as they could be the offending trigger.
- Standard monitoring with pulse oximetry, blood pressure and continuous three-lead ECG should be started as soon as possible to gauge response to treatment.

Adrenaline is immediately indicated only for severe life-threatening anaphylaxis:

- respiratory distress (stridor or severe bronchospasm)

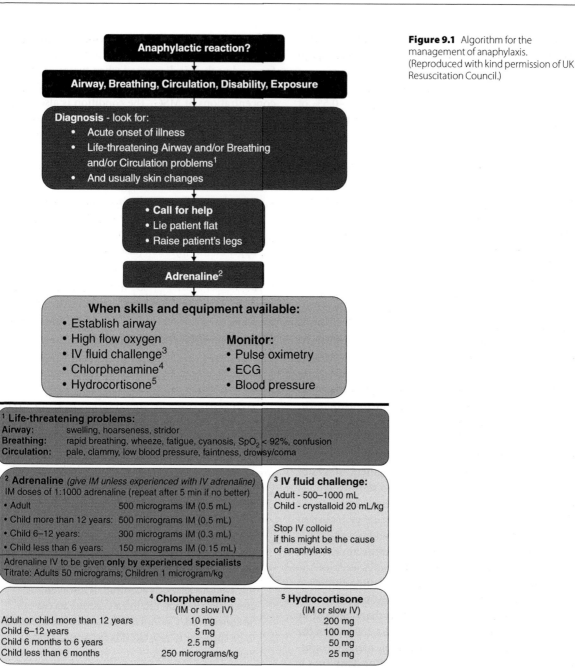

Figure 9.1 Algorithm for the management of anaphylaxis. (Reproduced with kind permission of UK Resuscitation Council.)

Anaphylactic reaction?

Airway, Breathing, Circulation, Disability, Exposure

Diagnosis - look for:
- Acute onset of illness
- Life-threatening Airway and/or Breathing and/or Circulation problems[1]
- And usually skin changes

- **Call for help**
- Lie patient flat
- Raise patient's legs

Adrenaline[2]

When skills and equipment available:
- Establish airway
- High flow oxygen
- IV fluid challenge[3]
- Chlorphenamine[4]
- Hydrocortisone[5]

Monitor:
- Pulse oximetry
- ECG
- Blood pressure

[1] **Life-threatening problems:**
Airway: swelling, hoarseness, stridor
Breathing: rapid breathing, wheeze, fatigue, cyanosis, SpO_2 < 92%, confusion
Circulation: pale, clammy, low blood pressure, faintness, drowsy/coma

[2] **Adrenaline** *(give IM unless experienced with IV adrenaline)*
IM doses of 1:1000 adrenaline (repeat after 5 min if no better)
- Adult   500 micrograms IM (0.5 mL)
- Child more than 12 years: 500 micrograms IM (0.5 mL)
- Child 6–12 years: 300 micrograms IM (0.3 mL)
- Child less than 6 years: 150 micrograms IM (0.15 mL)

Adrenaline IV to be given **only by experienced specialists**
Titrate: Adults 50 micrograms; Children 1 microgram/kg

[3] **IV fluid challenge:**

Adult - 500–1000 mL
Child - crystalloid 20 mL/kg

Stop IV colloid
if this might be the cause
of anaphylaxis

	[4] **Chlorphenamine** (IM or slow IV)	[5] **Hydrocortisone** (IM or slow IV)
Adult or child more than 12 years	10 mg	200 mg
Child 6–12 years	5 mg	100 mg
Child 6 months to 6 years	2.5 mg	50 mg
Child less than 6 months	250 micrograms/kg	25 mg

- hypotension (collapse or loss of consciousness).

Otherwise patients should be observed and monitored in an area where adrenaline and other resuscitation facilities are available.

Inappropriate administration of adrenaline can be dangerous, particularly in overdose or when given intravenously. In patients with a spontaneous circulation, intravenous adrenaline may cause:

- life-threatening hypertension
- tachyarrhythmias
- myocardial ischaemia.

The elderly or patients with ischaemic heart disease, hypertension or arteriopathies are at particular risk.

Based on current evidence, the benefits of giving appropriate doses of intramuscular adrenaline far exceed the risk, even in patients known to have ischaemic heart disease (grade C). As such, intramuscular adrenaline is the recommended route of administration.

The best site is the anterolateral aspect of the middle third of the thigh. Further doses can be administered at 5-minute intervals if the patient's condition fails to improve. Know the dose for emergency use!

Adrenaline IM dose – ADULTS
0.5 mg = 500 μg = 0.5 mL of 1:1000 adrenaline

Intravenous adrenaline is only recommended for those experienced in using it (e.g. anaesthetists, emergency physicians and intensive care doctors). Experience of administering intravenous adrenaline in cardiac arrest situations is *not* deemed sufficient experience. In the event of a cardiac arrest caused by an anaphylactic reaction, use standard treatment with IV adrenaline following ALS protocols.

Concerns in the past were raised regarding administering adrenaline to patients taking beta-blockers, due to the theoretical risk of unopposed alpha-adrenoceptor stimulation and reflex vagotonic effects leading to bradycardia, hypertension, coronary artery constriction and bronchoconstriction. However, the pharmacodynamic effect of adrenaline varies hugely between individuals. The Resuscitation Council UK now recommends that doses of adrenaline be titrated to effect, starting with a safe dose, giving higher doses if necessary.

Beta-blockers (including eye drops) should not be prescribed to patients with a history of anaphylaxis. A decision to start them should be made in conjunction with a cardiologist and allergy specialist.

Steroids may shorten the duration of the initial reaction and may prevent a biphasic reaction occurring.

Antihistamines speed resolution of skin changes associated with an anaphylactic reaction.

Bronchodilators can be used to treat persistent bronchospasm. IV aminophylline and magnesium sulphate can also be considered.

A catecholamine infusion may be required in patients who remain cardiovascularly unstable despite multiple doses of IM or IV adrenaline. These patients will subsequently require close monitoring in a high dependence area.

Patients who have had a genuine anaphylaxis reaction (i.e. life-threatening features) should be observed for at least 6 hours in an area with resuscitation facilities. A senior physician should be involved in the decisions regarding further treatment and total length of observation.

Investigations

The concentration of circulating mast cell tryptase (a protease) increases substantially during anaphylaxis. Levels may not rise significantly until 30 minutes or more after the onset of symptoms. They peak at 1–2 hours after onset and normalize after approximately 6–8 hours. The tryptase assay has a high specificity but relatively low sensitivity and some cases of anaphylaxis may be missed. Given the wide differential diagnosis of anaphylaxis a positive result can be very helpful, particularly if the diagnosis is in doubt.

Take time and date labelled blood samples (5–10 mL clotted blood) for mast cell tryptase as follows:

1. Initial sample as soon as feasible after resuscitation has started. Do not delay resuscitation to take sample.
2. Second sample at 1–2 h after the start of symptoms.
3. Third (baseline) sample either 24 h or in convalescence (e.g. in follow-up allergy clinic).

Liaise with laboratory and ensure safe delivery of the samples to the appropriate technician, as the diagnosis depends upon this test. Tryptase is a stable enzyme and can be stored overnight in a fridge if necessary.

Discharge from hospital

Unpredictable biphasic reactions can occur with quoted incidences of 1–20%. An experienced physician should therefore be involved in discharge decisions. It may be appropriate to keep patients under observation for up to 24 hours in some circumstances including:

- idiopathic triggers causing slow, severe reactions
- patients with brittle asthma or with a severe asthmatic component
- where continued absorption of the allergen is a possibility, e.g. foods
- patients with a history of biphasic reactions
- patients presenting in the evening or night, or those who may not be able to respond to deterioration.

On discharge, give clear instructions to return to hospital if symptoms return. A 3-day course of steroids and antihistamines should be considered.

Follow-up

All patients should be referred to an allergy specialist. If uncertain who to refer to, a list of clinics can be found on the *British Society for Allergy and Clinical Immunology (BSACI)* website. Clinics with a specialist interest in anaphylactic reactions during anaesthesia can be found on the *Association of Anaesthetists of Great Britain and Ireland* website.

Include in the referral:

- a detailed history regarding the pattern of events surrounding the reaction, with emphasis on timings of potential triggers
- a list of administered treatments
- copies of relevant patient records, e.g. ambulance records, observation charts, drug cards, etc.
- results of investigations already available or pending.

The allergy specialist will:

- attempt to identify the trigger
- educate the patient and general practitioner regarding future allergen avoidance
- provide the patient with a written management plan regarding future episodes of anaphylaxis, which may include the use of an adrenaline auto-injector.

The decision to prescribe an adrenaline auto-injector ideally should be made by an allergy specialist. An auto-injector is warranted following a severe, systemic reaction for an individual deemed to be at high risk:

- asthmatics
- reactions to trace allergens only
- repeat exposure cannot be avoided
- access to emergency treatment is difficult.

Patients or their caregivers also need to know how and when to use the device plus be physically able to. The patient's GP must also be informed. Only 50–75% of patients prescribed auto-injectors carry them around at all times. Of these, only 30–40% can correctly self-administer them.

Always take the opportunity to reinforce anaphylactic management plans with a patient or their caregiver.

Cephalosporins in patients with a penicillin allergy

Classic teaching is that 10% of patients with a history of penicillin allergy will have a cross-reaction to a cephalosporin. This 'observation' is based on studies from the 1960s and 1970s that had significant methodological flaws:

- Poor definition of 'allergy'
- Old drug-manufacturing techniques which commonly led to contamination of one drug with another

- Failure to take into account that a patient with an allergy to penicillin actually has a greater risk of allergy to *any* medication, irrespective of structural similarities.

In reality the risk of cross-reactivity between penicillin and cephalosporin has been reported as:

- ~0.5–2.5% for first and second generation cephalosporins which have side chains that are similar to penicillin
- near zero for third and fourth generation cephalosporins.

Therefore in a patient with a *documented IgE-mediated response to penicillin*, third and fourth generation cephalosporins can be used safely. First and second generation cephalosporins that have side chains similar to that of penicillin (i.e. cefaclor, cefadroxil, cefatrizine, cefprozil, cephalexin, cephradine) should be avoided.

References

1. Sheikh A, Hippisley-Cox, Newton J and Fenty. Trends in national incidence, lifetime prevalence and adrenaline prescribing for anaphylaxis in England. *JR Soc Med*. Mar 1, 2008; 101(3): 139–143.

2. Working Group of the Resuscitation Council (UK). Emergency treatment of anaphylactic reactions: guidelines for healthcare providers. Resuscitation Council; January 2008.

3. Ryder SA, Waldman C. Anaphylaxis. *Br J Anaesth CEACCP* 2004; 4(4): 111–113.

4. McLean-Tooke AP, Bethune CA, Fay AC, Spickett GP. Adrenaline in the treatment of anaphylaxis: what is the evidence? *BMJ* 2003; 327: 1332–1335.

5. Bernstein DI, Bernstein JA, Burks W, Feldweg AM, Fink JN, Greenberger PA, Golden DB, James, JM, Kemp SF, Ledford DK, Lieberman P, Sheffer AL. The diagnosis and management of anaphylaxis practice parameter: 2010 Update. *J Allergy Clin Immunol* 2010; 126 (3): 477–480e42.

6. Hoyer C, Hill MR, Kaminski ER. Angio-oedema: an overview of differential diagnosis and clinical management. *Br J Anaesth CEACCP* 2012; 12(6): 307–311.

Chapter 10

Anxiety/panic disorder

Stephen Haydock

Introduction

Anxiety is experienced by all of us at some time and is an appropriate response to stressful or worrying circumstances. Patients with an anxiety disorder experience anxiety that interferes with normal functioning and occurs without obvious provocation or is markedly out of proportion to the provoking stimuli. Such disorders can be extremely disabling, resulting in a marked reduction in quality of life, chronic high usage of health resources and reduced employment prospects. They are commonly not recognized and consequently many patients remain undiagnosed and do not receive appropriate treatment.

Classification

- Generalized anxiety disorder
- Panic disorder
- Stress disorders, e.g. post-traumatic stress disorder
- Phobic disorders
  - agoraphobia
  - social phobia
  - specific phobias, e.g. pentheraphobia (fear of one's mother-in-law!)

A physician involved in the acute medical take will commonly encounter and should have an understanding of generalized anxiety disorder and panic disorder. Generalized anxiety disorder (GAD) is common but frequently not recognized and treated. The UK Adult Psychiatric Morbidity in England Survey suggests that the disorder affects 4.4% of the population of which only 33% of patients with GAD reported any treatment or interventions [1]. Panic disorder is thought to affect 2% of the UK population but is more common among those accessing primary and secondary care for a range of medical problems.

It is important to remember that we will generally encounter patients with GAD and panic disorder through a presentation that may focus primarily on physical symptoms. The underlying anxiety disorder may not be apparent unless we delve more deeply into the circumstances surrounding the emergency attendance (see also Chapter 48).

History

The symptoms suggestive of an anxiety disorder may only be elicited on direct questioning.

An anxiety disorder is characterized by:

- uneasiness, fear or panic
- intrusive obsessive thoughts
- compulsive ritualistic behaviours
- poor concentration
- insomnia and nightmares
- rumination on/flashbacks to previous traumatic life events
- numbness/tingling of hands and feet
- urinary frequency; loose bowels
- dry mouth, nausea, palpitations, breathlessness, dizziness
- motor restlessness
- cold/sweaty palms.

In addition it is important to seek specific features of a co-morbid depressive illness:

- loss of interest in activities of life
- low mood and feelings of hopelessness
- sleep disturbance
- loss of appetite
- low self-esteem
- poor concentration
- thoughts of self-harm.

Acute Medicine, ed. Stephen Haydock, Duncan Whitehead and Zoë Fritz. Published by Cambridge University Press.
© Cambridge University Press 2015.

And co-morbid drug or alcohol use, including agents that can produce symptoms of anxiety:

- caffeine-containing preparations
- cocaine and amphetamines
- beta-agonists
- thyroxine
- corticosteroids.

A number of medical conditions can present with features of an anxiety disorder and should be considered and excluded:

- mitral valve prolapse
- tachyarrhythmias
- thyrotoxicosis
- phaeochromocytoma.

Examination

This should be essentially unremarkable but it must:

- appreciate that patients will commonly have co-morbid medical problems
- seek to identify any specific medical problems that can manifest with symptoms of anxiety.

Scenario 10.1

A 77-year-old woman is referred by the emergency department and is a known 'frequent flyer'. She is complaining of chest discomfort and palpitations. This is her third presentation in 3 weeks. The presentations are very similar and each time she has accessed medical care by dialling 999 in the late evening/early hours of the morning. Extensive investigation on a previous admission last year was unable to find a cause for her symptoms. The previous two admissions were overnight stays on the medical assessment unit and she was discharged home next morning with a 'diagnosis' of troponin negative chest pain. She lives alone (her husband died a year previously). She has no package of care. There is evidence of mild cognitive impairment.

We should be alert to the possibility that recurrent emergency attendances similar to that above might reflect an underlying generalized anxiety disorder. Such presentations are particularly common in the elderly and ethnic minorities where the principal focus of the presentation relates to concerns regarding the physical health of the patient or a family member.

Generalized anxiety disorder

- Usually presents around 20 years of age.
- Twice as common in men as in women.

- Affect about 4% of the UK population.
- Recognized genetic component (five times increased risk in first degree relatives).
- Chronic condition with poor remission rates.
- Fear, worry and apprehension that is out of proportion to the perceived stimulus.
- The worries are typically widespread, relate to everyday concerns, frequently shift focus and cannot be dispelled by the patient.
- Impair normal social and working life.
- Irritability, poor concentration, increased sensitivity to noise and insomnia.
- Somatic symptoms due to sympathetic overactivity.
- Muscle tension resulting in restlessness, inability to relax and muscle aches and pains (shoulders and back).
- Rarely an isolated condition and up to 90% may have another psychiatric condition
  - depression is very common (major depression and dysthymia)
  - panic disorder, phobias
  - somatization disorder
  - substance misuse.
- Co-morbid physical medical conditions are common.
- Presentation to primary or secondary care may focus on somatic problems due to anxiety or the co-morbid physical problems rather than the psychiatric manifestations.

GAD in the elderly

GAD has a peak onset around the age of 20 years and epidemiological studies have suggested a low prevalence in those over 55 years of age. However, it has also been suggested that there may be a major problem in the elderly population that has gone unrecognized, affecting 10–20% of older adults.

Symptoms of anxiety develop or recur with ageing due to:

- feeling of vulnerability brought on by increasing frailty and falls
- medical co-morbidities
- social isolation
- financial concerns.

Diagnosis can be difficult in elderly patients because:

- the condition is often not considered by the clinician

- elderly patients may not recognize or be prepared to discuss their anxieties
- the condition may be obscured by co-morbid depression, physical illness, polypharmacy and cognitive impairment
- the focus is on somatic manifestations rather than the psychological aspects.

It is important when seeing an elderly patient who is admitted to hospital to consider the existence of an anxiety disorder contributing to their presentation. Repeated presentation to hospital may mask such a disorder where hospital is seen as a safe and reassuring place compared to a cold, dark and lonely house.

Management

Aims to:
- provide symptomatic relief
- restore to normal function
- prevent disease relapse.

Principles of stepped care

NICE advocates a stepped care approach to the management of both anxiety disorders and depression. Such an approach attempts to control the patient's illness with the minimum restriction to the patient (minimum inconvenience, cost, side effects) whilst providing monitoring that permits a step-up of care if the patient's symptoms are not adequately controlled with the current level of support.

Such a stepped approach is typically:

Step 1 Education regarding illness and monitoring in primary care

Step 2 Self-help (books, CDs, internet, computer programs); guided self-help; psycho-educational groups in primary care

Step 3 More restricting approaches such as CBT, applied relaxation, pharmacotherapy in primary care

Step 4 Management using psychological therapies and pharmacotherapies in a secondary or tertiary care setting

Pharmacological treatment

- *Anxiolytics* such as benzodiazepines were previously used extensively but long-term use is associated with sedation, tolerance and dependence. *Now only used as a brief intervention (2–4 weeks) to reduce anxiety in certain circumstances.*
- *Antidepressants* require a treatment period of some weeks for symptom improvement:
  - tolerance and dependence do not occur
  - SSRIs (e.g. sertraline) (first line), SNARIs (e.g. venlafaxine, duloxetine) (second line) and tricyclics (e.g. amitriptyline) are all effective. Tricyclics not preferred due to risk in overdose.
- *Pregabalin* is a GABA analogue that binds directly to the N-type brain voltage-gated calcium channel and has relatively rapid onset; it is indicated for those patients unable to take antidepressant medications due to side effects or co-morbid psychiatric and physical illness.
- *Antipsychotics* are licensed only for refractory/treatment resistant disease.
- *Buspirone* is a partial agonist at the serotonin 5-HT$_{1A}$ receptor and is only licensed for short treatment durations.

Psychological treatment

- Various approaches are available based upon techniques of cognitive behaviour therapy. Such approaches may not be appropriate, however, for elderly patients with significant cognitive impairment.

Scenario 10.2

A 25-year-old woman has been brought into the emergency department after collapsing in the supermarket. She is complaining of chest tightness, breathlessness and palpitations associated with a tingling sensation around the mouth and in her hands. On examination she is tachypnoeic, has a marked tachycardia and is clearly very distressed. Investigations reveal a sinus tachycardia and a respiratory alkalosis with normal oxygen saturations. She reveals that similar less severe episodes have happened previously and she is becoming increasingly concerned about them.

Panic disorder

Peak onset is in the 20s and it is twice as common in women as in men. Patients present with recurrent attacks that are characterized by intense fear that peaks rapidly within 10 minutes of onset, are not due to substance abuse or co-morbid medical problems and are associated with:

- palpitations, pounding heart or accelerated heart rate
- sweating
- trembling or shaking
- sense of shortness of breath or smothering
- feeling of choking
- chest pain or discomfort
- nausea or abdominal distress
- feeling dizzy, unsteady, light-headed, or faint
- derealization or depersonalization (feeling detached from oneself)
- fear of losing control or going crazy
- fear of dying
- numbness or tingling sensations
- chills or hot flushes.

In addition, patient exhibits persistent anxiety regarding a further attack and its consequences. Attacks may occur without an obvious precipitant or in response to a particular situation/location or trigger such as injury, illness, bereavement or conflict.

Panic disorder frequently coexists with:

- other anxiety disorders, in particular agoraphobia
- somatoform disorders
- depression
- substance misuse

and is more common amongst medical patients presenting with cardiac and gastrointestinal disease.

Management

Long-term prognosis is good with two-thirds of patients entering remission within 6 months of treatment. Patients presenting to secondary care should be managed in accordance with NICE guidance:

- Establish if patient has ongoing treatment.
- Perform minimum investigation to exclude organic problem.
- Do not admit but discharge to primary care for further assessment and management.
- Provide written information on the condition and why referred to primary care.
- Provide written information about local and national voluntary self-help groups.

Subsequent management will involve:

- access to self-help materials and psychoeducational groups
- cognitive behaviour therapy
- drug treatment with SSRIs (first line) or tricyclic antidepressants (second line).

Reference

1. Health and Social Care Information Centre. Adult Psychiatric Morbidity in England – 2007, Results of a household survey. Published 27 January 2009, Available to download at www.hscic.gov.uk/pubs/psychiatricmorbidity07.

Further reading

NICE. *Generalised Anxiety Disorder in Adults: Management in Primary, Secondary and Community Care* (2011) National Clinical Guideline 113. National Institute for Health and Care Excellence. Available as a download from: www.nice.org.uk/nicemedia/live/11810/58247/58247.pdf.

Chapter

11

Blackout/collapse
Cardiac pacemakers

Stephen Haydock and Mark Dayer

Introduction

A range of pathological processes can damage the sinus node or interrupt the normal conducting pathway to the rest of the heart. Many such defects can be corrected by pacemaker implantation. The NHS performs 15 000–20 000 such procedures per year at a cost of £3,200, of which £1,500 is the cost of the device itself. Modern devices can also be selected which can improve cardiac function or treat tachyarrhythmias.

Scenario 11.1

Mr WHB, a 78-year-old man, presented to A&E with a syncopal event. He suddenly collapsed whilst in the garden. He was seen to be pale but came around quickly and was not confused. Examination was normal, except for a soft ejection systolic murmur. His ECG showed right bundle branch block. He recalled a previous episode 3 months before, when he had been admitted and monitored overnight. No rhythm problems were noted. An ECHO the following day showed good left ventricular function and mild aortic stenosis. He was discharged and underwent 72-hour heart rhythm monitoring as an outpatient, which was normal. An implantable loop recorder (ILR) was fitted and 2 months later he had a further syncopal event. His ILR showed bradycardia and 2:1 heart block (Figure 11.1). He was admitted and underwent implantation of a dual chamber pacemaker and subsequently had no further events.

Table 11.1 details the modern history of cardiac pacemakers [1].

Mechanism of operation

A modern 'permanent pacemaker' consists of an implantable pulse generator and insulated lead wires.

The implantable pulse generator contains the battery/power source (the opaque bit on the CXR near the shoulder) and the circuitry to control the sensing, output and telemetry functions. Lithium iodide batteries are used as they have a long operating life, 7–10 years, and a voltage output which decreases gradually with time, making a sudden battery failure very unlikely. The pulse generator is typically planted subcutaneously below the clavicle of the non-dominant arm (≈90% implanted on the left).

Insulated lead wires conduct electrical impulses from the pulse generator to the myocardium and conduct sensed electrical activity of the myocardium back to the pulse generator. The tip of the pacing lead in contact with the myocardium is the negative cathode. The positive anode is either a separate electrode on the lead (bipolar pacing system) or the pulse generator itself (unipolar pacing system). In either case, flow of current is from the cathode to anode via the myocardium, body tissues and fluids, which act as conductors to complete the circuit. The leads are usually passed via the subclavian vein (transvenous/endocardial leads). Epicardial leads are implanted on the outside of the heart (<5% lead placements). They are primarily used in paediatric cardiology or for patients in whom transvenous lead implantation is contraindicated.

Pacemaker classification

Modern pacemakers are capable of a range of functions. In order to standardize nomenclature across the world the *North American Society of Pacing and Electrophysiology* and the *British Pacing and Electrophysiology Group* have developed an internationally recognized five-letter system of classification (sometimes only I–III are needed) (Table 11.2).

Acute Medicine, ed. Stephen Haydock, Duncan Whitehead and Zoë Fritz. Published by Cambridge University Press. © Cambridge University Press 2015.

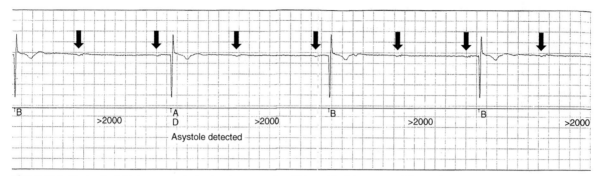

Figure 11.1 The implantable loop recorder tracing demonstrating 2:1 heart block (arrows mark P waves).

Table 11.1 History of development of implantable electronic cardiac devices

Date	Development
1952	First description of temporary electrical cardiac pacing for bradycardias
1958	First use of permanent transvenous pacing
Early 1960s	Asynchronous pacemakers (i.e. pacing without any regard to the electrical activity of the patient's heart)
Late 1960s	Introduction of single-chamber 'on demand' pacemakers that paced with regard to patient's own electrical activity
1979	First dual chamber (DVI) pacemaker introduced
1985	First rate-responsive pacemaker introduced
1990s	Implantable cardioverter defibrillators introduced
2000s	Cardiac resynchronization therapy (biventricular pacing) introduced
Today	Complex dual chamber pacemakers using rate-responsive pacing to provide pacing rate to match metabolic demands of the body. Complex algorithm to minimize right ventricular pacing. Many other features can permit remote monitoring including monitoring of activity and fluid levels, detection of sleep-disordered breathing, treatment of atrial and ventricular arrhythmias, etc.

Table 11.2 Internationally accepted pacemaker classificatory system

Code position	Functionality
I	Paced chamber (A = atria, V = ventricles, D = dual chamber)
II	Sensed chamber (A = atria, V = ventricles, D = dual chamber, 0 = none)
III	Response to sensing (T = triggered, I = inhibited, D = dual, both T and I, R = reverse, 0 = none)
IV	Rate modulation programmability (P = simple, M = multi-programmable, R = rate adaptive, C = communicating, 0 = none)
V	Anti-tachycardia function (P = pacing, S = shock, D = dual)

Most permanent pacemakers currently inserted are of the dual chamber variety (DDDR). Single chamber (VVI) pacemakers are often used for patients in permanent atrial fibrillation though, and can be useful in the acute setting of temporary transvenous pacing (discussed later). Although they have the advantage of simplicity due to the single lead placement they have been superseded in sinus rhythm because:

- Single atrial lead pacing does not provide back-up if A-V conduction is impaired
- Single ventricular lead pacing does not provide atrial and ventricular synchronization and in

patients in sinus rhythm, VVIR pacing seems to increase the risk of developing atrial fibrillation and can result in 'pacemaker syndrome':

- feeling of fatigue, dizziness and breathlessness
- more likely to occur in patients with low intrinsic heart rate and diastolic ventricular dysfunction (now commonly referred to as heart failure with a normal ejection fraction)
- can usually be managed by upgrading to a dual chamber pacemaker.

In addition, modern pacemakers can store a vast array of diagnostic information that can be subsequently downloaded if an event occurs (*pacemaker interrogation*).

Complications of pacemaker insertion

- *Pneumothorax* incidence depends on the experience of physician and technique used; it occurs during subclavian vein cannulation, typically in 1–3% of cases. Manage as per normal management of pneumothorax and inform the pacing team. Rarely a significant haemothorax requiring surgical drainage may develop.
- *Pericardial effusion* occurs in less than 1 in 200 implants, but can be life-threatening. It may present almost immediately, but commonly develops over 24–48 h. Pericardial drainage is usually sufficient, but may require surgery to repair the hole.
- *Arterial puncture* usually does not cause any significant complications.
- *Early electrode displacement* affects about 2% of leads.
- *Infection* occurs in ≈2% of pacemaker procedures. Typically within 3 months, but can occur at any stage after insertion. Local infection presents with tenderness and erythema at insertion site, and pus may be discharged. A bacteraemia (usually *Staphylococcus aureus*) may occur. Need to take blood cultures, start antibiotics according to local policy, and notify pacing physician. Pacing system will always need removal and subsequent replacement.
- *Generator erosion* through the skin, thought to be secondary to infection in most cases.
- *Wound site haematoma*: small haematomas are common, larger haematomas requiring evacuation are rare.

- *Incorrect lead placement* occurs more commonly than typically recognized. As transvenous pacing leads are placed in the right side of the heart, ventricular pacing is associated with conduction that gives the conducted complexes an effective left bundle branch block morphology on the ECG. If an RBBB (unless biventricular pacing) morphology is seen, then it suggests the pacing wire has passed to the left side of the heart, typically through a PFO or ASD, or is possibly placed in the coronary sinus (*usually by the registrar!*).
- *Diaphragmatic pacing* commonly occurs after biventricular pacing, but is otherwise rare. In most situations this can be alleviated by reprogramming the device. Lead repositioning is rarely required.

Pacemaker checks

Pacemakers need to be checked at regular intervals, initially fairly frequently, but typically annually from 6 months after implantation. In addition they should be checked/interrogated when patients are admitted to hospital for an event; the data stored on the pacemaker may be diagnostic or the pacemaker may need adjustment or rarely be malfunctioning.

Common pacemaker malfunctions

The fact that pacing spikes cannot be seen on the ECG does not mean that the pacemaker is not working. Pacemakers are designed to treat slow heart rates. Similarly, in a patient with a defibrillator, the fact that a patient remains in VT does not mean that the device does not work. They are carefully set up to treat rhythms that meet particular characteristics, and the rate of the VT may simply be lower than the rates the device is set up to treat.

- *Failure of sensing* is evident when pacing spikes are imposed on normal electrical activity of atria or ventricles. This may result from lead problems (dislodgement, breakage, insulation loss) or at the myocardium (poor intracardiac signal, or signal occurs in refractory period of pacemaker).
- *Oversensing* is when a pacemaker fails to pace when appropriate; there may be evidence of electrical background noise on ECG trace, most commonly the sensing of myopotentials or 'T wave oversensing'. It can result from detection of physiological intracardiac signals causing pacing inhibition or physiological extracardiac signals such as muscle potentials, shivering etc.,

or from electromagnetic interference (hospital equipment).

- *Failure of capture*: the pacing signal (spike on ECG) does not result in atrial or ventricular depolarization. Causes include problems with the pulse generator (inappropriately low programmed output or low battery); problems with leads (breakage, dislodgement or insulation loss); and problems with myocardium (increased stimulation threshold due to myocardial disease, metabolic disorders and some drugs).
- *No output*: the pacing spikes are absent from the ECG, which can be desirable if appropriately inhibited. Otherwise may be due to lead problems (wire breakage, loose connection to generator, component failure) or end of battery life.
- *Rapid paced rates* result in an inappropriate broad complex tachycardia; this may be due to a pacemaker driven tachycardia (PMT) in dual chamber pacing systems (where retrograde conduction to the atria is sensed and triggers ventricular activation via the pacemaker) or tracking of rapid atrial rates from sinus tachycardia, atrial fibrillation or atrial flutter.

Note: placing a magnet over the pacemaker prevents the sensing function and *usually* causes the pacemaker to revert to fixed rate pacing which will terminate the PMT or tracking tachycardia.

Indications for electronic cardiac device implantation

Permanent electronic cardiac device implantation is performed for three general indications:

1. Bradyarrhythmias and defects of intracardiac conduction
2. Resynchronization therapy for refractory cardiac failure
3. Defibrillators to treat rapid ventricular arrhythmias

Bradyarrhythmias/conduction defects

Introduction

Bradyarrhythmias can produce a range of symptoms:

- Asymptomatic
- Irritability, lassitude, poor concentration
- Fatiguability, reduced exercise capacity,

- Cardiac failure
- Dizziness, syncope and presyncope.

You will recall from undergraduate physiology that:

$$\text{Systemic blood pressure} = \text{cardiac output} \times \text{total peripheral resistance}$$

$$\text{Cardiac output} = \text{stroke volume} \times \text{rate}$$

Therefore a fall in heart rate may result in a fall in cardiac output that is manifest as a fall in blood pressure and cerebral perfusion. Symptoms will depend on the appropriate function of compensatory mechanisms, concurrent pharmacotherapy and the degree of existing structural heart disease. These factors determine whether the fall in cardiac output, due to the fall in heart rate, can be compensated for by a corresponding increase in stroke volume and total peripheral resistance. It is for this reason that bradyarrhythmias are well tolerated in young fit patients. Indeed very fit young people have a resting bradycardia that indicates their high level of cardiovascular fitness. This contrasts with the elderly patient with a significant degree of cardiac disease and burden of hypotensive drugs who may experience frequent syncope with a bradycardia that would be asymptomatic in a younger individual.

We are often faced with patients on the medical take who present with syncope thought to be due to a bradyarrhythmia or who have reduced exercise capacity or other symptomatology that might be attributed to a bradyarrhythmia:

- It can be difficult in such patients to decide if the problems are related to the bradyarrhythmia or coexisting co-morbid conditions, e.g. COPD.
- The bradyarrhythmia could be evidence of a high degree of cardiovascular conditioning.
- Always consider if the bradycardia is due to a potentially reversible or transient cause:
  - medication
  - acute myocardial ischaemia
  - electrolyte abnormalities
  - hypothyroidism
  - hypothermia.

For patients presenting with a syncopal episode the gold standard for diagnosis remains ECG confirmation of the rhythm disturbance during the syncopal episode and all attempts should be made to obtain such confirmation. In this context arrhythmias causing syncope can be thought of as:

- *Persistent* in patients presenting with a syncopal episode with ECG evidence of an underlying disturbance of cardiac rhythm likely to be causative
- *Intermittent* when a patient presents with a syncopal episode but without ECG changes, but an arrhythmogenic basis is suspected. Continuous cardiac monitoring is indicated depending on the frequency of syncopal episodes to confirm the clinical suspicion:
  - *Daily*: 24 h Holter monitor or inpatient telemetry
  - *Every 2–3 days*: 48–72 h Holter monitor
  - *Weekly*: 7 day Holter monitor or external loop recorder
  - *Monthly*: 14–30 day external loop recorder
  - *Less often than monthly*: implantable loop recorder, cardiac event recorder.

In addition to cardiac monitoring, attempts can be made to provoke the arrhythmia. Such provocation tests are discussed in Chapter 61 and include:

- carotid sinus massage
- tilt table testing
- exercise provocation.

Electrophysiological testing (EPS) may be indicated under certain circumstances.

EPS and provocation studies can be particularly useful in those patients in whom a rhythm disturbance is *suspected* but monitoring has failed to confirm an intermittent bradyarrhythmia or tachyarrhythmia as the cause.

Indications for permanent pacing

Persistent bradyarrhythmia

Dual chamber pacing is indicated for:

- management of persistent sinus bradycardia in *symptomatic* patients when a reversible (e.g. drug therapy) cause has been excluded
- third degree heart block
- second degree heart block type 2
- second degree heart block type 1 (Wenckebach) is more controversial but should be considered in *symptomatic* patients where there is thought to be risk of progression to complete heart block (e.g. evidence of conduction problem below bundle of His indicated by broad QRS complex).

Intermittent bradyarrhythmia

(Based on 2013 European Society of Cardiology guidelines [2].)

With documented (ECG) evidence
Dual chamber pacing is indicated for:

- Sinus bradycardia and prolonged sinus pauses following termination of a tachycardia in tachy-brady syndrome if symptomatic and unable to treat arrhythmia.

Dual chamber pacing may be appropriate for:

- Documented symptomatic intermittent sinus arrest or sino-atrial block in asymptomatic mild bradycardia (HR 40–50) (although this is controversial)
- Intrinsic sinus node disease associated with syncope and symptomatic pauses
- Intermittent AV block including paroxysmal atrial fibrillation and slow conduction even in absence of documentation
- Intermittent bradycardia and asystole in patients with reflex syncope 40 years or older with documented symptomatic pauses of greater than 3 seconds or asymptomatic pauses of greater than 6 seconds as pacing may reduce syncope burden. However, reflex syncope is a benign condition with regard to mortality. Pacemaker implantation therefore requires very careful consideration especially in young patients as there is not much evidence for actual benefit although there may be a strong placebo effect!

Suspected (no ECG evidence on monitoring)
- Bundle branch block
- Reflex syncope
- Unexplained syncope

Dual chamber pacing is indicated for:

- Syncope and bifascicular block – RBBB and LAD, LBBB or alternating LBBB and RBBB [3].
- Reflex syncope due to demonstrated carotid sinus hypersensitivity may benefit from pacing, especially if testing associated with prolonged (>6 seconds) asystole. However, this is a benign condition with respect to mortality. Pacing is being performed to reduce syncope frequency (up to 75% reduction) and consequent risk of physical injury.
- Patients with tilt table induced *vasovagal syncope with a cardio-inhibitory response* may benefit

from pacing, although the evidence is weak and there is a divergence of opinion. However, this is a benign condition commonly seen in young people. It would appear sensible to offer pacing to those patients with cardio-inhibitory vasovagal syncope over 60 years of age with recurrent physical injury due to syncope suggestive of a minimal prodrome.

Cardiac resynchronization therapy (CRT) in refractory cardiac failure

Introduction

Cardiac failure is thought to affect 2% of the adult population in developed countries. It is directly responsible for 1% of admissions and implicated in 4% of all admissions. These admission figures are likely to be a considerable underestimate of the true scale of the problem due to poor recognition and appropriate clinical coding. It is estimated that CRT could benefit 400 per million of the UK population. Implantation rates are currently less than half this (130 per million). CRT is particularly beneficial for:

- Female patients
- Cardiac failure due to cardiomyopathy of a non-ischaemic cause
- Broad QRS with LBBB morphology; the broader the QRS, the greater the benefit (>150 ms).

Indications

NICE issued guidance for the indications for implantable devices in patients with cardiac failure and/or risk of sudden cardiac death in June 2014 [4]. This relates to the use of cardiac defibrillators (ICDs), cardiac resyncronisation therapy (CRT-D) or cardiac resyncronisation therapy with pacing (CRTD-P). Such devices should be considered for patients with a left ventricular ejection fraction (LVEF) of 35% or less. The eligibility and specific type of device to be implanted is determined by the:

- NYHA status
- QRS duration
- Presence or absence of left bundle branch block.

Other indications for ICD implantation

ICD implantation is indicated as above for patients with an LVEF <35% with a narrow QRS complex and NYHA status I–III who are considered at risk of sudden cardiac death. In addition it is indicated:

- post VF or VT cardiac arrest without a treatable cause
- with spontaneous sustained VT with syncope or significant haemodynamic compromise
- those with a familial cardiac condition with a high risk of sudden death, such as long QT syndrome, hypertrophic cardiomyopathy, Brugada syndrome or arrhythmogenic right ventricular dysplasia
- previous surgical repair of congenital heart disease.

Temporary cardiac pacing

Describes the emergency implementation of cardiac pacing in the context of treatment of a life-threatening bradyarrhythmia or tachyarrhythmia until the arrhythmia resolves or until long-term definitive therapy can be initiated.

Traditionally in the UK transvenous emergency cardiac pacing has been performed out of hours by the on-call medical registrar and in the past was almost viewed as a 'rite of passage'. Increasingly this approach has been viewed as unsustainable due to:

- Significant reduction in the need for temporary cardiac pacing. Most registrars acquired their ability to perform transvenous cardiac pacing in the past in the context of complete heart block complicating an ST-elevation myocardial infarction. ST-elevation infarction is itself much less common than previously and when it does occur is usually managed out of hours by interventional cardiologists.
- Less experience with central venous cannulation as indications for such access and monitoring have declined.
- The European Working Time Directive and consequent reduction in out-of-hours on-call frequency further reduces exposure to patients with an urgent pacing requirement.
- The availability of brief external cardiac pacing.
- Increasing out-of-hours access to trained cardiologists on 24-hour cover.
- Much higher complication rate (especially infection) when performed by those not experienced in the procedure, which can delay definitive treatment and worsen outcomes.
- Significant radiation exposure associated with prolonged fluoroscopic screening during wire insertion and positioning.

Nevertheless this procedure remains a competency for trainees accrediting in Acute Internal Medicine. This is facilitated by the requirement for ACCS trainees to undergo 6 months training in both anaesthesia and ITU together with further experience at registrar grade, where they should become competent at placement of central venous catheters guided by use of ultrasound. It is not unreasonable that such individuals could develop the required competencies and maintain appropriate levels of experience with the support of cardiology colleagues. However, trans venous pacing wires are usually inserted by the radiology team in most medium-sized district general hospitals and bigger.

Indications for emergency temporary cardiac pacing [5]

In context of myocardial infarction:

- Symptomatic bradycardia (sinus bradycardia with hypotension, and Mobitz type 1 with second degree heart block unresponsive to atropine +/– isoprenaline infusion)
- Bilateral BBB (alternating BBB or RBBB with alternating LAHB/LPHB) if associated with symptomatic bradycardia
- Complete heart block (especially in context of anterior ischaemia) if symptomatic.

Bradycardia not associated with an acute MI:

- Second or third degree AV block with symptoms
- VT secondary to bradycardia unable to be controlled by other means.

  In addition temporary pacing may be performed:

- In cardiac surgery where use of implantable epicardial leads, which can be removed postoperatively, is routine
- Occasionally during angioplasty
- As overdrive pacing for some tachyarrhythmias.

  Other less clear indications exist.

Procedure for temporary transvenous pacing

This is a complex procedure and space permits only general considerations. It should only be attempted by those experienced in the technique or under the direct supervision of someone who is. Temporary wires are notoriously prone to infection and may make a patient pacing dependent in the long term when they might not have become so otherwise. There is rarely no time to discuss the appropriateness or otherwise with a cardiologist and every attempt should be made to do so.

The procedure for inserting pacing wire is shown in Box 11.1.

Box 11.1 Procedure for temporary transvenous pacing

- Ensure adequate resuscitation facilities are available including equipment permitting defibrillation and external cardiac pacing.
- Ensure continuous ECG monitoring (limb leads only).
- Conduct procedure with *full aseptic technique*.
- Cannulate the right internal jugular vein using Seldinger technique (ultrasound guidance is advised) and insert the pacing sheath. This approach is preferred as it permits a straight path for wire insertion; other routes include:
  - right subclavian vein, but carries risk of pneumothorax and denies the preferred route for permanent pacing
  - femoral veins carry the risk of DVT and increased infection risk but are easier to access and may be the optimal approach in the sick patient who may be unable to lie flat.
- Advance the electrode tip through the sheath under fluoroscopic guidance until it lies horizontally in right atrium with tip pointing to right.
- Rotate the wire between the index finger and thumb until it points to the patient's left.
- Advance the wire steadily through the tricuspid valve and along the floor of the right ventricle to the apex. Disturbances of cardiac rhythm are commonly seen as the wire crosses the valve and should be ignored if transient.
- When position looks satisfactory test for capture:
  - Set rate at a minimum of 10 beats per minute above patient's intrinsic ventricular rate (65–70 beats per minute is reasonable)
  - Set voltage as recommended by the manufacturer (usually about 3 volts) and check for capture so that each pacing spike is followed by a QRS complex
  - Check for the pacing threshold by gradually lowering the pacing voltage until there is loss of capture (should be <1 volt)

- - Set pacing voltage to twice the threshold
  - Check sensing by setting pacing rate at 10–20 beats per minute below intrinsic ventricular rate; pacing spikes should disappear.
- Carefully remove the pacing sheath.
- Suture the wire to the skin close to insertion and cover with dressing.
- Request CXR to confirm wire position and absence of pneumothorax.
- Ensure checked daily by experienced staff for threshold voltage, battery status, connections, wound site infection and underlying infection.
- The need for the device should also be reviewed on a daily basis. If it seems likely that permanent pacing will be required, then this should be arranged as soon as possible and preferably within 24 hours of insertion of the temporary wire.
- In many units prophylactic antibiotics are given and continued whilst the wire is in place.

External cardiac pacing

- Requires the use of large, high impedance electrodes directly applied to the chest wall of the patient.
- Significant discomfort and distress is caused to the patient if awake and so this should only be performed in the unconscious or sedated patient.
- It is only appropriate in emergencies.

References

1. Aquilina O. A brief history of cardiac pacing. *Images Paediatr Cardiol* 2006; 8(2): 17–81.

2. 2013 ESC Guidelines on cardiac pacing and cardiac resynchronization therapy. *Eur Heart J* 2013; 34: 2281–2329. Available to download at http://eurheartj.oxfordjournals.org/content/34/29/2281.full.pdf.

3. Moya A, Garcia-Civera R, Croci F et al. Diagnosis, management, and outcomes of patients with syncope and bundle branch block. *Eur Heart J* 2011; 32: 1535–1541.

4. Implantable cardioverter defibrillators and cardiac resynchronisation therapy for arrhythmias and heart failure. NICE Technology Appraisal TA314. Available online at: www.nice.org.uk/guidance/TA314/chapter/1-Guidance.

5. Gammage MD. *Heart* 2000; 83: 715–720.

Suggested reading

NICE. Dual-chamber pacemakers for symptomatic bradycardia due to sick sinus syndrome and/or atrioventricular block. NICE Technology Appraisal Guidance 88. Available to download at www.nice.org.uk/nicemedia/live/11552/33011/33011.pdf.

Breathlessness

Robert A. Stone

Introduction

Shortage of breath is one of the commonest presenting complaints. The symptom of breathlessness means different things to different people and there is no universally accepted definition.

Breathlessness develops when healthy persons undertake progressively increasing exercise and it finally causes them to stop or slow down. The same or a similar disagreeable sensation occurs in patients with a variety of underlying diseases at less than normal levels of activity and under these circumstances is pathological.

Dyspnoea is the sensation of breathing discomfort that, if perceived as disproportionate to the situation, may lead an individual to describe breathlessness. An array of different subjective sensations contributes to an individual's final experience.

The language of breathlessness is important to appreciate. Patients may describe their experience in very different terms to one another and this must be explored carefully within the medical history if accurate causation is to be established.

Pathophysiology

- Dyspnoea occurs if the respiratory system is subjected to increased drive or a mechanical load. Hypercapnia and resistive changes are the main drivers. Hypoxia, contrary to popular belief, is a less important stimulus. Most studies of dyspnoea have been undertaken in healthy individuals and many patients with chronic hypercapnia or hypoxia do not describe breathlessness at rest.
- Receptors within the upper airway and on the face can modulate dyspnoea (the rationale for using fans or cool air to alleviate breathlessness). Within the lung, rapidly adapting irritant receptors respond to mechanical and chemical stimuli, slowly adapting stretch receptors detect changes in lung inflation and C-fibres are nociceptive. Mechanoreceptors in the chest wall detect changes in load. Receptors in the carotid body, carotid artery and brainstem detect perturbations in arterial PO_2, PCO_2 and pH. The dyspnoeic effect of hypercapnia is probably mediated via its effect on pH sensitive central chemoreceptors. The role in mediating dyspnoea of receptors present within the heart, pericardium and pleura is unclear.

- Afferent sensory information integrates in the dorsal brainstem and is subject to considerable cortical influence. Individuals may react very differently to sensory input and the behavioural response is dependent upon circumstances, personality, anxiety levels or the presence of cortical brain disease.

- The upshot of increased afferent activity allied to its cortical modulation is heightened respiratory drive, which leads to breathlessness being reported if there is a perceived disconnect between the incoming information and the outgoing efferent response. Dyspnoeic sensations are not dependent upon an intact efferent pathway, however, as patients with high cervical lesions and those paralysed during mechanical ventilation report breathlessness in response to hypercapnic challenge.

Causes of breathlessness

Some causes of breathlessness are listed in Table 12.1. Patients may have more than one underlying condition and it is useful to ask oneself whether the cause(s) is

Acute Medicine, ed. Stephen Haydock, Duncan Whitehead and Zoë Fritz. Published by Cambridge University Press.
© Cambridge University Press 2015.

Table 12.1 Some causes of breathlessness (those conditions causing acute breathlessness are given in italicized bold)

System	Cause of breathlessness
Respiratory	
Upper airway	Infections: *epiglottitis*, tonsillitis, pharyngitis, deep neck infection *Foreign body* Tumour: laryngeal, pharyngeal Vocal cords: *bilateral vocal cord palsy*, crico-arytenoid rheumatoid, sub-glottic stenosis *Angio-oedema* *Anaphylaxis*
Lower airways	Mechanical obstruction: tracheal tumour, tracheomalacia, bronchial tumour, *foreign body*, bronchomalacia, amyloidosis, papillomatosis, Kaposi's sarcoma Obstructive airway diseases: *asthma*, *COPD*, bronchiectasis, cystic fibrosis, small airways disease/bronchiolitis Airway infiltration and inflammation: *aspiration*, endobronchial sarcoidosis, vasculitides, inhalation injury
Lung parenchyma	Lung infections: *pneumonia*, *diffuse lung infection*, parasitic infiltrations Volume loss: *lung collapse*, *lobar collapse* Interstitial lung diseases: acute pneumonitis, *adult respiratory distress syndrome*, idiopathic pulmonary fibrosis, drug-induced interstitial disease, occupational interstitial lung disease, hypersensitivity pneumonitis, paraquat poisoning, *non-cardiogenic pulmonary oedema*, *neurogenic pulmonary oedema*, *acute mountain sickness* Malignancy: metastatic disease, diffuse tumour infiltration, lymphangitis carcinomatosa
Pleura/chest wall	Pleural disease: pleural effusion, pleural tumour Skeletal problems: *fractured ribs*, kyphosis, kyphoscoliosis, ankylosing spondylitis, diffuse cutaneous scleroderma Neuromuscular diseases: *GBS*, amyotrophic lateral sclerosis, steroid myopathy, statin myopathy, polymyositis, polymyalgia rheumatica, dermatomyositis, post-polio, *myasthenia gravis*, paraneoplastic syndromes including Lambert–Eaton, mitochondrial myopathy, *diaphragmatic paralysis – unilateral and/or bilateral*
Disorders of pulmonary circulation	*Pulmonary embolism*: pulmonary hypertension, secondary and primary; pulmonary venous thrombosis; superior vena cava obstruction; pulmonary vasculitis
Cardiovascular	*Pulmonary oedema*
	Coronary circulation: *myocardial infarction*, *angina equivalent*
Dysrhythmia	*Atrial fibrillation*
Heart valves	Any valve disorder; *papillary muscle rupture*; *valve rupture*
Heart muscle	*Systolic left ventricular failure*; diastolic dysfunction; hypertensive heart disease; cardiomyopathies; myocarditis; right heart dysfunction
Pericardium	Tamponade; pericardial effusion or constriction
Congenital heart disease	Any defect leading to shunting or secondary pulmonary hypertension
Non-cardiorespiratory	
Acidosis	*Diabetic ketoacidosis*; kidney failure; liver failure; *salicylate poisoning*; *septicaemia*; *lactic acidosis*; malignancy; *organophosphate poisoning*; *methanol*; *ethylene glycol*; *carbon monoxide poisoning*
CNS lesions	*Brainstem lesions*; hypothalamic lesions; *neurogenic pulmonary oedema*; malignant hyperpyrexia
Anaemia	*Major blood loss*; chronic anaemia; haemolysis; sickle cell disease
Psychogenic	*Anxiety states*; *hyperventilation syndrome*
Obesity	Deconditioning
Thyrotoxicosis	
Abdominal fullness	Ascites; tumour; pregnancy
Rare causes of breathlessness	*Fat embolism*; *air embolism*; *amniotic fluid embolism*; eclampsia or pre-eclampsia

respiratory, cardiac, non-cardiorespiratory or potentially multifactorial. Take careful note of what the patient describes, how the symptom is related and link the history to a thorough examination and targeted investigations.

Scenario 12.1

A 40-year-old ex-soldier is referred to the MAU with breathlessness. He was previously a heavy smoker of 20–30 cigarettes per day since his teens. He stopped smoking shortly after his medical discharge 5 years previously due to breathlessness attributed to a combination of asthma and COPD. He is normally breathless on exertion and has noticed this to be gradually worsening. He has noticed some progressive weight loss. He has become much more breathless over the last 3 days associated with fevers and a cough productive of green sputum. On examination he is tachypnoeic, has early clubbing, bilateral late inspiratory crackles and signs of right mid-zone consolidation. ECG shows right axis deviation. The chest radiograph confirms a right middle zone pneumonia. Bloods are consistent with an acute bacterial infection.

Clinical assessment

Acute severe breathlessness dictates an immediate response. *Rapid assessment to determine the presence of potentially life-threatening allergic, upper airways, respiratory, cardiac, neurological or metabolic disease is a mandatory first step in the acutely breathless patient that will give way to a more detailed and systematic evaluation after the necessary remedial measures.*

History

General points

- Onset, duration, exacerbating factors, postural relationship, severity and impact of breathlessness.
- Medications and medication changes.
- A collateral history can be useful, as others will often date the circumstances and trajectory much more precisely. Patients themselves may describe breathlessness in different terms: 'trouble breathing', 'hard to breathe', 'difficulty breathing', 'running out of energy' and 'tiring out' are commonly used phrases. If the history seems vague, ask directly whether the patient feels short of breath or breathless.

Impact of breathlessness

- Objective measures such as the respiratory rate, oxygen saturation and arterial blood gases do not correlate with degree of dyspnoea.
- Assess how breathlessness actually affects activities of daily living such as washing, dressing, shopping, work, leisure time and sexual activity.
- The most widely used classification of breathlessness is the Medical Research Council (MRC) scale (Table 12.2), which permits a standardized approach to quantifying disability, although it is narrow in its outlook.

Specific situations

Acute physiological disturbances and poisonings

- Acidosis increases respiratory drive: diabetic ketoacidosis, hypercapnic respiratory failure, acute kidney failure, liver failure and lactic acidosis.
- Salicylate poisoning stimulates the respiratory centre directly whereas methanol and ethylene glycol do so via acidosis.
- Carbon monoxide may induce breathlessness either through impaired oxygen delivery or acute pulmonary oedema.
- Overdose of selective serotonin reuptake inhibitors is associated rarely with the serotonin syndrome, which may itself lead to hyperpnoea, agitation and breathlessness when severe. So too may the neuroleptic malignant syndrome.
- Patients with sepsis, malignancy and thyrotoxicosis may also report breathlessness.

Neurological and neuromuscular disease

- Acute brain injury may induce neurogenic pulmonary oedema and breathlessness.
- Brainstem and posterior fossa bleeds, hypothalamic or other central nervous system lesions leading to acute compression of the respiratory centre can cause extreme hyperpnoea; by contrast, these patients may not feel breathless.
- Neuromuscular conditions affecting the respiratory axis may induce breathlessness via ventilatory failure or chronic thoracic restriction.

Table 12.2 Medical Research Council (MRC) Breathlessness Scale

Grade	Degree of breathlessness related to activities
1	Not troubled by breathlessness except on strenuous exercise
2	Short of breath when hurrying or walking up a slight hill
3	Walks slower than contemporaries on level ground because of breathlessness, or has to stop for breath when walking at own pace
4	Stops for breath after walking about 100 m or after a few minutes on level ground
5	Too breathless to leave the house, or breathless when dressing or undressing

Respiratory diseases

- A history of aspiration, foreign body, toxin inhalation or ingestion, allergy and recent upper or lower airway infection should be sought if there is acute breathlessness.
- While breathing difficulty usually associates with pneumonia, abnormal respiratory sensation is not a universal experience in this situation and frail elderly patients in particular may be exceedingly unwell with pneumonia yet report no breathlessness.
- The current and past occupational history is especially important, detailing potential irritants, dusts or airway sensitizers that could associate with airways or parenchymal disease. Ask about domestic pets, especially birds, and recent changes in the home or work environment. Smoking should be detailed as current, previous (pack years) or never smoked.
- Breathlessness in asthma is generally episodic, the dyspnoea is associated with sensations of chest tightness and wheeze, is often worse in the mornings and may disrupt at night. The breathlessness of exercise-induced asthma occurs typically 15–20 minutes after exercise has ceased although asthmatic airways often constrict during exercise in cold air.
- Breathlessness in COPD is insidious, progressive and varies little from day to day. It is associated with cough, phlegm and wheeze. There may be a history of exacerbation, though patients with emphysema typically describe breathlessness in isolation and may become significantly disabled by sudden exertion, bending down and lifting. Emphysematous patients often feel full in the lungs, as if they can't breathe to the top.
- By contrast, patients with bronchiectasis produce significant sputum volumes. They may have a past history of childhood whooping cough, measles or pneumonia.
- Small airways disease (bronchiolitis) is often preceded by viral illness but is also associated with rheumatological disorders and smoking. Breathlessness that doesn't improve, or deteriorates, after respiratory viral illness should prompt consideration of bronchiolitis or carditis.
- Parenchymal lung diseases usually cause progressive decline though antigen exposure in patients with hypersensitivity pneumonitis may cause acute breathlessness. If occupational, this may be worse on first exposure during the working week and become more intrusive as the working week progresses. Idiopathic pulmonary fibrosis associates with unpleasant dry cough; 'flare-ups' cause breathlessness to deteriorate over days or weeks. Triggers include infection, oesophageal reflux, pulmonary embolism and medication changes. It is especially important to recognize the latter, as pre-existing interstitial lung disease may flare acutely in certain patients receiving agents such as amiodarone, methotrexate or biological therapy; patients with rheumatological disease and deteriorating breathlessness should always be asked about recent medication changes.
- Pulmonary embolism is almost always accompanied by breathlessness. The dyspnoea is due variably to V/Q mismatch, hypoxia, pulmonary infarction and alteration in small airways dynamics resulting in localized air trapping. The severity of breathlessness is an unreliable guide to the extent of embolism but there may be accompanying features of pulmonary infarction; some patients with major acute pulmonary embolism display evidence of circulatory distress yet appear relatively undisturbed by their breathing. The breathlessness of pulmonary hypertension, whether primary or secondary, is progressive, exertional and may become very severe. Syncope is a feature of advanced pulmonary hypertension.
- Pneumothorax causes acute breathlessness, often accompanied by pain. Although common in tall,

thin young males, it is imperative to consider pneumothorax, which may be bilateral, in patients with asthma or COPD who have become suddenly more breathless. Acute expansion of an emphysematous bulla can present similarly and careful thought is necessary when interpreting the X-ray in these cases; inappropriate intercostal drainage of a bulla that has been mistaken for a pneumothorax can lead to broncho-pleural fistula and persistent air leak.

- Pleural effusions cause breathlessness by restricting thoracic/diaphragmatic movement, compressing underlying lung and squeezing the mediastinum. Thoracic pain that accompanies breathlessness in patients with pleural effusion should alert to the possibility of underlying malignancy, empyema or pulmonary infarction.

- The restrictive effects of kyphosis (increasingly seen in older patients with degenerative bone disease), kyphoscoliosis and pain due to fractured ribs or chest injury can all lead to breathlessness. Patients with respiratory muscle weakness that affects the diaphragm (but also intercostal muscles) typically feel worse when lying flat (orthopnoea) or going beyond waist depth in water.

- Obesity is a common confounding factor that causes breathlessness via thoracic restriction and deconditioning. A thorough assessment for other potential causes of breathlessness should be undertaken in obese individuals before ascribing their weight as the sole association of the symptom. Obstructive sleep apnoea, itself a source of breathlessness, is common in this patient group.

Cardiovascular diseases

- Cardiovascular disease may be the sole cause or a significant co-factor in acute and chronic breathlessness. Any condition affecting heart function can cause breathlessness; it is associated with pulmonary oedema, heart failure, rhythm disturbance, valvular heart disease, coronary artery disease and pericardial problems (Table 12.1).

- Patients with left ventricular failure may describe paroxysmal nocturnal dyspnoea, sudden increases in breathlessness that typically wake them from sleep and needing air. Orthopnoea is respiratory discomfort when lying flat, often necessitating sleep in the bolstered or upright position. Although a cardinal symptom of heart failure, it

also occurs in patients with respiratory muscle weakness. Sleep-disordered breathing is common in patients with heart failure and may contribute to breathlessness via pulmonary hypertensive effects.

- Cardiologists often encounter breathless patients in whom the diagnosis of ischaemic heart disease has been overlooked. Breathlessness can be the sole symptom, 'angina equivalent', in some patients with significant coronary disease. It is a diagnosis to consider in the patient who describes chronic effort-related breathlessness of no clear cause.

- Pericardial effusion may cause acute or chronic breathlessness. Significant pericardial effusions causing acute or subacute tamponade are easy to miss and this is a diagnosis that should be kept in mind especially in those with malignant disease and unexplained breathlessness.

Anaemia

- Anaemia impairs tissue oxygen delivery. It usually presents insidiously and is a common co-factor in breathless patients with cardiorespiratory disease in whom it is important to recognize, as relatively small changes in haemoglobin may impact significantly upon function. Major blood loss or acute haemolysis may also lead to breathing difficulty and sickle cell disease is associated with breathlessness via pulmonary infarction, pulmonary oedema and rib infarction with underventilation.

Hyperventilation syndrome

- Hyperventilation syndrome can occur when there is an inappropriate increase in breathing without a clear physiological stimulus. The over-ventilation in this condition causes breathlessness, respiratory alkalosis and a variety of non-specific symptoms that include light-headedness, fatigue and paraesthesiae. Carpo-pedal spasm is rare. The diagnosis should only be ascribed with great care as significant cardiorespiratory or physiological perturbations may themselves induce hyperventilation. The syndrome seems commoner in anxious individuals and those struggling to maintain intense competitive sporting programmes. Patients may describe an inability to take satisfying breaths.

Pregnancy

- Pregnancy increases minute ventilation, reduces functional residual capacity and affects airway smooth muscle reactivity. There is an additional cardiorespiratory demand. Reflux may also heighten thoracic sensation. It is common for pregnant women to experience a degree of respiratory discomfort but investigation may be necessary if new onset breathlessness or a sudden change is reported. The differential diagnosis of breathlessness in pregnancy includes anaemia, thromboembolic disease, asthma, cardiac disease, diabetes and thyroid disorder. Amniotic embolism and air embolism are very rare causes of acute breathlessness and associated cardiovascular crisis.

Examination

- Observe the patient's general demeanour; determine whether there is respiratory distress, tachypnoea, hyperpnoea, stridor or wheeze. Signs of impending crisis include difficulty speaking, intercostal recession, confusion, agitation and dusky skin.
- The body should be exposed from the waist upwards. Observe the patient take a deep breath. This may reveal stridor, respiratory asymmetry, poor thoracic excursion, hyperinflation, use of accessory respiratory muscles, tracheal tug, intercostal recession and a displaced cardiac apex. Examine for peripheral stigmata including impaired tissue perfusion, evidence of anaemia, cyanosis, tremor, dehydration, finger clubbing, tar staining, lymphadenopathy, goitre and rheumatological disease. Look in the mouth, at the fauces and eyes. Concentrate all the while on the patient's breathing pattern; those with hyperventilation syndrome take rapid, shallow, predominantly upper thoracic, breaths.
- Systems examination may reveal relevant cardiovascular signs such as atrial fibrillation, abnormal pulse/blood pressure, raised jugular venous pressure (if raised, assess the wave-form carefully to determine if it is fixed, rises or falls on inspiration), cardiomegaly, a displaced apex beat, abnormal or added heart sounds (particularly the presence of a third heart sound or accentuated/delayed P2), cardiac murmurs, pericardial rub,

peripheral or sacral oedema. Pulsus paradoxus, an abnormally large decrease in systolic pressure (>10 mmHg) on inspiration, is a common but not universal sign in moderate to severe cardiac tamponade. It is not a reliable indicator in acute severe asthma.

- Respiratory examination should again pay particular attention to the presence of stridor, wheeze, tracheal deviation, and differences in expansion, percussion note and tactile vocal fremitus that might indicate pneumothorax, lung collapse, pleural effusion or consolidation. Auscultate carefully from top to bottom anteriorly and posteriorly, noting the character of breath sounds and the presence of added sounds; the fine crackles of interstitial lung disease (and pulmonary oedema) may be sparsely present and not necessarily basal. Pleural rubs are often transient and localize to the site of pleuritic discomfort. Asking the patient to lie flat will determine the presence of orthopnoea. Abdominal paradox, an inward movement of the abdominal wall with inspiration, is suggestive of diaphragmatic weakness.
- Stridor is a rasping sound that indicates fixed obstruction of a major airway, usually by tumour. It may be inspiratory (more often with upper airway and vocal cord lesions), expiratory (typically intrathoracic lesions) or heard throughout the respiratory cycle. Stridor is best detected over the anterior neck or with the stethoscope placed near to the opened mouth. Wheeze is an altogether more musical sound that occurs in either part of the respiratory cycle but doesn't extend throughout inspiration or expiration. Most wheezes clear with coughing though a fixed wheeze, present in the same place over the thorax and failing to clear with coughing, can indicate airway blockage from inspissated mucus, or impending obstruction from tumour.

Investigations

- If the cause of breathlessness is not clear after first appraisal, taking the history, examination and viewing first-line tests, it is best to seek senior opinion to plan subsequent investigation, rather than adopt a scattergun approach.
- Essential investigations include:

- oxygen saturation
- chest X-ray
- electrocardiogram (ECG)
- full blood count
- blood glucose
- blood lactate
- renal and liver chemistry
- peak expiratory flow
- arterial blood gases, which should be sampled if the oxygen saturation is unclear or below 96% on air.

Oxygen saturation

- Normal oxygen saturation may belie the presence of significant disease, particularly in younger patients or those with acute asthma.
- The saturation may appear low if there is poor peripheral perfusion, hypothermia, profound anaemia, venous congestion, and if the patient is wearing black, green or blue nail varnish. Placing the probe sideways on the finger can avert the latter situation.
- For ambulatory patients with unexplained breathlessness, assessing any changes in saturation after a corridor walk can be a useful rough guide to the presence of an underlying diffusion defect. Rapid falls in saturation may be observed in those with interstitial diseases and pneumocystis pneumonia.

ECG

- Systematic scrutiny of the current *and previous* ECGs is mandatory.
- Most breathless patients are tachycardic. Many have atrial fibrillation, evidence of underlying ischaemic heart disease or hypertension.
- Right axis deviation is useful to note when trying to differentiate between pulmonary or cardiac disease. P-pulmonale (in isolation or associated with right axis and thoracic lead abnormalities) may indicate cor pulmonale whereas poor R-wave progression may signify left ventricular disease.
- Pulmonary embolism associates with right axis changes, right bundle branch block and T wave changes in the right thoracic leads; a right ventricular strain pattern may occur in acute major embolism or chronic thromboembolic disease with

pulmonary hypertension (CTEPH). The often-quoted S1Q3T3 pattern is encountered rarely.
- If the ECG appears normal on first inspection, remember to look at QRS voltage size and shape and for subtle abnormalities in re-polarization, ST segments and T waves.

Chest X-ray

- If the chest X-ray appears normal at first glance, consider whether subtle abnormalities are present:
  - Look at the calibre of the trachea and major airways.
  - Is there a retrosternal goitre?
  - Is the mediastinum wide and what about the retrocardiac area? Left lower lobe collapse is easy to miss.
  - Dark lung fields or regional hypoperfusion occur in airways disease and pulmonary embolism.
  - Peripheral vascular pruning is seen in COPD.
  - Bronchi may appear thickened in asthma.
  - Look at the hila carefully to check for masses.
- Upper lobe blood diversion, septal lines, fluid in the fissures and peri-bronchial cuffing all point towards left ventricular failure. The radiological pattern of pulmonary oedema is often atypical in patients with emphysema, the disrupted anatomy leading to alveolar opacities in areas of preserved lung. It is especially important to look for septal lines in patients with emphysema, suggesting coexistent left ventricular failure.
- Plump pulmonary arteries may indicate underlying pulmonary hypertension due to airways or pulmonary vascular disease. Asymmetric pulmonary vascular enlargement favours embolic disease.
- The lungs often appear small in interstitial lung disease, chronic thromboembolism (band atelectasis may also be seen in this situation) and diaphragm paralysis. Unilateral diaphragm elevation can indicate phrenic nerve palsy.
- The cardiac contours should be noted, with particular reference to cardiothoracic ratio, left ventricular configuration, right heart border and cardiac silhouette.
- Small pneumothoraces are best viewed by flipping the image onto its side.

Routine blood tests

If anaemia is present, note whether it is normochromic, microcytic or macrocytic; this will prompt further assessment of the reticulocyte count and haematinics. Arterial blood gases should be measured if lactate, kidney function, liver chemistry or blood sugar is significantly impaired.

Arterial blood gases

- Breathless patients should have arterial blood gases measured if acidosis or respiratory failure is suspected, and where the cause of breathlessness is unclear. Acute hypoxia or hypercapnia cause dyspnoea though patients with compensated respiratory failure may not mention breathlessness. Hyperventilation may elevate the oxygen saturation yet be accompanied by the metabolic acidosis of serious systemic disease or respiratory alkalosis of over-breathing. Conditions in which breathlessness is accompanied by rapid respiratory rate and respiratory alkalosis include pulmonary embolism, pulmonary oedema, pneumonia, pulmonary fibrosis and hyperventilation syndrome.
- The A–a gradient, literally the difference between alveolar and arterial oxygenation, is useful in determining whether hypoxaemia or normoxia with respiratory alkalosis has a pulmonary origin (e.g. diffusion defect, V/Q mismatch or right to left shunt). It is readily calculated using an online calculator. PaO_2 (available by blood gas measurement) is subtracted from the PAO_2 (derived from the alveolar gas equation).
- An increased gradient demonstrates high respiratory effort relative to the achieved level of oxygenation. A raised A–a gradient could indicate a patient breathing hard to achieve normal oxygenation, a patient breathing normally and achieving low oxygenation or a patient breathing hard and still failing to achieve normal oxygenation.

Peak expiratory flow volume (PEFV)

- PEFV must be measured if the patient has known or suspected asthma. The value should be related to the individual's usual best or what is predicted. *The PEFV on admission relates to mortality in patients with acute asthma.*

Spirometry

- Spirometry is essential to diagnose and differentiate between obstructive and restrictive lung disease. It must be performed correctly. A submaximal effort may give an incorrect assumption of restrictive disease.
- Airflow obstruction is defined as an FEV_1/FVC ratio <70% and restriction as FEV_1/FVC >80%.
- Spirometry is best reserved for the outpatient or emergency clinic, though sequential FVC measurement is invaluable to the inpatient care of patients with Guillain–Barré syndrome or myasthenic crisis.
- The severity of airflow obstruction and exacerbation frequency should be noted in patients with COPD as these phenotypic features have prognostic implications.

CT scanning

- CT must be used appropriately. Requests must provide sufficient detail for the reporting radiologist. Patients must be able to lie flat and hold their breath for at least 10 seconds in order to achieve satisfactory images.
- *CT pulmonary angiography* is now the investigation of choice to diagnose pulmonary embolism though interpretation of subsegmental abnormalities, especially in those with CTEPH, is less accurate than for lobar or segmental clots.
- *High resolution thoracic CT* reveals the distribution and characteristics of interstitial disease. Ground glass abnormalities occur in active alveolitis although pulmonary oedema and haemorrhage can confuse; scanning the patient prone may discriminate. Tree-in-bud opacities signify small airways inflammation or infection; a mosaic pattern is seen if there is lobular gas trapping adjacent to normal areas, as in small airways disease and pulmonary embolism. Airway wall thickening and mucus-plugging occurs in asthma and COPD.

Echocardiography

- Echocardiography should not be requested initially in every case of suspected heart failure or pulmonary embolism. It is of course a useful diagnostic tool but should be reserved *at presentation* for suspected cardiac tamponade or major pulmonary embolism.

- Patients with tamponade usually have a moderate or large pericardial effusion and there may be evidence of impending chamber collapse or reversal of the normal respiratory variation in flows.
- Urgent echocardiography is particularly useful in patients with major pulmonary embolism, as it may be undertaken at the bedside. Patients with pulmonary embolism should undergo echocardiography if there are signs of cardiovascular compromise or pulmonary hypertension; observing intracardiac clot, pulmonary hypertension and features of right ventricular stress should prompt urgent senior review to consider thrombolytic therapy.

Lung function tests

- Full lung function tests are useful in patients with chronic breathlessness.
- The three components (spirometry, lung volumes and diffusion) differentiate between:
  - obstructive (e.g. COPD)
  - restrictive (e.g. lung fibrosis)
  - increased lung volumes by causing air trapping (asthma, emphysema)
  - reduced lung volumes by shrinkage/stiffening (lung fibrosis, pleural disease)
  - abnormal diffusion from alveolus to pulmonary circulation (pulmonary oedema, emphysema, lung fibrosis, pulmonary vascular disease).

Other tests

- Further relevant tests will be determined by the clinical scenario and include D-dimer, cardiac troponin, thyroid function, salicylate/paracetamol or carboxyhaemoglobin levels and detection of other potential toxins, brain natriuretic peptide (BNP), serum calcium/magnesium, creatine kinase, overnight oximetry, chest ultrasound for managing effusions, pleural fluid analysis, fluoroscopic screening to diagnose diaphragm paralysis, nasendoscopy and bronchoscopy.
- The D-dimer is fast becoming an over-requested test that should be requested only when

pulmonary embolism is considered within the differential diagnosis. It is of value in those with chronic as well as acute thromboembolic disease.
- Elevated BNP levels are not specific to left heart failure and may occur in pulmonary embolism and right heart strain. Elevated cardiac troponin is an adverse prognostic indicator in patients with significant pulmonary embolism.

Management

Managing breathlessness: *depends on situation and cause.*

Recognize and manage life-threatening disease

- Potentially life-threatening conditions should be identified rapidly and managed according to established professional guidelines.
- Imperatives are maintaining airway security, breathing, oxygenation, circulation, tissue perfusion, relief of bronchospasm and pulmonary oedema whilst addressing the underlying cause.
- In the patient with impending collapse, consider tension pneumothorax, cardiac tamponade, pulmonary embolism, dysrhythmia, acute severe asthma and pulmonary oedema.
- After immediate management it is important to *define the ceiling of further care*, and whether it is medically appropriate to escalate therapy beyond palliation of breathlessness to non-invasive or full ventilatory and circulatory support. *Experienced doctors should make such decisions.*

Provide oxygen for hypoxic patients

- The British Thoracic Society emergency oxygen guideline emphasizes that, while oxygen must be administered carefully in the emergency situation, patients with COPD and other risk factors for hypercapnia who develop critical illness should have the same initial target saturation as other critically ill patients, pending the results of blood gas measurements.
- Thus, non-rebreathing masks should be used to deliver high flow oxygen at 15 L/min.
- Thereafter, if blood gases show persisting severe hypoxia or hypercapnia with respiratory

acidosis, assisted ventilation or controlled oxygen therapy via Venturi mask may be necessary in patients with known or suspected COPD, neuromuscular disease or risk factors for hypoventilation. The target saturation should be between 88% and 92% for this group. Other patients should receive oxygen to achieve target saturation of 94–98%.

Manage upper airway or lower airway obstruction and lung collapse

- Relief of mechanical obstruction is a highly effective treatment for breathlessness. Early specialist opinion is recommended.
- Patients with suspected anaphylaxis, angio-oedema or upper airway obstruction should receive adrenaline (including nebulized) and steroids as necessary. Broad spectrum intravenous antibiotic should be given immediately for infection. All patients with stridor or impending major airway obstruction should be considered for urgent inspection of the airway. Patients with lung cancer may benefit from stenting or tumour debulking by laser or cryotherapy unless they are known to be in the end phase of their condition.
- Sudden lung or lobar collapse due to mucus impaction may cause acute breathlessness necessitating urgent bronchoscopy. Respiratory physiotherapy is an effective treatment in this situation for those who are able to undertake it. To aid expectoration the airways must be kept moist, using humidified oxygen, and the patient well hydrated.

Relieve bronchospasm

- The sensation of bronchospasm is unpleasant. It occurs in any condition associated with airways hyperreactivity, not merely asthma or COPD. Many breathless patients with pulmonary oedema or lung infection will also benefit from a bronchodilator. Beta$_2$-agonists, nebulized as necessary with ipratropium bromide, are the treatment of choice. High flow oxygen, at a minimum rate of 6 L/min to generate respirable particles, should be used to nebulize patients with acute severe asthma. Furosemide bonchodilates and venodilates: alongside bronchodilators it can be a potent treatment for breathlessness, especially if there is coexistent pulmonary oedema.
- Persistent bronchospasm must be managed actively in patients with asthma or COPD. If nebulizers prove manifestly ineffective, intravenous magnesium may be helpful in acute asthma. Intravenous theophylline remains a highly effective treatment for recalcitrant bronchospasm and should be considered judiciously in both asthma and COPD patients who fail to respond to nebulizers. Patients with COPD exacerbation are increasingly managed with non-invasive ventilation; *this is not a treatment for bronchospasm,* persistence of which is often under-treated in such cases.

Ventilatory support

- Continuous positive airways pressure (CPAP) allied to high flow oxygen is useful in patients with tracheobronchomalacia and pulmonary oedema. It increases intraluminal airways pressure and alreolar recruitment, so improving patency and favouring resorption of extravasated oedema.
- Bi-level positive airways pressure (BiPAP) provides inspiratory assistance as well as pressure support and is often termed non-invasive ventilation (NIV). It is indicated in respiratory failure associated with COPD exacerbation (if the pH is <7.35 after blood gases have been re-checked following removal of inappropriate high flow oxygen therapy), thoracic restriction, hypoventilation and neuromuscular disease. Oxygen may be safely entrained into the inspiratory circuit provided the machine is set to spontaneous/timed mode with a specified back-up breathing rate.
- Both modes of support may make the breathless patient feel claustrophobic. The mask and pressure settings should be applied and set by a trained professional in an area where the patient can be monitored effectively.

Manage pulmonary oedema

- The breathlessness of pulmonary oedema will improve with oxygen if there is hypoxia, stabilizing coronary blood flow if there is cardiac ischaemia, offloading the left ventricle with medications that reduce preload (diuretic, nitrate, opiate) or afterload (angiotensin-converting inhibitor), diuresis, management of bronchospasm and pressure support.

Manage infection, tissue perfusion and metabolism

- Breathlessness improves as tissue hypoxia and acidosis reduce. Antibiotics, judicious crystalloid fluid replacement and blood transfusion should be given as necessary to patients with suspected sepsis or significant anaemia.

Provide pharmacological relief

- Analgesics help breathlessness where it is exacerbated by painful breathing.
- Most medications that improve breathlessness also cause respiratory suppression, notably in patients with type 2 respiratory failure.
- Antidepressants (especially those which improve sleep) and anxiolytics may be particularly useful if low mood or anxiety is thought to be contributing to heightened perception of dyspnoeic sensation. Sublingual benzodiazepines can rapidly alleviate acute anxiety in malignant or end-stage heart and lung disease.
- Opiates, and notably morphine, given in oral liquid aliquots, intravenous boluses or via a syringe driver, are highly effective at relieving dyspnoeic sensations. Morphine venodilates and provides additional benefit to patients with acute left ventricular failure. Where palliative sedation is required, opiates may be combined in the syringe driver with medications such as midazolam or methotrimeprazine.
- The early involvement of a palliative care specialist is recommended in patients with breathlessness associated with malignant or terminal disease.

General measures

- Being breathless is both unpleasant and frightening. Patients should be informed that breathlessness in itself is not harmful. Patients who are chronically breathless may continue to exercise and must be given information about managing their symptom. Downloadable leaflets are available from patient organizations such as the British Lung Foundation.
- COPD patients with MRC grade 3 and above breathlessness should be offered pulmonary rehabilitation, which improves exercise tolerance and breathlessness control.
- The active cycle of breathing technique (ACBT) encourages shoulder relaxation and recruitment of the abdominal muscles to aid breathing in those with hyperventilation.
- Fanning the face with cool air is a useful remedial measure, and generally more effective than short burst oxygen therapy, which has little practical benefit for patients with longer-term breathlessness.
- Eating little and often reduces bloating and diaphragm splinting, as does maintaining regular bowel movement.
- Smoking cessation improves sputum production and airways irritability in patients with airways disease.
- Weight loss in overweight breathless individuals can make a major difference.

> **Scenario 12.1 continued**
>
> *This man improved with conventional antimicrobial and bronchodilator therapy. However, the weight loss and clubbing were clearly a cause for concern. Subsequent investigation led to a diagnosis of extrinsic allergic alveolitis. It transpired that his exposure had been during his time in the army when he had served with the household cavalry. He had been responsible for feeding and grooming the horses used on ceremonial occasions. The diagnosis can often be found hidden in the history!*

Further reading

British Cardiovascular Society Guidelines: www.bcs.com/pages/page_box_contents.asp?pageID=704.

British Lung Foundation: breathlessness: www.blf.org.uk/Conditions/Detail/Breathlessness.

British Thoracic Society Guidelines: www.brit-thoracic.org.uk/guidelines.aspx.

European Society of Cardiology guidelines: www.escardio.org/guidelines-surveys/esc-guidelines/Pages/GuidelinesList.aspx.

Scottish Intercollegiate Guidelines Network (SIGN): www.sign.ac.uk/guidelines/index.html.

Chapter 13

Bruising and spontaneous bleeding

Julia Czuprynska

Introduction

Defects in various parts of the haemostasis pathway can lead to bleeding problems of differing severity.

Primary haemostasis relates to the formation of a platelet plug at the site of injury. Defects in primary haemostasis usually manifest as mucocutaneous bleeding with epistaxis, oral blood blisters, gum bleeding, skin haemorrhage and bleeding into the GI tract. They can be due to the following:

- *Vessel wall abnormalities*
  - Senile purpura
  - Cushing's syndrome
  - Scurvy
  - Collagen disorders
- *Platelet abnormalities*
  - Thrombocytopenia – congenital or acquired (e.g. drugs or liver disease)
  - Congenital defects of platelet function
    - Glanzmann's thrombasthenia
    - Bernard Soulier syndrome
  - Acquired defects of platelet function
    - Antiplatelet drugs
    - Uraemia
- *Abnormalities of von Willebrand factor*
  - Von Willebrand's disease

Secondary haemostasis describes activation of the plasma clotting cascade to result in fibrin clot formation. Defects can result in bleeding into joints (haemarthrosis) and tissues and may be due to:

- *Clotting factor deficiencies*
  - Congenital e.g. haemophilia A
  - Acquired

- Disseminated intravascular coagulation
- Vitamin K deficiency
- Over-anticoagulation
- *Increased fibrinolysis*
  - Massive trauma
  - Liver disease
  - DIC

> **Scenario 13.1**
>
> *An 85-year-old woman with dementia is admitted from a care home following a fall. The nursing staffs are worried because she is thin and has numerous bruises, particularly on the forearms and lower legs. They are concerned that she is the victim of aggressive handling at the hands of the care home staff. Her medication includes aspirin 75 mg daily and prednisolone 7.5 mg daily for previous temporal arteritis. Investigations including platelet count and clotting studies were normal.*
>
> *Involvement of the multidisciplinary team confirmed that the care home in question had a reputation for a high standard of care.*

Bleeding can be a distressing symptom and a cause of much anxiety. Establishing if a bleeding disorder is present may be challenging. It can be difficult to distinguish between the constellation of features representing an underlying bleeding disorder and a subjective exaggeration of symptoms that are arguably within normal limits. At the same time it is important not to dismiss a history of seemingly minor bleeding as it could reflect serious underlying pathology. For example, a new onset of petechiae around the ankles may be the presenting symptom of thrombocytopenia secondary to bone marrow failure caused by acute leukaemia. Bruising can represent non-haematological conditions, such

Acute Medicine, ed. Stephen Haydock, Duncan Whitehead and Zoë Fritz. Published by Cambridge University Press.
© Cambridge University Press 2015.

as collagen disorders, e.g. Ehlers–Danlos syndrome. Non-accidental injury should also be considered in the differential diagnosis.

Bruising

Easy bruising is a common complaint amongst patients, most of whom do not have an underlying bleeding tendency. It can manifest as:

- *Petechiae*: very small (<3 mm), flat reddish purple lesions due to bleeding in the skin and mucous membranes that are usually not related to trauma
- *Purpura*: reddish purple lesions (>3 mm)
- *Ecchymoses*: larger areas of subcutaneous bruising that may be out of proportion to the associated trauma.

Senile purpura (age-related purpura): Skin turgor reduces with age, and cutaneous blood vessels become more fragile and susceptible to haemorrhage. Older patients often describe bruising secondary to minor trauma, which usually affects the hands, forearms and shins. It can be exacerbated by some common medications:

- antiplatelet agents (aspirin, clopidogrel) and NSAIDs
- anticoagulants
- corticosteroids (easy bruising is seen in Cushing's syndrome as well as in chronic corticosteroid use, as in the above scenario).

The bleeding history

A detailed bleeding history and examination are crucial in determining whether a bleeding disorder is present. The timing of onset and pattern of bleeding will give important clues as to the underlying haemostatic defect.

- *A congenital bleeding defect* is suggested by bleeding issues occurring in early childhood with a relevant family history.
- *Acquired bleeding defects* generally have a later onset.
- Disorders of *primary haemostasis* tend to present with mucocutaneous bleeding.
- Disorders of *secondary haemostasis* tend to present with bleeding into joints and tissues.

BUT

- Determining whether a bleeding disorder is congenital or acquired and whether the defect involves primary or secondary haemostasis can prove difficult.

- For example, a patient with von Willebrand's disease may not present with bleeding until this tendency is unmasked by a significant haemostatic challenge such as surgery in later life. Conversely, a child may develop an acquired problem such as immune thrombocytopenia.
- The pattern of bleeding may also be confusing – patients with acquired haemophilia (caused by an antibody to endogenous factor VIII) can have extensive, life-threatening mucocutaneous or soft-tissue bleeding as opposed to the haemarthroses seen in patients with congenital haemophilia.
- Some of the questions below will not be relevant in the acutely bleeding patient but will be invaluable in the assessment of the patient with a strong suspicion of an underlying bleeding disorder. These patients should then be referred to haematology for consideration of further investigations.

The *bleeding history* should include the following points (where relevant):

1. When did the bleeding *symptoms start*? Were there any recent significant events (e.g. blood transfusion a week ago in the case of post-transfusion purpura)?
2. Any bleeding during *infancy or childhood*?
3. Bleeding secondary to *haemostatic challenges*:
   a. *Tooth extraction* (ask more specific questions, e.g. did you need to go to hospital? Require stitches?)
   b. *Surgery*.

   - It is a good idea to list operations and describe whether any haemorrhagic complications occurred.
   - Did the bleeding start during/just after the operation or was it delayed?
   - Was the patient taken back to theatre?
   - Was a blood transfusion required?
   - Is there an operation note to which you could refer?
   - Was there a surgical cause for the bleeding, e.g. severed vessel?

   c. *Childbirth*. List the number of children and how each was delivered. Duration of bleeding? Was the bleeding immediate/delayed?

4. *Epistaxis*. Duration of bleeding? Did it stop with pressure alone? Was hospital attendance required? Was cauterization necessary?

5. *Menstrual losses*. This can be a challenging area to assess. It is difficult to subjectively quantify blood loss. The use of pads/tampons varies between women for a number of reasons and does not necessarily correlate with degree of menorrhagia. There may be associated iron-deficiency anaemia.

6. *Gum bleeding, intra-oral blood blisters?*

7. *Any bleeding into muscles or joints?*

8. *Does the bleeding onset coincide with commencement of any drug?*

- A detailed drug history is necessary as many drugs are associated with bleeding.
- There are multiple antiplatelet agents in use as well as novel oral anticoagulants, which may be unfamiliar to the person taking the history.
- As well as directly interfering with haemostasis, drugs can cause an antibody-mediated thrombocytopenia or liver failure (causing coagulopathy).
- It is important to ask about herbal and non-prescription drugs.
- Drugs associated with thrombocytopenia may have been given during a procedure and not be obvious on the drug chart when reviewing a patient (e.g. glycoprotein IIb/IIIa inhibitors during angioplasty).

9. *Family history?* This is subject to recall bias but can be useful.

- Think about von Willebrand's disease or X-linked diseases such as haemophilia A and B.
- Haemophilia A and B are X-linked disorders and therefore usually seen in men.
- In rare cases, it is possible for women to have haemophilia. Some female haemophilia carriers can experience increased bleeding.
- If considering autosomal recessive disorders, consider asking (sensitively) about consanguinity.

10. *General health*.

- It is important to ask about alcohol intake. Liver failure is associated with thrombocytopenia and reduced synthesis of clotting factors. Alcohol is directly toxic to the bone marrow.
- Ask about diet (think vitamin K deficiency or scurvy secondary to vitamin C deficiency).

- Are there other medical problems which could influence the risk of bleeding, e.g. renal failure?

There are specific so-called '*bleeding assessment tools*' available such as the International Society on Thrombosis and Haemostasis (ISTH) Bleeding Assessment Tool, which includes a questionnaire and an interpretation grid to score the severity of the bleeding symptoms [1]. These are more commonly used in clinical trials and haematology outpatient clinics.

Examination

The examination of a patient should include:

- Assessment of haemorrhagic phenomena (distribution of petechiae/purpura, size and age of bruises, presence of blood blisters of the oral mucosa/tongue, fundoscopy).
- A general examination for clues to potential causes. It is important not to miss meningitis in the case of a purpuric rash.
- There may be splenomegaly (splenic pooling of platelets causing thrombocytopenia), lymphadenopathy (lymphoma or other malignancy causing marrow failure) or signs of liver disease.
- Telangiectasia of the lips/fingertips can signal the presence of hereditary haemorrhagic telangiectasia.
- Scurvy may be indicated by the presence of perifollicular haemorrhages and 'corkscrew hairs'.
- There may be hyper-elasticity of skin or joint hypermobility as in Ehlers–Danlos syndrome.
- In rare cases, oculocutaneous albinism can be seen with several inherited platelet disorders.

Investigation

The approach to investigation differs depending on the clinical scenario. Initial tests should include:

- *Full blood count (FBC)* and *blood film*
- *Clotting screen* to including prothrombin time (PT), activated partial thromboplastin time (APTT) and fibrinogen (+/– thrombin time depending on lab)
- *Renal* and *liver function tests*.

The FBC and blood film

- The FBC may reveal *thrombocytopenia*. The test should be repeated in the first instance, as there may be a reason for a spurious thrombocytopenia such as a clot in the sample.

- The blood film may have features suggesting an underlying leukaemia, myelofibrosis, myelodysplasia or perhaps a rare congenital thrombocytopenia.
- In acute leukaemia, bleeding may be caused by thrombocytopenia or there may be an associated disseminated intravascular coagulation, as can be seen in acute promyelocytic leukaemia.
- An isolated thrombocytopenia with an otherwise normal blood count and blood film, in the absence of splenomegaly or other attributable causes, will most commonly be due to *immune thrombocytopenia*. However, it is imperative only to label a patient with this diagnosis after a process of elimination. Look hard for an alternative explanation first. Ensure that a blood film has been examined (call the haematology lab), and discuss with the on-call haematology team. If the bleeding is of a concerning severity, the patient may need admission and require further investigations or additional intravenous immunoglobulin therapy. In the case of mild/negligible bleeding, the haematology team may decide to discharge the patient on oral steroid therapy with early follow-up. The patient *should not be discharged without discussing with haematology* and appropriate follow-up being arranged.
- Extremely high platelet counts ($>1000 \times 10^9$/L) in myeloproliferative disorders may be associated with increased bleeding, which can be exacerbated by aspirin.
- An important diagnosis not to miss in the case of thrombocytopenia is a *microangiopathic haemolytic anaemia* (MAHA) [2]. This umbrella term comprises three main disorders:
  - *thrombotic thrombocytopenic purpura* (TTP)
  - *haemolytic uraemic syndrome* (HUS)
  - disseminated *intravascular coagulation* (DIC).

Haemolysis with elevated liver enzymes (HELLP) syndrome is also a thrombotic microangiopathy associated with pregnancy, normally in the third trimester.

- All MAHAs involve the process of intravascular haemolysis where erythrocytes are damaged as they pass through networks of fibrin or hyaline mesh within the vessels causing the red cells to break into fragments. These fragments, or schistocytes, seen together with low platelets, are the hallmark of MAHA on a blood film and are usually associated with the presence of earlier red cell forms (reticulocytes and erythroblasts) produced hurriedly by the bone marrow to meet demand.
- DIC is associated with prolonged clotting times (PT and APTT), low fibrinogen (which can be normal in the early stages) and a high D-dimer. The key element of management is aimed at treating the underlying cause. *TTP* is a haematological emergency and associated with a mortality of 90% if untreated.

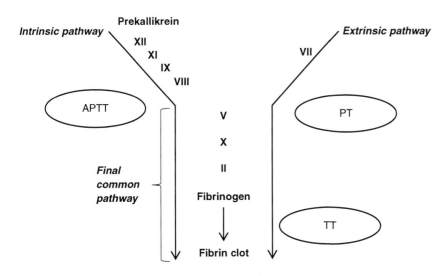

Figure 13.1 Simplified clotting cascade. APTT = activated partial thromboplastin time; PT = prothrombin time; TT = thrombin time.

- The mainstay of treatment of acquired TTP is plasmapheresis as soon as possible. This removes the causative autoantibodies, which are formed against ADAMTS-13 (an enzyme responsible for cleavage of ultra-large von Willebrand factor).
- Once TTP is suspected it *requires immediate involvement* of senior members of the on-call medical, haematology, ITU and apheresis teams.
- Platelet transfusion is contraindicated except in life-threatening haemorrhage, as it may precipitate thrombosis.

Clotting times

- Laboratory tests are subject to a number of 'pre-analytical variables', which means that the way in which samples are taken, handled, transported, etc. will affect the accuracy of the result.
  - Citrate (blue top) samples for coagulation tests must be adequately filled to ensure the correct ratio of citrate to plasma. Underfilled samples tested from a patient with normal clotting would produce prolonged clotting times.
  - A difficult venepuncture can activate the clotting cascade, giving rise to shortened clotting times.
  - Processing a sample with a high haematocrit will alter the ratio of citrate to plasma and produce prolonged clotting times. This is not representative of the clotting time in vivo, and the test will need to be modified.
- The *prothrombin time* (PT) measures the extrinsic pathway clotting factors, while the *activated partial thromboplastin time* (APTT) measures the intrinsic pathway clotting factors (Figure 13.1).
- The common pathway refers to the final part of the clotting cascade, which the first two pathways feed into. The common pathway factors are: II, V, X and fibrinogen. Deficiencies of any one of these can prolong both the PT and APTT (depending on the severity of the deficiency and the type of reagent used).
- Prolongation of both the PT and APTT will be due to either a mixed clotting factor deficiency (such as that seen with vitamin K deficiency, liver failure or DIC) or a deficiency of a single common pathway factor. Liver disease will cause prolonged PT and APTT due to reduced synthesis of multiple clotting factors, but the level of factor VIII is often not reduced but raised.

The PT and APTT vary in terms of which factor deficiencies they are sensitive to.

- The PT is sensitive to deficiencies of the common pathway factors mentioned above and factor VII (extrinsic pathway). It is used for monitoring warfarin therapy, where it is standardized to give an INR. As warfarin inhibits factors II, VII, IX and X (as well as protein C and S) it will also prolong the APTT.
- The APTT is sensitive to the common pathway factors mentioned above and factors VIII, IX and XI and XII. Hence the APTT will be prolonged in factor VIII and factor IX deficiency (haemophilia A and B, respectively). The APTT will also be prolonged with heparin use and in the case of acquired haemophilia A.
- It is important to remember that these are in vitro tests and do not necessarily reflect the in vivo situation. For example, patients with antiphospholipid syndrome and a lupus anticoagulant can have a significantly prolonged APTT but will be more prone to thrombosis. Factor XII deficiency will prolong the APTT but is not considered of any clinical significance.
- A rare cause of spontaneous severe bleeding, *acquired haemophilia* is another important cause not to miss [3] and is also associated with mortality of approximately 8–22%. It is more common in the elderly and can be associated with underlying malignancy or autoimmune disorders. Urgent discussion with haematology is advised as bypassing agents may need to be instituted. Treatment is based on immunosuppression to stop production of the culprit autoantibody.

Mixing studies

- In the case of a prolonged PT or APTT, it useful to perform 'mixing studies'. This means that patient plasma is mixed with reference plasma in a 1:1 ratio and the clotting test is repeated.
  - In the case of a clotting factor deficiency, the clotting time 'corrects' (significantly improves) with the addition of 'normal' plasma and clotting factor levels can be measured.

- In the case of acquired haemophilia, addition of normal plasma fails to correct the clotting time, indicating the presence of an inhibitory antibody.

Further investigation

In the case of a patient in whom there is a strong suspicion of an underlying bleeding disorder but where baseline tests have not resulted in a diagnosis, tests can be arranged with haematology input. These may include:

- PFA-100
- Platelet aggregation studies
- Assays for von Willebrand's disease.

Much of this will be organized in the outpatient setting.

Von Willebrand's disease [4] can be inherited but there is also an acquired form that is related to certain conditions such as lymphoproliferative disorders, cardiovascular disease (particularly aortic stenosis) and myeloproliferative disorders (associated with high platelet counts in essential thrombocythaemia) [5]. Cases should be discussed with haematology.

Systemic disorders

Clotting defects can result from systemic disease. Sepsis can lead to consumption of platelets and clotting factors as well as frank DIC. Liver failure is a common cause of acquired bleeding diathesis. Rare associations exist such as amyloidosis with secondary factor X deficiency (factor X adsorption onto the amyloid fibrils).

References

1. Tosetto A, Castaman G, Rodeghiero F (2013) Bleeders, bleeding rates and bleeding score. *J Thromb Haemost* 11 (Suppl.1): 142–150.

2. Scully M, Hunt BJ, Benjamin S, et al. (2012) Guidelines on the diagnosis and management of thrombotic thrombocytopenias and other thrombotic microangiopathies. *Br J Haematol* 158: 323–335.

3. Baudo F, Collins P, Huth-Kühne A, et al. (2012) Management of bleeding in acquired haemophilia A: results from the European Acquired Haemophilia (EACH2) Registry. *Blood* 120: 39–46.

4. Tiede A, Rand JH, Budde U, et al. (2011) How I treat the acquired von Willebrand Syndrome. *Blood* 117(25): 6777–6785.

5. Tefferi A (2012) Polycythaemia vera and essential thrombocythaemia: 2012 update on diagnosis, risk stratification and management. *Am J Hematol* 87: 284–293.

Further reading

Greaves M, Watson HG (2007) Approach to the diagnosis of mild bleeding disorders. *J Thromb Haemost* 5 (Suppl. 1): 167–174.

Hampton KK, Preston FE (1997) Clinical Review, ABC of haematology: bleeding disorders, thrombosis and anticoagulation. *BMJ* 314: 1026–1029.

Key N, Makris M, O'Shaughnessy D, Lillicrap D (2009) *Practical Hemostasis and Thrombosis*, 2nd edn. Wiley-Blackwell.

Vora A, Makris M (2001) An approach to investigation of easy bruising. *Arch Dis Child* 84: 488–491.

Cardiorespiratory arrest

Zoë Fritz

Introduction

'Life is a sexually transmitted condition and the mortality is 100%.' So said R. D. Laing, emphasizing the certainty of our own mortality, along with the risks of over-medicalizing death. In the UK:

- Around 60% of the population dies in hospital, and of those, 80% die with *Do Not Attempt Cardiopulmonary Resuscitation* Orders in place.
- In-hospital resuscitation has around a 15–20% survival rate for all those in whom it is attempted, but only 10% in the over 80s [1].
- The most recent National Cardiac Arrest Audit suggests 82% of in-hospital cardiac arrests do not involve a shockable cardiac arrhythmia, whereas most success is in those presenting with ventricular fibrillation.
- Out-of-hospital resuscitation has an even poorer survival rate of 7%.

Resuscitation is thus only attempted in a small proportion of the population and is successful in an even smaller proportion.

Surviving attempted resuscitation is more likely if:

1. There is early recognition that the patient is deteriorating and help is called quickly
2. There is rapid CPR and defibrillation
3. There is good post resuscitation care.

This has been summarized as the 'chain of survival' [2].

As a doctor, you can optimize the patient's outcome if you:

Maintain knowledge. It is a mandatory requirement that you hold a valid Advanced Life Support (ALS) certificate (and demonstrate willingness to undergo UK Resuscitation Council ALS course re-certification every 3 years). In addition you should be aware of the changing evidence base for best practice; this is particularly relevant for some of the peri-arrest scenarios

Develop good communication and leadership skills. It is critical that you are able to effectively ask for help with a deteriorating patient. It sounds simple, but ensure that you can succinctly present the clinical details of the situation to a colleague. At the end of the conversation, emphasize that the patient is unstable, and that you want another person to come to the bedside within minutes – *be explicit about the time frame!*

When leading an arrest, stand back and maintain the overall picture. You should be able to delegate specific tasks to colleagues equipped with appropriate competencies. Do not be afraid to ask for more help if those competencies aren't well represented.

When a patient is sufficiently unwell for you to be calling in a team of other doctors, you are aware that the patient's prognosis is poor. Ensure that you also delegate one of the nurses to let the patient's relatives know, to offer them the chance to come into hospital; if you are unable to help the patient medically, they may be comforted from having someone they know with them.

Scenario 14.1

You are urgently bleeped to review a 65-year-old man on one of the general medical wards. He was admitted earlier that day with pneumonia. Over the previous hour he has become increasingly dyspnoeic and tachycardic. On arrival he is struggling to breathe, sweating profusely and is clearly very unwell.

Acute Medicine, ed. Stephen Haydock, Duncan Whitehead and Zoë Fritz. Published by Cambridge University Press.
© Cambridge University Press 2015.

Pre-arrest – the deteriorating patient

The National Confidential Enquiry into Patient Outcomes and Deaths (NCEPOD) in 2005 recognized that non-VF cardiac arrests [3]:

- Commonly occur on non-monitored wards.
- Had the poorest survival.
- Often occurred after a period of slow and progressive physiological deterioration involving unrecognized or inadequately treated hypoxaemia and hypotension.

Regular review and observations

- Standardized documentation of physiological observations and the use of a 'track and trigger' (e.g. National Early Warning Score) are now widespread to facilitate early recognition of the deteriorating patient [4]. (See Addendum p. 101.)
- As doctors, when we assess an unstable patient on the wards or in the emergency department, we should:

  - Document a clear physiological monitoring plan. This should detail the parameters to be monitored and specify the frequency of observations [4].
  - Plan and document the time of the next medical review ('*I will review again/I have handed over for this patient to be reviewed again in 90 minutes*').
  - Have thought through and documented the next stage of the treatment plan: '*If this patient has not responded to initial treatment within 90 minutes, a referral to ICU will be made.*'

Recognizing and treating reversible contributors to cardiac arrest

When assessing a deteriorating patient, consider and treat all potential reversible causes of cardiac arrest [5]:

The four H's: hypoxia, hypovolaemia, hyperkalaemia (as well as hypokalaemia, hypocalcaemia and other metabolic abnormalities) and hypothermia

The four T's: thromboembolic, toxins, tension pneumothorax and tamponade.

All need to be considered and, if present, reversed to avoid cardiopulmonary arrest.

Practically speaking you should therefore rapidly perform:

1. An assessment of airways, breathing and circulation to ensure stability.
2. A quick history from the notes (try to keep to less than 5 minutes – it is an easy pitfall to spend ages over this) and the patient to determine their presenting complaint, past medical history and current problems.
3. A review of the drug chart to ensure that the patient's deterioration is not iatrogenic (e.g. allergic reaction to new antibiotics, opiate toxicity, Addisonian crisis from steroid withdrawal).
4. A physical examination, looking particularly for signs of respiratory and cardiac failure, and sources of sepsis (including the abdomen and the joints – don't miss septic arthritis).
5. An arterial blood gas to gain information not only about the patient's ventilation but also their electrolytes, haemoglobin, and acid/base status. Remember to check the lactate, as a sensitive (but not specific) indicator of a patient's physiological well-being.
6. A 12-lead ECG.
7. Secure IV access and send laboratory bloods including a full blood count, electrolytes, urea and creatinine, a magnesium, and, where appropriate, blood cultures or a group and save/cross match.

To do all of the above can take more than 30 minutes. Ask for help (e.g. from the outreach team) to ensure that some steps can take place in parallel, and the patient can be stabilized quickly.

Specific conditions

Hypoxia

- Reverse hypoxia with oxygen, remembering to assess whether the patient is or has been a smoker. Up-titrate oxygen to maintain appropriate saturations. Plan a repeat blood gas in an hour, to ensure that they are responding appropriately, and not retaining CO_2.

Consider new causes (pneumonia, heart failure, PE) for their hypoxia, and ensure appropriate treatment is started. Order a portable X-ray to help confirm the diagnosis (although do not allow to delay treatment).

Hypovolaemia

This is common post-surgery and trauma, but may also occur in patients with GI bleeds, sepsis or on diuretics. Intravascular volume should be restored rapidly with fluid. Refer urgently to the surgeons when haemorrhage is suspected.

Hyperkalaemia

- Urgent treatment is required if the serum potassium is ≥6.5 mmol/L

  or

- Hyperkalaemia is accompanied by ECG changes even in the presence of mild hyperkalaemia.

- Give 10 units Actrapid insulin with 50 g dextrose, and salbutamol nebulizers. Intravenous calcium chloride/gluconate is indicated (also in the presence of hypocalcaemia, and calcium channel-blocking drug overdose). Note that extravasation of high strength glucose solutions is extremely damaging to the skin and subcutaneous tissues (see Chapter 6).

Peri-arrest arrhythmias

Bradycardias

If the patient has adverse features (shock/syncope/heart failure/myocardial ischaemia):

- Give *atropine* 500 μg IV.
- This can be given up to six times up to a *maximum total dose of 3 mg.*

Where this is unsuccessful, or where there is risk of asystole (Mobitz type II AV block, complete heart block with broad QRS, ventricular pauses of more than 3 seconds or previous asystole):

- Give *isoprenaline* 5 μg/minute or *adrenaline* 2–10 μg/minute
- *or*
- *Transcutaneously pace* the patient as an *interim measure*, while transvenous pacing is arranged as an emergency (this is only useful in the very short term and sedation may be required).
- *Remember to check if the patient is on a beta-blocker or calcium channel blocker* and could have overdosed. In these situations *glucagon* is useful. IV calcium is useful in calcium channel blocker toxicity.

Tachycardias

- *If the patient has adverse features*: (shock/syncope/ heart failure/myocardial ischaemia), *give a*

synchronized DC shock. This can be attempted up to three times.
- Give *amiodarone* 300 mg IV over 10–20 minutes followed by amiodarone 900 mg over 24 hours.
- If the patient is stable, the next step is to determine the width of the complex, and the regularity of the beat. If the QRS is longer than 0.12 ms (three small squares on the standard ECG paper speed of 25 mm/s) then it is a broad complex. If it is less than 0.12 ms then it is a narrow complex.

Broad complex, irregular tachycardia

Seek urgent expert help. The differential includes:

- Polymorphic VT (e.g. torsades de pointes). Stop all drugs, correct electrolytes and give *magnesium* 2 g over 10 minutes.
- *Pre-excited AF* (e.g. patients with Wolff–Parkinson–White syndrome). Consider *amiodarone.*
- *AF with bundle branch block.* Treat as for narrow complex tachycardia below.

Broad complex, regular tachycardia

- *Ventricular tachycardia.* Treat with *amiodarone* 300 mg IV over 20–60 minutes, then 900 mg over 24 hours.
- *SVT with bundle branch block.* If this has been previously confirmed, give *adenosine* as with narrow complex tachycardia below.

Narrow complex, irregular tachycardia

Probable atrial fibrillation:

- Look for and treat precipitating causes (PE, ischaemic bowel, MI, infection, thyrotoxicosis).
- If within 48 hours of onset consider elective DC cardioversion.
- Treat with beta-blocker (e.g. *bisoprolol* 2.5 mg) or *diltiazem.*
- Consider digoxin or amiodarone if there is evidence of heart failure.
- Consider warfarinization for stroke prevention (use $CHADS_2VASC$ scoring system).

Narrow complex, regular tachycardia

- Sinus tachycardia
- Atrial flutter with regular AV conduction (often 2:1 block, often produces rate of 150)

- AV nodal re-entry tachycardia (AVNRT)
- AV re-entry tachycardia (AVRT due to WPW).

Try vagal manoeuvres, while on a monitor, in particular the Valsalva. (Listen for carotid bruits before doing carotid massage, and avoid if previous TIA/stroke.) Give adenosine 6 mg via rapid IV bolus (remember to warn the patient that they may feel dreadful, with a chest pain and a sense of doom), and repeat with 12 mg two times if necessary. Watch and record the rhythm strip during and following the adenosine, and look for atrial activity (e.g. flutter).

- *If sinus rhythm is not restored, seek help.* Atrial flutter is the likely diagnosis and a beta-blocker should be considered.
- *If sinus rhythm is restored,* diagnosis is likely to be re-entry paroxysmal SVT; record an ECG in sinus rhythm and consider choice of anti-arrhythmic prophylaxis (beta-blocker, calcium channel blocker, or flecainide if no ischaemic heart disease or structural abnormalities).

Special conditions in the emergency department

Part of the requirement of ALS and the core curriculum is that you can also treat less common arrests including those provoked by trauma, anaphylaxis, hypothermia, drowning and poisoning. Details of how to look after these particular conditions are beyond the scope of this chapter, but can be found in the ALS manual, and in the 2010 article by Soar et al. [6].

Cardiopulmonary arrest

Basic life support

A doctor should be confident not only in resuscitating individuals with a team and the resources of a hospital, but also in basic life support. In France, a medically qualified individual can be prosecuted if they do not offer assistance to a bystander; in the UK there has never been a case of someone being prosecuted for trying to help within their competence. Be familiar with BLS. In summary:

If you find an unresponsive individual, shout for help/use your mobile to call 999 (and ask for a bystander to see if an advanced emergency defibrillator is nearby).

A: assess airway, use simple manoeuvres – chin lift, and head tilt.

B: look, listen and feel for no more than 10 seconds for breathing – if breathing, put in the recovery position, and wait for the ambulance. If NOT breathing, start chest compressions.

C: perform 30 chest compressions at a rate of 100–120/minute.

Follow this with two breaths: maintain chin lift, pinch nose, close your lips around his mouth, and blow ensuring the chest rises and falls.

Continue with chest compressions and rescue breaths at a rate of 30:2.

Stop to recheck the victim *only* if he starts showing signs of regaining consciousness.

Advanced life support

1. Provide chest compressions at a rate of 100–120/minute and at a depth of 5–6 cm to maintain circulation of the blood throughout the arrest and keep these going with minimal interruptions (the 'preshock pause' should be less than 5 seconds).
2. Maintain the airway and oxygenation with basic airway management (jaw thrust, chin lift, oropharyngeal and nasopharyngeal airways as adjuncts) and laryngeal mask airway, i-gel supraglottic airway, or, if appropriate expertise is available, endotracheal intubation for a definitive airway. Use capnography to monitor effective ventilation and CPR.
3. Assess the rhythm and provide defibrillation if the patient is in ventricular fibrillation or ventricular tachycardia, along with amiodarone 300 mg after the third shock.
4. Give adrenaline 1 mg every 3–5 minutes to maintain the circulation.
5. Treat any reversible causes (as above with the peri-arrest approach).

Drugs

- Drugs should be given by the *intravenous route where possible* with the intraosseous route used as a second choice.
- The mainstay of drugs in CPR is adrenaline, supplemented by drugs to treat arrhythmias (amiodarone 300 mg, magnesium 2 g, and calcium chloride 10 mL of 10%).
- Giving sodium bicarbonate is NOT recommended, unless the arrest is associated with hyperkalaemia or tricyclic antidepressant overdose.

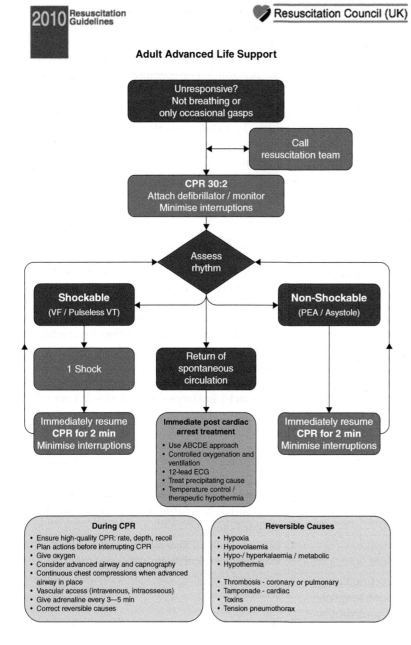

Figure 14.1 Adult advanced life support algorithm. Reproduced with the kind permission of the Resuscitation Council (UK).

Paediatric life support

You should also be familiar with paediatric life support, although you will not be expected to participate in paediatric resuscitations.

Critical differences from the adult protocol include:

- In *paediatric basic life support*, 5 rescue breaths are given first. Compressions to breaths are given at a ratio of 15:2.

- Compress the lower half of the sternum with one palm of one hand to a depth of one-third the depth of the child (with older children two hands will be needed).

In *paediatric advanced life support* – CALL FOR HELP – you are NOT expected to do this on your own.

For reference:

- The shock required is 4 J/kg.
- The appropriate adrenaline dose is 100 µg/kg.

Post cardiac arrest care

Successful return of spontaneous circulation (ROSC)

Once you have achieved *ROSC, do not relax*!

This is the point at which you can potentially minimize long-term physical and mental disabilities [7]. *Refer to intensive care*, and continue your care until the intensivists have clearly taken over; the two main goals are:

- Identifying the cause for the cardiac arrest, and instigating treatment
- Optimizing the physiological stability of the patient.

The following is therefore required:

- *Reduce hypoxaemia*. Keep SaO_2 at 94–98%. Ensure that your anaesthetist stays with the patient.
- *Consider myocardial ischaemia*. Consider angiography and percutaneous coronary intervention in ALL patients with known coronary disease, not just those with STEMI. Do a 12-lead ECG.
- *Maintain the blood pressure* to achieve urine output of 1 mL/kg per hour and decreasing lactate levels.
- *Maintain glucose levels* below 10 mmol/L but avoiding hypoglycaemia.
- *Treat hyperpyrexia* and consider therapeutic hypothermia.

Document the details of the arrest call in the notes, along with your suggested analysis of the cause for the arrest and the plan from this point. While you will not be expected to transfer the patient to ICU, you should have an understanding of what is necessary for such a transfer:

- Appropriate monitoring
- Drugs
- Clinical support.

Ensure that someone contacts the patient's next of kin to inform them of what has happened, and to answer questions as best as possible.

Unsuccessful cardiac arrest attempts

- In asystole, if no reversible causes for the cardiopulmonary arrest have been identified and there has been no change to the patient's rhythm following 20 minutes of ALS, then the chances of ROSC are very small, and the team leader should

check with their team if they agree that CPR should cease.
- This discussion can take place before 20 minutes (but generally after three cycles of attempted CPR) in cases where, from review of the patient's notes, it is clear that the prognosis is poor.
- In cases of ventricular fibrillation, CPR should continue for a prolonged period while reversible causes are addressed. If there is disagreement about whether to continue/cease CPR within the cardiac arrest team, then the team looking after the patient should be contacted and consulted before CPR is stopped.
- The details of the arrest call should be written in the notes.
- Deliberate self-poisoning in healthy patients is associated with very good outcomes despite prolonged resuscitation while the patient eliminates the ingested drug. *Stopping resuscitation in such circumstances requires very careful consideration.*

Informing the next of kin

- Either the person who has led the arrest call, or the team usually looking after the patient should tell the next of kin.
- Ideally they will have been phoned when the patient first deteriorated, but if not, it is best to bring them into hospital to tell them.
- If the next of kin directly asks a question on the telephone, ' has X died?', it is best to tell the truth; however, it is generally better not to volunteer this information on the phone, but to ask them to come into hospital quickly.
- As with all bad news, ensure that you have a private space, that you have handed over your bleep, and that there is the opportunity for questions. Having a nurse in with you is wise.

Team debrief

- While it is not always possible given the demands on the on-call, it is good practice to have a team 'debrief' and a cup of tea, following both successful and unsuccessful arrest calls.
- The arrest can be emotionally draining, and there may be members of the team for whom that arrest was the first exposure to CPR or even to death.

- At the very least, the team leader should thank those who were involved, and ask if there are any questions. It is also helpful to go over what happened, and see whether there were areas which were done well or badly, to improve the running of the next arrest call.
- A member of the resuscitation services should have been present at the arrest and will help ensure that the arrest was entered into the hospital audit.

Scenario 14.2

An 85-year-old man is admitted with a severe pneumonia. He has a history of cancer of the prostate and is known to have confirmed spinal metastases. He has been coping at home with his wife prior to this admission although his mobility is very limited. Both he and his wife have told the admitting house officer that they want all active treatment including cardiopulmonary resuscitation.

Ethical and legal framework around resuscitation decisions

The 2012 NCEPOD report 'Time to intervene? A review of patients who underwent cardiopulmonary resuscitation as a result of an in-hospital cardiorespiratory arrest' found evidence that many patients remain inappropriately 'for resuscitation', in the event of a cardiac arrest, and suggested that 'CPR status must be considered and recorded for all acute admissions, ideally during the initial admission process and definitely at the initial consultant review when an explicit decision should be made in this group of patients, and clearly documented (for CPR or DNACPR)' [8].

However, there are several factors which make decisions and discussions around resuscitation particularly challenging [9]:

- In the UK, patients have the legal right to refuse treatments, but not to request them. This applies to CPR, as it does to any other medical intervention, but CPR is often treated differently by the public and the press, partly because the result of not offering the treatment is immediate death.
- Widespread misunderstanding about survival rates: the public perception reflects what is shown on television dramas, namely a survival rate of around 67%, with many of them ' coming round' without a lengthy ICU admission.
- Evidence that DNACPR orders, despite being intended only to give instruction in the event of a

cardiac arrest, have a negative impact on the care patients receive; this contributes to the physician's discomfort in discussing or even making resuscitation decisions.
- Discussions about resuscitation necessitate both physician and patient confronting the possibility of death; in our society, this is still a subject we shy away from.

Discussions and decisions

Following the Tracey Judgement in June 2014 [10], there is a legal requirement for doctors to discuss DNACPR decisions with patients unless they think to do so would cause 'psychological or physiological harm'. The joint statement from the British Medical Association, the Resuscitation Council (UK) and the Royal College of Nursing, last published in 2007 [11], is about to be updated to reflect this.

There has been some consternation amongst the medical profession about this judgment, in particular about the time it will take to have meaningful discussions with patients about CPR.

The moral argument behind the judgement was strong, and can be summarised thus:

1. CPR is a potentially lifesaving treatment.
2. Doctors are unable to accurately predict whether attempting CPR will be of benefit.
3. If a patient is not informed that a decision about CPR is being made about them, they have no way of asking questions about the decision or requesting a second opinion.
4. To deprive them of the possibility of being involved in these decisions is in breach of article 8 of the European Convention on Human Rights, the right to family and private life.

Ideally resuscitation decisions should be made with the patient in the context of other treatment decisions. Instead of considering the 'CPR discussion' as a tick-box exercise to alleviate guilt/prevent litigation at having unilaterally made the decision, view resuscitation decisions as an opportunity to consider goals of care, find out about the patient's priorities, and plan appropriate treatments.

References

1. Meaney PA, Nadkarni VM, Kern KB, Indik JH, Halperin HR, Berg RA (2010) Rhythms and outcomes of adult in-hospital cardiac arrest. *Crit Care Med* 38: 101–108.

2. Nolan J, Soar J, Eikeland H (2006) The chain of survival. *Resuscitation* 71:270–271.

3. National Confidential Enquiry into Patient Outcome and Death. An acute problem? Available at: www.ncepod.org.uk/2005aap.htm (accessed 25 July 2013).

4. NICE. Acutely ill patients in hospital: recognition of and response to acute illness in adults in hospital, NICE Clinical Guideline 50. Available at: www.nice.org.uk/cg50 (accessed 25 July 2013).

5. Resuscitation Council UK. 2010 Resuscitation Guidelines. Available at: www.resus.org.uk/pages/guide.htm (accessed 25 July 2013).

6. Soar J, Perkins GD, Abbas G, et al. European Resuscitation Council Guidelines for Resuscitation 2010. Section 8. Cardiac arrest in special circumstances: electrolyte abnormalities, poisoning, drowning, accidental hypothermia, hyperthermia, asthma, anaphylaxis, cardiac surgery, trauma, pregnancy, electrocution. *Resuscitation* 2010; 81: 1400–1433.

7. Sunde K, Pytte M, Jacobsen D, et al. *Implementation of a Standardised Treatment Protocol for Post Resuscitation.* London: NCEPOD; 2005.

8. NCEPOD. Time to Intervene? A review of patients who underwent cardiopulmonary resuscitation as a result of an in-hospital cardiopulmonary arrest; 2012. Available at: www.ncepod.org.uk/2012cap.htm (accessed 24 July 2013).

9. Fritz Z, Fuld J (2010) Ethical issues surrounding do not attempt resuscitation orders: decisions, discussions and deleterious effects. *J Med Ethics* 36: 593–597.

10. Judgement Approved by for handing down in the case of Tracey v Cambridge University Hospitals and others (2014) Case No: C1/2013/0045 in the Court of Appeal (Civil Division) of the High Court of Justice, Queen's Bench Division Administrative Court. The judgment can be read online at www.judiciary.gov.uk/wp-content/uploads/2014/06/tracey-approved.pdf.

11. Decisions relating to cardiopulmonary resuscitation. A joint statement from the British Medical Association, the Resuscitation Council (UK) and the Royal College of Nursing, October 2007.

Addendum
ICU outreach teams

Wendy Chamberlain

Introduction

The ICU outreach role developed as a response to significant deficiencies identified in the care of patients on hospital general wards. The clinical deterioration of such patients was not resulting in an appropriate escalation in monitoring or intervention, resulting in delayed or preventable ICU admissions.

Many factors can be implicated in this clearly unsatisfactory situation:

- increased number of acutely ill patients in hospital who may be elderly with chronic co-morbid disease
- increased workload of medical teams with less time for supervision of junior staff
- Impact of the European Working Time Directive on junior doctor training
- decreased emphasis on and reduced exposure to acute illness in nursing training
- limited sharing of knowledge and skills by critical care with ward staff
- possible deskilling of ward staff, particularly in early recognition of deterioration, as sick patients are frequently cared for in critical care
- transfer of routine observations such as temperature, pulse rate and blood pressure to healthcare assistants, sometimes without proper supervision and decline of the monitoring of respiratory rate by ward staff as a sensitive but non-specific marker of deterioration.

In 2000 the Department of Health document *Comprehensive Critical Care: A Review of Adult Critical Care Services* recommended that all critical care units establish an outreach service and adopt a hospital-wide approach to critical care. This resulted in the 2002 publication *Guidelines for the Introduction of Outreach Services* by the Intensive Care Society. The importance of such developments was underlined by several investigations by recognized government bodies:

- 2005: NCEPOD, 'An Acute Problem'
- 2007: NHS National Patient Safety Agency, 'Safer care for the acutely ill patient: learning from serious incidents'
- 2007: NICE, 'Acutely Ill Patients in Hospital: Recognition of and response to acute illness in adults in hospital'.

These reports highlighted problems with the observation of vital signs and responses to deterioration in observed physiological parameters by nursing and medical staff. They made a number of recommendations regarding the frequency and nature of patient monitoring and advised that all hospitals should have a Track and Trigger early warning scoring system in place to cover all inpatients.

Early warning scores

The principal determinants of clinical outcome in patients with acute illness are:

- Early detection of deterioration
- Timeliness of clinical response
- Competency of clinical response.

A number of scoring systems have been developed and widely implemented by hospitals across the NHS (PAR, MEWS, MEOWS, PEWS). Measurable deterioration in clinical status as reflected in a rising score triggers a defined escalation from ward nursing staff, the outreach team and responsible medical staff.

The Acute Medicine Task Force recommended that the physiological assessment of all patients should be standardized across the NHS with the recording of a minimum clinical dataset resulting in an NHS early warning (NEW) score. This would provide a standardized record of illness severity and urgency of need, from first assessment and throughout the patient journey. It is based (like other systems) upon a scoring of the routinely measured physiological parameters:

- pulse
- temperature
- systolic blood pressure
- respiratory rate
- conscious level
- oxygen saturation
- whether the patient is receiving supplemental oxygen.

This would allow consistent assessment of illness severity across the NHS and provide a valuable baseline from which to evaluate the clinical progress of the patient. It would also enhance good clinical practice, support standardized recording of vital data and provide an important source of documentation for audit of the quality of patient care. However, many trusts that have adopted NEWS have found it too sensitive and have returned to their original Track and Trigger system.

What to expect of the outreach team (and what they expect of you!)

A call to the outreach team is usually triggered by an Early Warning Score or a general concern regarding a patient by nursing staff or medical staff. Outreach nurses (or less commonly physiotherapists) usually have had many years of experience in a senior ICU role. They understand the immediate needs of a sick patient in order to rapidly restore normal physiological parameters. They are able to complete an assessment, request investigations, interpret the results and instigate a management plan. They should work with you in the manner of a highly skilled diplomat. Good interpersonal skills and communication are vital for success in this role. This is not to say that they will not challenge you but it should always be in an appropriate manner.

In many Trusts the outreach team will carry and update a register of all the sick patients in the hospital, across all specialties. Discussion of these patients during clinical handovers at the end and start of clinical shifts (especially out of hours) provides a valuable opportunity to prioritize clinical resources and plan the review and management of such patients.

You can expect the outreach team to be skilled in:

- requesting and venesecting the patient for basic blood tests including blood cultures
- requesting plain radiology
- venous cannulation (may include use of ultrasound in difficult cannulations)
- arterial blood sampling
- administering/titrating oxygen therapy
- commencement and titration of non-invasive ventilatory support (BiPAP/CPAP).

When receiving a call, the outreach team will expect you to be able to provide the following clinical information:

- a full ABCDE assessment
- the clinical observations including urine output
- conscious level (AVPU ('alert, voice, pain, unresponsive') or GCS)
- arterial blood gas result (if appropriate)
- whether the patient has had a senior clinical review (specialist registrar or consultant)
- whether there is a treatment plan in the notes
- agreed level of escalation including resuscitation decision.

If there is no clear decision regarding escalation, then whilst the patient is receiving treatment, a senior review will be required by the registrar within the hour. There is a definite hierarchy in medicine and junior doctors may be reluctant to involve seniors. The outreach team endeavour to have a good relationship with all senior clinicians. They will call consultants at home during the night if appropriate, and this should be welcomed. If a difficult decision needs to be made then the correct person to do this is the consultant in charge of the patient.

The outreach team obviously has a close working relationship with the critical care unit and may be able to refer the patient directly or facilitate your interaction. The critical care team reviewing the patient will expect to have senior involvement from the responsible clinical team.

Concluding remarks

Critical care outreach is now an integral part of acute care in the NHS. Whilst there will be local variations in service delivery, the wealth of experience that senior outreach nurses possess enables them to rapidly assess a clinical situation and initiate investigation and management. The relationship between medical staff and outreach is extremely important and is particularly true for the specialist registrar out of hours. The hospital at night is a busy place with fewer clinicians. The medical staff and outreach can share the workload to optimize patient care. This, however, needs trust and understanding of each other's roles and abilities. Good communication is paramount so get to know and establish a good working relationship with your outreach team!

Further reading

Acutely Ill Patients in Hospital: Recognition of and response to acute illness in adults in hospital. 2007. Published by the National Institute for Health and Care Excellence. Available as a download from www.nice.org.uk/nicemedia/live/11810/58247/58247.pdf.

Guidelines for the Introduction of Outreach Services (2002) Published by the Intensive Care Society. Available as a download from www.anaesthesiaconference.kiev.ua/Downloads/ICU_standards-outreach_2002.pdf.

National Early Warning Score (NEWS) Standardising the assessment of acute illness severity in the NHS (2012). Published by the Royal College of Physicians. Available as a download from www.rcplondon.ac.uk/sites/default/files/documents/national-early-warning-score-standardising-assessment-acute-illness-severity-nhs.pdf.

Chapter 15

Chest pain

Stuart Walker

Scenario 15.1

*You are called down to 'resus' in the emergency depart-
ment to see a 65-year-old man with chest pain. He has a
past medical history of type 2 diabetes and had a myocardial infarction and subsequent coronary stenting
3 months ago. He presents with left-sided chest pain that
came on 'just like that' when he was walking to his part-
time job. He describes it as sharp, but it is not pleuritic
in nature. The pain goes through to his back and is the
worst he has ever experienced; even worse than his previous MI. He looks very unwell, he is clearly in pain and he is
sweaty. His blood pressure is elevated. His ECG shows left
bundle branch block but he reports that his ECG always
looks funny when he comes into hospital.*

Introduction

Chest pain is one of the most common acute medical
presentations in the UK, resulting in a high number
of emergency department attendances and hospital
admissions. Patients with chest pain may have an
immediately life-threatening condition, or, more commonly, a benign (and sometimes non-identifiable)
cause. Many have underlying coronary artery disease
but most do not. This makes the management of the
patient with chest pain challenging. It is essential not
to miss the patient with a life-threatening disorder, but
admission and invasive investigation of every patient
is inappropriate. It should also be borne in mind that
the patient finding themselves on the medical take
with chest pain will be anxious regarding possible life-
threatening causes. Always ensure you provide *clear
information to them and their loved ones*, including
reassurance when you are confident to do so. If you plan
further outpatient investigation and follow-up, explain
why you are doing this and the likely time frame.

Clinical assessment

Aims of the assessment

The competent medical assessment of the patient with
chest pain should:

- Quickly identify the patient at immediate risk
- Produce a *differential diagnosis that relates to that
  patient's symptoms*
- Risk stratify the patient according to standard criteria
- Identify an appropriate investigation and
  subsequent treatment strategy
- Decide where the patient should be managed, by
  whom and in what time frame
- Ensure that the patient and their relatives are fully
  informed of the situation.

Key initial steps

- Resuscitate the patient, according to standard
  ABCDE principles, if required.
- In parallel (with the help of nursing staff):
  - obtain a brief history (less than 3 minutes!)
  - consider immediate venous cannulation,
    analgesic/antiemetic requirements and oxygen
    administration
  - obtain a 12-lead ECG as soon as possible.
- If the ECG demonstrates diagnostic criteria for a
  new ST-elevation myocardial infarction (STEMI)
  then an *immediate* referral for consideration of
  primary angioplasty, according to local protocols,
  is required:
  - give aspirin 300 mg
  - consider clopidogrel/prasugrel/ticagrelor
    according to local guidelines

Acute Medicine, ed. Stephen Haydock, Duncan Whitehead and Zoë Fritz. Published by Cambridge University Press.
© Cambridge University Press 2015.

- give GTN as soon as practicable.
- Diagnostic criteria for a potential STEMI are:
  - ST elevation in two leads (>2 mm in leads V1–6 or >1 mm in limb leads)
  - ST depression compatible with posterior infarction
  - definite new LBBB (or presumed new LBBB) with a good history of significant, sustained cardiac pain.
- If a STEMI is not identified then a process of differential diagnosis and risk stratification is required.

Differential diagnosis

History

Take a full history at this stage. Consider asking the patient:

- Timings of presenting chest pain – When did it come on? How long did it last? How many times has it come back?
- Circumstances of pain – what were you doing when it came on? How quickly did it start? Did you have any other associated symptoms like breathlessness, palpitations, sweatiness, dizziness, cough and haemoptysis? How bad was it? What was it like?
- Is there a relationship to posture, movement, exertion, eating or breathing?
  - Pleuritic chest pain is often described as a stabbing pain or catching on inhalation; musculoskeletal chest pain may also be aggravated by breathing.
  - Pericarditic pain is often a central stabbing chest pain aggravated by lying down and eased by leaning forwards.
  - Gastro-oesophageal reflux is frequently brought on or worsened by lying down.
- What is the most exercise you can do? Do you get the pain on this exercise?
- Have you had this pain before? If so what caused it?
- What medication are you taking?
- Risk factors for thromboembolic disease – immobility, recent surgery, OCP.
- Do you have a prior history of coronary artery disease, hypertension, peripheral vascular disease, thromboembolic disease, stroke, diabetes, hypercholesterolaemia, smoking, family history of early onset vascular disease?

Examination

- Most importantly here – does the patient look unwell? Many of the patients with one of the immediately life-threatening causes of chest pain will show it. Is the patient well perfused or are they cold, clammy, pale and perspiring? Are they breathless at rest? Do they look anaemic?
- What are the basic observations – heart rate, blood pressure, oxygen saturation, respiratory rate? Are all the major pulses present?
- Is there chest wall tenderness (makes cardiac pain less likely but does not discriminate causes of pleuritic pain such as pulmonary embolism)?
- Is there a rash, as herpes zoster may be overlooked?
- Is there a heart murmur or evidence of cardiac decompensation (resting tachycardia, gallop rhythm, high JVP, chest crackles)?
- Is there a pericardial rub (pericarditis) or pleural rub (pulmonary embolism, pneumonia)?
- Is there a focal lung abnormality?

Basic investigation

Electrocardiogram

- Does the ECG show specific features of an acute coronary syndrome (ACS):
  - dynamic ST depression of >0.5 mm
  - hyperacute T wave peaking
  - T wave inversion (often >2 mm)
  - transient ST elevation.

Don't forget to repeat the ECG regularly after admission: if you are at all unsure of the ECG, ask for repeats at 5 and 10 minutes to assess for dynamic changes.

- If no features of ACS, is the ECG otherwise normal or does it have 'other' useful clues, e.g.:
  - LVH
  - atrial fibrillation
  - RV strain
  - RBBB or right axis deviation
  - S1Q3T3 (very rare).

Chest radiograph

Examine the chest X-ray carefully and systematically and ask yourself:

- Is the heart enlarged?
- Are there features of LVF?
- Are the lung fields normal?
- Are the pulmonary arteries of normal size?

- Is there mediastinal widening?
- Is the aortic knuckle normal?
- Is there a hiatus hernia?
- Is the skeleton normal? (Metastases, myeloma and pathological fractures may be missed.)

Blood tests

- FBC, U&E, LFT, clotting, glucose.
- Measure a baseline troponin on arrival and again after 6–12 hours according to local protocol.
- Consider other tests as appropriate:
  - D-dimer
  - Arterial blood gases.

Subsequent management

- Depends upon the outcome of this clinical and baseline-investigation assessment.
- See Table 15.1.

But at this stage always consider the 'Vascular Big 3': acute coronary syndrome (ACS), pulmonary embolism or acute aortic syndrome.

If you think this may be the case then ask yourself: 'What do I need to do about that, right now?' Then do it, and seek more senior advice as necessary.

Condition-specific considerations

Acute coronary syndrome

Causes of a raised troponin

Elevated serum troponin is evidence of injury or necrosis of the myocardium (but remember false positives and negatives occur). This may occur in a number of clinical scenarios. The diagnosis of myocardial infarction requires that the myocardial injury is secondary to a vascular cause. This is usually due to the formation of thrombus on a ruptured coronary arterial plaque, but can also result from:

- Coronary artery stenting
- Coronary artery vasospasm
- Coronary arteritis
- Coronary artery dissection
- Myocardial bridges (compression of a coronary artery that is surrounded by myocardium and flow can be restricted by myocardial contraction).

Other causes may be non-vascular, but regardless of the cause a raised troponin is associated with a poorer prognosis and is of importance.

Non-vascular causes of a raised troponin include:

- 'Demand:supply imbalance' caused by tachycardia or hypotension, e.g. GI bleed, significant anaemia, primary cardiac arrhythmias
- Myocarditis
- Takotsubo cardiomyopathy
- Sepsis
- Pulmonary embolism
- Acute respiratory failure
- Significant AKI or CKD
- Significant valvular heart disease.

The interpretation of a raised troponin is therefore entirely dependent upon the clinical circumstances in which the test was undertaken. Common sense must be applied to troponin testing in the seriously ill if valuable information is to be obtained.

Risk stratification of patient with suspected ACS

This should be undertaken in order to determine the appropriate subsequent treatment pathway. The risk assessment may include:

- Presence/absence of ongoing pain
- Presence/absence of ECG changes of ACS
- Formal risk scoring with a validated tool (e.g. GRACE risk score)
- Significant troponin elevation.

Low risk patients can be identified by:

- Pain that has fully resolved
- Normal ECG
- GRACE risk score low (e.g. <3% death at 6 months)
- Normal troponin.

Lower risk patients should be considered for a non-invasive coronary artery disease (CAD) exclusion test to prevent hospital admission, e.g. exercise test/CT coronary angiography.

Intermediate or high risk ACS patients should normally:

- Undergo invasive coronary angiography unless contraindicated with revascularization if appropriate.

The role of invasive investigations in other patients:

- Lower risk ACS patients in whom non-invasive testing shows a potential significant coronary problem may undergo invasive testing as appropriate.

Table 15.1 Differential diagnosis in chest pain – key differentiating features

	History	Exam	ECG	CXR	Troponin	Other blood tests	Other comments
ACS	'Typical' cardiac pain – mostly central chest with left arm, neck or jaw radiation Back/right arm radiation possible but uncommon	Often normal unless in pain	Dynamic change is key: ST depression, T wave inversion/ peaking, transient ST elevation	Often normal, may be increased heart size or LVF	Usually raised from baseline – but may not be	Nil specific	Further investigation as appropriate – with exercise tolerance test, CT angiogram, perfusion scan, coronary angiography
PE	Pleuritic pain common in small/ moderate PE Association with breathlessness very common Pain in massive PE may be less specifically pleuritic	Tachycardia, high respiratory rate, features of RV strain – high JVP, gallop rhythm, tricuspid regurgitation	Right axis deviation, RBBB, anterior T wave inversion, non-specific ST changes are all common S1Q3T3 neither sensitive nor specific	Pulmonary oligaemia often quoted but difficult to identify! Hilar PA enlargement can be characteristic	Often raised, possibly markedly so	Raised D-dimer sensitive but not specific	Usual diagnostic test now CTPA V/Q scan used rarely – e.g. in contrast allergy, renal failure or pregnancy. V/Q SPECT increasingly used
Aortic syndromes	Pain often of sudden onset (commonly within <1 minute) Radiates to back, abdomen, even legs Often described as 'the worst pain I have ever had' Often associated with 'collapse'	Absent pulses, ischaemic legs, BP difference in arms all helpful when present – but mostly pulse examination is normal Aortic valve regurgitation can be noted in some with type A dissection. Hypertension is the most consistent finding	Often LVH from underlying hypertension Inferior MI from right coronary artery occlusion happens but is rare	May be normal However, most will show enlarged mediastinum and/or enlargement/ double shadow of aortic knuckle Can also show pleural effusion/ LVF	Often raised	Possible renal failure from renal artery involvement	CT chest/abdomen with and without contrast now mandatory for most suspected aortic syndromes Transoesophageal echo less useful, other than in some borderline cases after CT or pre-surgery
Respiratory – pneumonia/ pleurisy	Pain altering with respiration is key – also cough, phlegm, high temperature, dyspnoea	Focal lung changes – consolidation, crackles, effusion, rub (often at site of greatest pain)	Often normal AF common ?RV strain of cor pulmonale	Focal features of diagnosis – note lower left lobe collapse is easily missed	Often raised in significant sepsis	High WCC, D-dimer, CRP	

Table 15.1 (cont.)

	History	Exam	ECG	CXR	Troponin	Other blood tests	Other comments
Gastrointestinal	A number of key features of GI pain are recognized – pain at night, when lying flat, acid brash, dyspepsia, dysphagia	Epigastric tenderness is common and not specific for a GI cause of chest pain	Normal	Usually normal – possible hiatus hernia	Usually normal – GI bleed can be associated with troponin raise if severe	?Anaemia, renal/liver assessment mandatory, amylase and calcium may be useful	Some patients with both proven angina and oesophageal reflux cannot differentiate between their own pains – so it may not be possible for clinicians to do so either!
Musculoskeletal	Key feature is whether the pain has a movement-related or postural component. Has there been an unusual activity that may have contributed to the underlying damage?	Pain often reproducible with alterations in position, e.g. after neck/back/limb movement. May be features of costochondral joint tenderness	Normal	Normal	Normal	Nil specific	Nil specific
Anxiety or hyperventilation	Associated feeling of impending doom/panic/anxiety. Peri-oral/digital paraesthesia. Dyspnoea often a marked feature	Patient may still be showing anxiety signs (e.g. agitation, tachycardia) or be hyperventilating	Hyperventilation can cause ECG changes of both T wave inversion (often in 1 lead only) or ST depression	Normal	Normal	Alkalosis, hypokalaemia, hypocapnia, hyperoxaemia, hypocalcaemia	ECG changes usually recover immediately on cessation of hyperventilation

- In patients with chronic stable angina it is reasonable to undertake an initial non-invasive strategy based upon secondary risk reduction and symptom control, before consideration of invasive investigation and treatment.

Non-invasive investigation strategies

- A number of tests are available for the non-invasive exclusion of CAD. These include:
  - Exercise testing
  - Perfusion scanning (dobutamine stress echo, nuclear scanning and perfusion MRI)
  - Coronary CT angiography.

Exercise testing remains a mainstay of many chest pain assessment services. This is despite a relatively low sensitivity and specificity for the identification of CAD, and many patients' inability to undertake a diagnostic level test due to the presence of co-morbidities.

- Its popularity is based upon a historical reliance on exercise testing (and thus familiarity).
- It is relatively simple to perform and provides good stratification on prognostic terms in those patients with known coronary artery disease, even if it has weaknesses at a diagnostic level.
- Current *NICE guidelines* do not recommend the use of exercise testing for diagnosis of coronary artery disease and in fact state: 'Do not use exercise ECG to diagnose or exclude stable angina for people without known coronary artery disease.'
- However, the *2013 European Society of Cardiology Guidelines* still advocate exercise testing as the first-line investigation for diagnostic purposes in patients with chest pain in the absence of known coronary disease with a pretest probability of 15–65% if they are able to exercise, anti-ischaemic drugs are stopped and resting ECG does not show changes that make the test uninterpretable (LBBB, paced rhythms and WPW) (evidence grade IB).

Perfusion scanning via echocardiography, nuclear or MRI is increasingly used to replace exercise testing. NICE approved tests include MRI perfusion scanning with SPECT, stress echocardiography, first pass contrast-enhanced MR perfusion or MR imaging for stress-induced wall motion abnormalities. Clearly all these tests have inherent strengths and weaknesses. There are a number contraindications to MRI scanning, including renal impairment, claustrophobia, metallic fragments in the orbits, other implants (many pacemakers, for example) and an inability to lie flat for a relatively prolonged period. Contraindications to dobutamine stress echocardiography would include obesity with poor echocardiographic windows and concerns about dobutamine administration (e.g. if prone to VT). Nuclear scanning can give very useful results but is very dependent upon high volume service provision and can give less reliable data in females or in the presence of LBBB.

CT angiography is increasingly used to diagnose coronary artery disease – both luminal (i.e. obstructive) and non-luminal. CT can also be used to give an assessment of LV function. A number of caveats are associated with its use: To obtain satisfactory images a slow steady heart rate is required (<60 bpm), the patient must be able to breath hold for ~15 s and must have sufficient renal function to allow radiographic contrast administration. It has a very high negative predictive value for CAD exclusion and a high positive predictive value for CAD identification. Whilst CT angiography is good at identifying the severity of mild CAD it is not yet so good at differentiating moderate from severe CAD.

The best strategy to assess lower risk ACS patients for CAD is therefore individualized by most centres according to their pre-test risk level, co-morbidities, size, ability to undertake exercise, etc.

Initial therapy for higher risk ACS group

If, on the basis of the initial assessment, an intermediate or high risk ACS is diagnosed then the patient should be given appropriate therapy according to local guidelines. This could include:

- Oxygen (maintain saturations at 94–98%, unless contraindicated)
- GTN sublingual if in pain, or by IV infusion if pain persists
- Aspirin 300 mg stat
- Clopidogrel/prasugrel/ticagrelor according to local policy
- Analgesia/antiemetic as required
- Beta-blockade/statin/ACE inhibition if appropriate
- Heparin or fondaparinux as per local policy
- Consideration given to glycoprotein IIb/IIIa antagonist therapy/direct thrombin inhibitor (e.g. bivalirudin) as per local protocols and in discussion with cardiology team.

The patient should then be considered for referral to the local cardiology team and placement in a cardiac-specific treatment area:

- Coronary care unit for highest risk patients (GRACE risk >6% mortality at 6 months, heart failure, hypotension, ongoing pain, ST changes, diabetes, etc.)
- Cardiology ward for intermediate risk.

Most high risk ACS patients would undergo invasive coronary assessment with diagnostic angiography as an inpatient, and then be revascularized if necessary, with stenting/coronary artery bypass grafting as appropriate.

Management of chest pain after prior coronary stenting

Consider:

- Is the new pain suggestive of repeat ischaemia?
- Is the pain the same as the prior 'angina' (and did the 'angina' improve with stenting at all)?
- Is there new ECG change – is it dynamic/different from the post-stenting routine ECG?
- Is there a 'trend' change in troponin – i.e. is it rising longer than expected post-stent (remember a troponin may be raised for over 1 week post ACS or stenting).

It is important to be aware that:

- Stent thrombosis is usually early (hours/days post stent) with dramatic, high risk, large MI but can sometimes occur later when patients stop antiplatelet agents prior to surgical or dental procedures.
- Stent pain is usually mild-moderate, different to angina and settles within hours of stenting procedure (although may persist for a few days, or rarely longer).
- Stent re-stenosis is usually longer term (6–12 months) and presents with stable angina, medium risk ACS or MI.
- ACS after 1 year is more often new disease rather than an issue related to the stent.

Complications of ACS

The commonest complications of acute coronary syndromes with significant myocardial damage indicated by a large troponin rise are:

- Left ventricular failure causing pulmonary oedema.
- Papillary muscle rupture and resulting valvular incompetence.

- Ischaemic ventricular septal defect if not revascularized.
- Cardiac arrhythmias; the early defibrillation of VF and pulseless VT of patients post MI is why coronary care units were developed.
- Depression is common post MI and can easily be overlooked by the physician.

Discharge arrangements

When patients are discharged who have had confirmed ACS, they should be prescribed secondary preventative medications in the form of:

- ACE inhibitors
- beta-blocker
- high dose statin
- aspirin
- clopidogrel (dependent on findings and bleeding risk)
- GTN sublingually prn.

Lifestyle advice should not be forgotten: taking regular exercise with a graduated increase in duration and intensity, and weight management (if appropriate). Smoking cessation must be stressed and advice regarding local smoking cessation support issued. Diabetic management should be reviewed in all diabetics. Patients should be advised to reduce dietary saturated fats. The Mediterranean diet has been shown to have benefits and can be supplemented further with omega 3 fish oils.

Often cardiac rehabilitation classes are arranged on discharge with specialist nurses and physiotherapists to help patients to regain their confidence and build up their exercise tolerance.

Pulmonary embolism

Pathophysiology of pulmonary embolism

The majority of pulmonary embolisms originate from clot in the large deep veins of the legs; in fact a significant number of patients diagnosed with a deep vein thrombosis will have concurrent pulmonary emboli at diagnosis (see Chapter 38).

General approach to the patient with suspected pulmonary embolism

Pulmonary embolism has a broad spectrum of clinical presentation – including cardiac arrest, collapse with severe haemodynamic compromise, acute chest pain with breathlessness, isolated pleuritic chest pain and isolated (i.e. pain-free) breathlessness including reduction in exercise tolerance. Although the diagnosis of PE is rising, it continues to be the most common unexpected finding at post-mortem, and a low threshold for excluding PE is required. First consideration should be given to 'massive' or immediately life-threatening PE management. A system for risk stratification and case identification should be adopted for other patients with PE.

'Massive' PE and consideration of thrombolysis

If a patient is seen with a potential 'massive' PE then thrombolysis should be considered and urgent CT scanning of the pulmonary arteries undertaken. Thrombolysis is the first-line treatment for massive PE and may be instituted on clinical grounds alone if cardiac arrest is imminent (BTS guideline [1]).

Indications for thrombolysis in CT-confirmed PE include a number/all of:

- Tachycardia with heart rate >100 bpm
- Blood pressure <100 mmHg systolic
- Arterial oxygen saturation of <94%
- Raised jugular venous pressure
- Dyspnoea at rest
- Significantly abnormal ECG.

Thrombolysis has significant risks and the decision on whether to thrombolyse a patient with a significant PE should usually be made by a senior clinician; patients who are hypotensive and unstable are likely to benefit more, but risk factors for stroke need to be balanced against this. Current usual thrombolytic of choice is alteplase followed by 48 hours IV heparin, although local protocols may vary. Current studies are taking place to determine clearer guidelines for thrombolysis of PE and to assess the risk of stroke in this population against the benefit of preventing long-term pulmonary hypertension.

Diagnosis of the non-life-threatening PE

The initial assessment of the possible medium to low risk PE patient should include history, full examination, ECG, CXR and arterial blood gas analysis. The patient can then be classified as having 'likely' PE or 'unlikely' PE using the Wells score as per NICE guidelines:

Clinical signs of DVT	3 points
An alternative diagnosis is less likely	3 points
Heart rate >100 bpm	1.5 points
Immobilization for >3 days or surgery in <30 days	1.5 points
Previous DVT	1.5 points
Haemoptysis	1 point
Malignancy	1 point

A score of ≤4 makes PE unlikely

- Normally proceed to D-dimer testing.
- If the D-dimer is normal (<0.5 mg/mL) then PE would normally be considered excluded.
- If the D-dimer is raised proceed to CT pulmonary angiography or V/Q SPECT.

A score of >4 makes PE likely

- Normally proceed direct to CT pulmonary angiography or V/Q SPECT after baseline anticoagulation.

D-dimer testing (see Chapter 38) is sensitive for detection of pulmonary emboli, but not specific as it can be abnormal in:

- Malignancy
- Pregnancy
- Sepsis
- Inflammation.

Imaging in pulmonary embolism

CT pulmonary angiography remains the most common imaging modality for diagnosing or excluding PE with around 90% sensitivity and 95% specificity. It has the potential to identify other significant pathology accounting for the presentation of chest pain: pneumonic consolidation, tumours, aortic dissection, rib fractures. It can demonstrate right heart dilation suggestive of massive PE and assess the clot burden. Contraindications include renal impairment and previous allergy to IV contrast media and in such patients ventilation perfusion imaging combined with single photon emission computed tomography (V/Q SPECT) is preferred. CTPA is more difficult in younger patients, shorter circulation times making good opacification of the pulmonary arteries more difficult. Scanning is associated with a radiation exposure of 2.2–7 mS, which is considerably higher than that resulting from V/Q or V/Q SPECT scanning. This underlies NICE advice also to consider the latter imaging modality as an alternative to CTPA taking into consideration the patient's age, history of cancer and increased risk of exposing dividing cells to radiation. The latter is a particular consideration in pregnancy in relation to radiation exposure to dividing breast tissue. It is hard to determine the actual risk to the mother in such circumstances. It has been suggested that the actual lifetime increased risk of breast cancer for a mother receiving a CTPA whilst pregnant is of the order of 11%, whilst late menopause and nulliparity each confer a 40% increased lifetime risk.

Nuclear medicine scanning. Traditionally the investigation of choice, V/Q scanning became less popular due to ready availability of CTPA in and out of hours and the high percentage of equivocal scans especially in the elderly and patients with coexistent lung disease. V/Q SPECT is a newer imaging modality that allows tomographic (3D imaging) rather than the planar images of older V/Q scanning. This results in equivalent or possibly higher sensitivities and specificities to CTPA. It is not available in all centres. If available it is an appropriate alternative first-line investigation in those in whom CTPA is contraindicated or in those who are young or when radiation exposure is of particular concern.

Echocardiography can be useful in the acute setting to look at the right heart chambers and pressures that can help inform the decision regarding urgent thrombolysis. Follow-up imaging can be used to exclude or monitor the development of pulmonary hypertension and guide both medical and surgical interventions for this condition.

Treatment of pulmonary embolism (excluding thrombolysis)

Patients with suspected pulmonary embolism should receive anticoagulation with treatment dose low molecular weight heparin pending investigation, unless they have significant bleeding risk in which case a clinical decision based on risk versus benefit is required; prompt scanning is frequently the safest strategy to avoid unnecessary risk.

- Fluid resuscitation may be required for the hypotensive patient in the acute phase. Do not be put off by distended neck veins. Increased filling pressure will be needed to overcome the increased resistance of the clot burdened pulmonary vascular bed.
  - Once a pulmonary embolism is confirmed: *either*
  - Continue LMWH and start an oral vitamin K antagonist, e.g. warfarin; LMWH can be discontinued once the INR is consistently above 2.0 *or*

- Commence the Xa inhibitor rivaroxiaban. Continued treatment with LMWH is not required. This is the only one of the newer agents licensed for the treatment of pulmonary embolism in the UK at time of going to press (see Chapter 38), although other product licences are likely to be granted soon.
- There are some patients who will need to remain on LMWH rather than switching to an oral anticoagulant. These include patients with active malignancy, those who use intravenous drugs, and those who are pregnant (note different dosing regime).
- The decision regarding duration of warfarin depends upon a balance of risk versus benefit – i.e. is related to both the PE recurrence risk and anticoagulation-related bleeding risk. In general though:
  - 3–6 months warfarin duration for 'provoked' PE with reversible risk factors
  - consideration for lifelong warfarin if massive/life-threatening PE, unprovoked PE, recurrent PE.

Investigating underlying cause and long-term follow-up

Long-term follow-up would normally include:
- Repeat clinical assessment plus
- Echocardiographic assessment for pulmonary hypertension (often at 3 months post-PE).

In patients who have an unprovoked PE (recent surgery/immobility, high BMI/pregnancy/known malignancy), screening tests need to be conducted to aid early diagnosis of possible causes of hypercoagulability.

- Full physical examination (including breast for women and PR/testicular exam for men)
- Chest X-ray
- Blood tests (full blood count, serum calcium and liver function tests and PSA in men)
- Urinalysis (with particular attention to proteinuria and haematuria).

In addition NICE recommends that we should consider further investigations for cancer in patients over 40, specifically:
- CT scan of abdomen and pelvis for both men and women
- Mammography for women.

The role of screening for malignancy in patients with unprovoked pulmonary embolism has long been a subject of controversy. There are no good adequately powered randomized controlled trials that address this issue.

- It remains *unclear* that earlier detection of malignancy in the context of venous thromboembolic disease significantly improves outcome in terms of mortality, morbidity or quality of life.
- There is a risk of inducing malignancy later in life due to radiation exposure.
- There are considerable cost and resource implications.
- There is a risk of causing stress, psychological and physical harm due to the detection and subsequent investigation of lesions that are not life-threatening (see Chapter 34).
- Many clinicians would request further imaging on the basis of 'red flags' for malignancy identified on history, examination and initial baseline tests.

Acute aortic syndromes

This term refers to:

Aortic dissection when blood enters the aortic wall through an intimal tear.

Intra-mural haematoma when blood enters the aortic wall from an in-situ bleed, in the absence of an intimal tear.

- Both are immediately life-threatening medical emergencies, with evidence suggesting a rising incidence.
- Dissections involving the ascending aorta are termed Stanford type A; those restricted to the descending aorta are termed type B.
- Death in aortic syndromes is related to aortic rupture, tamponade, heart failure and end-organ hypoperfusion (e.g. brain/kidneys). It is estimated that 40% of patients with an acute aortic syndrome die suddenly. The remainder are said to have a 1% hourly mortality rate in the early stages, confirming the need for rapid intervention for these patients. Advanced age and important co-morbidity add significantly to the mortality risk of aortic dissection.
- Dissection is more common in patients with:
  - hypertension

- connective tissue disorders (such as Marfan's/ Ehlers–Danlos syndromes)
- aortic vasculitis/pre-existent aneurysm.

When to suspect acute aortic dissection

Aortic dissection is relatively rare and can mimic other causes of chest pain so is easily missed. However, when it occurs, early suspicion and diagnosis is essential.

History

Listen to the patient: they will give you the diagnosis – the patient in the scenario that starts this chapter is trying to tell you he has a dissection. Did you listen to him?

- The quality of the pain – often described as tearing.
- The pain is often described as very severe – 'the worst pain I have ever had'.
- The pain may radiate from the chest to the back (or vice versa), and to the abdomen, or even to the legs in dissection of the whole aortic length into the iliac vessels.
- The index event is often of very sudden onset (but not always so) and can be associated with syncope/collapse.

Examination

- Hypertension is common.
- Aortic regurgitation may occur in type A dissection.
- Hypotension is a poor sign and may indicate incipient tamponade or rupture.
- The classical feature of blood pressure difference in the arms occurs, but in a minority of patients, and an equal blood pressure in each arm should not be taken as reassurance that a dissection is not present.
- Look at the ECG and CXR – the combination of LVH on the ECG and a wider mediastinum on the CXR should raise suspicion although neither is specific or sensitive

Investigation for an acute aortic syndrome

- Aortic dissection or intra-mural haematoma can be diagnosed by contrast CT, aortic MRI or transoesophageal echocardiography.
- It is also occasionally diagnosed by invasive aortogram (usually during an attempted primary angioplasty for an occluded right coronary actually caused by the dissection).

- Of these modalities the most commonly used is CT due to its high diagnostic accuracy and widespread availability.
- MRI can be used (and is viewed by some as the 'gold standard' investigation) but due to a relatively longer scanning time, higher number of contraindications and less availability is not yet ubiquitous.
- Transoesophageal echocardiography is generally used for pre/perioperative assessment or assessment of unclear CT outcomes rather than initial diagnosis in the presence of widespread CT availability.

Treatment of acute aortic syndromes

- The outcome of type A dissections managed medically is poor with a very high mortality rate, despite aggressive medical intervention to lower blood pressure (see below).
- In this group surgery is recommended for root repair/grafting if possible (dependent upon the patient's age/co-morbidities).
- Discussion with a cardiac surgeon is essential.
- Type B dissections/haematomas are usually best managed medically (surgery does not affect overall outcome in this group).
- Emergency treatment is with rapid, titratable beta-blockade; labetalol is commonly used.
- Aggressive blood pressure lowering is then mandated, using a combination of therapies such as calcium antagonists, ACE inhibitors (if good renal function) and alpha-blockers.
- Some patients benefit from subsequent aortic endovascular repair (stenting). Indications for stenting include:
  - evidence of aortic leakage
  - evidence of a contained aortic rupture
  - progressive false lumen dilation

- compromise of essential arterial supply (e.g. renal arteries) from false lumen.

Reference

1. British Thoracic Society Standards of Care Committee Pulmonary Embolism Guideline Development Group. British Thoracic Society guidelines for the management of suspected acute pulmonary embolism. *Thorax* 2003; 58: 470–483. doi:10.1136/thorax.58.6.470.

Further reading

2013 ESC guidelines on the management of stable coronary artery disease. The Task Force on the management of stable coronary artery disease of the European Society of Cardiology. *European Heart Journal* 2013; 34, 2949–3003.

Davies JM. The Pathophysiology of Acute Coronary Syndromes. *Heart* 2000; 83: 361–366.

GRACE calculator available at: www.outcomes-umassmed.org/grace/acs_risk/acs_risk_content.html (accessed 12 December 2013).

Granger CB, Goldberg RJ, Dabbous O, Pieper KS, Eagle KA, Cannon CP, Van de Werf F, Avezum Á, Goodman SG, Flather MD, Fox KAA, for the Global Registry of Acute Coronary Events Investigators. Predictors of hospital mortality in the Global Registry of Acute Coronary Events. *Arch Intern Med* 2003; 163: 2345–2353.

NICE. Chest pain of recent onset (CG95). http://guidance.nice.org.uk/CG95 (accessed 12 December 2013).

NICE. Unstable angina and NSTEMI: the early management of unstable angina and non-ST-segment-elevation myocardial infarction (CG94). http://egap.evidence.nhs.uk/unstable-angina-and-nstemi-cg94 (accessed 12 December 2013).

NICE. Venous thromboembolic diseases: the management of venous thromboembolic diseases and the role of thrombophilia testing (CG144). www.nice.org.uk/nicemedia/live/13767/59720/59720.pdf (accessed 14 December 2013).

Chapter 16

Confusion/acute delirium

Peter M. F. Campbell

Introduction

Delirium is a very common condition and seen in up to 50% of older hospitalized patients. It is often distressing to the doctors, but it is *always distressing to families and friends* to see their loved ones in a confused state.

Patients may present directly with delirium or develop features during their hospital stay. Although more common in older patients, it can be seen in the young. It is a *serious acute neuropsychiatric syndrome characterized by global cognitive dysfunction and inattention*. There are multiple causes for delirium and it can trigger a spiral of descent into functional decline, institutionalization or death. Affected individuals are more likely to have a longer hospital stay and to suffer complications of hospitalization, including falls and pressure ulceration.

Although it is a common problem, with potentially dreadful outcomes, we often underplay the importance of the condition to ourselves and also to patients and families. Those affected are not to be labelled as a 'social admission' or 'acopia', they are extremely unwell. If we recognize this and address the condition appropriately, we can improve outcomes.

The term delirium has long been the term used to describe confusion associated with fever and head injury and dates back to the first century AD, being derived from the Latin *de lira ire*, 'to go out from the ploughed furrow'. (When talking to people with delirium you can imagine that you are in a different furrow or path to them. This can be frustrating when you are trying to establish the facts – but stay calm!) It is an imprecise term and more recently other terms have been used synonymously:

- 'acute brain syndrome'
- 'organic brain syndrome'
- 'acute confusional state'
- 'acute cerebral insufficiency'.

These newer terms are also imprecise and so we have tended to revert back to delirium.

Prevalence

- 1–2% prevalence in community dwelling older folk
- 30% incidence in medical inpatients
- >50% incidence in particularly susceptible populations, such as those with hip fracture
- 70–87% incidence in elderly patients requiring intensive care support

These figures may underestimate the true extent of the problem as we know that we underdiagnose delirium, especially hypoactive delirium (we can miss it in up to 70% of cases). It is a diagnosis to search for as recognition and effective treatment does alter outcome.

> **Scenario 16.1**
>
> An 82-year-old woman is referred by the ED. She was found by her daughter after she rang her mother and could get no answer. She went to the house and found her mother still in bed in a confused and agitated state. She might have been in bed for more than 24 hours and had been incontinent of faeces and urine. The daughter rang 999 for her to be taken to the ED.
>
> The ED assessment was brief. Her daughter was not present. They stated that they had no history from Mrs Smith. She was confused and agitated. They were unsure of past medical history or medication. Her chest was clear and her neurology was 'grossly intact'. She smelled strongly of urine. They felt this was a likely urinary tract infection and diagnosed an 'acute trimethoprim deficiency'. She was referred to the MAU.

Acute Medicine, ed. Stephen Haydock, Duncan Whitehead and Zoë Fritz. Published by Cambridge University Press. © Cambridge University Press 2015.

The Trust has an electronic discharge summary system. She had been in 4 months previously with an episode of confusion possibly due to a UTI (no MSU on the pathology system from that admission). She is known to have mild cognitive impairment (but not dementia), congestive cardiac failure and an MI 3 years previously, falls, CKD stage 3 and osteoporosis. There was no record of medication.

This is a very familiar picture and illustrates a number of important points:

- A collateral history is needed from the daughter regarding normal level of functioning and antecedent events.
- A comprehensive physical examination has not been performed.
- Urinary tract infection has been diagnosed on the basis of minimal evidence and this has stopped the ED from looking for other causes.
- A detailed drug history must be obtained, in particular recent changes and drugs with anticholinergic or hypoglycaemic agents.
- Discharge summaries often do not contain a full past medical history and other important co-morbidities may be missed.
- Investigation is required to find the multiple causes for this patient's delirium.
- Consideration should be given to alternatives to acute admission.

It is important to view the causes of delirium for each individual patient as multifactorial and an interaction between existing risk factors (e.g. age, cognitive function, drugs, co-morbidities) and the acute insult(s) (e.g. new medications, infection). Our assessment should aim to identify and address where possible *all factors* that could be contributing to the confusional state

Non-modifiable risk factors

I am sure that if you close your eyes you can picture the patients you have seen with delirium in the assessment unit. They are likely to have had some non-modifiable risk factors that, if present, put a patient at increased risk:

- Dementia (found in two-thirds of cases of delirium)
- Age over 65
- History of delirium, stroke, neurological disorder or falls

- Chronic renal or hepatic disease
- Fractured neck of femur
- Multiple co-morbidities.

When you meet the next patient with these factors you should assess them for delirium.

Predisposing factors

It is the interplay between the risk factors above and other, possibly modifiable, factors that is thought to result in delirium. As these are potentially modifiable you must look for these and try to intervene. The following list is not exhaustive (we would fill this entire book if it were – and you would not read it):

- Intercurrent illness (infection, dehydration, trauma, anaemia, stroke, myocardial event – you need to go looking for these as the patient won't tell you)
- Medications (almost any so search to find out what has been started or stopped recently – including over-the-counter preparations – especially those that have a central effect or are known to have anticholinergic side effects)
- Metabolic derangement (again almost any can cause delirium)
- Surgery
- Change in environment
- Pain
- Distress
- Sleep deprivation.

In stark contrast to *young person medicine*, which is usually single organ pathology, the development of delirium, and all of the other *geriatric giants*, is usually *multifactorial*. A patient who is well and independent, but susceptible, has multiple insults that summate and these converge on the common endpoint of delirium. We need to identify and address each of these strands to take the patient back to their premorbid self. The underlying pathophysiology of why such diverse pathologies produce a final common endpoint of the syndrome is not fully understood. There are a number of possible mechanisms relating to:

- neurotransmission (especially the cholinergic system)
- inflammation
- stress responses
- neuronal injury
- anatomical changes.

Table 16.1 The *Diagnostic and Statistical Manual for Mental Disorders*, fourth edition (DSM-IV), provides the current standard for diagnosing delirium. This has four key features that characterize delirium

DSM-IV criteria for delirium
1   Disturbance of consciousness (i.e. reduced clarity of awareness of the environment) with reduced ability to focus, sustain or shift attention.
2   A change in cognition or the development of a perceptual disturbance that is not better accounted for by a pre-existing, established or evolving dementia.
3   The disturbance develops over a short period of time (usually hours to days) and tends to fluctuate during the course of the day.
4   There is evidence from the history, physical examination or laboratory findings that the disturbance is caused by the direct physiological consequences of a general medical condition.

Table 16.2 The Confusion Assessment Method (CAM) diagnostic algorithm. The diagnosis of delirium by CAM requires the presence of features 1 and 2 and either 3 or 4

Feature 1	*Acute onset or fluctuating course.* This feature is usually obtained from a family member or nurse and is shown by the following questions: Is there evidence of an acute change in mental status from the patient's baseline? Did the behaviour fluctuate during the day, or increase and decrease in severity?
Feature 2	*Inattention.* This feature is shown by the following question: Did the patient have difficulty focusing attention, for example, being easily distractible, or having difficulty keeping track of what was being said?
Feature 3	*Disorganized thinking.* This feature is shown by the following question: Was the patient's thinking disorganized or incoherent, such as rambling or irrelevant conversation, unclear or illogical flow of ideas, or unpredictable switching from subject to subject?
Feature 4	*Altered level of consciousness.* This feature is shown by any answer other than 'alert' to the following question: Overall, how would you rate this patient's level of consciousness? (alert is normal)

Clinical evaluation

The delirious patient has suffered a significant medical insult and is unwell. However, they may not appear unwell beyond the features of delirium and so this may be the only clue that they are sick and need your attention (Table 16.1).

Delirium can be subdivided into three main groups according to the patient's psychomotor status:

- *Hyperactive* delirium is relatively easy to spot as patients are agitated, restless and often make themselves known to staff.
- *Hypoactive* delirium is much harder to spot and is often missed as patients are withdrawn, quiet, apathetic and appear sedated. They are less intrusive on the ward, hence the risk of overlooking the diagnosis, but they equally need recognition and effective treatment.
- *Mixed* delirium has features of both hyperactive and hypoactive delirium and can oscillate from one to the other.

Making the diagnosis

The history is the key to diagnosis combined with examination and cognitive evaluation. As the patient may not be able to provide an accurate story, a good collateral history is vital. We look for the cardinal features of:

- cognitive impairment
- fluctuation
- onset over hours to days.

There is no blood test or scan that will give you the answer.

The Confusion Assessment Method (CAM or short CAM) has both a high sensitivity of 94–100% and a specificity of 90–95% (Table 16.2).

The systems examination should be as full as possible and the investigations extensive, in order to identify treatable factors. *Remember – it is usually a combination of insults that lead to delirium, so do not just stop when you find the first possible explanation.*

- If unable to complete examination due to the patient's non-compliance or fatigue, then try to return at a later time to complete your evaluation.
- If you are not able to return then state what hasn't been done so people who follow you know.
- *You must* get a set of physical observations, look at skin integrity, assess hydration and search for possible infection.

Older people often do not have a classical presentation of conditions, for example septic patients may not have a fever, and they may even have hypothermia. It can be argued that older people do have a predictable presentation of ill health (in the form of delirium or falls) – it is just not what we are taught at medical school.

In certain circumstances, such as in non-verbal patients on intensive care, we need to use alternative validated tools such as the CAM-ICU. It is recognized that delirium in patients on ICU leads to increased mortality, length of stay, cost and many other negative outcomes. It is important to diagnose, understand prognostic implication and look for modifiable factors as we would in any other patient.

There are many standardized tests for cognition. There is no consensus as to which test to use. It is important to recognize that these are not diagnostic and represent how someone is at a point in time (it is similar to a random glucose in diabetes – it is not a dynamic measure nor a tool that tells us what has happened over time). We can use tools such as the Mini-Mental State Examination (MMSE) or Abbreviated Mental Test Score (AMTS) on the wards (Table 16.3).

Investigations

Given the vast number of potential causes, there are lots of tests that may be appropriate to do. It is best to keep an open mind until more clues come to light. The following tests are almost always needed:

- full blood count
- urea and electrolytes

Table 16.3 Abbreviated Mental Test Score. More than two errors suggest cognitive impairment

Abbreviated Mental Test Score
1. How old are you?
2. What is the time (to the nearest hour)?
3. Give the patient an address (such as '42 West Street') for recall at the end of the test
4. What year is it?
5. What month is it?
6. What is the name of this place?
7. What was the date of your birth?
8. When was the Second World War?
9. Who is the present prime minister?
10. Count down from 20 to 1.
(No errors, No cues, No half marks)

- liver function test
- glucose
- calcium
- blood cultures
- urinalysis (and possibly culture)
- ECG
- CXR.

Other tests may be required on a patient by patient basis:

- Thyroid function tests
- B_{12} and folate
- Other cultures (sputum, swabs)
- Arterial blood gas analysis can be useful and can support diagnoses such as pulmonary emboli, sepsis and hepatic failure. Remember that it hurts the patient to do this (if the patient didn't like you examining them they will like this even less).
- Neuroimaging with *CT is usually unhelpful*. It should be preserved for people with a suspected intracranial lesion. Consider it where there are:
  - focal neurological signs
  - confusion following head injury or falls
  - evidence of raised intracranial pressure

  and reconsider if the patient doesn't progress as we would expect from our initial review.
- Lumbar puncture is not useful as changes in the CSF in patients with delirium are non-specific, unless conditions such as meningitis or encephalitis are suspected. Remember these conditions may not present as they would in a younger person and sometimes we need to exclude them when we can't find another cause.
- The EEG is usually abnormal in delirium and shows non-specific diffuse slow wave activity and doesn't alter our management. Nonetheless non-convulsive status epilepticus is under-recognized in older people and EEG should be performed if this is suspected.

Management

Patients may not be able to consent fully to treatment and we may use implied consent to treat serious illness. We need to be careful that we assess capacity and involve families to be sure we are acting in the patient's best interests. If there is doubt then second opinions can be sought. It can be useful to involve your hospital ethics group.

Treating the cause

There is nothing magical about treating delirium but it can be complicated as you are usually treating more than one condition. Treating one may exacerbate the other (e.g. pain and constipation). It is also possible that you are at risk of causing more harm than good (e.g. treating mild heart failure and causing incontinence with diuretics). There is a useful saying: *'The science of medicine is knowing what to do. The art of medicine is knowing when not to do it.'*

Create a plan that addresses the major contributors and recognizes those that you will not address. The plan will need reviewing as the patient progresses. You should remember triggers such as pain, and have a low threshold to prescribe analgesia (expression of pain can be impaired in patients with dementia and delirium and paracetamol can be effective and is well tolerated – it can be as effective in calming behaviour as neuroleptics).

You may need to stop/withdraw causative drugs, whilst remembering they were started for a reason. They may need replacing with a less toxic alternative.

If the patient is malnourished or abuses alcohol then thiamine should be administered, initially intravenously.

Preventing complications

To add to the complexity of treating the cause, you also need to work to monitor for and prevent complications of delirium, namely:

- falls
- dependency
- pressure sores
- incontinence
- drowsiness
- malnutrition.

Falls. This is a frail group who were at risk of falls before they developed a delirium. They will require a falls assessment and review by a physiotherapist. They should be nursed in an appropriate setting. You should avoid medication that may further increase the risk of falling. The use of restraints has not been shown to reduce the risk of falls and can worsen agitation. You should follow local guidance on the use of restraint. It is often better to manage the patient on a low bed or a mattress on the floor. If you explain this to the patient's family they will understand but they may be surprised otherwise.

Pressure sores. Check for pressure damage on admission and regularly thereafter. The patient should have a formal risk assessment (such as Waterlow score) and have appropriate pressure relief (such as air mattresses). Early mobilization is important but may increase the risk of falls. *ALL pressure sores are preventable.*

Continence. Patients should be assessed for incontinence. Catheters should be avoided due to the risk of local trauma, infection and long-term effects on continence.

Dependency. A multidisciplinary approach with therapy input improves physical and functional status on discharge. This is vital and should take place alongside medical treatments.

Malnutrition. Confused patients may struggle to eat adequate amounts to maintain their nutritional state. They will require prompting and a team that supports them with meals. If the patient has foods that they particularly like then the family should be able to bring these in for them. Methods such as nasogastric feeding are rarely used. This is practically difficult and it is vital that we assess fully to make sure we are acting in the patient's best interests.

Managing the symptoms of delirium

Non-pharmacological

We should always first seek a non-pharmacological approach to treating the confusion and agitation in the patient with delirium. Milder symptoms can respond to environmental changes. It can be very difficult to treat patients in the traditional ward setting with noise, poor lighting and little in the way of orientating features. Bed moves further worsen the confusion. Confused patients require:

- reassurance
- reorientation
- contact from familiar people.

This should be provided in a unit that has staff with an interest in dealing with frail patients and is designed to provide an environment that is conducive to recovery.

Pharmacological

If there is a risk of harm to the patient or excessive agitation then we may use medication to augment behaviour. This may be required to permit investigation or to relieve profound agitation in patients. Sedation is not a means of restraint. Harm can be caused by increasing risk of falls or causing further delirium. We need to be certain that we are acting in the best interests of the patient. It is good to discuss with relatives before initiating medication as it is important for them to understand our actions; it also gives them the opportunity to challenge them. If we initiate pharmacological behavioural control then it should be time limited and the effect regularly reviewed. We would hope to stop medication within 48 hours of initiation. Whatever agent is used we should start with a low dose and titrate slowly – *start low and go slow*.

There is limited evidence as to what the best agent for behavioural control is and you should consult local policy.

Neuroleptics. Haloperidol (in low doses such as 0.5 mg) is the first-line agent. The newer, atypical neuroleptics, such as risperidone, olanzapine and quetiapine, have been shown to have a cleaner side effect profile but they are less useful in delirium. Recently there has been concern about the risk of cerebrovascular events when risperidone and olanzapine have been used for behavioural control in the elderly. The extrapyramidal side effects of neuroleptics require us to use alternatives in patients with Lewy body dementia or Parkinson's disease.

Benzodiazepines such as lorazepam (in low dose such as 0.5 mg) have a faster onset of action than neuroleptics. Their profound sedating effect means they are usually used in people who would not tolerate neuroleptics or are withdrawing from alcohol.

Recovery

The inpatient mortality rate can be as high as 18% and is around twice that of matched controls without delirium and is associated with:

- increase in hospital length of stay
- increased dependency on discharge
- increased risk of care home admission
- increased risk of dementia (three-fold).

Patients who recover may take weeks to get better. They often don't get back to their premorbid state and this can be very distressing to all involved. Patients usually have increased care requirements on discharge and should have their discharge planned carefully by the multidisciplinary team.

Delirium is often the first presentation of a permanent cognitive dysfunction. Patients with delirium should be considered for review by a geriatrician or an old age psychiatrist for further evaluation.

Although we consider delirium to be reversible it can be the start of a spiral of descent for the patient.

Further reading

British Geriatrics Society. Guidelines for the prevention, diagnosis and management of delirium in older people in hospital (2006). Available as a download at www.bgs.org.uk/index.php/clinicalguides/170-clinguidedeliriumtreatment.

British Geriatrics Society. Quality care for older people with urgent and emergency care needs. 'The Silver Book' (June 2012). Available as a download at www.bgs.org.uk/campaigns/silverb/silver_book_complete.pdf.

Fong TG, Tulebaev SR, Inouye SK. Delirium in elderly adults: diagnosis, prevention and treatment. *Nature Reviews Neurology* 2009; 5(4): 210–220.

NICE. Delirium: diagnosis, prevention and management. Clinical Guideline 103 (July 2010). Available as a download at www.nice.org.uk/nicemedia/live/13060/49909/49909.pdf.

Cough

Robert A. Stone

Introduction

Coughing protects our airways against unwanted inhalation. It aids removal of material arising from the constant interaction between our respiratory tract and the outside environment. Two forms of response are recognized:

- An immediate reflex response generated from the larynx in 'emergencies' that is virtually impossible to suppress and akin to the closely allied laryngeal expiration reflex produced by touching the area around the vocal cords.
- A more usual intermittent and often casual forced expiration against a closed glottis that occurs as part of normal mucus clearance and in the presence of airways or other pathology.

The cough reflex

The cough reflex develops early in life, with a typical adult response present by 35 weeks of gestation. It remains potent throughout life but is less effective with advanced age and where corticobulbar function is reduced (e.g. stroke disease, degenerative neurological conditions and dementia).

The reflex is triggered by mechanical, chemical or osmotic stimuli, pH changes and alterations in anionic content within the airway surface liquid. The cough reflex is recruited predominantly by activation of sensory nerve endings situated beneath and between the epithelium of the larynx and tracheobronchial tree (Figure 17.1). It is served by afferent branches of the vagus and superior laryngeal nerves. 'Cough-sensitive' endings throughout their distribution can trigger coughing, and this is important when considering the patient with cough of unidentified cause. No single 'cough receptor' has been identified but the following are implicated:

- A major excitatory contribution arising from rapidly adapting endings on myelinated Aδ-fibres.
- Slowly adapting stretch receptors within the lung substance facilitate and intensify the afferent cough response (relevant to the generation of cough in acute asthma).
- Excitatory unmyelinated nociceptive C-fibres.
- C-fibres may also have a modulating role as their stimulation during concomitant mechanical irritation of the larynx attenuates cough.

The reflex is modulated centrally in the dorsal medulla under the influence of several neurotransmitter systems, notably opioid, NMDA/GABA and serotoninergic. It is subject to significant cortical influence. Thus, although reflex coughing is hard to control, the ability to suppress cough during wakefulness is possible and those with chronic persistent cough are observed to do so predominantly during waking hours.

The efferent response is transmitted to the respiratory muscles and diaphragm via the phrenic and intercostal nerves. The inherent sensitivity of an individual's cough reflex, i.e. how likely they are to cough, therefore represents a balance between:

- excitatory afferent inputs
- inhibitory afferent inputs
- cortical influence.

The reflex can either become less sensitive (e.g. neurological disease) or more sensitive (e.g. lung disease or chronic persistent cough). Powerful coughing can be provoked by the smallest of physical or chemical stimuli.

Acute Medicine, ed. Stephen Haydock, Duncan Whitehead and Zoë Fritz. Published by Cambridge University Press.
© Cambridge University Press 2015.

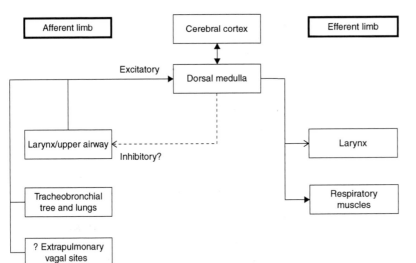

Afferent limb · Cerebral cortex · Efferent limb

Excitatory → Dorsal medulla

Larynx/upper airway ← - - - - Inhibitory? → Larynx

Tracheobronchial tree and lungs → Respiratory muscles

? Extrapulmonary vagal sites

Figure 17.1 *The cough reflex:* afferent responses are mediated via the vagus and superior laryngeal nerves. *Triggering:* stimulated by rapidly adapting irritant receptors in larynx and airways, nociceptive C-fibres in airways and lung (also have an inhibitory effect); slowly adapting stretch receptors in lung facilitate the intensity of coughing. Extrapulmonary vagal receptors (e.g. heart) may also modulate cough. *Integration:* occurs in nucleus of tractus solitarius, is subject to cortical influence under control of several neurotransmitter systems. *Efferent response:* motor to larynx and respiratory muscles. May also be efferent non-adrenergic/non-cholinergic output within airways, associated with local inflammation.

Scenario 17.1

A 60-year-old man attends the MAU ambulatory clinic. He has been referred by the emergency department which he attended the previous week with a transient loss of consciousness after a 'coughing fit'. This happened in the context of a persistent, irritating cough for the previous 3 months. He stopped smoking a year ago. The cough is becoming a considerable problem to him. He is also concerned that he has been told not to drive by the ED doctors until he has been seen in clinic. He is sure that fainting after a coughing fit shouldn't stop him driving. How should this man be investigated and does he really need to stop driving?

Clinical assessment

Cough is the commonest indicator of respiratory disease and has many causes (Table 17.1). It can occur in isolation but commonly with other symptoms such as breathlessness, wheeze, chest tightness, chest discomfort and chest pain. It is allied closely to upper or lower airway, cardiovascular and gastrointestinal disorders. Successful management depends upon establishing its duration, its context, identifying the cause if possible and then removing or treating the provoking factor(s). A thorough history is especially important and patients may have more than one provoking factor.

History

Cough is somewhat arbitrarily classified as:

- *Acute* (less than 3 weeks duration, with 'hyperacute' coming on within hours)

Table 17.1 Some conditions associated with cough

Anatomical region	Associated condition
Upper airways	Upper respiratory tract infection
	Rhino-sinusitis
	Post-nasal drip
	Pharyngitis
	Laryngitis
	Tumours/foreign bodies
	Infiltrative conditions
Thoracic airways	Tracheitis
	Acute/chronic bronchitis
	Adult pertussis
	Asthma
	'Cough-variant' asthma
	Eosinophilic bronchitis
	Small airways disease/obliterative bronchitis
	Airways infiltration (e.g. sarcoidosis)
	Bronchial tumour/foreign body
	Bronchiectasis
Lung parenchyma	Pneumonia/lung infection
	Interstitial lung disease
	Tumour/lymphangitis
	Pulmonary oedema
	Pulmonary infarction
Pleura	Pneumothorax
	Pleural effusion
	Tumour/pleural infiltration

Table 17.1 (*cont.*)

Anatomical region	Associated condition
Cardiovascular disease	Heart failure
	Pericardial disease
Pulmonary vascular disease	Pulmonary embolism
	Pulmonary infarction
Mediastinal disease	Lymphoma
	Mediastinal masses
	Mediastinitis
Gastrointestinal disease	Gastro-oesophageal reflux (acid and/or volume)
	Microaspiration
	Achalasia
Medications	ACE inhibitor therapy

- *Subacute* (3–8 weeks)
- *Chronic* (>8 weeks).

Although most acute coughs are benign some may be the first manifestation of significant systemic disease. Patients often find it hard to date the onset of their cough. A systematic approach should be adopted, considering common causes, but thinking around the other possibilities and most particularly excluding malignancy.

Acute cough

By far the commonest cause of acute cough is upper airway or tracheobronchial infection, associated with the typical features of acute viral or bacterial illness. Hyperacute cough with onset over hours also occurs commonly with infection but also enquire regarding:

- occupational exposure
- toxin inhalation
- allergen exposure
- pre-existing airways disease or hypersensitivity pneumonitis.

Sudden onset of coughing typically occurs in:

- infection
- after exposure to airway toxins
- aspiration or foreign body inhalation.

Some patients with a history of chronic persistent cough and a sensitized cough reflex may experience extreme paroxysms of coughing after seemingly innocuous activities such as:

- taking a deep breath
- encountering aerosol sprays

- entering a warm or cold room
- switching on the car air-conditioning.

Severe coughing paroxysms can lead to retching, vomiting or even syncope (see below).

Chronic cough

Significant disease is more likely to be associated with coughing that develops gradually over weeks or longer. Ask about:

- potential triggers such as recent upper/lower respiratory infection
- changed work/domestic environment and potentially relevant exposures (chemicals, pets, dusts, occupational history)
- if the cough dates to a particular point in time – consider foreign body inhalation
- relation to medication (e.g. ACE inhibitors)
- smoking history
- systemic features of disease.

Sputum production

It is useful to discriminate between productive and dry coughing although the presence of the former does not exclude potential causes of the latter. Productive cough occurs predominantly in:

- lung and/or airways infection
- COPD
- bronchiectasis.

  Ascertain *sputum colour and volume.*
  Ask about *blood in the phlegm,* which can occur in:

- malignancy
- infection
- pulmonary infarction
- bronchiectasis.

  A *change in the character of a smoker's cough* is also a pointer towards possible malignancy.

Timing of cough

Cough that is worse in the morning, especially if productive, favours overnight accumulation of mucus due to:

- upper airway disease
- bronchiectasis
- COPD.

Sleep-disruptive cough is also caused by sputum accumulation but suggests:

- unstable asthma
- heart failure
- oesophageal reflux.

Night-time coughing is generally indicative of underlying disease.

Associated features

Throat clearing and sneezing are common in upper airways disease. Patients with post-nasal drip syndrome or chronic rhinosinusitis often describe a sensation of something trickling down from the back of the nose. Patients with ear disease may experience cough due to stimulation of Arnold's nerve within the auditory canal. Asthma is commonly associated with cough, usually accompanying wheeze and chest tightness. It often occurs at night.

Cough-variant asthma is characterized by:

- cough without significant wheeze, chest tightness or peak flow variability
- airways that are hyper-responsive to inhaled challenge with constrictors such as methacholine.

Eosinophilic bronchitis is a similar syndrome with:

- cough without airway hyper-responsiveness
- significant (>3%) sputum eosinophilia
- often subsequent development of asthma or chronic airflow limitation.

Cough related to left ventricular failure is often non-specific but may be:

- postural
- night-time predominant
- associated with paroxysmal nocturnal dyspnoea.

Reflux

- Reported in up to 30% of patients with chronic cough and cough may be the only feature, occurring in the absence of heartburn.
- A history of acid or volume reflux should be sought in all patients presenting with unexplained cough.

Chronic persistent cough of unidentified cause

- Much commoner in middle-aged women.
- May associate with upper airways disease, reflux or inflammatory airways disease.
- Such individuals develop an abnormally sensitive cough reflex, akin to a state of airways hyperalgesia.

Examination

- Is the patient actually coughing? (Is the cough causing discomfort or distress?)
- Is the airway competent?
- Is there stridor or large airways noise?
- Does the cough appear moist or dry?
- Assess the tongue, the dentition, the tonsils and check for foreign bodies.
- Take note of oral mucosal quality, moistness and secretions.
- Examine ears for any pathology.

Undertake a careful and systematic physical examination to detect features of respiratory, cardiovascular, systemic or associated disease. In particular look for clubbing and auscultate front and back to detect crackles that might indicate pulmonary oedema, lung fibrosis or bronchiectasis.

Investigation

First-line investigations

- Chest X-ray is mandatory and aids diagnosis of:
  - lung cancer
  - interstitial lung disease
  - infections
  - bronchiectasis
  - pleural disease
  - cardiac failure.
- Also note:
  - hyperinflation (asthma or small airways disease)
  - hilar/para-tracheal adenopathy (sarcoidosis/lymphoma)
  - mediastinal widening (lymphoma)
  - suggestion of upper gastrointestinal disease (visible hiatus hernia or enlarged gastric bubble in achalasia).
- Note the oxygen saturation, peak flow and consider checking spirometry.
- Sinus X-rays are unhelpful.
- Basic blood tests, including assessment of inflammatory markers such as CRP.

- If productive, send sputum for microbiological analysis.

Second-line investigations

The cause of most acute coughs will be apparent after history, examination and first-line tests have been performed. If cough persists, it is advisable to consult a respiratory specialist in order to plan further second-line tests specific to each individual case.

Bronchoscopy will usually be necessary if malignancy is suspected. Inspection of the upper and lower airways can also reveal:

- nasal disease
- post-nasal drip
- laryngeal reflux
- continuing infection
- endobronchial infiltration (e.g. sarcoidosis)
- foreign bodies.

Adult pertussis is difficult to diagnose. Close contact or a high index of suspicion during an outbreak may be sufficient but otherwise nasopharyngeal swabs and serology are necessary, if not wholly reliable.

Other tests that may prove useful include:

- D-dimer (pulmonary embolism) and BNP (cardiac failure)
- echocardiography (left ventricular function)
- full lung function testing (interstitial/airways disease)
- high resolution chest CT scanning (bronchiectasis/interstitial disease/airways disease)
- CTPA (pulmonary vascular disease)
- sinus CT (chronic sinusitis)
- oesophageal pH/manometry (reflux and motility disorders)
- airways reactivity testing (cough-variant asthma)
- induced sputum analysis (eosinophilic bronchitis), not routinely available outside specialist 'cough clinics'.

Management of cough

General advice

The management depends on the underlying cause(s) but airway protection is paramount:

- Avoid cough-provoking factors at home/work
- Avoid ACE inhibitors

- Keep well hydrated
- Moist inhalations are useful.

There is limited evidence for the efficacy of proprietary cough remedies, although patients with chronic cough often report benefit from catarrh pastilles and menthol-containing lozenges.

Anti-tussives

A lack of detailed understanding of the homeostasis of cough has resulted in a paucity of useful non-opioid anti-tussives devoid of respiratory suppressant effects.

- Opiate-based anti-tussives are useful in cough with no identifiable cause but CNS effects and constipation are common.
- Dextromethorphan and pholcodine seem better tolerated.
- Morphine is most potent (but associated with more side effects) and is especially useful for patients with cough due to malignancy or interstitial disease.
- Avoid methadone due to risk of accumulation.
- No compelling evidence to suggest nebulized opiates are effective in cough.
- Recent small trials have suggested gabapentin may help those with cough of unidentified cause.

Specific situations

Post-infective cough usually settles spontaneously but may persist for many weeks (as sensitivity of the cough reflex reduces). Cough following upper respiratory infection may be accompanied by post-nasal drip, which is treated with nasal corticosteroids and/or antihistamines. Patients with post-viral cough develop transient increases in airways reactivity, which occasionally responds to inhaled corticosteroid or anticholinergic medications. Coughing may become prolonged if airway infection has not been fully eradicated and antibiotics should be considered on a case-by-case basis. They are useful if there is deemed to be ongoing bacterial bronchitis or accompanying sinusitis.

Cough due to adult pertussis is treated with a macrolide or co-trimoxazole but good results depend upon starting therapy within 2 weeks of onset of symptoms.

ACE inhibitor cough is reported in 10–30% of patients. It can occur at any time during treatment and these should be withdrawn in patients with unexplained coughing. The cough reflex may take weeks to settle and 3-month abstinence is suggested. Angiotensin receptor blockers are a suitable alternative.

Upper airways disease related cough is managed according to cause: nasal corticosteroids, antihistamines, leukotriene antagonists and nasal anticholinergic therapy are of variable use in allergic, non-allergic and vasomotor rhinitis. Start with a combination of nasal steroid and antihistamine, though treatment may be necessary for several months. Patients with suspected rhinosinusitis may require lengthy courses of antibiotics and follow-up by an ear, nose and throat specialist.

Asthma and allied disorders usually respond to initiating or escalating doses of inhaled corticosteroids. Leukotriene receptor antagonists may improve cough-variant asthma. A short course of oral prednisolone is a very effective treatment for these conditions when cough is severe and disruptive. Prednisolone is not recommended as a long-term treatment for cough due to airways disease but it can be a useful remedial measure if the cough reflex is too sensitive to permit effective use of inhaled steroids.

COPD and bronchiectasis result in sputum production that may confound coexistent causes of cough in this group of patients. Sputum volume and expectoration is improved by:

- adequate hydration
- infection control
- mucolytic agents to reduce viscosity
- chest physiotherapy, which when correctly taught and practised regularly is a very effective management for troublesome sputum
- hand-held 'flutter devices' that aid mucus break-up and clearance by producing expiratory oscillations within the airway.

Gastro-oesophageal reflux related cough generally responds to:

- Modification of the provoking factor (e.g. diet, alcohol, smoking, weight, excess caffeine).
- Raising the head of the bed by four inches.
- Proton pump inhibitors – the mainstay of treatment. A high dose trial for at least 8 weeks is suggested.
- Non-acid reflux may respond to motility agents such as metoclopramide.

Persistent reflux-related coughs are followed up by a respiratory physician or gastroenterologist with an interest in this problem.

Chronic unexplained cough can be very difficult to manage as the cough reflex becomes abnormally sensitive, akin to a state of airways sensory hyperalgesia (demonstrable by an augmented cough response to inhaled capsaicin). Identify a provoking factor or association if possible, and then remove the cause until the cough reflex settles down. Respiratory physicians should manage chronic unexplained cough. Available management guidelines and algorithms are highly variable and informed by a poor evidence base.

Smokers who report a change in the character or quality of their cough should be investigated carefully to exclude bronchial carcinoma. Blood-staining of sputum in smokers should also raise the suspicion of malignancy. Many smokers report an improvement in sputum volume when they quit, although the coughing may initially become more intense and irritating.

Offer smoking cessation advice at every opportunity and enlist hospital or community services (practice nurse or smoking cessation practitioners). Patients are more likely to quit if they are well motivated and offered support in a non-judgemental manner. For those with partners who smoke, a dual approach can be helpful.

Cough syncope (as per chapter scenario). Coughing generates swings in intrathoracic pressure of up to 300 mmHg. Significant fluctuations in venous return may lead to syncope in those with severe cough. UK rules provided by the DVLA advise driving must cease for 6 months (increased to 12 months if multiple attacks) for Class 1 licence holders, though reapplication may meantime occur if the cause is well controlled, smoking ceases, reflux is treated and BMI <30 kg/m^2. Class 2 licence holders must cease driving for at least 5 years, though reapplication may occur after 1 year if the same criteria are met and confirmed by specialist opinion.

Referral to respiratory physicians

Refer patients with troublesome cough in whom there is associated respiratory/systemic disease or no clear underlying cause – it is far better to refer than miss significant disease.

It is very helpful to discuss the case with the respiratory team when referring from the ambulatory clinic, so that any relevant tests can be planned before the initial respiratory consultation.

Indications for admission to hospital

Admission for coughing alone is unusual and more often there are associated symptoms or significant

- faecal impaction, suggesting overflow diarrhoea
- abnormal anal sphincter tone suggesting potential faecal incontinence
- rectal mass lesion or cancer.

Investigations

Baseline serological tests

- FBC
- U&Es
- LFTs
- TFTs
- Magnesium
- Phosphate
- Coeliac serology
- Amylase
- CRP/ESR
- Ferritin
- B_{12}/folate

Faecal tests

- Stool microscopy: for ova and cysts and culture sensitivity
- *C. difficile* toxin
- Faecal elastase: to exclude pancreatic insufficiency
- Faecal calprotectin (not universally available): a faecal calprotectin level of <50 µg/g excludes significant bowel inflammation of any cause, but especially Crohn's disease and ulcerative colitis

Endoscopic evaluation

- *Rigid sigmoidoscopy*: can be considered as a bedside test in case of bloody diarrhoea for rapid diagnosis. Rectal and sigmoid biopsies can be obtained. It is rarely used these days due to easy and rapid access to flexible sigmoidoscopy.
- *Flexible sigmoidoscopy*: particularly useful for investigating (bloody) non-infective diarrhoea. Allows visualization of bowel mucosa and colonic biopsies. If severe colitis is suspected, flexible sigmoidoscopy should be performed without enema preparation.
- *Oesophagogastroduodenoscopy and duodenal/ jejunal biopsies*: to diagnose coeliac disease and obtain jejunal aspirate and biopsies in suspected small bowel bacterial overgrowth or giardiasis.

- *Colonoscopy*: with colonic biopsies to diagnose inflammatory bowel disease and microscopic colitis. If there is an acute risk of toxic megacolon (possible perforation) or the presence of acute kidney injury (risk of hypovolaemia from bowel preparation), then colonoscopy and the necessary oral bowel cleansing preparations should be avoided.

Radiological evaluation

- *Chest film*: an erect CXR is useful in suspected perforation.
- *Abdominal film*: to exclude faecal loading causing overflow diarrhoea, identify mucosal oedema or toxic dilatation in acute severe colitis.
- *CT scan*: if renal function is acceptable, then CT colonography is an alternative to colonoscopy although histological analysis of biopsies or polyps is not possible. It also requires full oral bowel cleansing. For elderly patients and those with impaired renal function, using oral senna tablets as bowel preparation and tagging stool with Gastrografin is safer albeit with loss of sensitivity.
- *MRI scan*: to investigate the small bowel using enterography with oral contrast.
- *Barium studies*: although largely superseded by endoscopic techniques, small bowel follow-through or small bowel enema still has a role in diagnosing small bowel pathology.

Other tests

- *Glucose or lactulose hydrogen breath test*: to diagnose small bowel bacterial overgrowth.
- *SeHCAT scan*: to diagnose bile salt malabsorption (23-seleno-25-homo-tauro-cholic acid is a taurine conjugated bile acid analogue).

Management

General principles

- Establish severity including dehydration, electrolyte disturbances and systemic features of an acute abdomen (may occur in acute colitis) requiring immediate medical and/or surgical attention.
- Severe cases of diarrhoea require hospitalization for correction of fluid and electrolyte imbalance and isolation until infectious causes are ruled out.

Indication for urgent surgical review

Urgent surgical consultation is requested in the following conditions:

- toxic bowel dilatation or perforation on the abdominal or chest X-rays
- diarrhoea with signs of acute abdomen such as abdominal tenderness, guarding and rebound tenderness
- suspected acute severe ulcerative colitis in conjunction with the gastroenterology team
- diarrhoea with profuse rectal bleeding.

Once the clinical condition is stabilized, further management depends upon individual circumstances.

Some specific causes of diarrhoea

Infective colitis

- Most common cause of acute diarrhoea in developing countries. It is usually benign with moderate symptoms and is self-limiting with conservative management. Severe cases require hospital admission.
- It can be bloody or non-bloody depending upon the underlying infective agent.
- *E. coli* is the most common cause worldwide followed by *Shigella* and *Campylobacter*.
- *C. difficile* related diarrhoea is common in elderly patients exposed to antibiotics.
- Adequate hydration with correction of electrolyte imbalance is the key to the management.
- Antibiotics such as ciprofloxacin (500 mg twice a day for 5 days) are considered in severe cases of infective colitis caused by *Shigella*, *Salmonella* and *E. coli*. *Campylobacter* may be treated with a macrolide such as azithromycin (250 mg daily for 5 days) although most cases resolve without antibiotics. Consult local prescribing guidelines before prescribing.

Clostridium difficile related colitis

- *C. difficile* is the most common cause of antibiotic related diarrhoea especially in older and hospitalized patients.
- Antibiotics disturb the normal colonic microbiota leading to colonization by *C. difficile* with release of toxins causing mucosal inflammation and damage.

- Presents with bloody or non-bloody diarrhoea, abdominal discomfort, malaise, dehydration and electrolyte disturbance.
- Diagnosis is made by detecting endotoxins A and B using enzyme immunoassay, which has 80% sensitivity and 95% specificity. Other diagnostic tests include:
  - stool cytotoxin test
  - polymerase chain reaction (PCR) assay
  - stool culture
  - glutamate dehydrogenase enzyme immunoassay.
- Endoscopy can show the presence of raised, yellowish plaques adherent to inflamed mucosa known as pseudomembranes.
- Stopping the causative antibiotic is the key to management. Asymptomatic cases require no treatment while mild to moderate cases are treated with metronidazole 400 mg tds for 7–10 days. Severe cases require addition of oral vancomycin 125 mg qds for 7–10 days.
- Relapse rates are up to 25% in treated cases, which require additional vancomycin and/or metronidazole. Other treatment options are quinolones, rifaximin, probiotics, intravenous immunoglobulin or faecal transplant. Specialist advice should be sought from Gastroenterology and Microbiology in resistant or relapsed cases.
- Surgical input may be needed if toxic megacolon develops.

Drug induced

Other drugs such as laxatives, antacids, proton pump inhibitors, and antineoplastic agents can lead to diarrhoea that can continue for a few weeks despite stopping the causative drug (see Table 19.1).

Inflammatory bowel disease

- Chronic remitting, relapsing inflammatory diseases of the gastrointestinal tract, which include:
  - ulcerative colitis (UC, mucosal inflammation remains confined to the colon)
  - Crohn's disease (CD, transmural and patchy inflammation, affecting any segment of bowel from oral cavity to anus).
- Usually presents in a younger population 12–40 years old with chronic diarrhoea +/– blood

Table 19.1 List of medications causing diarrhoea

Osmotic
Citrates, phosphates, sulphates
Magnesium-containing antacids and laxatives
Sugar alcohols (e.g. mannitol, sorbitol, xylitol)

Secretory
Anti-arrhythmics (e.g. quinine)
Antibiotics (e.g. amoxicillin/clavulanate (Augmentin))
Antineoplastics
Biguanides
Calcitonin
Cardiac glycosides (e.g. digitalis)
Colchicine
Non-steroidal anti-inflammatory drugs (may contribute to microscopic colitis)
Prostaglandins (e.g. misoprostol (Cytotec))
Ticlopidine

Motility
Macrolides (e.g. erythromycin)
Metoclopramide
Stimulant laxatives (e.g. bisacodyl (Dulcolax), senna)

Malabsorption
Acarbose (Precose; carbohydrate malabsorption)
Aminoglycosides
Orlistat (Xenical; fat malabsorption)
Thyroid supplements
Ticlopidine

Pseudomembranous colitis (Clostridium difficile)
Antibiotics (e.g. amoxicillin, cephalosporins, clindamycin, fluoroquinolones)

(usually in UC), abdominal pain, bloating, weight loss and anaemia (predominantly CD) along with features of systemic illness.

- Diagnosis is made on clinical assessment and confirmed by endoscopy, histology and radiology such as CT/MRI (in case of small bowel involvement).
- Specialist advice should be sought from Gastroenterology as soon as a diagnosis has been made.
- Severe cases (both UC and CD) require hospitalization and:
  - treatment with steroids (usually IV hydrocortisone 100 mg qds)
  - venous thromboembolism prophylaxis as these patients are at high risk for PE/DVT
  - gastroenterology specialist input at the earliest opportunity with transfer to a specialist GI ward and ideally shared care with a GI surgeon

- addition of immunosuppression when symptoms of ulcerative colitis do not improve and CRP at day 3 is >48, using IV ciclosporin although surgery is another option preferably before complications such as perforation or toxic megacolon develop
- in CD, anti-TNF therapy such as infliximab may be used to induce remission when severe disease does not settle clinically using intravenous steroids but only under GI supervision
- all benefit from seeing a dietitian (many are malnourished) and a specialist IBD nurse if available.
- Mild to moderate cases of confirmed CD and UC should have outpatient management with early review (2–4 weeks) in a gastroenterology clinic.
  - UC should respond well to high dose 5-amino-salicylate preparations (5-ASA) using mesalazine at 2.4 g twice a day along with topical treatment with mesalazine enemas and/or suppositories.
  - For CD, 5-ASA preparations are less effective for anything except colonic disease so oral steroids may be required. Budesonide (start at 9 mg/day for 1 month then reduce by 3 mg every month) is the preferred steroid when treating terminal ileal CD due to the first pass effect although prednisolone (start 30–40 mg/day and taper down by 5 mg every week) is an alternative but this requires co-prescription of a calcium and vitamin D preparation to minimize bone loss. Steroid responsive cases will require long-term immunosuppression such as azathioprine (2.5 mg/kg, check TPMT (thiopurine methyl transferase) level) as maintenance treatment.

Irritable bowel syndrome

- Irritable bowel syndrome (IBS) causes diarrhoea in a significant number of cases (along with abdominal pain, bloating and excessive wind). It usually affects a younger population (predominantly females 2:1 ratio) and results in significant morbidity (see Chapter 2).

Diverticular disease

- Diverticula (sac-like protrusions of the colonic wall) are an age-related wear-and-tear phenomenon. They are a well-known cause of recurrent diarrhoea in the older age group and can be diagnosed by radiological imaging or endoscopy.

- Treatment consists of dietary modification using fibre supplements and antibiotics for complications such as diverticulitis. More severe cases or the presence of complications such as colonic bleeding, intussusception and perforation require colectomy.

Microscopic colitis

- Microscopic colitis, including both:
  - collagenous colitis
  - lymphocytic colitis.
- An infrequent but important cause of non-bloody diarrhoea, which usually affects an older population with female predominance.
- Bowel mucosa is macroscopically normal at endoscopy with colonic biopsies from right and transverse colon showing:
  - thickened subepithelial collagen layer in collagenous colitis
  - increased number of subepithelial lymphocytes in lymphocytic colitis.
- Treatment consists of oral steroid using budesonide (as above), 5-ASA medications and anti-diarrhoeal medications such as loperamide. NSAIDs and sometimes PPIs are considered to be a causative factor and should be stopped.

Bacterial overgrowth

- The small bowel lumen normally contains very few bacteria. Colonization of the small bowel with bacteria (due to previous small bowel surgery, blind gut loop, radiation exposure, etc.) is an important cause of chronic diarrhoea, weight loss and deficiency of micronutrients (particularly vitamin B_{12} and fat-soluble vitamins A, D, E and K).
- Diagnose on clinical assessment and glucose hydrogen breath testing.
- Treatment requires empirical antibiotics with anaerobic and aerobic cover. This usually involves cyclical courses of antibiotics using tetracycline, quinolones, co-amoxiclav and more recently rifaximin. Probiotics show little benefit.

Bile salt malabsorption

- Disturbance of the enterohepatic circulation of bile due to underlying condition including cholecystectomy (excessive bile production), ileal resection or enteropathy due to radiation (inability to reabsorb bile salts), which lead to irritation of the colon and cause diarrhoea, abdominal bloating and urgency.
- Diagnosis is based on clinical suspicion and confirmed by SeHCAT scan.
- Treated with bile salt resins such as cholestyramine (4 g daily, can increase up to 12–24 g/day), colestipol (5 g 1–2 times/day, can increase to 30 g/day) or colesevelam (2.5–3.75 g/day).

Coeliac disease

- This is a common condition caused by gluten sensitivity with a prevalence of about 1/100 population. Patients present with diarrhoea, abdominal bloating, pain, tiredness and anaemia.
- Diagnosis is made serologically by testing for anti-tissue transglutaminase antibodies with a sensitivity of more than 98%. Confirmation is made using duodenal biopsies, which show villous atrophy and presence of intraepithelial lymphocytes.
- Treatment is with gluten-free diet and correction of nutrient deficiencies including folate and iron, which requires referral to an appropriately trained dietitian.

Colon cancer

- Third most common cause of cancer-related death in the UK with approximately 30 000 new cases and 16 000 deaths, per year.
- Usually presents with altered bowel habit in people >50 years old with rectal bleeding mixed with stool, tiredness, low appetite and loss of weight. In rare instances, presentation is with pain due to local invasion or symptoms of intestinal obstruction.
- Diagnosis is made by colonoscopy to obtain histological confirmation with staging CT scan of the chest, abdomen and pelvis.
- Dukes classification is used to stage the disease: *Dukes A*: tumour confined to mucosa or submucosa

Dukes B: tumour completely penetrates smooth muscle reaching the serosa
Dukes C: tumour invaded to the local lymph nodes
Dukes D: tumour with distal metastases.

- Surgery is curative for localized tumour (Dukes A and B). Metastatic lesions can be present in about 30% of patients undergoing curative surgery so neoadjuvant chemotherapy after curative surgery is considered in Dukes C. Patients with a single hepatic or pulmonary metastatic lesion of <3 cm can also be considered for surgical resection of their secondary. More advanced cases require a palliative approach.

VIPoma

- VIPomas are exocrine pancreatic tumours, which cause profuse diarrhoea. Diagnosis is made by raised serum VIP levels (>75 pg/mL); this is taken as a fasting gut hormone – see biochemical department advice about taking the sample and transporting to the lab.
- Management includes correction of fluid and electrolyte imbalance and octreotide subcutaneously for symptom control. Surgery is considered curative in about one-third of cases.

When to seek specialist advice

Diarrhoeal disease ranges in severity and aetiology. The majority of cases with simple non-bloody diarrhoea can be managed conservatively; however, situations where early specialist advice should be sought are:

- Cases of probable acute ulcerative colitis where both colorectal surgeons and the gastroenterology team should be involved early as chances of colectomy are high. Stoma nurses should be involved in such cases due to the high colectomy rate to give the patient and their family an opportunity to ask questions and understand the devices used.
- Severe *C. difficile* colitis patients need close liaison with gastroenterology and microbiology teams and consideration of colectomy in severe disease.
- Malnourished patients require early assessment using your hospital malnutrition screening tool (such as MUST) with appropriate dietetic input.
- The majority of cases where admission is required to manage chronic diarrhoea require early referral to Gastroenterology to streamline investigation and management.

Multidisciplinary approach

- A multidisciplinary approach involving surgeons, gastroenterology, radiology, microbiology and dietetics is key to the management of severe and complex cases of diarrhoea due to inflammatory bowel disease or *C. difficile* colitis.
- Colon cancer management will additionally involve oncological input. Colorectal specialist nurse input is invaluable for patients and their families who struggle to come to terms with such diagnoses. For patients where treatment options may be very limited due to extensive disease, support from the palliative care team for symptomatic relief is essential.
- Early involvement of these specialists should be sought in selected complex cases.

Infection control measures

- Each hospital in the UK has its own infection control policy and these measures should be followed while managing patients with diarrhoea in order to prevent cross-contamination. Infection control measures should be strictly observed until infectious causes are excluded. The basic principles of infection control are:
  1. *Isolation*: the patient should be isolated and apron and gloves should be worn before and changed after each patient contact.
  2. *Cleaning*: thorough cleaning by removing all visible dirt is an effective way of minimizing cross-contamination and spread of infection.
  3. *Hand hygiene*: the hand hygiene policy should be followed strictly, i.e. washing hands before undertaking invasive procedures, before and after patient contact, after removal of gloves, after procedures likely to cause contamination and after using the toilet.
  4. *Disinfection and sterilization*: is a process of destroying microorganisms by using different chemicals and physical cleaning.

Further reading

Beaugerie L, Soko H. (2013) Acute infectious diarrhoea in adults: epidemiology and management. *Presse Med* 42: 52–59.

Boynton W, Floch M. (2013) New strategies for the management of diverticular disease: insight for the clinician. *Therap Adv Gastroenterol* 6: 205–213.

Brown WR, Tayal S. (2013) Microscopic colitis: a review. *J Dig Dis*: 14: 277–281.

Ciclitera PJ, Dewar DH, McLaughlin SD, et al. (2010) The management of adults with coeliac disease, British Society of Gastroenterology Guidance. www.bsg.org.uk/images/stories/clinical/bsg_coeliac_10.pdf.

Gore JI, Surawicz C (2003) Severe acute diarrhoea. *Gastroenterol Clin North Am* 32: 1249–1267.

Johnson I, Nolan J, Pattni S, et al. (2011) New insight into bile salt malabsorption. *Curr Gastroenterol Rep* 13: 418–425.

Mowat C, Cole A, Windsor A, et al. (2011) Guidelines for the management of inflammatory bowel disease, British Society of Gastroenterology. *Gut* 60: 571–607.

Pacheco SM, Johnson S. (2013) Important clinical advances in the understanding of *Clostridium difficile* infection. *Curr Opin Gastroenterol* 29: 42–48.

Spiller R, Aziz Q, Creed F, et al. (2007) Guidelines on the irritable bowel syndrome: mechanisms and practical management, British Society of Gastroenterology. *Gut* 56: 1770–1798.

Thomas P, Forbes A, Green J, et al. (2003) Guidelines for the investigation of chronic diarrhoea, 2nd edition. *Gut* 52: 1–15.

Dyspepsia

Paul D. Thomas

Scenario 20.1

You are asked to review a 57-year-old man on MAU who was initially sent up by his GP with chest pain. Serial troponins and ECG have been normal. On questioning, he in fact describes retrosternal and epigastric discomfort that appears to be related to meals rather than exercise. He thinks that he may have 'lost a bit of weight' but he's not sure how much. He is a smoker and drinks 2–3 pints of beer per day. He has no other significant past history. There is nothing to find on examination, except mild epigastric tenderness. Other investigations are unremarkable except for a mild microcytic anaemia.

Definition and terminology

Dyspepsia (literally 'bad digestion') is a symptom not a diagnosis and one for which there is no universally agreed definition. This has led to difficulties in conducting clinical trials and in establishing its prevalence in differing populations.

United Kingdom guidelines for the management of dyspepsia, e.g. NICE, include both upper abdominal/epigastric discomfort and gastro-oesophageal reflux (GORD) symptoms such as heartburn in the definition, whereas some authorities (e.g. the Rome Group) exclude the latter as reflux is regarded as a separate condition [1]. However, this distinction is difficult to make in clinical practice as there is considerable overlap between 'dyspeptic' and 'reflux' symptoms. Furthermore, the diagnosis of GORD is not straightforward as the most widely used investigation, endoscopy, shows no abnormality in the majority of cases. This chapter will include GORD in the discussion on dyspepsia. There have been recent attempts to reclassify dyspeptic symptoms (Rome III criteria) but here

we apply a broad definition of chronic or recurrent upper abdominal discomfort which includes:

- Postprandial pain
- Fullness
- Early satiety
- Heartburn.

Prevalence and aetiology

- Prevalence in Western populations approaches 40%.
- Prevalence is 20–30% when heartburn is excluded.
- Only 25% will present to primary care.

Very few studies have investigated aetiology based on community presence of dyspepsia so the exact frequency of causes is unclear. However, findings at endoscopy show:

- Normal or minor changes: 60%
- Oesophagitis: 19%
- Gastric ulcer: 5%
- Duodenal ulcer: 5%
- Gastric cancer: 2%
- Oesophageal cancer: 1%
- Miscellaneous: 5%.

Normal findings at endoscopy represent:

- Functional dyspepsia
- Endoscopy negative gastro-oesophageal reflux (also called 'non-ulcer dyspepsia').

Together with objective evidence of gastro-oesophageal reflux (oesophagitis) these two diagnoses account for 80% of presentations.

Malignancy only accounts for 3–5% of endoscopic findings. However, this represents a major diagnostic concern given the large symptom burden of

Acute Medicine, ed. Stephen Haydock, Duncan Whitehead and Zoë Fritz. Published by Cambridge University Press.
© Cambridge University Press 2015.

predominantly benign disease. Unfortunately gastric and oesophageal cancer is often symptom-free until advanced and this in part accounts for the very poor survival in patients with these tumours (5-year survival of 15% and 13%, respectively).

Clinical assessment

History

Symptoms rather than abdominal findings are usually most helpful in indicating the likely diagnosis. Consider other possible causes of abdominal pain:

- Quality
- Site
- Pattern of abdominal pain or discomfort
- Alleviating and aggravating factors.

Although pain is poorly localized in the abdomen there is a broad association between pathology site and pain localization.

- Visceral pain from obstruction or spasm is typically cramping, colicky and intermittent.
- Malignant disease typically causes dull, gnawing, poorly localized pain.
- Peptic ulcer pain may be related to eating but can be relieved or aggravated by food.
- Pain due to pancreatic pathology and mesenteric ischaemia is also frequently exacerbated by eating.
- A response to acid suppressant medication is suggestive of a peptic cause.

There are three main patterns of symptoms in dyspepsia:

- 'Peptic' – epigastric pain typically after eating
- 'Functional' – upper abdominal discomfort/ fullness, early satiety and bloating
- 'Reflux type' – heartburn and retrosternal pain.

However, the ability of these symptoms to discriminate underlying causes of dyspepsia is poor and clinical diagnosis without investigation is unreliable. A clinical diagnosis will miss 50% of peptic ulcer cases and a provisional diagnosis of peptic ulcer is only confirmed in a third of cases. Therefore, *symptom assessment cannot be used reliably for diagnosis in patients with dyspepsia.*

Other history

- A full drug history should be obtained. Common medications that contribute to dyspepsia include:
  - non-steroidal anti-inflammatory drugs (NSAIDs)
  - aspirin
  - bisphosphonates
  - steroids
  - erythromycin and other antibiotics
  - metformin
  - digoxin
  - calcium antagonists
  - theophyllines.

Many other drugs have the potential to cause dyspepsia and a temporal relationship to starting medication along with reference to the *British National Formulary* should be made.

- Family history. Gastric cancer is more common in individuals who have a first degree relative affected. Hereditary syndromes include:
  - hereditary non-polyposis colorectal cancer
  - hereditary diffuse gastric cancer
  - Peutz–Jeghers syndrome
  - Breast cancer genes *BRCA1* and *BRCA2* increase the risk of developing stomach cancer.

Alarm features

The following symptoms in association with dyspepsia are regarded as indicators of possible malignancy and mandate further assessment (NICE [2] and National guidance). However, the ability of these symptom criteria to predict major pathology is very limited. The current UK 'FastTrack' referral process for suspected upper gastrointestinal malignancy has a positive yield of only 4% [3].

- Iron deficiency anaemia
- Unexplained weight loss
- Persistent vomiting
- Dysphagia
- Abdominal mass

Examination

Clinical examination is often unrevealing in patients with dyspepsia. Epigastric tenderness is a very non-specific finding and does not necessarily indicate pathology. Careful palpation of the abdomen for an abdominal mass should be performed along with assessment for organomegaly and lymphadenopathy.

Differential diagnosis

1. *Biliary colic* typically causes intermittent severe right upper quadrant pain sometimes radiating

to the back, often associated with vomiting. The patient remains well between episodes. Ultrasound scanning of the upper abdomen should be performed if suspected.

2. *Cardiac disease*. Elderly patients in particular may present atypically with cardiac disease reporting symptoms of epigastric or lower retrosternal discomfort, often with 'functional' type symptoms of belching.

3. *Pancreatic disease*. Chronic pancreatitis is rare without a history of recurrent acute pancreatitis or chronic alcohol use. Pancreatic malignancy occurs typically over the age of 55 with a higher risk in male smokers. Pain is typically dull and constant, sometimes radiating to the back. If pancreatic disease is suspected, a CT abdomen is the investigation of choice.

4. *Mesenteric ischaemia*. Pain typically occurs 30–60 minutes after eating and is a deep gnawing pain that leads to a fear of eating and hence weight loss. This is usually associated with arterial disease elsewhere but can rarely be associated with anatomical abnormalities such as the median arcuate ligament syndrome. CT mesenteric angiography will clarify.

5. *Small bowel disease*. Small bowel enteropathy, e.g. coeliac disease, is often asymptomatic. Small bowel malignancy is extremely rare but can cause persistent abdominal discomfort, sometimes associated with colicky pain if a degree of obstruction is present.

6. *Colonic*. Rarely invasive tumours of the transverse colon can lead to epigastric discomfort or pain. Advanced pathology such as this will normally be evident on CT scanning.

7. *Abdominal wall/costochondral*. Abdominal wall herniation can cause localized pain. Costochondral and xiphisternal inflammation can cause constant discomfort in the epigastric area and mimic peptic pain. Examination reveals localized tenderness over the cartilage along the lower rib border.

Management of uninvestigated dyspepsia

Not all patients require endoscopic investigation and this is usually inappropriate for younger patients. The obvious concern is to exclude underlying malignancy and 'alarm symptoms' should be sought, accepting the limited value of these symptoms in predicting cancer.

Age is an important consideration in deciding whether to investigate further.

- Gastrointestinal malignancy is rare below the age of 50.
- Guidelines have suggested mandatory endoscopy in the presence of dyspepsia at various ages (45–55). However, the merits of this approach have not been formally studied despite widespread adoption.
- There is evidence to suggest that uncomplicated dyspepsia may be *negatively* associated with malignancy [3] and a systemic review [4] found no evidence that empirical treatment without endoscopy for simple dyspepsia was harmful compared with prompt endoscopy.

Empirical treatment is a reasonable option in the younger patient without alarm features. There are two main strategies:

1. Testing for *Helicobacter pylori* and treating if positive
2. Empirical proton pump inhibitor (PPI) therapy.

The strong association between *Helicobacter* and peptic ulcer disease has led to recommendations to adopt a test and treat strategy for dyspepsia. The merits of this approach are influenced by:

- Cost
- Prevalence of the organism in any given population
- Risk of serious disease such as gastric cancer.

Test and treat for *Helicobacter pylori* has been found to be as safe and effective as endoscopy in managing patients less than 55 with uncomplicated dyspepsia and is the preferred strategy adopted by the British Society of Gastroenterology and Scottish Intercollegiate Guidelines Network (SIGN) [5] (Figure 20.1). NICE guidance recommends *either* test and treat *or* empirical treatment with a PPI. These approaches are less invasive and costly than endoscopy.

Investigation

Upper gastrointestinal endoscopy (gastroscopy) is the investigation of choice for dyspepsia as it:

- is more sensitive and specific than barium meal
- allows biopsy of any mucosal lesion.

Approximately 1% of the UK population undergo gastroscopy annually. Diagnostic gastroscopy is a safe procedure with less than one in 1000 risk of complications. For diagnostic gastroscopy in patients with

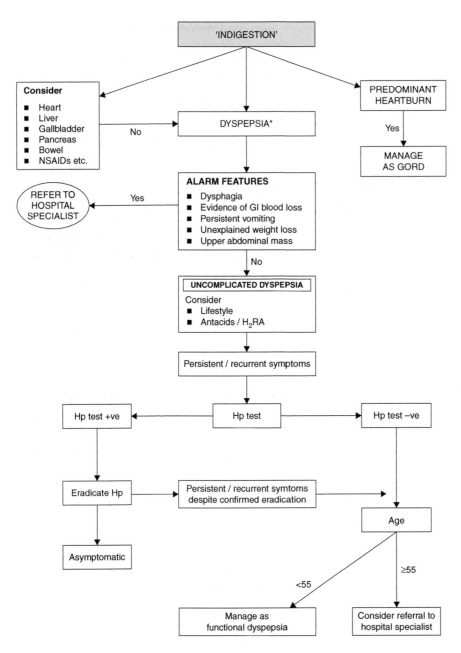

Figure 20.1 Algorithm for the investigation and management of dyspepsia (SIGN Guidelines [5]). Hp, *Helicobacter pylori*. H2RA: H2-receptor antagonist.

'INDIGESTION'

Consider
- Heart
- Liver
- Gallbladder
- Pancreas
- Bowel
- NSAIDs etc.

No → DYSPEPSIA*

PREDOMINANT HEARTBURN

Yes

MANAGE AS GORD

ALARM FEATURES
- Dysphagia
- Evidence of GI blood loss
- Persistent vomiting
- Unexplained weight loss
- Upper abdominal mass

Yes → REFER TO HOSPITAL SPECIALIST

No

UNCOMPLICATED DYSPEPSIA
Consider
- Lifestyle
- Antacids / H₂RA

Persistent / recurrent symptoms

Hp test +ve ← Hp test → Hp test –ve

Eradicate Hp → Persistent / recurrent symtoms despite confirmed eradication →

Asymptomatic

Age

<55 → Manage as functional dyspepsia

≥55 → Consider referral to hospital specialist

* Rome II definition

low morbidity, this risk is less than one in 10 000. These risks include:

- perforation
- bleeding
- aspiration pneumonia (particularly in frail elderly inpatients).

Other investigations include:

- full blood count, biochemistry, liver function tests
- ferritin B₁₂ folate (if anaemia)
- *Helicobacter pylori* testing (as per Figure 20.1)
- ultrasound scan of the biliary tree and pancreas if endoscopy is negative and symptoms do not respond to acid suppressant treatment.

Peptic ulceration

The two predominant risk factors for peptic ulcer disease are:

1. *Helicobacter pylori*
2. NSAIDs.

Helicobacter pylori

Around 80% of gastric ulcers and 95% of duodenal ulcers are associated with *Helicobacter* and can be cured by its eradication. *Helicobacter* is also associated with gastric cancer. *Helicobacter pylori* can be identified by:

- serology
- breath tests
- stool antigen
- biopsy for culture and urease test on a biopsy sample.

The population prevalence varies from 20% in Sweden to 40% in the United Kingdom to 80% in South America.

For patients with proven peptic ulceration:

- *Helicobacter pylori* eradication therapy should be offered if the organism is present.
- A 3- to 7-week course of PPI therapy should follow to ensure ulcer healing after the one-week treatment course for *Helicobacter*.
- Retesting for *Helicobacter* is not routinely recommended. However, if required, the C14 or C13 urea breath test is the investigation of choice with an accuracy of 95%. Serology is not recommended for retesting given the long period of time required for antibody titres to fall.

Non-steroidal anti-inflammatory drugs (NSAIDs)

- Up to 25% of patients taking NSAIDs will develop peptic ulceration and 2–4% will bleed or perforate. Age over 65 and the use of high dose NSAIDs significantly increase the risk of ulceration (odds ratio 4.7 and 8 respectively).
- These drugs should be used with caution in elderly patients and those with a past history of peptic ulceration.
- NSAIDs should be stopped where possible in patients with a diagnosed peptic ulcer and full dose PPI therapy should be given for 2 months.

- If *H. pylori* is present then this should be eradicated. This reduces the risk of ulcer recurrence but does not aid healing.

If patients need to take NSAIDs after a peptic ulcer has healed, this should be used with caution and if possible NSAIDs should be prescribed on an as required basis in minimal doses. Studies have shown ibuprofen and naproxen to be the least ulcerogenic NSAIDs. If NSAIDs need to be continued patients should be co-prescribed a PPI for gastric protection or consideration should be given to switching to a Cox-2 inhibitor.

Low dose aspirin is associated with a two- to four-fold increased risk of gastrointestinal bleeding. Furthermore, a large proportion of patients taking aspirin are elderly, have multiple co-morbidities and may be co-prescribed NSAIDs or anticoagulants. In patients admitted with bleeding peptic ulcers with coexistent cardiac disease necessitating the use of antiplatelet agents (e.g. cardiac stents), aspirin should be discontinued for as short a time as possible until bleeding has stopped and ideally less than 3 days. Low dose aspirin can then be recommenced with ongoing PPI therapy.

Gastro-oesophageal reflux (GORD)

Gastro-oesophageal reflux is one of the more common conditions encountered by both gastroenterologists and primary care physicians. The prevalence is approximately 10–20% in the Western world with troublesome heartburn seen in about 6% of the population. The classic symptoms of GORD are:

- heartburn
- regurgitation

but the condition can also lead to:

- dysphagia
- atypical chest pain
- chronic cough
- asthma
- laryngitis.

GORD may also contribute to dyspeptic symptoms such as:

- epigastric pain
- nausea
- belching
- bloating.

Diagnosis

A presumptive diagnosis of GORD can be made on the basis of the typical presentation with heartburn with or without regurgitation. Response to empirical treatment with a PPI is supportive evidence for the diagnosis. However, as has been seen previously, a symptom-based diagnosis and response to a PPI may not be reliable. One meta-analysis suggested sensitivity of 78% and a specificity of 54% for this approach.

Endoscopy has an excellent specificity for the diagnosis of GORD when oesophagitis is present. Unfortunately the large majority of patients will have 'non-erosive' GORD and an unremarkable endoscopy. Therefore the role of endoscopy in GORD is primarily to:

- exclude other diagnoses
- assess the severity of oesophagitis
- diagnose Barrett's oesophagus.

It is also helpful in assessing for any anatomical predisposition to reflux such as hiatal hernia and in the assessment of atypical chest pain with suspected GORD. Therefore endoscopy should be used selectively in the following patients:

- those with alarm symptoms
- elderly patients
- those at high risk of Barrett's oesophagus
- those with non-cardiac chest pain
- patients unresponsive to PPI.

Endoscopic evidence of oesophageal inflammation (oesophagitis) can be classified using the Los Angeles (LA) grading system with the least severe inflammation grade A and the most severe grade D. The more severe grades C and D may require maintenance therapy with a PPI to maintain healing whilst the lesser grades can be treated with short PPI courses (e.g. 4–8 weeks).

Barium studies of the oesophagus are unable to detect oesophagitis or Barrett's oesophagus and have largely been superseded by endoscopy. However, they remain helpful in the assessment of patients with dysphagia and oesophageal reflux to assess for dysmotility and oesophageal stricturing.

Ambulatory oesophageal pH monitoring is the investigation with greatest sensitivity and specificity for GORD. This can be performed either with a trans-nasal catheter, which is left in place for 24 hours, or with a telemetry capsule that is clipped to the distal oesophagus during an endoscopy. This can record for 48–96 hours. Patients record symptoms in a diary and this is correlated with reflux events. This is useful to ascertain whether reported symptoms are actually due to reflux episodes. pH monitoring has a important role in clarifying a diagnosis of GORD:

- When there is diagnostic doubt.
- When symptoms are refractory to PPI treatment.
- Before embarking on endoscopic or surgical therapy in patients with non-erosive GORD. In this situation it is usually combined with oesophageal manometry testing to exclude oesophageal dysmotility (e.g. achalasia), which would be a contraindication to surgical fundoplication. A number of endoscopic procedures have been developed to increase lower oesophageal pressure and treat GORD including injection of bulking agents at the lower oesophageal sphincter and radiofrequency ablation. Further data is required on the effectiveness of these approaches, which have not yet been accepted into routine practice.

Management

Uninvestigated patients with reflux type symptoms should be managed as for uninvestigated dyspepsia.

Lifestyle changes. Certain foods such as chocolate, caffeine, alcohol, acidic or spicy foods can lead to GORD through mechanisms that include lower oesophageal sphincter relaxation and delayed gastric emptying. Weight loss is recommended for patients who are overweight or who have had recent weight gain and the elevation of the head of the bed and avoidance of meals 2 hours before bedtime can help in patients with nocturnal GORD.

For patients with minor oesophagitis (LA grade A and B) or endoscopy negative patients with typical GORD symptoms, a 1- to 2-month course of a PPI should be offered.

- There is no major difference in efficacy of different PPIs and response is largely dose related.
- For patients with a partial response, increasing the dose (e.g. from 20 mg to 40 mg omeprazole) should be considered.
- PPI therapy will heal oesophagitis in approximately 80% of cases compared with 40% in patients taking H2-receptor antagonists.
- If symptoms recur following treatment then a maintenance PPI at the lowest dose necessary to control symptoms should be used. This may include using PPI therapy on an as required basis with patients managing their own symptoms.

It should be emphasized that GORD is a chronic relapsing condition (60–80% of patients will relapse within a year if treatment is discontinued) and many patients will require ongoing treatment to control their symptoms.

For patients with severe oesophagitis (LA grade C and D) and/or oesophageal stricturing due to reflux-induced inflammation, maintenance therapy is often required to prevent recurrent inflammation and further complications. Some patients with an inadequate response to a PPI may benefit from the addition of an H2-receptor antagonist or a prokinetic (e.g. domperidone) to PPI therapy.

Helicobacter pylori. The relationship between *Helicobacter* infection and GORD is controversial. Theoretically, *Helicobacter*-induced gastritis and achlorhydria should reduce reflux and eradication may increase the tendency to acid production but in practice this does not seem to occur. There is also concern about patients with *Helicobacter* receiving long-term maintenance therapy for GORD because of the risk of atrophic gastritis and its association with gastric cancer. For this reason European guidelines recommend eradication of *H. pylori* in this situation although American guidelines do not.

Surgical therapies for GORD. These include:

- laparoscopic fundoplication
- bariatric surgery in the obese.

A 12-year follow-up study of patients randomized to fundoplication or omeprazole showed approximate equivalence between these two options with 50% remaining in remission [6]. Surgery can be considered for patients who:

- do not wish to continue medical therapy
- develop side effects with drugs
- have volume regurgitation due to a large hiatal hernia
- have oesophagitis refractory to medical therapy.

Surgical therapy is *NOT* recommended in patients who:

- do not respond to PPI therapy
- have atypical symptoms such as non-cardiac chest pain
- do not have documented oesophagitis
- do not have evidence of reflux on ambulatory pH monitoring.

Barrett's oesophagus

This occurs when metaplastic columnar epithelium replaces the normal oesophageal stratified epithelium as a result of chronic acid exposure. The significance is that this change can predispose to oesophageal

adenocarcinoma with an annual incidence of 0.5% per year. However, most patients who have Barrett's oesophagus are undiagnosed and the risk for individuals undergoing endoscopic screening is significantly less than this. Furthermore the impact on life expectancy for an individual is very low and most patients with Barrett's oesophagus do not develop oesophageal malignancy.

Risk factors for Barrett's oesophagus

- Age greater than 50
- Male sex
- Caucasian
- Symptoms of chronic GORD
- Increased BMI

In this group there is a case for endoscopic screening for Barrett's oesophagus whereas general population screening is not recommended. Patients with documented Barrett's change should undergo endoscopic surveillance although the interval at which this should occur is controversial. Historically in the UK this has been biannually although recent American guidelines have recommended a 3- to 5-year surveillance interval.

Surveillance by endoscopic biopsies of the Barrett's segment can detect dysplasia which may predispose to oesophageal cancer. Dysplasia can be difficult to assess histologically, especially in the presence of inflammation, and so the presence of dysplasia should be confirmed by two pathologists following treatment of any associated inflammation.

- Low-grade dysplasia should undergo repeat assessment with multiple endoscopic biopsies within a 6- to 12-month period.
- High-grade dysplasia has a higher risk of a coincidental adenocarcinoma and patients should be considered for oesophagectomy or local ablative treatment.

Patients with Barrett's oesophagus should be maintained on a PPI although there is no evidence to suggest this reduces progression or cancer risk.

Functional dyspepsia

Functional dyspepsia is pain or discomfort centred on the upper abdomen for which no organic cause can be found. Functional dyspepsia is thus a diagnosis of exclusion that presupposes investigation of the patient, most commonly by endoscopy. This is important given the poor discrimination of symptom-based diagnoses in excluding significant pathology. The Rome III criteria subdivide functional dyspepsia into two syndromes:

- 'Epigastric pain syndrome' comprising intermittent pain and burning in the epigastric area
- 'Postprandial distress syndrome', which includes postprandial fullness and early satiety after meals.

It remains unclear whether these distinctions have any practical implications in terms of pathophysiology or treatment. Functional dyspepsia does overlap with non-erosive GORD and together they comprise the great majority of patients seen in both primary and secondary care with dyspeptic symptoms.

The mechanisms underlying functional dyspepsia include:

- delayed gastric emptying
- visceral hypersensitivity
- impaired fundic accommodation to meals
- duodenal hypersensitivity
- psychosocial factors.

Patients should be reassured and a full explanation of their symptoms given.

Management of symptoms can be difficult. There is probably a small benefit in eradicating *H. pylori* in functional dyspepsia but a Cochrane review indicated the number needed to treat was 17. PPI therapy is more effective, with a number needed to treat of 9. Prokinetic therapy may be of benefit but studies have been small and at present the evidence is inadequate. Low dose tricyclic antidepressants (e.g. amitriptyline) may be effective.

Scenario 20.1 continued

Cardiac pain can present atypically especially in the elderly; however, it is likely that this man is describing dyspeptic symptoms. He has a number of alarm features to his history: he has lost weight, has a microcytic anaemia and is over 50 years of age. He warrants an urgent endoscopy to exclude an upper GI malignancy combined with symptomatic treatment.

References

1. Rome III diagnostic criteria for functional gastrointestinal disorders 2006. www.romecriteria.org/criteria/

2. NICE. Dyspepsia: Managing dyspepsia in adults in primary care. NICE guidance 17. August 2004. Revised June 2005. www.nice.org.uk/nicemedia/live/10950/29460/29460.pdf.

3. Kapoor N et al. Predictive value of alarm features in a rapid access upper gastrointestinal cancer service. *Gut* 2005; 54(1): 40–45.

4. Ofman JJ, Rabeneck L. The effectiveness of endoscopy in the management of dyspepsia: a qualitative systematic review. *Am J Med* 1999; 106: 335–346.

5. Scottish Intercollegiate Guidelines Network (SIGN). Dyspepsia Guideline No 68. March 2003. www.sign.ac.uk/guidelines/fulltext/68/.

6. Spechler SJ, Lee E, Ahnen D, et al. Long-term outcome of medical and surgical therapies for gastroesophageal reflux disease: follow-up of a randomized controlled trial. *JAMA* 2001; 285: 2331–2338.

Further reading

American Gastroenterological Association. Technical review on the evaluation of dyspepsia. *Gastroenterology* 2005; 129: 1756–1780.

Katz PO, Gerson LB, Vela MF. Guidelines for the diagnosis and management of gastroesophageal reflux disease. *American Journal of Gastroenterology* 2013; 108: 308–328.

Talley NJ, Vakil N. Guidelines for the management of dyspepsia. *American Journal of Gastroenterology* 2005; 100: 2324–2337.

Chapter 21

Dysuria

Sathish Thomas William

Scenario 21.1

A 25-year-old male is seen in the ambulatory clinic. He complains of malaise, generalized joint aches and pains that move around. In particular his left knee and right elbow are painful and swollen. On careful questioning he admits having pain in the urethra on passing urine. He has had unprotected sex several times with a new girlfriend that he met 3–4 weeks previously.

Introduction

Dysuria is the sensation of pain or burning on urination. Dysuria is a common presentation seen in primary and secondary care. It is commonly due to infection and can manifest with:

- urethritis
- prostatitis
- epididymo-orchitis
- cystitis
- pelvic inflammatory disease
- upper urinary tract infection involving the kidneys and ureters.

Urinary tract infection (UTI) causing dysuria is one of the most common infectious diseases in community and hospital settings, with a high morbidity and high economic cost.

Aetiology

Dysuria could be related to infectious, inflammatory, malignancy, structural and sometimes unknown cause (Table 21.1).

Community-acquired urinary tract infections

- Most are due to ascending urethral infection and therefore much more common in women, with prevalence increasing with age.
- They are particularly common in pregnancy with sometimes adverse outcomes [2]:
  - Anatomical uterine changes cause pressure on ureters and anterior displacement of bladder.
  - Resulting urine stasis predisposes to infection.
  - Adverse outcomes: low birth weight, preterm delivery and neonatal mortality.

- *Escherichia coli* and *Staphylococcus saprophyticus* account for about 80% of infections, particularly in women under 50 years of age. *E. coli* is found to colonize the urinary tract more easily due to its presence in the intestinal flora and can cause ascending infections leading to pyelonephritis.
- Other pathogens include *Klebsiella* spp., *Proteus mirabilis*, *Enterococcus* species.
- Complicated urinary tract infections occur in patients with functional or anatomical abnormalities of the genitourinary tract and are associated with a broader range of infecting organisms (including multiple organisms) and increased risk of antibiotic resistance. Risk factors include:

  - male sex
  - elderly
  - hospital-acquired infection
  - pregnancy

Acute Medicine, ed. Stephen Haydock, Duncan Whitehead and Zoë Fritz. Published by Cambridge University Press.
© Cambridge University Press 2015.

Table 21.1 Common causes of dysuria (modified and adapted from Bremnor JD et al [1])

Infection	Conditions	Common causes
Non sexually transmitted	Urinary tract infection, pyelonephritis, cystitis, urethritis, prostatitis	*E. coli, S. saprophyticus, Proteus* spp., *Klebsiella* spp., *Haemophilus, Enterococcus* spp.
Sexually transmitted	Urethritis, epididymo-orchitis, cervicitis, pelvic inflammatory disease, prostatitis, sexually acquired reactive arthritis, disseminated gonococcal infection (rare)	Chlamydia, gonorrhoea, mycoplasma, ureaplasma, herpesvirus, *Trichomonas vaginalis*
Inflammatory	Drug-induced cystitis, eosinophilic cystitis Atrophic vaginitis, lichen sclerosus, spondyloarthropathies	NSAIDs, danazol, cyclophosphamide, acetyl salicylic acid Hypo-oestrogenaemia Reiter's syndrome
Malignancy	Urogenital malignancies	Bladder, prostate, vulval, vaginal, penile cancers
Miscellaneous	Trauma Psychogenic Urological malformations	Honeymoon cystitis, catheterization Anxiety and stress disorders, somatization disorders, hysteria Urinary outflow obstruction, benign prostatic hyperplasia, stones, diverticula

- indwelling catheters
- recent urinary tract intervention
- functional or anatomical abnormality of the urinary tract
- recent antimicrobial use
- symptoms for >7 days at presentation
- diabetes mellitus
- immunosuppression.

Sexually transmitted infections

- Dysuria secondary to lower genital tract infections in younger age groups is *strongly associated with sexually transmitted infections (STI)* with associated urethral discharge and testicular pain in males, and vaginal discharge, lower abdominal pain, dyspareunia and postcoital bleeding in women.
- The most common STIs in patients presenting with dysuria are chlamydia and gonorrhoea. Untreated these infections could cause a number of complications including pelvic inflammatory disease (PID), infertility, chronic pelvic pain, epididymo-orchitis and disseminated infections with high morbidity and cost.
- The most affected age groups are 16–25 years (females > males in the 15–19 year age group). Chlamydia and gonorrhoea comprised 64% and 54% of diagnoses made in this age group attending UK genitourinary medicine clinics in 2012.

- Recent significant increase in the diagnosis of gonorrhoea is seen within men having sex with men in the UK, including a 37% increase in gonorrhoea and 8% increase in chlamydia diagnoses in 2011 compared with the previous year.
- Rates of acute STI diagnoses vary according to the area of residence. In the UK highest rates are seen in urban areas, socially deprived and certain ethnic groups such as Black African and Black Caribbean. Cultural, economic and behavioural factors are also important.
- Sexually related urethritis causing dysuria is gonococcal, when *Neisseria gonorrhoeae* is detected and non-gonococcal (NGU) when *Neisseria gonorrhoeae* is not detected. The most common causes of NGU include:
  - *Chlamydia trachomatis* (40%)
  - *Mycoplasma genitalium* (25%)
  - *Ureaplasma urealyticum* (5–10%).
- Less commonly NGU may be due to other bacteria, e.g. *Neisseria meningitidis*, coliforms, *Haemophilus influenzae*; viruses, e.g. adenovirus, herpesvirus; protozoa, e.g. *Trichomonas vaginalis*; and fungal, e.g. candidiasis. In a small proportion of patients no obvious cause is found.
- Dysuria secondary to vulval or perineal lesions in women (e.g. from vulvovaginitis or herpes simplex virus infection) can be painful when lesions are exposed to urine.

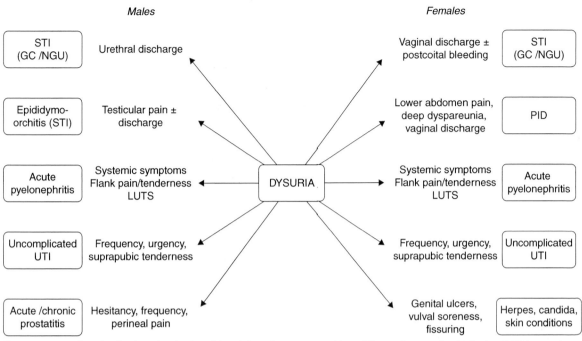

Figure 21.1 An algorithm for clinical evaluation of dysuria based on symptoms/signs. STI: sexually transmitted infection; LUTS: lower urinary tract symptoms; GC/NGU: gonococcal/non-gonococcal urethritis; PID: pelvic inflammatory disease; UTI: urinary tract infection.

Other causes

Inflammatory causes include urethral strictures, irritation, foreign bodies, allergic reactions, medications, spondyloarthropathy, renal stones and urogenital malignancies. In older men urinary symptoms secondary to benign prostatic hyperplasia can be a cause.

Clinical presentation

The evaluation of a patient with dysuria should be led by careful history correlated with examination findings and relevant investigation. A sexual history is important to know the likelihood of a sexually related infection and timing of infection. A clinical examination should include looking for systemic signs of disseminated infection or upper urinary tract infection. Vital signs should be recorded. A genital examination should be performed (see Chapter 25). Figure 21.1 gives an algorithm for clinical evaluation of dysuria.

The site and timing of pain often leads to the cause of dysuria. Pain felt in the distal urethra and during micturition suggests anterior urethral pathology. *Suprapubic with post-micturition pain* suggests posterior urethral or bladder pathology.

Systemic features of pyrexia, rigors and loin pain are seen in acute pyelonephritis.

Urinary frequency is most often caused by decreased bladder capacity or painful bladder distension. Less commonly it may be due to overflow secondary to BPH, urethral pathology and central or peripheral neurological disorder.

Urinary hesitation and slow urination are most commonly caused by urethral obstruction or decreased bladder contractility.

Urinary urgency occurs as a result of inflammation of the bladder (cystitis) and trigonal or posterior urethral irritation caused by stones or tumour. Urgency and frequency with systemic symptoms is usually a marker of upper urinary tract infections.

A bloody discharge, as distinct from haematuria or haematospermia, raises concern about urethral carcinoma, an uncommon condition.

Women with vaginal soreness can present with dysuria when urine passes by the site. Therefore it is important to differentiate if the pain is external or internal while passing urine. Vulval or vaginal soreness is seen with candidiasis, ulcerations due to herpes and non-infectious inflammatory skin conditions.

Gonorrhoea or NGU in men is characterized by urethral discharge and dysuria.

- Incubation period for gonorrhoea is shorter (3–7 days) than for *Chlamydia trachomatis* (around 2 weeks).
- Gonorrhoeal discharge is typically yellowish green and copious.
- >80% of men with gonorrhoea are symptomatic compared to 50% of women.
- Infections due to chlamydia or other NGU-related organisms cause a mucoid or clear discharge. Early morning discharge with or without dysuria is also seen with these organisms.
- Co-infections with both gonorrhoea and chlamydia are not uncommon.
- Presence of tender epididymis or testis in men and of deep dyspareunia in women with lower abdominal pain suggests epididymo-orchitis and PID, respectively, a complication of gonorrhoea or chlamydia infection.
- Intermenstrual bleeding or menorrhagia is not associated with gonorrhoea.

Disseminated gonoccocal infection is rare and presents with skin rash, arthralgia, tenosynovitis, arthritis and lower urinary tract symptoms.

Acute and chronic bacterial prostatitis presents with perineal pain, lower urinary tract symptoms including frequency, dysuria and hesitancy and swollen or tender prostate. (Prostatic massage is contraindicated in acute prostatitis due to risk of sepsis.)

Sexually acquired reactive arthritis (SARA) is an immune inflammatory response, commonly due to chlamydia that presents with a triad of urethritis, conjunctivitis and arthritis. Other manifestations include psoriasiform rash affecting palms and soles, tenosynovitis, enthesitis and circinate balanitis.

Dysuria secondary to herpes simplex virus is disproportionately severe compared with the amount of discharge seen. Regional lymphadenopathy and constitutional symptoms usually coexist.

Trichomonas vaginalis is a relatively uncommon cause of dysuria in men and is more prevalent in Black African ethnic groups. The urethral discharge is scanty and may be associated with tingling sensation of the urethra.

Ureteric stones could present with colic pain, haematuria and sometimes dysuria.

A detailed drug history is important to rule out drug-induced cystitis.

Management

Investigation

Investigation should be tailored towards the most likely cause.

- Urinalysis and a mid-stream urine sample is indicated in non-STI-related infections.
- The sensitivity of urine dipstick to diagnose UTI is around 80% if positive for white cells or nitrites and with one or more symptoms. A negative urine dipstick does not rule out an infection. A recent review article found only positive nitrite had a significant likelihood ratio to detect UTI (LR 7.5–24.5) and a negative leucocyte esterase ruled out UTI (LR 0.2).
- A positive urine culture usually has a colony growth of 10^5; however, lower values are equally sensitive and specific with ongoing symptoms. In the presence of symptoms, a colony forming unit of $\geq 10^2$ has high sensitivity and specificity [3]. Sterile pyuria may be present in patients with prostatitis, nephrolithiasis, urological neoplasms, and fungal or mycobacterial infections. Recent advances in PCR technology (sensitivity and specificity >99%) have simplified testing for chlamydia and gonorrhoea. A first catch urine in males and a vulvovaginal swab (self taken) or endocervical swab should be sent for chlamydia and gonorrhoea in patients with sexual risks.
- Routine testing for mycoplasma or ureaplasma is not available in all centres in UK.
- In men with urethral discharge, a Gram stain urethral slide (sensitivity 90–95%) and in women an endocervical slide (sensitivity <50%) make an immediate diagnosis of gonorrhoea [4].
- Cultures for gonorrhoea are gold standard and although sensitivity is low, in view of increasing resistance to many antimicrobials, it should be sent in PCR-positive cases or before treatment in suspected cases.
- NGU is diagnosed microscopically (urethral smears with >5 polymorphs per high power field).
- In women with external dysuria, cultures for candidal infection or a swab for herpes simplex

Table 21.2 Treatment for dysuria

Community-acquired lower UTI	Trimethoprim 200 mg bd 3 days or Nitrofurantoin 50 mg qds 3 days
Acute pyelonephritis	Ciprofloxacin 500 mg bd 7 days or Co-amoxiclav 625 mg bd 14 days
Non-gonococcal urethritis	Azithromycin 1 g PO stat or Doxycycline 100 mg bd 7 days
Gonorrhoea	Inj ceftriaxone 500 mg IM stat with azithromycin 1 g PO stat
Acute or chronic bacterial prostatitis	Ciprofloxacin 500 mg bd for 28 days or Ofloxacin 200 mg bd for 28 days If allergic to quinolones: trimethoprim 200 mg bd for 28 days

PCR with syphilis serology in the presence of genital ulcerations should be considered.

- Systemically unwell and/or immunocompromised patients would need a blood culture.
- Radiological imaging of the renal tract in recurrent infections or non-responders to antibiotics should be considered to rule out:
  - focal infections
  - anatomical anomalies
  - obstruction
  - prostatic involvement.

Treatment

Treatment of dysuria depends on the likely diagnosis (Table 21.2). The current guidelines [5] suggest:

- Empirical treatment with an antibiotic for otherwise healthy women aged less than 65 years of age presenting with severe or >3 symptoms of lower UTI (LUTI).
- In non-pregnant women a 3-day course of trimethoprim or nitrofurantoin is indicated or a 7-day course of ciprofloxacin if upper urinary tract infection is suspected.
- In pregnant women a 7-day course of amoxicillin, cephalexin or nitrofurantoin is recommended. In men with uncomplicated UTI, the antimicrobial recommendations are similar to women.
- In acute pyelonephritis and prostatitis, fluoroquinolones are recommended.

- In areas with >10% resistance to first-line agents, alternative drugs should be considered.
- With increasing incidence of MRSA and *C. difficile*, broad spectrum antibiotics should be avoided in uncomplicated LUTI.
- If recurrent symptoms of dysuria, antibiotics need to be modified based on culture reports or local microbiology advice.
- If STI is suspected, a single dose of azithromycin 1 g would treat chlamydia, mycoplasma and ureaplasma.
- Gonorrhoea has shown resistance to penicillins, sulphonamides, quinolones and tetracyclines. There is evidence of increasing minimum inhibitory concentration to cephalosporin and therefore current guidelines recommend a third generation cephalosporin with azithromycin (Inj ceftriaxone 500 mg intramuscular stat dose with azithromycin 1 g PO stat). Partner treatment is important to avoid reinfection of the patient and to treat undiagnosed STI in the community. A referral to sexual health or genitourinary clinics would facilitate the partner notification, treatment and test of cure. A general counselling on safe sex and avoidance of sexual intercourse for at least 1 week and until partners are treated is recommended for gonorrhoea and NGU. Non-infectious causes of dysuria need managing with other relevant specialties.
- Referral to urology is required if a diagnosis of urological malformation, urodynamic dysfunction is made.

Prevention of recurrent urinary infection

Recurrent urinary infections can be a significant problem in women. Management includes:

- Avoiding diaphragm/spermicide methods of contraception
- Switching from tampons to pads
- Cranberry juice may be beneficial
- Good toilet hygiene and postcoital voiding
- Elderly women may benefit from vaginal oestrogen creams
- Low dose antimicrobial prophylaxis
- Patient-directed antimicrobial therapy at symptom onset.

References

1. Bremnor JD, Sadovsky R. Evaluation of dysuria in adults. *Am Fam Physician* 2002; 65(8): 1589–1596.

2. Krcmery S, Hromec J, Demesova D. Treatment of lower urinary tract infection in pregnancy. *Int J Antimicrob Agents* 2001; 17(4): 279–282.

3. Meister L, Morley EJ, Scheer D, et al. History and physical examination plus laboratory testing for the diagnosis of adult female urinary tract infection. *Acad Emerg Med* 2013; 20(7): 631–645.

4. Barlow D, Phillips I. Gonorrhoea in women: diagnostic, clinical and laboratory aspects. *Lancet* 1978; i: 761–764.

5. Scottish Intercollegiate Guidelines Network (SIGN). Management of suspected bacterial urinary tract infection in adults. Edinburgh: SIGN; 2012. (SIGN publication no. 88). (July 2012). Available from www.sign.ac.uk.

Chapter

22

Falls

Lucy Pollock

Introduction

Falls in the elderly are common. Every year, over 500 000 older people attend the ED in the UK following a fall. Falls produce injury, distress and fear, and often lead to loss of functional independence.

It is useful to consider the concept of *'life space diameter'* – how much space a person moves through as they carry out the activities of their day. For the fit and affluent, life space diameter is unlimited, and surfing in Sumatra is a realistic possibility. With increasing frailty, this diameter shrinks. For an active elderly woman, a hip fracture may mean she never takes another walking holiday. Later, after a fall whilst shopping she loses the confidence to use public transport. A fall in the garden renders her housebound. Finally after another hip fracture, she moves into a nursing home, where her space has diminished to the triangle of bed, chair and commode.

Presentation to hospital represents an opportunity to intervene in this unhappy progression. The risk of future falls (and fractures) can be reduced, as can loss of confidence and function. A fall is usually produced by a combination of impairment in several physiological systems at once, often with interplay of social and environmental factors. These patients deserve a methodical approach.

Elderly patients who have fallen recover better, with a reduced risk of further falls, if they are managed using a multifactorial falls risk assessment. This approach is mandated by NICE, recognizing that comprehensive geriatric assessment improves outcomes for older patients in many settings. To the hard-pressed junior doctor in ED or MAU, the idea of tackling a comprehensive assessment is daunting, but we serve the patient well by looking beyond the presenting injury, considering why the fall happened and what can be done to prevent future events. Doctors assessing patients who have fallen should be familiar with local services such as falls or syncope clinics, together with mechanisms for access to social work and therapy assessment in hospital and on discharge.

> ### Scenario 22.1
>
> *Mrs F, an 84-year-old woman, is referred by the emergency department to MAU following a fall. She was found on the kitchen floor. She has hip pain, but X-rays in the ED show no fracture. The ED notes mention that she is 'vague' and 'smells strongly of urine'. Her observations are stable.*

This scenario feels familiar. The easy diagnosis of urinary tract infection is tempting. However, stale urine, infected or not, smells strong, and an episode of incontinence certainly does not indicate infection. It's likely that a UTI, if present, is only part of the picture. A more complete history and examination will reveal other factors contributing to the fall.

History

Remember that confusion, acute or chronic, can be easily overlooked. Always check whether the patient is cognitively intact – if not, is this a delirium or a dementia picture?

- Use a validated tool to document cognition, even in those who appear cognitively intact: the 10-point AMTS (see Chapter 16) is an easy quick test. Otherwise you will be caught out at some point by a charming elderly patient with an excellent social facade, who answers your questions fluently but turns out to be living in a parallel universe on the consultant ward round.

Acute Medicine, ed. Stephen Haydock, Duncan Whitehead and Zoë Fritz. Published by Cambridge University Press. © Cambridge University Press 2015.

- In the cognitively intact patient, a validated score makes an invaluable baseline, should a delirious illness develop later.

What is the key information?

- What was the mechanism of the fall?
- Were there any symptoms prior to her fall?
- Might she have lost consciousness? Were there witnesses? What did she look like? How long did it take for her to recover?
- Amnesia for syncope is recognized – ask if she remembers actually hitting the floor.
- Did she get her hands out to break her fall?
- Broken glasses or facial injuries suggest transient loss of consciousness.
- What is her usual mobility like?
- Has she any conditions that predispose to falls, e.g. cerebrovascular disease, Parkinson's disease, diabetes or arthritis?
- Current medication? Recent changes?
- Alcohol history? ('Do you usually have a glass of wine or something like that?' is more likely to elicit a frank response than 'How much alcohol do you drink?' – then ask tactful questions to clarify quantity.)
- Has she fallen before? How often, and why?
- What is her social situation?
- Has she lost confidence?

How do we obtain this information?

- The patient may be able to give a complete history.
- Witness accounts are valuable, especially when confusion or syncope is present.
- A phone call to a residential or nursing home pays dividends, especially as you can also establish whether there are concerns about the patient being discharged.
- Her GP may supply details, including a medication history.
- Whenever possible, look at old notes, previous discharge summaries or clinic letters.

Mechanical fall: try to avoid using this phrase *without a specific description of the event*. It is an over-used expression, implying that no further thought is necessary about the cause of the fall or what can be done to prevent further events! Always clarify what you mean. Consider two patients with Colles' fracture, both labelled as 'mechanical fall'. One had a single fall due to ice on the way to her Zumba class, and is otherwise active and independent. She is a completely different kettle of fish from the next patient, who has tripped over a rug, walks with a stick, has fallen twice in the last 6 months and is rapidly losing confidence.

> **Scenario 22.1 continued**
>
> *She has type 2 diabetes, hypertension, a total knee replacement, and had a stroke with mild residual weakness several years ago. Her vision is limited and her daughter worries that she may have had 'hypos'. She has felt dizzy for months, and has had two other falls in recent weeks. Her medication includes ramipril, amlodipine, clopidogrel, metformin, gliclazide, furosemide, bendroflumethiazide, betahistine and co-codamol. She is unsure whether she lost consciousness, or whether she simply lost her balance – she certainly hit her head as she fell.*

Dizziness is common, and produces grave misunderstanding between patients and doctors. Doctors often assume that dizziness means 'vertigo', but patients, especially the elderly, are rarely referring to true rotational vertigo. They more often mean:

- They feel unsteady (specifically that their balance is poor), or
- They feel light-headed.
- Sometimes, 'I feel dizzy' is more non-specific: it may mean 'I'm frightened of falling' or 'I don't want to leave my house in case something bad happens'.

Elicit the details of dizziness in a careful order: if you start by asking 'Do you mean everything's moving around you?' you will probably get a false positive response:

- Ask first whether the patient feels unsteady or off balance when they stand.
- Then ask 'Do you ever get a light-headed feeling when you stand, as if you might be going to faint?'
- Finally ask 'Do you ever feel that the room's spinning around you, as if you stepped off a playground roundabout?'
- You are much more likely to find that your patient has poor balance or feels light-headed, than true vertigo.

True vertigo, whilst rare, is important and presents a diagnostic challenge. Broadly, we need to decide whether the patient has a

- *peripheral cause*, e.g. benign paroxysmal positional vertigo or vestibular neuritis
- *central cause*, e.g. cerebellar stroke.

The detailed assessment of the patient with vertigo is discussed in Chapter 63.

Transient loss of consciousness (TLoC) or syncope is discussed in Chapter 61. In the elderly remember that 'vasovagal' episodes (true faints) account for a lower proportion of TLoC: cardiac syncope and postural hypotension should be considered. TLoC should not be called 'vasovagal' without presence of all the '3 P's':

- *Positional* – fainting happens whilst standing; TLoC whilst sitting is not a faint.
- *Provoked* – for example, by pain or strong emotion, not happening 'out of the blue'.
- *Prodrome* should be present – the patient describes how they felt bad for a few seconds before losing consciousness.

If in any doubt, refer to a geriatric, cardiology, or TLoC clinic for further investigation.

- Older patients with pulmonary embolism may present with syncope. Don't ignore low oxygen saturation results unless they are explained by other known pathology.
- The patient with unexplained loss of consciousness is *NOT* allowed to drive until investigations either suggest a very low risk of recurrence or allow a cause to be treated. This often causes upset and should be explained tactfully.

Medication review

Medications are implicated in many falls, and rigorous review is necessary. To reduce the risk of further falls, each medication must be scrutinized, and its benefit weighed up against potential side effects. Pay particular attention to the following:

Postural hypotension

- All antihypertensive drugs (including alpha-blockers like doxasozin or tamsulosin prescribed for benign prostatic hyperplasia)
- Antianginals
- All antidepressants (even small doses of common SSRIs can cause symptomatic postural hypotension)
- Antiparkinsonian drugs (a 'double whammy' as Parkinson's itself is associated with autonomic neuropathy).

Extrapyramidal side effects (parkinsonism)

- All antipsychotic medications can produce extrapyramidal side effects, as can
- Some unexpected but commonly prescribed medicines such as metoclopramide (Maxolon) and prochlorperazine (Stemetil)
- Most antiepileptic drugs (watch for gabapentin or pregabalin prescribed for neuropathic pain)
- Lithium.

Weakness (asthenia)

- Oral steroids can produce profound myopathy.
- Calcium channel blockers such as amlodipine are culprits, and can also provoke tremor.

Hypoglycaemics

- Elderly patients with tight diabetes control fall over four times more frequently than those allowed to run higher sugars.
- Metformin can be associated with B_{12} deficiency and neurological deficit.

Sedatives

- These include opiates and sleeping tablets.
- Look for opiate patches – often they are not amongst the boxes of medicines with the patient.

There is overlap with medications that cause delirium: *if a drug stops someone thinking straight, they won't be able to walk straight either!*

Stopping some drugs abruptly can provoke important withdrawal effects. Getting medication right requires skill and experience, and the 'complex' faller is likely to need a review by a geriatrician.

Scenario 22.1 continued

In Mrs F's case, we now wonder whether her dizziness has been due to postural hypotension, a result of her multiple cardiac medications, or whether she's been having hypoglycaemic events as her daughter suspects – or both.

Mrs F's Abbreviated Mental Test Score is 9/10. Her JVP is visible but not raised; her heart sounds are normal and her chest clear. She has ankle oedema. Abdominal examination is unremarkable. Her cranial nerves are intact; she has mild left-sided weakness, with limitation due to pain in her hip, and her left plantar is up-going. There's no sensory level. Her knee joints are arthritic and she has hallux valgus and corns. There's a non-blanching area of redness over her sacrum. She is able to stand with help but doesn't feel able to walk. Her blood pressure drops from 140 systolic to 115 when she stands: she feels very unsteady.

Examination

What are we looking for?

Given the myriad contributors to falls in the elderly, and given that many of these will coexist, *our patient clearly needs a thorough systems examination*. As well as looking for *causes* of her fall, we must check for *consequences* too. Pay particular attention to the following:

Neurological examination

- Has a stroke caused her to fall?
- Has the fall resulted in a subdural haematoma?
- A spinal cord lesion could either produce or result from a fall.
- Check visual acuity by covering each eye in turn, making sure the patient can read large print and hasn't got a significant field defect.

Musculoskeletal examination

- Is there joint instability that caused her to fall?
- Has she sustained a fracture?
- Look at her feet, and her footwear.

Examine the gait: If the patient can get out of bed, always ask to see them walk. You're looking for:

- Parkinsonism or ataxia
- Generalized or focal weakness, and pain
- You will see how confident your patient is, and will quickly get a feel for whether it's likely to be safe to discharge her directly from the ED or MAU.

(*Neurological and musculoskeletal examinations* should be performed when a patient is unable to walk steadily unaided. You may not be able to perform a textbook assessment, but listen to the history carefully and try not to miss signs of cord compression, stroke or fracture.)

Skin examination

- Examination of the skin is important, and often omitted.
- Our scenario patient has been on the floor for some time and already has a grade 1 sore (unbroken skin but non-blanching erythema). Given her age, immobility and cardiac failure, she's at high risk of skin breakdown.
- Always check skin, especially heels and sacrum, and highlight your findings to nurses so that they can provide a pressure-relieving mattress and heel lift boots, and turn her regularly.

- The development of a pressure sore can be compared to reversing a car hard into a wall: the cost and complexity of resolving the problem is much greater than the time it takes for the initial injury. *But* the analogy ends there, as the human cost of a pressure sore is infinitely greater than that of a damaged car, and a sore that develops over a few hours in the Emergency Department can prove fatal: *80% of elderly patients with a grade 4 pressure sore will be dead within 6 months.*

Cardiovascular examination

(See syncope and presyncope, Chapter 61.) In particular watch out for:

- Hypotension
- Cardiac murmur of aortic stenosis (with low volume and slow rising pulse)
- Carotid sinus massage in the ED or MAU can be performed in those with TLoC: reproduction of symptoms with a pause of 3 or more seconds, or the development of AV nodal block, in the context of a history of syncope, is a class A indication for pacing.

Postural blood pressure: there is no agreed standard for this:

- Lie the patient flat if possible, for 20 minutes before baseline blood pressure.
- Measure blood pressure on standing *and* after 2 or 3 minutes.
- If it continues to fall, keep re-measuring until a nadir is reached.
- A systolic drop of at least 20 mmHg, or to below 90 mmHg, or a diastolic drop of 10 mmHg, is significant, *especially accompanied by symptoms.*
- Absence of a postural drop on a single occasion doesn't mean that the patient does not get postural hypotension.

Generalized weakness (common)

- Concurrent illness
- Malignancy
- Electrolyte imbalance
- Medications (especially high dose steroids, which can rapidly produce a proximal myopathy, and drugs known to cause asthenia or weakness)
- Nutritional deficiencies. There are no good studies of vitamin C status in the elderly, but those with a poor diet must be at risk, and certainly some frail patients with muscle weakness seem to respond

very well simply to being fed properly, with or without vitamin supplements.

Continence

- Incontinence is associated with falls (and fractures).
- Often shared pathology such as neurodegenerative disease, or treatment with alpha-blockers producing both postural hypotension and sphincter weakness.
- Having to rush for the toilet and struggling with pads puts the vulnerable patient into situations where the ability to remain upright is overwhelmed.
- Every incontinent patient deserves a proper assessment: you can start the process with a brief targeted history and examination, urinalysis and bladder scan to assess post-void residual volume. Refer your patient to the local continence service.

Investigations

Investigations should be guided by the clinical picture. Sometimes none at all are required: *The fit 76-year-old who slipped whilst ice skating with her grandchildren does not need blood tests!*

If the cause of the fall is unclear, or the patient has repeated falls, sensible investigations would include the following:

Blood tests

- FBC
- Glucose
- Urea and electrolytes (plus creatinine)
- LFTs
- TFTs
- Calcium

Mild derangements are common and may not be significant, e.g. chronic mild hyponatraemia, but note that *even mild hypokalaemia can contribute to muscle weakness.*

Urine dipstick

- Results should be interpreted cautiously as blood and protein are common findings and do not indicate infection.
- Negative results for both leucocyte esterase and nitrites rule out urinary tract infection with 95% sensitivity.

- Specificity rates are lower, so a positive result for either does not reliably indicate infection.

Electrocardiogram

- Particularly useful in the context of syncope.

Investigations to avoid

These include D-dimer and troponin measurements without a high clinical suspicion of thromboembolic disease or myocardial infarction. Unless the patient has new hypoxia, cardiac chest pain or evolving ischaemic ECG changes, these tests have high false positive rates, and can initiate a damaging spiral of unnecessary investigation and treatment.

Radiological investigations

- May include a chest X-ray depending on the clinical picture, and X-rays to exclude bony injury.
- Remember that hip fractures are not always visible on initial films, 3–4% being occult.
- Offer magnetic resonance imaging (MRI) if hip fracture is suspected despite negative anteroposterior pelvis and lateral hip X-rays.
- If prompt MRI is not available or is contraindicated, consider computed tomography (CT).

When is a CT head necessary?

The incidence and mortality rate of subdural haemorrhage and other intracranial bleeding increase with age. However, not everyone who has had a fall needs scanning.

Urgent CT head is indicated in:

- those with new focal neurology following a fall.

Consider CT head in:

- delirium after a fall when no other cause for acute confusion is apparent.

Have a lower threshold for scanning in:

- anticoagulated patients (look out for novel oral anticoagulants such as rivaroxaban, dabigatran and apixaban)
- those with a bleeding tendency such as thrombocytopenia or raised INR
- those with a previous intracranial bleed.

Avoid CT head (especially repeated imaging):

- in patients with dementia who have fallen *unless there is* a history of a noticeable step down in cognition not explained by disease progression, infection, medication or environmental change

- in the very frail, consider whether the findings of a CT scan will alter management: an honest conversation with family members may reasonably lead to a plan to avoid investigations that are not going to improve the patient's well-being.

Management and ensuring safe discharge

In addition to management of specific problems identified during the clinical assessment, address the following points.

Analgesia

- When needed, prescribe paracetamol (regularly in the cognitively impaired, who do not ask for medication).
- If using opiates always co-prescribe a regular laxative, and be prepared for delirium.
- Use NSAIDs cautiously and avoid if possible in renal impairment, congestive cardiac failure, microcytic anaemia or upper GI disease.

VTE prophylaxis

- Evidence in the frail elderly is limited [1].
- Try to weigh up the risk of VTE and balance that against the burden of treatment, especially in those near the end of life. A thin, very demented woman covered in bruises is not likely to benefit from daily enoxaparin injections.

Treating osteoporosis

- In fragility fracture, it's usually best to ask the patient and their GP to consider osteoporosis treatment: there are many options, with side effects and compliance issues requiring a tailored approach.
- Arrange a DEXA bone scan for under-75s.
- Make use of the fracture liaison service if you have one available.

Therapy assessments

- Early therapy assessment in the ED or MAU is effective. Therapists facilitate early discharge and

can initiate rehabilitation for those who need admitting. They can often judge whether the patient needs assessment by a geriatrician whilst still an inpatient and what outpatient follow-up should be offered (falls clinics, therapy and support at home).
- The OPAL (Older Patients Assessment and Liaison) model of care, offering early multidisciplinary assessment for frail patients, has been demonstrated to reduce length of stay [2]. (See also Chapter 33.)

Same day discharge

Many patients who present following a fall can be safely discharged the same day from the ED or MAU with appropriate follow-up. These include:

- Patients with transient loss of consciousness/syncope: following a full recovery, the patient may go home with prompt follow-up in a falls or TLoC clinic. Exceptions include those with exertional syncope, recent MI or a history of malignant arrhythmia who should be discussed with a cardiologist or admitted.
- Patients who are mobile, cognitively intact and confident.
- Patients who come from a nursing or residential home, who are back to their usual level of mobility (but see pitfalls explained below).
- Some patients with dementia and good social support.

Pitfalls in discharging patients who have fallen

- *Do not discharge* a patient who is haemodynamically unstable.
- *Do not discharge* home a patient who is unable to get out of bed and walk safely, unless you have had a detailed conversation with the family and carers about the level of support available. Families caring for a patient who is very frail, or has terminal illness or dementia, may be rightly keen to avoid admission. They may be able to manage at home, but you must ensure that they have adequate support. Assessment by an OPAL-type team may help. Urgent referrals to social services, palliative care teams, and community therapy teams may be needed. Document family conversations and referrals carefully and ensure

the GP has a prompt, informative discharge summary – a phone call is usually gratefully received.

- *Discharging a patient back to residential care* can be tricky. It is frustrating when a home refuses to take back a resident on the grounds that their mobility isn't good enough, but staffing levels are lower in residential than in nursing care, and there are legal constraints which mean that residential homes are not permitted to care for people beyond a certain level of dependency. A patient needing the help of two people to transfer from bed to chair will not usually be able to return to a residential home. We may need to arrange a period of rehabilitation (think community hospital, intermediate care, or a step-up bed in a nursing home). If the history is of a gradual decline, without a reversible cause, referral to social services starts the assessments for transfer to a nursing home.

Recognizing falls as a sign of neglect or abuse

- Occasionally, a fall may reflect neglect or abuse. A demented husband may be struggling to care for his frail, unsteady wife. He cancels care because of concerns about cost, and refuses adaptations to their home that would make her safer.
- Most hospitals have a staff member responsible for safeguarding adults: contact them, or refer to social services.
- Where there is concern about care in a residential or nursing home, document carefully all signs that could be consistent with poor care, such as general cleanliness of the patient and her clothing, the state of pressure areas, the age and distribution of bruises.
- *Don't jump to conclusions*: very unsteady wandering patients may fall repeatedly in the best homes, a pad will be wet after a few hours in ED, bruises on wrists and shins may reflect senile purpura (see Chapter 13), *but highlight your concerns to a senior and to social services*.
- Rarely, a fall may reflect criminal activity by family, carers or strangers. If you are worried, talk to the safeguarding team, social services or the police.

Arranging appropriate follow-up after discharge

- Many hospitals have an established pathway from ED/MAU to falls clinics which provide multifactorial assessment, strength and balance training and home hazard assessment and intervention.
- Use this pathway or refer to Care of the Elderly for outpatient review. Patients who are well and have sustained a single, clearly explained fall, and those who are extremely frail may not benefit – but it's usually best to make a referral including as much detail as possible so that the falls team can decide what to offer. Consider referral for social care assessment.

Communication with GPs and other agencies

- Include all relevant information in your discharge summary, highlighting medication changes and any need for further action such as clinic referrals and osteoporosis assessment.
- Give the patient a copy.

Support for the patient on discharge

- Explain plans carefully, and provide written information about measures the patient can take to prevent further falls, and where they can seek further advice and assistance.

And finally!

Coming to hospital with a fall is a life-changing event for many older people. On leaving your care, the patient or their family should feel confident that you have found out why they fell, and done everything possible to prevent another event.

That's hard work, but rewarding: it makes a real difference.

Scenario 22.1 continued

Mrs F's gliclazide, betahistine, amlodipine and furosemide are stopped, and ramipril is halved. Her 'dizziness' resolves. She is discharged home with the support of a community rehabilitation team who work to improve her balance and core strength. Her confidence improves and she is able to resume her weekly shopping trip with her daughter.

References

1. Greig M, Rochow S, Crilly M, Mangoni A (2013) Routine pharmacological venous thromboembolism prophylaxis in frail older hospitalised patients: where is the evidence? *Age and Ageing* 42: 428–434.

2. Harari D, Martin F, Buttery A, O'Neill S, Hopper A. (2007) The older persons' assessment and liaison team 'OPAL': evaluation of comprehensive geriatric assessment in acute medical inpatients. *Age and Ageing* 36: 670–675.

Further reading

NICE Clinical Guideline CG161 (2013) Falls: assessment and prevention of falls in older people. Available to download at www.nice.org.uk/nicemedia/live/14181/64166/64166.pdf.

NICE Clinical Guideline CG124 (2011) The management of hip fracture in adults. Available to download at www.nice.org.uk/nicemedia/live/13489/54919/54919.pdf.

Chapter

23

Fever

Daniel E. Greaves and Sani H. Aliyu

Introduction

Fever is one of the most common presenting complaints both on the wards and in the MAU. Patients may present with other symptoms and signs which point towards the cause, but often this is not the case. A thorough history and careful examination, alongside knowledge of the common causes of fever and their differentiation, are important to allow the most relevant investigations to be selected. It is equally important to rapidly identify febrile patients who are very unwell and need urgent treatment, as well as those who pose an infection risk to others and therefore require isolation.

Pathophysiology of fever

Prostaglandin E2 (PGE2) release in the hypothalamus is stimulated by:

- *Endogenous pyrogens*: cytokines including IL-1, IL-6 and TNF, which are released in response to inflammation, infection and trauma.
- *Exogenous pyrogens*: either present on the coat of bacteria (lipopolysaccharide present on all Gram-negative bacteria) or secreted as toxins (by Gram-positive bacteria such as *Staphylococcus aureus* and *Streptococcus pyogenes*).

Elevated PGE2 levels in the anterior hypothalamus (the body's thermostat) stimulate a systemic response to raise body temperature.

- *Vasoconstriction* diverts blood away from the peripheries and leads to the cold sensation associated with fever which may result in shivering ('rigor'), which raises body temperature further.
- *Non-shivering thermogenesis* in fat and muscle whereby uncoupling of the oxidative phosphorylation pathway switches ATP production to heat production.

Antipyretics, such as paracetamol and NSAIDs, work by inhibition of cyclo-oxygenase, the enzyme which produces prostaglandins from arachidonic acid derived from membrane phospholipids. This results in re-setting of the hypothalamic thermostat to the normal range. Sweating and vasodilation may result as the body aims to cool itself back to the normal temperature range.

Causes of fever

- Infections:
  - bacterial infection (pyogenic, mycobacteria and atypical/intracellular bacteria)
  - viral infection
  - fungal infection (mainly immunocompromised patients)
  - protozoal infections

- Malignancy
- Inflammatory/autoimmune conditions
- Tissue damage due to trauma, burns or cerebral haemorrhage
- Thromboembolic disease
- Drug fever
- Inherited: familial Mediterranean fever, etc.

Clinical approach to the febrile patient

As with all acute medical presentations, *the history is particularly important.*

Acute Medicine, ed. Stephen Haydock, Duncan Whitehead and Zoë Fritz. Published by Cambridge University Press. © Cambridge University Press 2015.

History

Description of fevers

- Discrete episodes or a swinging pattern
- Prolonged, recurrent or periodic episodes
- Association with rigors

Other associated symptoms

- Night sweats and weight loss (usually a feature of chronic infection/malignancy)
- Rash (bacterial, viral, parasitic, drugs)

Travel and exposures while overseas

(See below in 'Approach to the febrile returning traveller' section.)

Sexual history

(See Chapter 25 for how to take a full sexual history.)

Environmental exposure

- Water
- Animals/pets
- Occupational
- Unwell contacts

Past medical history

- Immunosuppression: iatrogenic (chemotherapy, steroids, biologics, organ transplant), haematological malignancy, HIV
- Relevant infections: e.g. TB
- Dental work
- Recent surgical procedures, metal prostheses, etc.

Drug history

- Antibiotics given, e.g. by GP
- Recreational drug use – especially intravenous drug user

Examination

Perform a careful examination with particular attention to:

Rash/skin abnormality

- Maculopapular rash (viral infections)
- Purpura (disseminated sepsis with DIC, especially meningococcal septicaemia, vasculitis)
- Cellulitis – discrete red, hot, tender area which may enlarge relatively rapidly in severe disease
- Insect bites – especially an eschar
- Tattoos – classically associated with hepatitis B
- Peripheral stigmata of endocarditis – splinter haemorrhages, Janeway lesions, Osler's nodes (rare)

Lymphadenopathy (see Chapter 40)

- *Localized*: mainly due to adjacent bacterial infections (consider also TB, toxoplasma, lymphoma)
- *Generalized*: lymphoma, HIV and EBV

Initial investigations

Routine blood tests

- FBC (note neutrophilia, lymphopenia and eosinophilia).
- U&E.
- LFT.
- Inflammatory markers: usually CRP. Expect CRP to be highly elevated in acute bacterial and fungal infection (often >200 mg/L) and much less so in viral infection (often 10–50 mg/L). ESR is useful in defining an underlying inflammatory process but generally lacks specificity.
- Arterial (or venous) blood gas: chiefly to check lactate in this setting but also oxygenation status if presenting with severe respiratory symptoms.

Microbiological tests

- Blood cultures
- Other cultures guided by history, e.g. urine, sputum, stool, throat swab, wound swab

Plain radiology

- Chest X ray

Management (see also 'Sepsis', Chapter 55)

Resuscitation

- Use standard ABCD approach.
- Many febrile patients are dehydrated, so IV fluids are often appropriate even if blood pressure and renal function are within normal ranges.

Antibiotics

- If clinical assessment and initial investigations suggest a likely cause for the fever (e.g. pneumonia or a UTI) then empirical antibiotics may be appropriate after cultures have been taken (consult local hospital guidelines).
- If the source of fever is not clear and the patient's vital signs are stable, then avoid blindly prescribing empirical antibiotics, as the vital opportunity to observe the patient in hospital and take further cultures may be lost. Exceptions to this rule are if the patient is systemically septic with evidence of shock or if they are neutropenic (see below). If in doubt consult a senior colleague or an infection specialist.

Level of care

- Consider this at an early stage.
- Is it safe to send the patient to a general medical ward or is a higher level of care required?

Infection control

- Can the patient remain in an open bay or should they be isolated in a side room and barrier nursed?
- Indications for isolation (pending culture results):
  - Acute diarrhoea or suspected *C. difficile* colitis
  - Suspected pulmonary TB
  - Suspected varicella zoster infection (chickenpox or shingles) or viral exanthema (measles)
  - Suspected influenza or other severe viral respiratory illness, e.g. MERS CoV (Middle Eastern respiratory syndrome associated coronavirus)
  - Known/suspected MRSA colonization
  - Known/suspected colonization with ESBL (extended spectrum beta-lactamase) producing or other multidrug resistant bacteria
  - Suspected meningococcal meningitis
  - Febrile returning traveller (until diagnosis established).

Pyrexia of unknown origin (PUO)

- *Definition* (as proposed by Petersdorf and Beesen in 1961):
  - fever >38.3°C on at least three occasions
  - duration of fever of >3 weeks
  - no diagnosis despite *1 week of inpatient investigation*.
- True PUO is rare and the term is overused in patients who have had only minimal investigations performed.
- Patients are often also considered to have a PUO despite antibiotics being started – these can mask the source of a deep-seated infection such as an abscess or osteomyelitis.
- Always go back to the history as a first measure and make sure no exposures (travel, pets, sexual encounters, occupation, drugs, etc.) have been missed. In general, remember that the patient with PUO is more likely to have an uncommon presentation of a common disease (e.g. prolonged fever) than a rare disease (Table 23.1).

Some common and important presentations

Approach to the febrile returning traveller

Scenario 23.1

A 25-year-old medical student presents to the ED with fever and abdominal pain. He had returned from a 6-week medical elective in Ghana 5 days earlier and had been unwell for 2 days. He was taking doxycycline as malaria prophylaxis. On examination he is febrile and mildly tachycardic with a clear chest and globally slightly tender abdomen.

Remember that returning travellers are just as likely to present with infections which can be acquired within the UK (e.g. influenza, community-acquired pneumonia, bacterial gastroenteritis) as they are to present with imported illnesses.

Travel history

- *Dates of travel and duration*: useful when considering incubation period of infections (see below).
- *Places travelled to*: rural versus urban.
- *Exposures while abroad*: insect bites, animal contact, fresh/sea water exposure, unwell contacts, foods, drinking tap water, sexual contacts.
- *Prophylaxis and vaccines*: e.g. malaria.

Table 23.1 Common causes of pyrexia of unknown origin (PUO) and appropriate diagnostic investigations

Diagnosis	Investigations
Subacute bacterial endocarditis (SBE)	Duke's criteria: both echo and microbiological criteria are required Blood cultures (3 sets from different sites taken at different times) Transthoracic echo (TTE) Transoesophageal echo (if TTE non-diagnostic and suspicion of SBE still high) Urinalysis – blood and protein Serology (in culture negative SBE – *Bartonella*, *Coxiella* (Q fever), *Chlamydia*)
Tuberculosis	Pulmonary TB: CXR, sputum microscopy (request stain for acid fast bacilli (AFB) specifically) and culture Extrapulmonary TB: 3 × early morning urine (100 mL each – 3 consecutive days), lumbar puncture (for tuberculous meningitis), CT scan – for abdominal/lymph node TB, TTE (for pericardial disease), biopsy – e.g. of LN, pericardium or other masses – is crucial for diagnosis and antimicrobial susceptibility testing Consider an HIV test
Occult abscess or osteomyelitis	Blood cultures Imaging: USS of abdominal organs (liver is common site of occult abscess) CT chest, abdomen and pelvis. MRI spine if back pain Radiolabelled leucocyte scan/PET scan Biopsy: for culture and histology once lesion identified. Patient should be off antibiotics for minimum 2 days beforehand to maximize yield
EBV	Bloods: lymphocytosis and thrombocytopenia Deranged LFTs (hepatitic pattern) Heterophile antibody test positive Serology: raised IgM in early disease, followed by IgG Virus can be detected in blood by PCR – not necessary in acute illness
HIV	Have a low threshold for performing an HIV test in a PUO situation (with patient consent). Refer all new positive cases to infectious diseases or genitourinary medicine for urgent assessment In advanced HIV disease may present with opportunistic infection (e.g. PCP, cerebral toxoplasmosis, TB, cryptococcal meningitis) or malignancy (lymphoma, Kaposi sarcoma)
Lymphoma	Bloods: raised serum lactate dehydrogenase Imaging: CT neck, chest, abdomen and pelvis for disease staging. Lymph node biopsy – crucial for diagnosis
Renal cell carcinoma	Bloods: anaemia or erythrocytosis, thrombocytosis, hypercalcaemia Imaging: abdominal USS or CT Biopsy is diagnostic
Vasculitis	Bloods: leucocytosis and raised ESR, acute kidney injury Proteinuria, active urine sediment ANCA positive (note that negative ANCA does not rule out vasculitis) Low complement (C3 and C4) Biopsy is diagnostic – e.g. of artery (temporal arteritis), lung or kidney
Still's disease	History: high fever once/twice per day and accompanying salmon pink rash Bloods: anaemia and leucocytosis, high CRP and ESR, high ferritin
SLE	Bloods: pancytopenia, raised ESR (CRP often normal), acute kidney injury Positive ANA, anti-dsDNA and anti-Sm antibodies Proteinuria Low complement (C3 and C4) Biopsy of skin or kidney may be helpful
Drug fever	Diagnosis of exclusion. Patient looks well Common causes: antibiotics (beta-lactams, nitrofurantoin), anticonvulsants (phenytoin, carbamazepine), allopurinol, unfractionated heparin Bloods: leucocytosis and eosinophilia (often absent) Trial discontinuation of drug may help

Investigations

- Stop chemoprophylaxis while investigating for malaria.
- Malaria film (×3 on 3 separate days) plus HRP dipstick test (detects histidine rich protein of *Plasmodium falciparum*).
- Blood cultures – for enteric (typhoid) fever and other bacterial pathogens.
- HIV test (patient consent required).
- Serologies: dengue, hepatitis, rickettsia, schistosomiasis, strongyloides – less appropriate for acute physicians.
- Discuss need for additional tests with local microbiologist or infectious diseases physician. In particular, *undertake a risk assessment for viral haemorrhagic fever in all febrile patients returning from an endemic area within the past 21 days.*

Initial management

- Empirical treatment with anti-malarials or antibiotics is usually *NOT* indicated *before* results of initial blood tests taken in the ED/MAU (including malaria film) are known.
- Antibiotics should be discussed with a senior colleague. Seek advice from an infection specialist.
- Fluid resuscitation if clinically dehydrated or hypotensive.
- Antipyretics and analgesia as appropriate.
- If acute bacterial sepsis is likely (based on clinical history plus raised CRP and neutrophils) consider a broad spectrum antibiotic with activity against typhoid fever, e.g. ceftriaxone.

Common causes of undifferentiated fever in the returning traveller

Malaria

- Distribution: throughout tropics.
- Incubation period: 1–3 weeks for *P. falciparum*. May be months for *P. vivax, P. ovale* or *P. malariae*.
- Key symptoms are generally non-specific: fever, malaise, abdominal pain.
- May also present very unwell with impaired consciousness or acute respiratory distress syndrome.
- Investigations: malaria blood film/dipstick test. Parasitaemia >2% indicates severe disease.

- Treatment: depends on species, location acquired and disease severity. Quinine, atovaquone-proguanil (Malarone) and artemisinin derivatives may all be used. See UK Malaria treatment guidelines in the Further reading section.

Enteric fever (typhoid)

- Distribution: developing countries globally, especially southeast Asia.
- Incubation: 7–18 days.
- Key symptoms: generally non-specific – fever, myalgia, headache, constipation. On examination: rose spots on abdomen and hepatosplenomegaly (both may be absent).
- Investigations: blood culture, stool culture.
- Treatment: ceftriaxone. Ciprofloxacin may be used pending culture results but emerging resistance is of concern.

Amoebic liver abscess

- Distribution: throughout developing countries worldwide.
- Incubation period: 8–20 weeks.
- Key symptoms: abdominal pain and RUQ tenderness – very similar to a bacterial abscess.
- Investigations: USS liver, amoebic serology, aspiration if diagnosis uncertain.
- Treatment: metronidazole followed by paramomycin. Drainage not usually required.

Arbovirus infection (dengue fever and chikungunya)

- Distribution: throughout tropics, especially southeast Asia and South America.
- Incubation: 4–8 days.
- Key symptoms: fever, erythematous maculopapular rash over chest and back, myalgia and bone pain, lethargy.
- Investigations: serology – IgM if symptomatic for >5 days. Blood PCR for early presentation.
- Treatment: supportive.

Rickettsial infection

- Distribution: mainly sub-Saharan Africa (game parks).
- Incubation: 4–7 days.
- Key symptoms: maculopapular rash, eschar and localized lymphadenopathy.

- Diagnosis: serology.
- Treatment: doxycycline.

Acute schistosomiasis (Katayama fever)

- Distribution: sub-Saharan Africa.
- Incubation: 4–6 weeks.
- Key symptoms: exposure to fresh water, itchy skin thereafter (swimmer's itch), urticarial rash, cough and wheeze, myalgia and arthralgia.
- Diagnosis: eosinophilia on FBC, serology, ova seen on microscopy of stool or urine in later stage of disease.
- Treatment: praziquantel.

Viral haemorrhagic fever (VHF; rare but important)

- Distribution: sub-Saharan Africa (rural areas).
- Incubation: up to 3 weeks.
- Key symptoms: initially non-specific – fever, malaise, cough, sore throat. Progression to hepatitis, encephalopathy, haemorrhage and shock.
- Investigations: blood samples should NOT be processed in routine lab if VHF is suspected (infection risk). Contact infectious diseases or microbiology urgently for advice.
- Treatment: mainly supportive in an ITU setting.

Management of acutely unwell septic patient (meningitis)

> **Scenario 23.2**
>
> *A 52-year-old woman is brought in by ambulance having been found unconscious by her husband. She was last seen awake 6 hours previously and had been complaining of fever, headache and generalized malaise at the time. She had seen her GP a few days earlier for left-sided ear pain. On examination she is febrile, tachycardic and hypotensive. She responds appropriately to a painful stimulus but not to voice alone. You note that she has a stiff neck…*

History

- May not be possible to get history from the patient if they are obtunded: Think of accompanying relatives, paramedic documentation, etc.
- Seek other clues as to the underlying source:
  - *Recent hospitalization*: history of dental procedures, sinusitis, head trauma, immunosuppression, injected drugs.
  - *Recent travel*: As above but don't forget meningitis as a cause of imported fever and severe sepsis.
  - Past medical history of prosthetic material in situ: metallic or tissue heart valves, joint prostheses, pacemaker, indwelling central catheters.
  - *Symptoms preceding the deterioration* may be helpful, e.g. ear pain indicating possible intracranial spread of infection (otitis media) with meningitis, as in this case.

Examination

- *General assessment*: ABCD approach to patient.
- *Signs of hypotension*: mottling or reduced capillary refill time.
- *Signs of CNS infection*: meningism (stiff neck, Kernig's and Brudzinski's signs), unequal pupils (may indicate space-occupying lesion), extensor plantars.
- *Signs of an acute abdomen*: board-like rigidity, rebound tenderness.
- *External sources of sepsis*: indwelling long lines, urinary catheters.
- *Others*: petechial rash of meningococcal septicaemia, zoster or herpetic rash, extensive skin or soft tissue infection, ear discharge or inflamed tympanum, mastoiditis.

Initial investigations

- As for previous investigation of fever, *but* also include
- Measure arterial blood lactate: important measure of organ perfusion.
- Check clotting: essential if invasive procedures are being considered or if suspect DIC.

Management

- See also Chapter 55.
- *Antibiotic administration*: should be given within 1 hour of presentation for a patient with septic shock. It is extremely important that blood culture samples are taken *before* antibiotics are commenced provided this does not delay the administration of antibiotic within the hour. Give parenteral antibiotics at the earliest opportunity in children and young people with a petechial rash (or immediately if the rash is spreading or becomes purpuric). *Note: lumbar puncture should not delay the administration of antibiotics for suspected meningitis.*

- *Antibiotic choice*: general principle is to start with broad empirical cover which can be rationalized over the next 24–48 hours pending culture results. Aim to cover Gram-positive, Gram-negative and anaerobic infections. *Refer to local hospital guidelines.*
- *Undifferentiated sepsis/septic shock*:
  - *CNS infections*: antibiotics with good CNS penetration, e.g. ceftriaxone or cefotaxime.
  - *Chest sepsis*: beta-lactams (e.g. co-amoxiclav) plus additional macrolide cover against atypical infections, e.g. *Legionella.*
  - *No defined source*: extended spectrum beta-lactams, e.g. piperacillin-tazobactam. Consider additional Gram-negative or anti-pseudomonad cover with aminoglycosides for neutropenic patients.
  - *Beta-lactam allergic patient*: combination therapy, e.g. vancomycin (Gram-positive cover), ciprofloxacin/gentamicin (Gram-negative cover), metronidazole (anaerobic cover).
  - *Carbapenems*: overprescribed. Not usually indicated as empirical cover unless patient has a known history of multi-resistant Gram-negatives (e.g. ESBL-producing *E. coli* from urine).
  - *Aminoglycosides*: bolus of gentamicin (3–5 mg/kg) may help for suspected Gram-negative bacteraemia. Caution in acute renal failure.

Performing a lumbar puncture (LP) (Box 23.1)

An LP is an important diagnostic tool for bacterial, viral, mycobacterial and fungal meningitis/encephalitis (Table 23.2). Also used for other infectious and neurological conditions: e.g. subarachnoid haemorrhage (if not diagnosed on CT scan), Guillain–Barré syndrome, multiple sclerosis, CNS malignancy and paraneoplastic syndromes, cerebral toxoplasmosis, CNS syphilis, neuroborelliosis.

Contraindications

- Raised intracranial pressure.
- Coagulopathy – platelets >50 or INR >1.4 or active anticoagulation (e.g. with LMWH). Discuss with a haematologist.
- Suspected spinal epidural abscess.
- Skin infection over the LP site.

CT head and lumbar puncture

- Considered standard practice to do CT head before LP in patients with suspected acute meningitis. However, this results in delay of LP and therefore reduces diagnostic yield.

Indications for CT head prior to LP

- Altered consciousness
- Seizures
- History of immunocompromise
- Focal neurological deficit
- Papilloedema

Consent for LP

Mention the following complications:

- *Infection*: at puncture site.
- *Bleeding*: haematoma can cause local nerve compression.
- *Nerve injury*: leading to numbness or pain.
- *Post-LP headache*: 10–30% of patients (minimize by lying flat for 6 hours and drinking a caffeinated beverage).
- *Cerebral herniation*: this can happen even with *normal CT* scan.

Box 23.1 Procedure for performing a lumbar puncture

- Positioning – lie the bed completely flat. Ask patient to lie on their side with their head bent forward and knees bent up as far as possible. A pillow held between the knees increases comfort. Ensure their low back is level with the side of the bed facing you. Both their shoulders and hips must be in vertical alignment. Feel between spinous processes of L4–5 and L5–S1 until the space between two spinous processes is identified.
- Clean the area using chlorhexidine and apply a sterile drape with a hole over the puncture area.
- Anaesthetize the puncture site using 5–10 mL of 1% lidocaine (orange needle for skin, then green needle for deeper tissue).
- Lumbar puncture: ensure needle is bevel up and pointing towards the patient's umbilicus (i.e. slightly towards their head) but also completely horizontal. Advance the needle through subcutaneous fat (minimal resistance) and the spinal ligaments (gritty feeling). Remove stylet at this point to check for flow of CSF.

- Once CSF flowing, attach manometer to measure opening pressure (normal 10–15 cm H_2O). Collect approx. 10 drops per universal container. Replace the stylet before removing the needle. Apply dressing to puncture site.
- Remember to take a venous blood sample for measurement of plasma glucose. CSF samples must be conveyed urgently to the lab as cell count may not be reliable if refrigerated overnight.

Interpretation of Lumbar puncture results

See Table 23.2 for representative CSF findings in patients with suspected meningitis.

Management of suspected acute bacterial meningitis

- *Antibiotics*: ceftriaxone or cefuroxime are first choice agents (refer to local prescribing guidelines). Ideally give after LP done, although give pre-LP if it will be delayed by >30 minutes (e.g. by CT head).
- *Supplemental antibiotics*: addition of ampicillin/amoxicillin if *Listeria* is suspected (>55 years old or immunocompromised). Addition of vancomycin if penicillin-resistant pneumococcus is suspected (recent travel to areas of known high prevalence of pneumococcal penicillin resistance, e.g. southern Europe and North America). Note: Advice from a microbiologist or infectious disease physician should be sought before these antibiotics are added.
- *Steroids*: improve outcomes in pneumococcal meningitis only, but no detrimental effect on meningococcal meningitis. Therefore give if any suspicion of pneumococcal disease – e.g. adult patient, history of ear or sinus disease.
- *Senior input*: inform seniors early. HDU/ITU input may be required for septicaemic patients.

Fever in the immunocompromised patient

Scenario 23.3

You are asked to review a 50-year-old woman on the MAU who has self-referred with suspected 'neutropenic sepsis'. She has recently completed her second cycle of chemotherapy for small cell lung cancer. She has recorded a temperature of 38°C at home and feels generally unwell.

Immunocompromise may be congenital or acquired.

Congenital (all are rare): e.g. chronic granulomatous disease, common variable immune deficiency.

Acquired (common):

- Infectious: HIV
- Metabolic: diabetes mellitus
- Iatrogenic (most important emerging group):
  - solid organ transplantation
  - bone marrow transplantation
  - chemotherapy
  - biological therapy, e.g. anti-TNF drugs for rheumatological conditions
  - steroids and steroid sparing agents.

Infections to which immunocompromised individuals are predisposed depend on the type of immune deficit.

Neutropenia (e.g. post chemotherapy, haematological malignancy, during bone marrow allograft):

- Bacterial infections (bacteraemia) – *Pseudomonas aeruginosa*, other aerobic Gram-negatives
- Invasive candidiasis (candidaemia and disseminated infections)
- Invasive mould infections (e.g. pulmonary aspergillosis).

T-cell-mediated: immunocompromise (e.g. HIV, solid organ and bone marrow transplant, haematological malignancy, biological therapy, steroid therapy):

- Mucosal candidiasis
- Pneumocystis pneumonia (PCP)
- Viral infections: adenovirus, BK and JC virus
- Reactivation of latent infection:
  - toxoplasmosis
  - cytomegalovirus (CMV)
  - Epstein–Barr virus (EBV)
- Mycobacterial infection: TB and atypical mycobacteria.

Be aware that *common bacterial infections (e.g. pneumonia) are more common in all immunocompromised patients* and must not be forgotten. Presentation of such infections may be unusual, however, as the host response may not be typical.

Clinical approach to the febrile neutropenic patient

- Neutropenia is defined as a blood neutrophil count of $<1 \times 10^9$/L. Profound neutropenia is $<0.5 \times 10^9$/L.

Table 23.2 Interpretation of lumbar puncture results

Diagnosis	Neutrophils (cells/mm³)	Lymphocytes (cells/mm³)	Gram stain	Protein (g/L)	Glucose	Comment
Normal values	<5	<5	Negative	0.1–0.45	~2/3 of serum glucose measured simultaneously	
Bacterial meningitis	>100 NB: may be replaced by lymphocytes following antibiotic treatment	10–50	Positive in 60–90%. Commonly: Gram-positive cocci in pairs (pneumococcus), Gram-negative diplococci (meningococcus), Gram-positive bacilli (listeria)	0.5–1.0	<1/2 serum	Culture positive in 75–85%. PCR for meningococcus and pneumococcus can be used if culture negative (discuss with microbiology)
Viral meningitis	10–50 (may be normal)	>100	Negative	Normal	Normal or slightly low	PCR is diagnostic test: enterovirus commonest, followed by HSV and VZV
Tuberculous meningitis	50–100 (highly variable)	>100	Negative	>2.0 Usually higher than bacterial meningitis	<1/2 serum Usually lower than bacterial meningitis	Acid-fast bacilli are rarely seen on auramine/ZN stain. Culture has higher sensitivity. Consider TB PCR if suspicion is high (discuss with microbiology)
Cryptococcal meningitis	10–50 (may be normal)	>100 (may be normal)	Negative	0.5–1.0	<1/2 serum	Rarely seen in HIV negative patients. Opening pressure may be very elevated. India ink stain positive but cryptococcal antigen (CRAG) is more sensitive

- Fever is common in neutropenic patients: Initial assessment of severity may be misleading; therefore antibiotics are usually started empirically pending culture results.
- *Patients can deteriorate very rapidly*, therefore rapid assessment is important.
- *Patients will require protective isolation* (see below).
- Localizing the source of sepsis may be very difficult from the history due to minimal symptoms (other than fever). Likewise on examination signs of inflammation may be subtle. It is therefore important to perform a careful physical examination, including:
  - *Head and neck*: signs of meningism.
  - *Mouth and throat*: mucositis, oral candidiasis.
  - *Chest*: signs of consolidation.
  - *Abdomen*: tenderness may indicate typhlitis (neutropenic enterocolitis). This can lead to perforation so get a surgical review. CT scan of the abdomen will likely be required.
  - *External genitalia and peri-anal region*: look for erythema, tenderness around the anus and haemorrhoids. *Digital rectal examination is contraindicated* due to the risk of damaging the rectal mucosa and introducing infection.
  - *Indwelling central line sites*: erythema and discharge may indicate a site infection, likewise tenderness along the vein may indicate thrombophlebitis. Note that *absence of inflammation around the line exit site does not exclude a line infection* as a bacterial biofilm may be coating the lumen.
- In the first instance the microbiological investigations are similar to any other febrile patient in whom the source of sepsis is not clear – i.e. cultures of blood, urine, stool (if diarrhoea) and sputum (if coughing). Separate cultures from indwelling central lines should be sent along with peripheral cultures.
- *Start antibiotics promptly after a full septic screen has been performed.* Aim to deliver the first dose of antibiotic within one hour of the patient's arrival. Refer to local hospital guidelines for antibiotic choice. Commonly used agents are either a carbapenem (such as meropenem) or anti-pseudomonal penicillin (such as piperacillin-tazobactam) with the possible inclusion of vancomycin if a central line infection is suspected.

- In neutropenic patients who remain febrile despite empirical antibiotics and in whom cultures are negative, invasive fungal infection must be considered. *Aspergillus* sp. is a much feared cause of chest sepsis in neutropenic patients. This is usually diagnosed by a combination of imaging appearance on CT chest and bronchoscopic samples showing fungi either on histological preparation or fungal culture. Assays to detect *Aspergillus galactomannan*, a fungal antigen, and *Aspergillus* PCR are also used in some centres. Management of invasive fungal infection is difficult and best supervised by a microbiologist or infectious disease physicians. Mortality may be over 40% despite antifungal treatment.

Infection control and antibiotic prophylaxis

> **Scenario 23.4**
>
> *A 75-year-old woman is admitted for a total knee replacement. Five days post procedure she is noted to have a warm and tender knee with some discharge from the wound site. Multi-site swabs are positive for MRSA. Fluid cultured from a washout of the knee replacement also grows MRSA…*

Infection control aims to reduce the incidence of healthcare-acquired infection through simple measures such as screening and isolation of patients.

Identifying patients carrying resistant pathogens, such as MRSA, allows appropriate prophylaxis and treatment to be given to reduce the risk of complications.

MRSA: Screening and decolonization

- All patients are screened for MRSA using a multi-site swab on admission to hospital or if elective surgery is planned.
- Certain areas also screen for other resistant pathogens, e.g. ESBL or vancomycin resistant enterococci (using rectal swabs) depending on the local prevalence and degree of vulnerability of the patients (e.g. oncology and intensive care units).
- Decolonization of MRSA is with a combination of antibiotic nasal ointment, shampoo and body wash. The exact agents used will vary between hospitals.
- Following decolonization, serial MRSA multi-site swabs are sent. *The patient is no longer considered to be colonized if three consecutive swabs each taken*

a week apart are negative. They can then be nursed in an open ward.

Isolation

- Can be divided into *source isolation* (of an infectious patient to prevent spread of infection) or *protective isolation* (of a vulnerable patient to prevent spread of infection from the hospital environment – e.g. neutropenic patients).
- *Prioritization of side rooms* (for commonly encountered pathogens):
  1. *C. difficile* diarrhoea
  2. MRSA colonization/infection
  3. Multi-resistant Gram-negative colonization/infection (e.g. ESBL producing *E. coli*)
  4. Vancomycin-resistant enterococci colonization/infection.
- *Other important pathogens requiring isolation*:
  - Bacterial or viral gastroenteritis (e.g. *Salmonella* or norovirus).
  - Meningococcal meningitis – side room plus masks until 24 hours of antibiotics given.
  - Pulmonary TB (sputum smear positive and no risk factors for multidrug resistance) – side room plus masks until 2 weeks of treatment given with satisfactory response.
  - Highly infectious/dangerous pathogen (e.g. multidrug resistant TB, VHF) – negative pressure side room. VHF requires transfer to special secure unit.

Hand washing

- Good hand-washing practice is essential to reduce the spread of hospital-acquired infection. A thorough hand wash, ensuring no areas of skin are missed, may take 15–30 seconds.
- Hands should be washed before any clinical procedure and after contact with a patient or any item at their bedside.
- If no visible dirt is present on the hands then alcohol gel may be used instead of washing. Note, however, that the gel is ineffective against spores of *C. difficile* and norovirus: soap and water must be used after glove removal when caring for these patients.

Antibiotic prophylaxis (general principles)

- Prophylaxis is given prior to surgery to reduce the incidence of surgical site infection. A single dose of antibiotic, given just before the start of the procedure, is usually sufficient.
- In broad terms, prophylaxis is most important when the risk of infection is high (e.g. when handling the gut) or when the consequences of infection are potentially disastrous (e.g. neurosurgery with implantation of foreign material or joint replacement surgery). The choice of antibiotic should reflect the likely bacteria which may contaminate the wound: e.g. for abdominal surgery cover must include Gram-negatives and anaerobes. Always refer to local guidelines. The presence of multi-resistant organisms known to be colonizing the patient, such as MRSA, must also be taken into account.

Notification of infectious diseases

- Doctors are required by law to inform the local Health Protection Unit (HPU) of any patient they suspect of having a notifiable infectious disease.
- Speed of notification is more important than accuracy: Hence the HPU should be informed if the diagnosis is suspected rather than waiting for the results of diagnostic tests.
- A comprehensive list of notifiable diseases, which is beyond the scope of this book, is available on the Public Health England website (see Further reading).

Further reading

Fever in the returning traveller

British Infection Authority. UK Malaria Treatment Guidelines: www.britishinfection.org/drupal/content/clinical-guidelines.

Johnston V, Stockley JM, Dockrell D, et al. Fever in returned travellers presenting in the United Kingdom: Recommendations for investigation and initial management. *Journal of Infection* 2009; 59: 1–18.

Management of the systemically unwell patient

British Infection Authority UK Meningitis Treatment Guidelines: www.britishinfection.org/drupal/content/clinical-guidelines.

Dellinger RP, Levy MM, Rhodes A, et al. Surviving Sepsis Campaign: International Guidelines for Management of Severe Sepsis and Septic Shock: 2012. *Intensive Care Med* 2013; 39:165–228.

Antibiotic prophylaxis

Scottish Intercollegiate Guidelines Network (SIGN):
Guideline 104 – Antibiotic Prophylaxis in Surgery.
Published July 2008.

Notification of infectious diseases

Public Health England website (formerly known
as the HPA – Health Protection Agency):
www.hpa.org.uk/Topics/InfectiousDiseases/
InfectionsAZ/NotificationsOfInfectiousDiseases/
ListOfNotifiableDiseases.

Fits and seizures

Christopher J. S. Price

Introduction

Neurology as a specialty has a reputation for mystery, a misinterpretation fostered in our undergraduate training [1]. On the medical admissions unit (MAU), acute neurological presentations account for 12% of all admissions, of which a quarter involve blackouts of some kind [2]. As a trainee on the MAU you are therefore challenged to deal with something you may not be comfortable with, but cannot avoid. This chapter complements those on syncope and cardiac dysrhythmias, and aims to arm you with the appropriate tools to be effective in making a diagnosis, and having made it, adopt the correct management strategy. This will require the employment of your core skills, in particular that of *history taking*. This is both a science and an art. Without doubt, this area challenges a clinician's attitudes to uncertainty.

For the purposes of this chapter a seizure is defined as an '*abnormal excessive or* synchronous neuronal activity *in the brain*'. Where recurrent this is referred to as *epilepsy*. *Non-epileptic attacks* can take on astonishingly similar appearances, but have no underlying electrical correlate.

Scenario 24.1

A 25-year-old female factory worker presents to the MAU having collapsed at work and having made some recovery in the ambulance. She has a history of moderate alcohol consumption. She has no background risk factors for epilepsy. The ambulance staff reports she had been a bit shaky but was not incontinent. They could get no sense out of her until she arrived in the emergency department (ED). Examination of her cardiovascular system was normal; she has a Glasgow Coma Scale (GCS) score of 15/15; full neurological examination was normal.

Clinical assessment

Box 24.1 outlines the *differential diagnosis*. The task of the admitting physician is to discriminate between these.

Box 24.1 Brief overview of the differential diagnosis of transient loss of consciousness

Syncope
  Cardiac
  Non-cardiac
Seizure
Psychogenic
Hypoglycaemia
Parasomnia

1. What are the key points to be covered in the history?

You must first try and get a precise account of the event.

Learning point: the value of a witnessed account, even from trained professionals, varies [3]. What may seem like crucial details to the expert epileptologist are often missed. Obtaining a witnessed account is, however, superior to no objective account and is sometimes better than that obtained from paramedics who have a tendency to overcall. A witnessed account should hence be avidly sought.

2. What value should you place on the clinical pointers?

The process of making a diagnosis from a blackout scenario is purely clinical. A number of key features are sought. With respect to the three commonest present-

Acute Medicine, ed. Stephen Haydock, Duncan Whitehead and Zoë Fritz. Published by Cambridge University Press.
© Cambridge University Press 2015.

Table 24.1 Core features of the most common blackout types (+ refers to frequently seen, +/– indicates variably seen, – indicates infrequent or rare)

	Tonic–clonic seizure	Syncope	Non-epileptic attack
Precipitant	Variable, sleep related	Pain, fright, standing, blood/needles; rarely lying down	Variable, usually in company
Premonitory symptoms	Rarely identified	Dizziness, sweating, nausea, visual and hearing changes	Variable
Duration	Usually 0.5–3 minutes	Seconds	Minutes
Eyes	Open	Open or closed	Variable
Rigidity	+	+/–	Usually not sustained
Clonic movements	Usually 60–90 seconds, violent	Brief, usually less than 30 seconds	Flailing, not jerks Variable intensity
Colour change	Often blue	Marked pallor	–
Breathing change	+	–	–
Self-injury	Bitten side of tongue	Variable	Does not exclude; may bite front of tongue
Incontinence	Non discriminatory	Non discriminatory	Non discriminatory
Post-ictal confusion	10–30 minutes; often waking in ambulance or A&E department	Brief, <2 minutes; often 'tired'	–

Table 24.2 Sensitivity, specificity and odds ratio of listed clinical features in favour of seizure or syncope [4]

	Sensitivity	Specificity	Odds ratio
Seizure			
Cyanosis	0.29	0.98	16.9
Tongue biting	0.45	0.97	16.5
Head turning	0.42	0.95	13.5
Post-ictal delirium	0.85	0.83	5
Muscle pain	0.16	0.95	3.4
Unconscious >5 minutes	0.68	0.55	1.5
Syncope			
Prolonged upright	0.4	0.98	20.4
Sweating	0.36	0.98	18
Pallor	0.81	0.66	2.8

ations (syncope, seizure and non-epileptic attacks), core features to these are outlined in Table 24.1.

Importantly, no single feature is taken in isolation: shaking is seen in both syncope and seizure (although often less violent in syncope) and incontinence can be seen in either.

A number of these specific pointers can be expressed in terms of sensitivity, specificity and odds ratio (OR) in Table 24.2 [4].

3. What antecedent risk factors increase likelihood of seizure?

a. History of learning difficulties
b. Previous brain injury of any kind
c. Alcohol
d. Drug usage
e. Family history of epilepsy

Traumatic brain injury (TBI) confers a particularly significant risk; in this instance relative risk can rise as high as 9 in severe cases.

Making the correct diagnosis at this stage remains very important. For neurologists, making an incorrect diagnosis of seizure and/or epilepsy is considered more damaging for the patient than a correct diagnosis delayed. This is because epilepsy remains a stigmatizing illness with implications for:

1. Driving
2. Occupation
3. Family
4. Lifelong exposure to potentially toxic drugs.

It is important to appreciate that there are:

Epilepsy mimics: conditions that look like epilepsy but aren't, e.g. parasomnia
Chameleons: conditions that don't look like epilepsy but are, e.g. frontal lobe seizures.

One key diagnostic step is to establish whether they are all the same, i.e. stereotyped. Where the diagnosis remains unclear, it is most appropriate to label them as 'attacks'.

Overall, if you cannot reach a firm conclusion, seek help but do not be ashamed of your uncertainty.

Scenario 24.1 continued

It was decided to contact the employer for a description of the event. A direct witnessed account clearly states she was upright, went stiff, had eyes open, and was very sweaty and convulsed violently for 4–5 minutes. No clear colour change was observed. On investigation she was found to have a long QTc of >450 ms and was referred to a cardiologist; following cardiac investigation she was commenced on a beta-blocker. However, she went on to have further clearly described seizures and was commenced on lamotrigine to good effect. Neurological investigations were all normal.

---

4. Having made the diagnosis of a seizure, what kind of seizures are they?

Where possible a classification of a seizure should be attempted on MAU. The main classification groups of seizures are shown in Box 24.2.

Box 24.2 Brief summary of seizure classification from Panayiotopoulos [5]

Generalized seizures

- Tonic–clonic (in any combination)
- Absence (not to be confused with complex focal seizures)
- Absences with special features
- Myoclonic absence
- Eyelid myoclonia
- Myoclonic/atonic /tonic
- Clonic
- Tonic
- Atonic

Focal seizures, e.g. temporal or frontal lobe
Secondary generalized after focal onset

It is not really acceptable to label attacks just as 'seizures' as different types of seizure:

- have different causes
- require different investigations
- require different treatments.

Some typical features of focal onset seizures according to brain location include:

Frontal: these look bizarre. They often occur from sleep, and may involve head turning. They may appear in various postures, e.g. fencing or even cycling. This type of seizure is easily interpreted as non-epileptic.

Temporal: deja/jamais vu, epigastric 'aura' (butterflies), ictal fear (sometimes very difficult to distinguish from panic attacks); transient epileptic amnesia, ictal spitting and vomiting; strange tastes or smells.

Parietal: rare, sensory.

Occipital: also rare, the main differential is migraine. Epileptic phenomena are colourful, brief and formed; they don't tend to evolve. Migraine visual aura is more often monochromic, linear and evolves over minutes/hours.

All of the above can go on to generalize into the classical tonic–clonic seizure, often with very little warning.

Having made the diagnosis of seizure, what has caused it?

Broadly speaking, causes of epilepsy fall into three groups:

Symptomatic: relates to a known cause, summarized in Table 24.3.

Idiopathic: relates in general to a genetic cause (there is debate about the term), e.g. tuberous sclerosis.

Cryptogenic: where no cause is identified.

A *seizure threshold* is primarily dictated genetically but may be influenced by a variety of factors, for example:

- alcohol
- fasting
- recreational drugs
- prescription drugs, e.g. metronidazole

Table 24.3 An outline of common aetiologies in secondary or symptomatic epilepsies

Vascular	Neoplastic	Infectious	Toxic/metabolic	Other	Inflammatory
Previous stroke	Any primary or	Travel related, e.g.	Alcohol	Traumatic brain	Vasculitis
Cerebral vein thrombosis	secondary tumour	malaria	Recreational drugs	injury	Multiple sclerosis
	Paraneoplastic or	Encephalitis	Low Na, Mg or		
	autoimmune limbic		glucose		
	encephalitides				

- sleep disturbance
- 'stress'.

  Two clinical scenarios require specific mention:

Alcohol-related seizures

- The problem of alcohol-related seizures is a common one.
- They occur in the context of alcohol dependence and care must be taken *not to overestimate* its contribution to the problem.
- A high proportion of patients have other risk factors, e.g. prior head injury or a history of epilepsy preceding their dependence [6].
- Alcohol-related seizures are perhaps *best considered a diagnosis of exclusion.*
- An alcohol history should be taken in all patients presenting with blackouts. Although alcohol is thought to have a directly toxic effect, a more frequent presentation is that of withdrawal. Some patients may even present in status epilepticus.

Management

- Those presenting with focal onset or in status should have further investigations.
- The management of alcohol-related seizure should begin with ensuring patients are not hypoglycaemic.
- One should also *have a low threshold* for other investigations such as imaging and urine toxicology tests.
- Thiamine has no direct anticonvulsant effect but should be administered to all patients in withdrawal.
- Benzodiazepines remain the short-term treatment of choice; lorazepam with a longer duration of action versus diazepam is the treatment of choice but care must applied when used over the longer term [7].
- Long-term use of anticonvulsant drugs remains controversial; such patients are often non-compliant and there is evidence that abrupt withdrawal from drugs such as phenytoin is harmful. If, however, there is evidence of structural brain disease, i.e. symptomatic epilepsy in the context of alcohol, or if there are clear EEG abnormalities, then long-term therapy may be justified.
- For the purposes of driving, alcohol-related seizures are not considered provoked, nor are those attributed to a structural abnormality or sleep disturbance. Provoked seizures are caused by trauma, documented metabolic derangements, e.g. hypoglycaemia, or causes that are unlikely to recur, e.g. subarachnoid haemorrhage (see section on driving).

Seizures in pregnancy

- Blackouts presenting in pregnancy are common. Most are syncopal. However, seizures presenting in pregnancy require particular care.
- Three broad diagnostic groups are recognized:
    - those that have an established diagnosis of epilepsy (non-pregnancy related)
    - those that have symptomatic epilepsy from a new and 'common' problem, e.g. hypoglycaemia causing seizure
    - those that have seizure in the setting of a rare clinical neurological problem:
        - eclampsia
        - intracranial haemorrhage (ICH)
        - cerebral vein thrombosis (usually presents with headache)
        - reversible cerebral vasoconstriction syndrome (RCVS)
        - posterior reversible encephalopathy syndrome (PRES)
        - thrombotic thrombocytopenic purpura (TTP).
- Specialist advice in diagnosis and management should be sought early especially where these rare scenarios are suspected.
- Seizures are more common in PRES than RCVS and such patients require prompt imaging with MRI as CT can be normal [8].

Investigation

Having attempted classification of a seizure, and considered a cause, investigations can be tapered accordingly:

ECG: an ECG is a mandatory test in all cases of blackout [9]. Ensure that your machine has the facility to check the PR interval and that the corrected QT interval (QTc) is calculated according to Bazett's formula.

Blood tests: in an emergency setting checking electrolytes, in particular glucose, sodium and magnesium, is required in almost all cases. Serum assays of anticonvulsant drug levels need to be considered on a case-by-case basis. Three particular instances when this is indicated are: when toxicity is considered, in pregnancy when levels may fluctuate and when compliance is deemed to be an issue. For only a small number of drugs, namely phenytoin and phenobarbital, will the result return in time to make acute decisions based upon them.

The peripheral white cell count will often be raised following a seizure. This is a non-specific 'stress' reaction and needs to be interpreted with caution. Perhaps of more importance than the absolute numbers is the pattern over time; most raised white cell counts in seizures will resolve; those that do not should trigger other investigations. Pyrexia should also be considered. A low threshold for further investigation, to include imaging and lumbar puncture, should be maintained particularly where encephalitis or meningitis is suspected (see Chapter 23).

In general the use of prolactin is not encouraged despite some evidence that a raised level >10–20 times baseline is helpful [10]. This test is not a substitute for taking a good clinical history and is difficult to interpret in certain types of epilepsy, e.g. focal onset.

Urinalysis: maintain a low threshold of sending urine for toxicology, particularly in younger patients. Be aware of a number of drugs that can lower seizure threshold, e.g. quinolone antibiotics or psychotropic medication. The effects of selective serotonin reuptake inhibitors (SSRIs) are probably overestimated.

A full list is available at: http://professionals.epilepsy.com/page/table_seniors_drugs.html.

Imaging: in adults presenting with a first seizure, *imaging is required in all cases*. Optimal imaging in epilepsy is almost exclusively MRI but practical resource-based constraints mean that CT, at least initially, is usually done. If CT is normal in that context, an MRI wherever possible should be arranged thereafter. MRI is a very helpful tool in focal onset epilepsy but a much less useful one in primary generalized epilepsies.

In those patients presenting to MAU with an established diagnosis of epilepsy (and you are satisfied with it), reimaging is required only when:

(a) there is a suspicion of new pathology, e.g. encephalitis

(b) there are new focal neurological signs.

EEG: this is an over-requested investigation and should really be discussed with a neurologist or neurophysiologist first. An EEG is indicated in cases of focal seizure, especially in non-symptomatic cases. EEG is a tool that assists diagnosis only in exceptional circumstances, e.g. non-convulsive status and in specialist hands. In the context of non-epileptic attack disorder (NEAD) it can be useful when performed soon, i.e. within hours of an attack. It is often non-specifically abnormal in the elderly and those with neurodegenerative disease.

EEG can be used to aid classification and prognosticate. EEG is a key tool in making a diagnosis of idiopathic generalized epilepsy where particular tools, e.g. photostimulation, are used. On an intensive care unit (ICU), it has a role in the management of status epilepticus.

Management of the first seizure

Having made the diagnosis of a first seizure, and put in place some investigations, it remains important to give the patient some more information. Patients should be aware that:

- The patient should not drive and should inform the DVLA. In the UK, *this is the patient's responsibility but clear documentation of this advice must be made in the medical notes*. DVLA guidance changes regularly and should be consulted frequently: www.dft.gov.uk/dvla/medical. For a first seizure, this usually involves not driving for a period of 6 months. There is an Access to Work government scheme in the UK to assist those affected in their ability to continue to work; the number to ring is 03452688489.

- Cause, provocation, imaging and EEG may all guide prognosis and risk of a second seizure, and hence epilepsy. The MESS study outlined that there was *no benefit to early treatment after a single seizure* but prognosis was influenced by a number of factors; long-term remission, however, was not affected. Hence *non-symptomatic first seizures are in general not commenced on anticonvulsants* [11]. Symptomatic seizures require a different approach, often involving a lower threshold for treatment than non-symptomatic cases [12].

- Individual institutions will most often have their own care pathway for the assessment and management of a first seizure (that of Musgrove Park is shown in Figure 24.1).

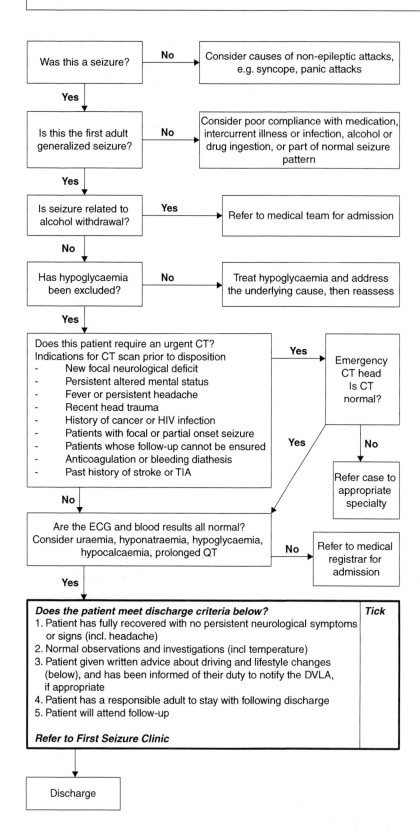

Figure 24.1 An algorithmic guide to first seizure management.

Management of the known epileptic presenting to MAU with seizures

- This is a common scenario. The first task is to ensure the diagnosis is secure and hence *a review of the old notes is the key*. Other aspects to consider are: recent intercurrent illness (often infection) and any other factor that may lower seizure threshold (drugs, sleep disturbance, alcohol). In particular there should be specific enquiry about drug compliance.
- Beyond these factors, assuming unprecipitated seizures, there remains the option to alter drugs over the longer term. *A neurologist or specialist nurse should be involved at this point.*
- In the author's opinion, an epilepsy specialist nurse is a pivotal component to service provision to such patients. Whilst their role between organizations may vary, there remains a core of supporting activities carried out. These include provision of, in no strict order:

  - continuity of care
  - reduced misdiagnosis
  - empowerment
  - awareness and education for patient and staff
  - risk management
  - employment advice
  - reduced epilepsy-related morbidity and mortality.

Principles of anticonvulsant prescription

A number of clear principles guide prescription of anticonvulsant medications. This is something that an epilepsy specialist (nurse or doctor) should lead on but you should be aware of some of the issues:

- *Security of diagnosis.* Significant harm is done when patients are prescribed anticonvulsants inappropriately. Every effort must be made to secure the correct diagnosis. This may take time, and neurologists are familiar with pressures sustained when uncertainty prevails. Care must be taken to explain the risks of an incorrect diagnosis in terms of lifestyle, occupation, driving, drug toxicity risks and the psychological burden of living with a long-term condition.
- *Classification.* It remains clear that certain types of seizure and epilepsy respond to different anticonvulsants. For example, unless there is a clear background diagnosis of epilepsy, purely alcohol-related seizures might require benzodiazepine therapy only, in conjunction with abstinence. Perhaps the key step is to discriminate generalized seizures from those of focal onset (with or without secondary generalization). A full description of drugs used in different types of epilepsy can be found in the NICE guideline [13]. Of note, certain drugs may worsen myoclonic (jerky) episodes (especially carbamazepine).
- *When to commence anticonvulsant therapy.* A large number of factors are involved in a discussion with the patient about starting therapy. These include classification, frequency and impact of seizures (quality of life and function), symptomatic or non-symptomatic cause, EEG changes, driving, plans for contraception, potential for interaction and the risk of sudden unexpected death in epilepsy (SUDEP) (to name but a few). A bespoke approach to each patient is required; hence the need to involve either a neurologist or specialist nurse.
- *Side effect profile.* This involves an experience of commonly used anticonvulsant drugs in order to find the appropriate balance between effectiveness

Table 24.4 Common side effects of the most frequently used anticonvulsants.

Drug	Main side effects
Phenytoin	Neuropathy, ataxia (cerebellar atrophy), gum hypertrophy, bone marrow suppression, drug-induced lupus, Stevens–Johnson syndrome, cardiotoxicity, osteoporosis
Phenobarbital	Drowsiness, cognitive impairment, anaemia, folate deficiency (also phenytoin), reduced libido, osteoporosis
Sodium valproate	Teratogenicity, tremor (parkinsonism), cognitive impairment, hair loss, deranged liver function tests, weight gain, thrombocytopenia
Carbamazepine	Tiredness, drowsiness, ataxia, diplopia, marrow suppression, skin reactions, cardiac
Lamotrigine	Rash (increased if recent or current valproate), aseptic meningitis
Levetiracetam	Irritability, depression, paraesthesia, pharyngitis

and tolerability. In general, older drugs have provided effective treatments for epilepsy but often at a cost, e.g. phenytoin may cause neuropathy or ataxia, carbamazepine drowsiness and ataxia and barbiturates in particular are sedative drugs. These drugs are therefore most often reserved for second- or third-line drugs. The main side effects of commonly used drugs are included in Table 24.4.

- *Epilepsy in women of childbearing age*. This area warrants particular attention. In general pregnant patients are not advised to stop taking medication during pregnancy. This is based upon the risks both to the mother and unborn child. An evolving dataset is now available on the teratogenicity risks of anticonvulsants to the unborn child, both in terms of major malformations and in the more subtle but equally important area of cognitive development [14]. Sodium valproate is thought to carry particularly high risks to the unborn child. Optimal management should include planning ahead, getting patients onto lower risk drugs, and folate supplementation in conjunction with joint neurological/obstetric care.
- *Speed of titration*. In oncology patients, for example, rapid titration is often required. Drugs such as carbamazepine and lamotrigine cannot be titrated rapidly.
- *Drug interactions*. A full set of interactions between different drugs is provided in the *British National Formulary* (BNF). In particular, care about contraception should be taken with all enzyme-inducing drugs; lamotrigine also affects levels of ethinylestradiol used for contraception.

Status epilepticus (convulsive)

- The definition of convulsive status epilepticus, distinguished from non-convulsive status, is evolving; traditionally this has been thought of as '*20 minutes of convulsive or repeated convulsions with minimal or no interval recovery of consciousness*'.
- Most seizures lasting greater than 5 minutes do not stop spontaneously.
- In animal models permanent neurological damage often occurs prior to the 20-minute threshold. Management is therefore 'expectant'.

- Mortality is as high as 38% in those older than 60 years and morbidity is often high.
- A local protocol for the diagnosis and management of status epilepticus is shown in Figure 24.2.
- Imaging in such cases, where practical, should be considered particularly in refractory status or where focal signs are evident.
- A low threshold for lumbar puncture, assuming no contraindications, should also be adopted.
- The role of continuous EEG monitoring is controversial and poorly supported by evidence.
- Toxicology should be considered and done early in the admission.
- Early referral to the intensive care unit (ICU) remains mandatory.
- Where cases diverge from existing guidelines, especially in refractive cases, recommendation is made for liaison with neurology services, intensive care teams and on occasions the regional neurological ITU.

Non-epileptic attack disorder (NEAD)

- NEAD is challenging to diagnose and difficult to manage.
- The causes may remain obscure but are likely to relate to a complex set of psychosocial factors.
- They are frequently seen in the context of a secure diagnosis of epilepsy and may be almost impossible for the patient, relatives or indeed physicians to discriminate.
- Their diagnosis, where not clear (see Table 24.1), may require further investigation such as video EEG. Neither injury, nor occurrence from sleep, confidently excludes them.
- *Their management requires expert neuropsychiatric input*.

Sudden unexpected death in epilepsy (SUDEP)

- This catastrophic event is increasingly recognized in epilepsy patients.
- Formal guidance has been provided that all patients with epilepsy should be counselled about SUDEP, although this remains controversial [15].
- Acute and emergency physicians should be aware of the risk factors for this:

(Doses are approximate and should be calculated according to weight)

0–5 min

Treat as medical emergency:
- Secure airway; administer high flow oxygen
- Call for help
- Monitor vital signs, including temperature and glucose
- Establish IV access: bloods for FBC, glucose, LFT, U & E, Mg, Ca, toxicology and anticonvulsant levels

If concerns re hypoglycaemia, poor nutrition or alcohol, give 250 mg of thiamine IV (pair of Pabrinex ampoules), followed by 50 mL of 50% glucose

5–15 min emergent

- Administer 4 mg IV lorazepam (0.1 mg/kg)
- If lorazepam not available:
  - Clonazepam 1 mg IV (0.015 mg/kg) or
  - Diazepam 10 mg IV (0.15 mg/kg)
- If IV access not possible:
  - Buccal midazolam 5–10 mg (0.1 mg/kg)
  - Rectal diazepam 10 mg (0.15 mg/kg)

Increasing pharmacoresistance

Consider discussion with neurologist or neurological ICU

30 min

- Give phenytoin 18 mg/kg at 50 mg/min
  - If phenytoin unavailable or contraindicated, consider:
    - 2 g IV sodium valproate (30 mg/kg, max. 400 mg/min) or
    - 2.5 g IV levetiracetam

Refractory

- Intubate, general anaesthesia, admit to ITU
- If not possible consider phenobarbital 10 mg/kg at 100 mg/min max (NB risk of cardiorespiratory depression)

Figure 24.2 A guideline used in the diagnostic work-up and management of convulsive status epilepticus in adults in hospital.

- nocturnal seizures
- living alone
- poorly controlled epilepsy
- multiple antiepileptic drugs.

Conclusion

In this chapter, an overview of the admissions unit approach to diagnosis, investigation and management of seizures and epilepsy is provided. This area tests a number of skills, in particular that of history taking. Often further information is required and there remains a clear role for the emergency physician, armed with some of the science provided above, to start to make sense of things. In particular that role should include getting a clear witnessed account of events as soon as possible. Throughout, a sceptical and inquisitive approach to this scenario is to be encouraged.

References

1. Ridsdale L, Massey R, Clark L. Preventing neurophobia in medical students, and so future doctors. *Pract Neurol* 2007; 7(2): 116–123.

2. Maxwell G, James J, Archibald N, Bateman D. Acute neurology in the district general hospital: the role of the acute neurologist. *J Neurol Neurosurg Psychiatry* 2012; 83(Suppl 2): A30.

3. Mannan JB, Wieshmann UC. How accurate are witness descriptions of epileptic seizures? *Seizure* 2003; 12(7): 444–447.

4. Sheldon R, Rose S, Ritchie D, Connolly SJ, Koshman M-L, Lee MA, et al. Historical criteria that distinguish syncope from seizures. *J Am Coll Cardiol* 2002; 40(1): 142–148.

5. Panayiotopoulos CP. The new ILAE report on terminology and concepts for the organization of epilepsies: critical review and contribution. *Epilepsia* 2012; 53(3): 399–404.

6. Rathlev NK, Ulrich AS, Delanty N, D'Onofrio G. Alcohol-related seizures. *J Emerg Med* 2006; 31(2): 157–163.

7. D'Onofrio G, Rathlev NK, Ulrich AS, Fish SS, Freedland ES. Lorazepam for the prevention of recurrent seizures related to alcohol. *N Engl J Med* 1999; 340(12): 915–919.

8. Edlow JA, Caplan LR, O'Brien K, Tibbles CD. Diagnosis of acute neurological emergencies in pregnant and post-partum women. *Lancet Neurol* 2013; 12(2): 175–185.

9. Westby M, Davis S, Bullock I, Miller P, Cooper P, Turnbull N, Beal R, Braine M, Fear J, Goodwin M,

Grünewald R, Jelen P Pawelec J, Petkar S, Pitcher D, Pottle A, Rogers G, Swann G, et al. *Transient loss of consciousness ('blackouts').* National Institute of Health and Care Excellence. 2010; August 10: 1–429.

10. Sandstrom SA, Anschel DJ. Use of serum prolactin in diagnosing epileptic seizures: report of the Therapeutics and Technology Assessment Subcommittee of the American Academy of Neurology. *Neurology* 2006; 67(3): 544–545.

11. Marson A, Jacoby A, Johnson A, Kim L, Gamble C, Chadwick D, et al. Immediate versus deferred antiepileptic drug treatment for early epilepsy and single seizures: a randomised controlled trial. *Lancet* 2005; 365(9476): 2007–2013.

12. Powell R, McLauchlan DJ. Acute symptomatic seizures. *Pract Neurol* 2012; 12(3): 154–165.

13. National Institute of Health and Care Excellence. *The Epilepsies.* 2012; 1–636.

14. Lindhout D. Antiepileptic drugs during pregnancy and cognitive outcomes. *Lancet Neurol* 2013; 12(3): 219–220.

15. Leach JP. SUDEP discussions with patients and families. *Pract Neurol* 2012; 12(2): 103–106.

Chapter 25

Genital discharge and genital ulceration

Sathish Thomas William

Introduction

Genital discharge in women is one of the commonest presentations seen in sexual health clinics and primary care (for urethral discharges in men see 'Dysuria', Chapter 21). Many women will have already self-treated for these symptoms before seeking medical help. It is occasionally reported in patients presenting to acute medicine, either being volunteered by the patient, or more commonly in response to direct questioning. It may be physiological or pathological. It may be related to, or incidental to, the primary presentation. It can be a significant symptom resulting in considerable distress and needs to be appropriately addressed. Pathological vaginal discharge potentially can lead on to:

- pelvic inflammatory disease
- vaginal cuff cellulitis following surgery

    and especially problematic during pregnancy:

- prematurity
- low birth weight
- postpartum endometritis.

Genital ulcer diseases (GUD) are a common presentation in genitourinary medicine clinics. However, they can present in other settings including primary care, emergency departments and medical specialties. It is important to understand the causes, investigations and management of these conditions as they can be very distressing to the patients and have public health implications if due to sexually transmitted infection.

Taking a sexual history

The British Association for Sexual Health and HIV published guidelines for consultations requiring sexual history taking in 2013 [1].

Key components of the sexual history include:

For men

- Urethral discharge
- Dysuria
- Genital skin problems
- Peri-anal/anal problems (MSM)

For women

- Change in vaginal discharge
- Vulval skin problems
- Lower abdominal pain
- Dysuria
- Menstrual irregularities:
    - date of last menstrual period
    - contraceptive history
    - cervical cytology history

For both sexes

- Details of last sexual interaction including:
    - timing
    - partner gender
    - sites of exposure
    - condom use
- Previous sexual interactions (detailed as above)
- History of sexually transmitted diseases
- Risk history for HIV, hepatitis B and C
- Establish mechanism to feed-back test results
- Competency/child protection concerns if under 16 years of age

Examination

This should include a genital examination (in company of a chaperone) looking for:

- enlarged inguinal lymph nodes
- presence of urethral discharge

Acute Medicine, ed. Stephen Haydock, Duncan Whitehead and Zoë Fritz. Published by Cambridge University Press. © Cambridge University Press 2015.

- testicular tenderness in men

and in *women*:

- assessment for suprapubic tenderness
- vulval/vaginal soreness
- genital ulcerations
- vaginal discharge should be considered
- A bimanual examination in the presence of dyspareunia or pelvic pain to rule out PID is essential.

Scenario 25.1

A 30-year-old woman is referred for investigation of pleuritic chest pain. She is to be discharged following exclusion of any significant pathology. When it has been explained that investigations are normal and that she can go home, she quietly mentions that she has a troubling vaginal discharge that is causing her distress and embarrassment. She asks if you can 'sort this out' before she goes home as she doesn't want to see her own GP as they 'don't get on'.

Pathophysiology of vaginal discharge

Physiological

Is the commonest cause in women of childbearing age. Alterations in the oestrogen and progesterone levels during a menstrual cycle lead to changes in the cervical secretion, misperceived as a pathological vaginal discharge. Preovulation, the discharge is thin and clear (oestrogen effect) and post ovulation it becomes thick and sticky (progesterone effect).

Infectious

Bacterial vaginosis is the commonest infectious cause and is non-sexually transmitted [2]. The lining of the vaginal squamous cells is rich with glycogen. Lactobacilli, which are the normal flora of the vagina, convert this into lactic acid, thereby lowering pH and inhibiting the growth of other organisms. Alteration of this pH can result from:

- vaginal douching
- presence of STI
- smoking
- change of sexual partners.

The most common causative organisms for bacterial vaginosis include:

- *Gardnerella vaginalis*
- *Prevotella* spp.

- *Mycoplasma hominis*
- *Mobiluncus* spp.

It is associated with:

- increased risk of HIV acquisition
- pregnancy complications
- pelvic inflammatory disease.

Vaginal candidiasis is a frequent presentation in this age group and around 75% of women would have had it once in their lifetime [3]. Risk factors include:

- prior broad spectrum antibiotics
- pregnancy
- hyperoestrogenaemia
- immunosuppression.

Sexually transmitted infections: Chlamydia and gonorrhoea are the leading causes of STI-related vaginal discharge in the UK. They cause infection of the lining cells of the endocervix and urethra (see Chapter 21). Trichomoniasis (*Trichomonas vaginalis*, flagellated protozoan) is another important STI [4] that infects the vagina, urethra and paraurethral glands. Globally it is the most prevalent curable STI and in the UK is more common among Black Africans. It is associated with low birth weight, preterm delivery and increased HIV acquisition.

Non-infectious

Non-infectious causes are:

- retained tampon
- foreign body
- uterine malignancies
- cervical ectopy.

Clinical features

- *Chlamydia and gonorrhoea* usually produce a mucopurulent discharge with dysuria, lower abdominal pain, contact bleeding, postcoital bleeding or deep dyspareunia. Presence of these symptoms should lead to evaluation of the recognized complication of pelvic inflammatory disease.
- *Bacterial vaginosis* causes a thin white homogeneous discharge with a fishy odour and seen coating the vaginal walls. Itching or inflammation is not seen.
- *Candidiasis* produces a thick white curdy discharge associated with itching, vulval/vaginal soreness, fissuring, external dyspareunia, external dysuria and satellite lesions.

Table 25.1 Management of common causes of vaginal discharge (these recommendations are consistent with UK National Guidelines published by BASHH and those of the International Union Against Sexually Transmitted Infections (IUSTI) [5])

Bacterial vaginosis	Oral therapies: Metronidazole 400 mg PO bd for 5–7 days Metronidazole 2 g PO stat Intravaginal therapies: Intravaginal metronidazole gel (0.75%) od for 5 days Intravaginal clindamycin cream (2%) od for 7 days
Vulvovaginal candidiasis	Oral therapies: Fluconazole 150 mg PO stat Itraconazole 200 mg PO bd for one day Intravaginal therapies: Clotrimazole vaginal pessary 500 mg stat or 200 mg od for 3 days Miconazole vaginal ovule 1200 mg stat Econazole vaginal pessary 150 mg stat
Trichomoniasis	Metronidazole 400 mg PO bd for 7 days Metronidazole 2 g PO stat Tinidazole 2 g PO stat
Chlamydia	Azithromycin 1 g PO stat Doxycycline 100 mg PO bd for 7 days In pregnancy: Erythromycin 500 mg PO bd for 10–14 days
Gonorrhoea	Inj ceftriaxone 500 mg IM stat with azithromycin 1 g PO stat Second line: Cefixime 400 mg PO stat Azithromycin 2 g PO stat

- *Trichomoniasis* causes mild to profuse white frothy discharge with vulval itching and vaginitis. The pathognomonic 'strawberry cervix' is seen in 15% under colposcopy. Dysuria is infrequent.
- *Retained tampon or foreign body* causes offensive discharge and could lead to toxic shock syndrome.
- *Atrophic vaginitis and lichen sclerosus* cause minimal discharge and are associated with visible thinning of vulval architecture and external dyspareunia.

Management

NICE review recommends treatment for bacillary vaginosis and vaginal candidiasis based on clinical features alone if there are no risks of other serious infections.

Laboratory investigations include:

- Vaginal pH.
- High vaginal swab microscopy for causative organisms of bacillary vaginosis, clue cells, candidal hyphae/spores and candida culture.
- PCR nucleic acid amplification tests for chlamydia and gonorrhoea from a self-collected vulvovaginal or endocervical swab is highly sensitive and specific (>99%).
- Gonococcal culture and sensitivities if high clinical suspicion and before antibiotic treatment.
- If facilities exist, immediate diagnosis of gonococcus by microscopy of endocervical swab has <50% sensitivity.
- Trichomoniasis is detected on a vaginal wet film in around 70% cases. The gold standard for *Trichomonas vaginalis* diagnosis is culture but recent molecular diagnostics (PCR/antigen-based tests) have improved the sensitivities.

For STIs, referral to genitourinary medicine clinics facilitates partner notification and treatment. A general counselling on safe sex and avoidance of sexual intercourse for at least 1 week and until partners are treated is recommended for chlamydia, gonorrhoea and trichomoniasis.

Treatment for the above conditions is included in Table 25.1. Local guidelines should also be consulted. In about 30% of the cases no apparent cause is found and may require reassurance or referral to appropriate specialties based on clinical features.

Scenario 25.2

A 20-year-old woman is referred by the emergency department. She has been unwell for 3–4 days with fever, headache and general malaise. Meningism is elicited on examination. She is suspected of having a viral meningitis. On the MAU she develops painful retention of urine. During catheterization, ulceration of the genitalia is noted by the nursing staff.

Pathophysiology of genital ulceration

Among STIs, *genital herpes* (HSV) then *syphilis* are the most common cause of GUD worldwide. *Chancroid, donovanosis,* and *lymphogranuloma venereum* (LGV) are more prevalent in developing countries but are relatively rare in the UK. Since 2003 a significant increase in LGV has been seen within MSM in the UK. Other causes include:

Infectious

- Fungal (candida)
- Secondary bacterial infection
- EBV.

Non-infectious

- Behçet's disease
- Aphthous ulcers
- Malignancy
- Inflammatory skin conditions
- Allergic reactions
- Trauma
- Fixed drug eruptions:
  - sulphonamides
  - tetracycline
  - quinolones
  - non-steroidal anti-inflammatory drugs.

GUD is recognized as an important co-factor for acquisition of HIV. It increases HIV shedding and acquisition of HIV and other STIs.

Clinical features

Genital herpes

Is caused by herpes simplex virus type 1 and 2 and has increased by 90% in the past decade in the UK. This may be partly due to increased detection through polymerase chain reaction (PCR) tests and changes in sexual practices [6]. The incubation period for HSV is 4 days (range 2–9 days). Ulceration could be a primary or recurrent episode. It especially affects young people (15–24 years) with women more commonly presenting than males, although the prevalence is increasing among MSM.

- Primary episodes are more severe than recurrences and present with prodromal symptoms such as temperature, myalgia and headaches followed by blisters forming tender multiple ulcers. Acute onset often present to the ED.
- Tender regional lymphadenopathy is common.
- May be associated with neuropathic pain and sacral radiculopathy leading to urinary retention requiring catheterization.
- Symptoms and signs last for 2–3 weeks without treatment and around 1–2 weeks with treatment.
- There is an increased risk of recurrences soon after a primary episode.
- Aseptic meningitis (Molleret's) may occur.

Infectious syphilis

Caused by the spirochaete *Treponema pallidum* [7], there has been a twelve-fold increase in the last decade. Ninety per cent of cases in the UK are in men. Most of the increase is seen in white MSM (67%), aged 25–34 years; around 27% are co-infected with HIV, although there is a small increasing number of young/adolescent heterosexuals. Risk factors for infection include:

- unsafe sexual behaviour
- social deprivation
- high turnover of sexual partners.

'*Primary chancre*' forms around 4–6 weeks after acquisition (range 9–90 days).

Classically:

- there are non-tender, single or multiple, indurated, shallow to deep ulcers (Figure 25.1)
- regional lymph nodes are commonly involved and are non-tender, rubbery and discrete
- it is highly infectious and without treatment self-resolves in 2–3 weeks.

It can present atypically with:

- painful, superficial, purulent and self-destructive ulcerations.

Any anogenital ulcer should be considered to be due to syphilis unless proven otherwise.

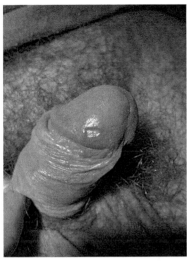

Figure 25.1 Characteristic penile ulcer of syphilis.

During the secondary stage of syphilis, mucocutaneous lesions involving the genitalia, condylomata lata (moist papular growth in mucocutaneous regions), can be mistaken for genital ulcers.

Lymphogranuloma venereum

- *Chlamydia trachomatis* serovars L1, 2, 3
- Transient erosive ulceration on the genitalia
- Tender inguinal and/or femoral lymphadenopathy
- Usually presents with proctitis in MSM rather than genital ulceration.

Chancroid

- *Haemophilus ducreyi*
- Painful shallow ulcers with granulomatous bases and purulent exudates

- The ulcer edge is typically ragged and undermined
- Tender, fluctuant regional lymph nodes (buboes) are seen.

Donovanosis

- *Klebsiella granulomatis*
- Disease of tropics
- Ulcers are well-defined, granulomatous, friable and bleed easily
- Regional lymph nodes are involved, sometimes ulcerating into the overlying skin.

Candidal genital ulcerations

- Tender, itchy, erythematous, fissures
- Associated with thick vaginal discharge in women.

Behçet's disease

- Important non-infectious cause of genital ulceration [8]
- Recurrent systemic inflammatory disorder of unknown origin causing genital ulcers in around 70–90% cases
- Tender, recurrent ulcers involving scrotum or vulva leaving a residual scar are seen
- Multisystem disease characterized by cutaneous lesions, uveitis, retinal vasculitis, parenchymatous brain lesions and vascular thrombosis.

Inflammatory skin conditions

(Usually also involve extragenital sites.)
- Psoriasis

Table 25.2 Treatment of common sexually transmitted infection causing GUD (these guidelines are consistent with UK National Guidelines published by BASHH)

Herpes simplex 1 and 2	Aciclovir 400 mg tds for 5 days Valaciclovir 500 mg bd for 5 days
Primary/secondary syphilis	Inj benzathine penicillin 2.4 MU intramuscular (IM) stat Inj procaine penicillin G 600 000 units IM od for 10 days Second line: Doxycycline 100 mg bd for 14 days Azithromycin 2 g PO stat or 500 mg od for 10 days Erythromycin 500 mg PO qds for 14 days
Lymphogranuloma venereum	Doxycycline 100 mg bd for 21 days
Chancroid	Azithromycin 1 g PO stat Ceftriaxone 250 mg IM stat Ciprofloxacin 500 mg PO stat

- Lichen sclerosus:
  - more common in women and particularly affects the vulval region
  - itchy white patches that may undergo erosion and become painful
- Bullous pemphigus.

Malignancy

The commonest malignancy is squamous cell carcinoma.

- Eroding ulcer with everted edges that may bleed on contact
- Common with increasing age
- Inguinal lymphadenopathy is commonly present.

Management

- Swabs for HSV1 and 2; PCR has very high sensitivity in the early stages of the infection.
- HSV serology is of limited use and should be used with caution. If suspected, treatment should be initiated pending confirmatory results to reduce distress and complications.
- Serological testing for syphilis *is mandatory*.
- Dark ground microscopy can identify *Treponema pallidum* but is often only done in genitourinary clinics.
- Recently multiplex PCR tests from genital swabs can test for HSV1 and 2, *Treponema pallidum* and *Haemophilus ducreyi* subject to local availability.
- Partner notification and follow-up should be arranged with the local genitourinary medicine clinic.
- Recommended treatments for common infectious causes are included in Table 25.2. Local Trust guidelines should also be consulted.
- Diagnosis of Behçet's disease is based on clinical criteria in liaison with rheumatologists. Increase in *inflammatory markers, cytokines and a positive pathergy test adds to the diagnosis*.
- Investigation and management of other causes of genital ulcers are based on history, examination and with involvement of relevant specialties.

References

1. 2013 UK national guideline for consultations requiring sexual history taking. Clinical Effectiveness Group, British Association for Sexual Health and HIV. Available to download at www.bashh.org/BASHH/Guidelines/Guidelines/BASHH/Guidelines/Guidelines.aspx.

2. Donders G. Diagnosis and management of bacterial vaginosis and other types of abnormal vaginal bacterial flora: a review. *Obstet Gynecol Surv* 2010; 65(7): 462–473.

3. Odds FC. *Candida and Candidosis: A Review and Bibliography*, 2nd edn. London: Baillèire Tindall; 1988.

4. Coleman JS, Gaydos CA, Witter F. *Trichomonas vaginalis* vaginitis in obstetrics and gynecology practice: new concepts and controversies. *Obstet Gynecol Surv* 2013; 68(1): 43–50.

5. 2011 European (IUSTI/WHO) Guideline on Management of Vaginal Discharge. Available to download at www.iusti.org/regions/Europe/pdf/2011/Euro_Guidelines_Vaginal_Discharge_2011.Intl_Jrev.pdf.

6. Adams HG, Brown ZA, Corey L, et al. Genital herpes simplex virus infections: clinical manifestations, course, and complications. *Ann Intern Med* 1983; 98(6): 958.

7. Goh BT. Syphilis in adults. *Sex Transm Infect* 2005; 81(6): 448–452.

8. Geri G, Pineton de Chambrun M, Wechsler B, et al. New insights into the pathogenesis of Behçet's disease. *Autoimmun Rev* 2012; 11(10): 687–698.

Further reading

British Association of Sexual Health and HIV. UK National Guideline for the Management of Bacterial Vaginosis 2012 (Clinical Effectiveness Group). Available to download at www.bashh.org/documents/4413.pdf.

British Association of Sexual Health and HIV. UK National Guideline on the Management of Vulvovaginal Candidiasis (2007) (Clinical Effectiveness Group). Available to download at www.bashh.org/documents/1798.pdf.

British Association of Sexual Health and HIV. UK National Guideline on the Management of *Trichomonas vaginalis* (2007) (Clinical Effectiveness Group). Available to download at www.bashh.org/documents/87/87.pdf.

British Association of Sexual Health and HIV: UK National Guideline on the Management of Genital Herpes (2007) (Clinical Effectiveness Group). Available to download at www.bashh.org/documents/115/115.pdf.

British Association of Sexual Health and HIV: UK National Guideline on the Management of Syphilis (2008) (Clinical Effectiveness Group). Available to download at www.bashh.org/documents/115/115.pdf.

Chapter

26

Haematemesis and melaena

Gareth Corbett and Ewen Cameron

Introduction

Acute upper gastrointestinal (GI) haemorrhage is the commonest life-threatening GI emergency and a common presentation on the medical take. It has an incidence of 100 cases per 100 000 of the population per year in the UK, where it is associated with over 9000 deaths per annum [1].

Patients present with the following symptoms:

- *Haematemesis* is the vomiting of fresh blood
- *Coffee ground vomiting* is the vomiting of altered blood
- *Melaena* is the passage of black altered blood per rectum
- *Haematochezia* is the passage of fresh blood per rectum in cases with very brisk upper GI bleeding.

Patients may also have haemodynamic compromise, depending on the severity of haemorrhage, and require early volume resuscitation to prevent death from hypovolaemic shock and its sequelae. Upper GI haemorrhage is usually classified according to whether the underlying cause is:

- *variceal* bleeding
- *non-variceal* bleeding.

The medical management of each is different, and with good clinical assessment the type of bleeding can often be predicted prior to endoscopy. Although the final goal of therapy is definitive endoscopic therapy, ***optimal pre-endoscopic resuscitation is imperative.***

Scenario 26.1

A 68-year-old man is admitted to the medical assessment unit directly via ambulance after collapsing at home. He is with his wife, who reports that he has been having tarry black stool for the past 24 hours. He has not vomited, but feels nauseated and has no appetite. He is tachycardic, hypotensive and appears pale.

This patient is showing signs of shock and the management aims are to:

- provide early resuscitation
- elicit a detailed history and physical examination
- arrange appropriate definitive therapy.

Early resuscitation should follow the standard principles of resuscitation.

- For those patients with haematemesis or coffee ground vomiting who are at risk of aspiration, ensure the airway is clear and examine for signs of aspiration (particularly if drowsy due to hepatic encephalopathy).
- Assessment of the severity of haemorrhage can be performed by estimating the proportion of circulating volume lost using basic vital sign observations (Table 26.1) and this can be used to determine appropriate fluid resuscitation.
- Volume replacement is best achieved using large bore intravenous cannulae inserted into each antecubital fossa and blood should be drawn for biochemistry, haematology, a coagulation screen, group and save, and possibly cross matching.
- Volume replacement should be performed using rapid boluses of intravenous fluid followed by reassessment with the size of bolus dependent on the clinical condition and co-morbid conditions such as cardiac and renal failure.
- Occasionally central venous monitoring can be helpful in guiding resuscitation in those patients with significant co-morbidity

---

Acute Medicine, ed. Stephen Haydock, Duncan Whitehead and Zoë Fritz. Published by Cambridge University Press. © Cambridge University Press 2015.

Table 26.1 Classification of acute haemorrhage (Advanced Trauma Life Support (ATLS), American College of Surgeons)

Class of haemorrhage	Proportion of circulating volume lost	Physical signs	Treatment required
1	Up to 15%	No change in vital signs	Usually none
2	15–30%	Tachycardia, narrowing in blood pressure, peripheral vasoconstriction leading to pallor and cool peripheries	Crystalloid intravenous fluid
3	30–40%	Tachycardia, hypotension, increased capillary refill time, reduced cognitive function	Intravenous crystalloid or colloid resuscitation plus red cell transfusion
4	>40%	Hypotension, reduced conscious level or coma, possibly bradycardic. High risk of cardiac arrest due to hypovolaemia	Aggressive volume replacement with crystalloid or colloid plus blood products required

BUT

- the risks associated with insertion are greater at times of hypovolaemia
- long thin catheters result in lower maximum flow rates than wide bore peripheral cannulae.
- There is no evidence to support the use of colloids rather than crystalloid in this situation. (The use of blood products is described later in the chapter.)
- For those likely to require large volumes of fluid and blood products, resuscitation fluids should be pre-warmed to prevent hypothermia and the associated risk of end-organ failure and coagulopathy.

Having stabilized the patient's physiology, the physician then has time to fully assess the patient.

Interpreting blood tests

Full blood count (FBC)

Remember that after haemorrhage:

- Level does not fall until haemodilution occurs such that in those with significant bleeding the initial result may underestimate the degree of blood loss.
- Bone marrow response may lead to an increase in mean corpuscular volume (MCV) due to a reticulocytosis.
- There is often a coexistent thrombocytosis and leucocytosis which does not necessarily reflect the presence of sepsis. (The C-reactive protein is usually normal in this setting.)
- A low MCV is suggestive of chronic rather than acute blood loss.

- A low platelet count should alert the physician to the possibility of portal hypertension (due to hypersplenism) and hence the possibility of variceal haemorrhage.

Urea and electrolytes

- Blood urea concentration rises in upper GI haemorrhage as a result of rapid protein metabolism and breakdown caused by blood in the GI tract. Whenever large quantities of amino acids are presented to the liver, protein formation begins rapidly. Haemoglobin is rich in valine and leucine but lacks the essential amino acid isoleucine. This means there is failure of protein formation and the peptide chains that have been formed are broken down again. The waste product of protein degradation is urea and blood urea concentration increases. In addition, hypovolaemia, if present, leads to reduced renal perfusion and a pre-renal acute kidney injury. A urea level disproportionately higher than creatinine is a useful indicator of an acute upper GI haemorrhage.

Liver biochemistry

- A patient can be cirrhotic and have normal liver biochemical tests.
- A patient without cirrhosis can have grossly deranged liver biochemistry.
- Patients with more advanced cirrhosis will tend to have an elevated serum bilirubin and reduced serum albumin concentrations.

Clotting screen

- The most common reason for deranged clotting in this setting is warfarin therapy.
- Prothrombin time can also be prolonged in patients with liver disease and rarely in patients with clotting factor deficiencies.
- Increasing numbers of patients are being treated with low molecular weight heparin and the newer anticoagulants (e.g. rivaroxaban, dabigatran, apixaban). Clotting studies *do not reflect* the level of bleeding tendency in these patients.

Causes of upper gastrointestinal haemorrhage

The next step in the management of the patient in the scenario is to determine the aetiology of their melaena. It is most likely to be upper gastrointestinal in origin, although occasionally small intestinal vascular lesions, caecal lesions or Meckel's diverticulum can lead to significant haemorrhage and produce melaena stool. Here we consider the upper GI causes primarily.

Differentiation between probable variceal and non-variceal haemorrhage is crucial to the management of these patients.

Clues to variceal haemorrhage include:

- History of chronic liver disease or cirrhosis
- Stigmata of chronic liver disease such as jaundice, spider naevi, thrombocytopenia and a prolonged prothrombin time
- Whilst a history of excess alcohol intake is a risk factor for cirrhosis, the majority of heavy drinkers presenting with GI haemorrhage do not have varices.

If the patient is likely to have a *variceal haemorrhage* (11% of all patients with upper GI bleeding) *early medical and endoscopic intervention is required* to improve outcomes.

Non-variceal upper GI haemorrhage has a number of causes which include (frequently found on endoscopy):

- Peptic ulcer (36%)
- Oesophagitis (24%)
- Gastritis (22%)
- Duodenitis (13%)
- Mallory–Weiss tear (4.3%)
- malignancy (3.7%)
- Vascular lesions such as angiodysplasia, gastric antral vascular ectasia (GAVE) or Dieulafoy lesions (2.6%)
- Occasionally haematemesis is the result of ingested blood from epistaxis and the high emetogenic nature of blood results in vomiting.

Not all reported coffee ground vomiting is due to GI haemorrhage. This is particularly true in the absence of melaena or signs of blood loss on blood tests. Specifically look for evidence of sepsis and intestinal obstruction in these patients.

Upper GI tract erosive disease is by far the most common cause of upper GI haemorrhage. This is commonly associated with the use of

- Aspirin
- Non-steroidal anti-inflammatory drugs (NSAIDs).

Other drugs which are associated with upper GI ulceration and bleeding include

- Corticosteroids
- Bisphosphonates
- SSRI antidepressants
- Doxycycline.

Anticoagulant medications do not cause upper GI haemorrhage; however, 7% of patients are on warfarin at the time of their GI bleed and anticoagulants *will increase the severity* of bleeding when this occurs.

Helicobacter pylori is an important cause of peptic ulcer disease, with a 10–20% lifetime risk of a peptic ulcer and 1–2% risk of gastric cancer in infected individuals.

Mallory–Weiss tears often present with the patient describing sequential vomiting followed by an episode of haematemesis. They usually heal spontaneously, although endotherapy is occasionally required.

Gastric antral vascular ectasia (GAVE) is sometimes referred to as 'watermelon stomach' due to the endoscopic appearance which is similar to the cut surface of a watermelon. It is associated with portal hypertension, chronic kidney disease and collagen vascular disorders.

A Dieulafoy lesion is a large and tortuous superficial mucosal arteriole (first described by the French surgeon Paul Georges Dieulafoy in 1898). A superficial erosion will lead to significant haemorrhage, which can be difficult to diagnose as they are only easily seen when actively bleeding.

Rarely an *aorto-enteric* (usually in the context of an infected vascular graft) or *aorto-oesophageal* (usually

Table 26.2 Rockall score parameters

Variable	Score 0	Score 1	Score 2	Score 3
Age	<60	60–79	>80	
Shock	No shock	Pulse >100 SBP >100	SBP <100	
Co-morbidity	Nil major		Congestive heart failure, IHD, major morbidity	Renal failure, liver failure, metastatic malignancy
Diagnosis	Mallory–Weiss tear	All other diagnoses	GI malignancy	
Evidence of bleeding	None		Blood, adherent clot, spurting vessel	

in the context of mediastinal neoplasia or radiotherapy) *fistula* may occur resulting in life-threatening haemorrhage.

Risk scoring

The mortality associated with upper GI haemorrhage is approximately:

- 7% for new admissions (primary haemorrhage)
- 26% for current inpatients (secondary haemorrhage).

Use of risk scoring is not universally adopted in acute medical units; however, it can serve two key purposes:

- Allows early identification of low risk patients who might be discharged for ambulatory management
- Assists in the recognition of high risk patients.

There are two widely used validated scoring systems.

The Rockall score (Tables 26.2 and 26.3) was developed following the 1993/4 audit of upper gastrointestinal haemorrhage in the UK [2]. It has pre and post endoscopy parameters, and predicts risk of rebleeding and mortality. It is relatively simple to use and does not require blood results but has the disadvantage of requiring an endoscopy before a full score can be calculated.

The Glasgow-Blatchford score (Table 26.4) predicts the need for medical intervention (e.g. blood transfusion or endoscopic therapy) without the need for endoscopy and is therefore a useful tool for determining patients who might be suitable for ambulatory care [3].

- A score of 0 means the patient is unlikely to need intervention and is therefore considered low risk.
- A score of 1 or more places the patient into a higher risk category and these patients should generally be offered endoscopy prior to discharge.

Some units elect to include patients with a score of 1 in their ambulatory service although these patients

Table 26.3 Risk of rebleeding and mortality according to Rockall score

Rockall score	Risk of rebleeding	Risk of mortality
0	5	0
1	3	0
2	5	0
3	11	3
4	14	5
5	24	11
6	33	17
7	44	27
8 or more	42	41

carry a higher risk. It is likely that further refinement of this scoring system will identify a larger group of patients suitable for ambulatory management. A score of 6 or more is associated with a greater than 50% risk of intervention.

The other scoring system commonly used in upper gastrointestinal bleeding is called the 'Forrest Classification' [4], which was described in 1974. It uses an endoscopic classification to determine the risk of rebleeding from ulcers (Table 26.5).

Medical therapy in non-variceal upper GI haemorrhage

The drive for definitive therapy in upper GI bleeding via endoscopic haemostasis often leads to the relatively straightforward medical interventions being forgotten. Referrals for urgent upper GI endoscopy in patients who have not been provided with adequate volume resuscitation or blood product replacement are unfortunately commonplace. The management priorities for patients with non-variceal haemorrhage should be:

- Check ABC and intervene as necessary

Table 26.4 Glasgow-Blatchford score parameters

Admission risk marker	Score component value
Blood urea (mmol/L)	
≥6.5 to <8.0	2
≥8 to <10.0	3
≥10 to <25.0	4
≥ 25	6
Haemoglobin (g/L) for men	
≥120 to <130	1
≥100 to <120	3
<100	6
Haemoglobin (g/L) for women	
≥100 to <120	1
<100	6
Systolic blood pressure (mmHg)	
100–109	1
90–99	2
<90	3
Other markers	
Pulse ≥100	1
Presentation with melaena	1
Presentation with syncope	2
Hepatic disease	2
Cardiac failure	2

- Risk stratification
- Correct blood loss
- Assess and treat for coagulopathy
- Determine whether high dependency or intensive care is required
- Refer for definitive endoscopic therapy
- Post endoscopy medical therapy.

Correcting blood loss

Determining the blood products required to treat haemorrhage can often be difficult. Using the classification of acute haemorrhage, patients with class 3 or 4 haemorrhage will definitely require blood products, therefore by using observations of vital signs a decision can be made regarding which blood products and how much to request. For those patients with major haemorrhage not responding to initial fluid resuscitation, many hospitals now have 'major blood loss protocols' which ensure that patients receive the appropriate mix of blood, platelets and fresh frozen plasma to prevent the development of transfusion-related coagulopathy. *Early senior review is mandatory in these patients.*

Recent studies have suggested possible negative outcomes with early blood transfusion in upper GI haemorrhage and some now advocate a relatively restrictive transfusion strategy.

Coagulopathy

- Population studies show that 7% of patients with non-variceal upper GI haemorrhage will be taking anticoagulant medications.
- Severe haemorrhage may result in coagulopathy due to blood loss.
- Patients with variceal haemorrhage are likely to have underlying liver disease putting them at risk of coagulopathy. It is essential to take a detailed medication history to check whether the patient is on anticoagulant or antiplatelet drugs.

Patients with active bleeding and coagulopathy should have the coagulopathy reversed.

- There are very few occasions where the risk of thrombosis is greater than the risk of bleeding in the immediate peri-haemorrhage period.

Table 26.5 Forrest classification of bleeding upper gastrointestinal ulcers

Forrest Class	Description	Risk of rebleeding without endoscopic therapy
Forrest I (active bleeding)	IA – spurting vessel	85–100%
	IB – oozing	10–27%
Forrest II (signs of recent haemorrhage)	IIA – visible vessel	50%
	IIB – adherent clot	30–35%
	IIC – haematin covered flat spot	<8%
Forrest III (no signs of haemorrhage)	III – clean base ulcer	<3%

- Vitamin K is used for patients on warfarin, but it does not immediately correct the clotting so prothrombin complex or fresh frozen plasma should also be used. The former is more effective.
- Coagulopathy should ideally be corrected prior to endoscopic intervention.
- The decision as to when to restart anticoagulation will depend on the indication and the severity of haemorrhage. If required early, clinicians will often use unfractionated heparin as this can be reversed much more rapidly than low molecular weight heparins in the event of recurrent haemorrhage.

Patients with thrombocytopenia with platelets <50/mm^3 should be considered for platelet transfusion following discussion with a haematologist. Increasing numbers of patients are encountered on newer antiplatelet drugs such as clopidogrel. Clopidogrel, like aspirin, is an irreversible platelet inhibitor but also has a long half-life such that *transfused platelets may be inhibited*. A decision to stop and reverse this drug will depend on the severity of the bleeding and the indication for its use. For example, the risk of stent thrombosis is very high in patients with drug-eluting coronary stents particularly in the first year after placement. In this setting, decisions should be taken in conjunction with a cardiologist.

Determining level of care

Most patients with acute upper GI bleeding in the UK are managed on a general medical ward. However, some require high dependency or intensive care unit care. The risk scores described above can help to identify patients more likely to need intervention, and therefore can form the foundation of determining which patients to consider managing in higher level care areas. These decisions should be taken following discussion with a senior physician responsible for the patient.

High dependency care should be considered for patients with:

- high risk scores
- haemorrhage requiring ongoing transfusion.

Referring for definitive endoscopic therapy

The role of endoscopy in patients with upper GI haemorrhage encompasses:

- diagnosis (differentiating between variceal and non-variceal haemorrhage)
- haemostasis.

Referral for endoscopy is a key part of the management plan in these patients but should not occur at the expense of resuscitation.

- Only half of acute trusts in the United Kingdom provide 24-hour emergency endoscopy services, but most patients do not require endoscopy out of hours.
- If a patient can be haemodynamically stabilized they can usually undergo endoscopy during a designated theatre slot during the working day.
- The standard of care for most patients is endoscopy within 24 hours.

Emergency endoscopy should be considered when:

- Resuscitation is unsuccessful
- If patients rebleed after initial resuscitation
- If variceal haemorrhage is strongly suspected or if aorto-enteric fistula is suspected (along with contrast-enhanced CT).

Endoscopic therapy has been shown to reduce rebleeding, mortality and need for surgery in patients with active bleeding and non-bleeding visible vessels. Initial therapy is usually with epinephrine (adrenaline) injection. A second modality of therapy (thermal or endoscopic clipping) has been shown to produce additional benefit.

Haemostatic powders which can be sprayed onto a bleeding lesion and promote clot formation are emerging as a potential new treatment in this patient group. This treatment may be useful for patients with severe uncontrollable bleeding to prevent the need for surgery or angiography. One potential benefit of these technologies is the lower degree of expertise required for use compared to traditional haemostatic techniques.

Patients who have required endoscopic intervention should be cared for by a gastroenterologist. For those with ongoing bleeding, treatment options include:

- Repeat endoscopic therapy
- Surgery
- Mesenteric angiography with coil embolization (specialist centres).

Post-endoscopy medical therapy

The discovery of *Helicobacter pylori* in 1982 and the introduction of proton pump inhibitors (PPIs) in 1989 revolutionized the management of peptic ulcer disease. Prior to this many patients would require surgical intervention, including partial gastrectomy to treat peptic ulcer disease. There is now good evidence that giving intravenous PPIs (high dose bolus followed by 72 hour infusion) after endoscopic therapy reduces the rate of rebleeding from around 35% to 10%, but has no effect on overall mortality.

Ongoing controversy relates to the use of PPIs prior to endoscopic therapy. Current guidelines in the UK suggest withholding PPIs prior to endoscopy. These guidelines are based on a lack of evidence of benefit in terms of important outcomes (rebleeding, mortality and need for surgery) when used indiscriminately. Several studies have suggested a lower rate of lesions requiring endoscopic therapy so their use would certainly be appropriate in cases where there is likely to be a significant delay before endoscopy.

Whilst many gastroenterologists will stop antiplatelets for some time after an upper GI haemorrhage, there is emerging evidence of higher mortality in those not continuing aspirin. A decision on when to restart these drugs should take into consideration the indication for antiplatelets and the severity of haemorrhage but it is probable that these should be restarted early in many patients. Given the irreversible inhibition of platelet function by aspirin and clopidogrel, some would advocate not stopping them at all.

Patients with gastric ulcers should have a repeat endoscopy to confirm healing and exclude a neoplastic cause of the ulcer.

Testing for *Helicobacter pylori* and providing eradication therapy when positive is mandatory in patients with peptic ulcer disease to prevent recurrence. It is diagnosed by:

- Breath test
- Urease test on a gastric biopsy (*Campylobacter*-like organism or CLO test)
- Histology of gastric biopsy
- Faecal antigen test
- Blood serology.

The first-line eradication regime usually consists of a PPI given twice daily, alongside amoxicillin 500 mg bd and clarithromycin 500 mg bd all given for a week. The amoxicillin can be changed to metronidazole 400 mg bd in penicillin-allergic patients. Second and third line treatment regimens are usually initiated and supervised by a gastroenterologist and are sometimes guided by culture and sensitivity testing. As eradication regimes are at most 90% effective, it is imperative that success of eradication

is determined using a post-treatment confirmatory test, such as repeat breath test or faecal antigen.

Variceal haemorrhage

Acute haemorrhage from varices of either the oesophagus or stomach usually results in large volume fresh haematemesis. Variceal haemorrhage should be suspected in any patient presenting with haematemesis and/or melaena with signs of chronic liver disease. In the UK, portal hypertension usually develops on the background of cirrhosis, but can also be associated with other causes such as portal vein thrombosis. Thrombosis of the splenic vein is associated with the development of gastric varices. The overall mortality from an acute variceal haemorrhage is 15% for all patients and 41% for current inpatients.

These patients are managed differently to those with non-variceal haemorrhage. Acute variceal haemorrhage can lead to sequelae other than those of hypovolaemia, including hepatic encephalopathy. The management priorities in patients with variceal haemorrhage are:

- Airway protection
- Fluid resuscitation
- Assess and correct coagulopathy
- Vasopressin therapy
- Early endoscopic intervention
- Broad spectrum antibiotics
- Options if haemostasis has failed.

Airway protection and fluid resuscitation

These patients are at particularly high risk of complications and should be managed at least in a high dependency unit. The combination of large volume haematemesis and reduced conscious level due to hepatic encephalopathy make these patients particularly at risk of aspiration. In this setting, endoscopy is most safely performed after the patient has been intubated. Fluid resuscitation follows the same principles as in non-variceal haemorrhage, and coagulopathy should be corrected as described above although care should be taken not to over-transfuse these patients as this can precipitate rebleeding.

Vasopressin therapy

Terlipressin is an intravenous vasopressin analogue given in boluses three to four times per day. It has been shown to reduce mortality from variceal haemorrhage by 34%. It should therefore form a standard part of the acute management of bleeding varices. Because of its vasoconstrictive effect, care should be taken in patients with arterial disease.

Early endoscopic intervention

Bleeding from varices requires early intervention, and is one of the indications for out-of-hours upper GI endoscopy. Haemostasis is usually achieved with variceal band ligation with further sessions performed to eradicate the varices. Reduced complication rates and more rapid eradication have meant that this has superseded injection sclerotherapy.

Gastric varices cannot be ligated in the same way, and injection with agents such as cyanoacrylate glue is used to achieve haemostasis.

After endoscopic band ligation of varices the patient should be prescribed a PPI and sucralfate to reduce the risk of bleeding from the ulcers formed when the banded mucosa sloughs away.

An emerging endoscopic therapy for bleeding oesophageal varices which cannot be controlled with band ligation is a fully covered stent providing tamponade. This is an alternative to the Sengstaken–Blakemore tube.

Intravenous broad spectrum antibiotics

Bacterial infections occur in around 20% of patients presenting with acute variceal haemorrhage. Infections are associated with increased rates of rebleeding and mortality. Prophylactic antibiotics have been shown to significantly improve short-term survival. Fluoroquinolones, such as ciprofloxacin, are recommended based on published studies; however, antibiotic choice is usually based on local unit guidelines.

Failure to control haemorrhage

Balloon tamponade is the first-line treatment when haemorrhage cannot be controlled endoscopically. A Sengstaken–Blakemore tube is a tamponade device designed specifically for controlling variceal haemorrhage.

- It should be inserted into patients who have a protected airway and *should only be inserted by those experienced in their use* as failure to insert correctly can result in fatal complications (e.g. oesophageal perforation).

- The tube has two balloons (gastric and oesophageal) and two aspiration ports (gastric and oesophageal).
- It is inserted orally into the stomach before filling the gastric balloon with water.
- The tube is then pulled against the fundus to tamponade the variceal inflow. This is usually adequate, but occasionally inflation of the oesophageal balloon is also required.
- The oesophageal balloon should never be inflated prior to inflation of the gastric balloon.
- The aspiration ports should be used regularly to check for bleeding distal to the tube.
- It should be inflated for no longer than 24 hours initially.

This is only a temporizing measure as around 50% of patients rebleed when the tube is deflated and leaving the balloons inflated will lead to ischaemic damage.

Transjugular intrahepatic porto-systemic shunt or TIPSS is the other option but is usually only performed in specialist centres. It involves introducing a catheter into the inferior vena cava via the jugular vein and placing a stent trans-hepatically between portal and hepatic veins. This technique has been shown to stop bleeding, and improve mortality in certain patient groups. It has the disadvantage of causing encephalopathy in some patients.

Secondary prophylaxis

Preventing further episodes of variceal haemorrhage is a priority for this group of patients. There is a significant reduction in rebleeding and mortality when beta-blockers are prescribed. Propranolol is usually used. After endoscopic eradication of varices, the patient should also be offered a programme of variceal surveillance and prophylactic band ligation if they recur as this has been shown to reduce the risk of rebleeding and mortality.

Further investigation

A cohort of patients presenting with melaena will have normal initial upper GI endoscopy. If the patient shows continuing signs of bleeding they should be kept in hospital for further investigation, until the diagnosis is made. If the history of melaena is definite and the patient was anaemic, but stabilized without intervention, then outpatient investigation is acceptable, usually within 2 weeks of discharge. The investigations to be considered include:

- *Colonoscopy* to look for bleeding proximal colonic lesions (tumours, polyps or vascular lesions)
- *CT abdomen/CT mesenteric angiogram* to localize the site of bleeding in the GI tract and usually obviate the need for formal *mesenteric angiography*
- *Wireless capsule endoscopy* to identify the site of bleeding in the small intestine
- Other investigations such as red cell scintigraphy and Meckel's scans are occasionally useful.

Key points

- Upper GI haemorrhage is the commonest GI emergency.
- Early resuscitation using the ABC approach is vital.
- There is no strong evidence for PPIs prior to *timely* endoscopy.
- Definitive endoscopic therapy should be delivered after resuscitation, ideally within 24 hours.
- Emergency endoscopy is indicated in patients not responding to resuscitation or those that rebleed.
- 72 hours of PPI following endoscopic therapy reduces the rate of rebleeding.
- Variceal haemorrhages are treated differently, with early endoscopy mandated.
- Other interventions such as interventional radiology could also be considered to achieve haemostasis.

References

1. Hearnshaw SA, Logan RF, Lowe D, Travis SP, Murphy MF, Palmer KR. Acute upper gastrointestinal bleeding in the UK: patient characteristics, diagnoses and outcomes in the 2007 UK audit. *Gut* 2011; 60(10): 1327–1335.

2. Rockall TA, Logan RF, Devlin HB, Northfield TC. Risk assessment after acute upper gastrointestinal haemorrhage. *Gut* 1996; 38(3)316–321.

3. Stanley A, Ashley D, Dalton H, Mowat C, Gaya D, Thompson E, Warshow U, Groome M, Cahill A, Benson G, Blatchford O, Murray W. Outpatient management of patients with low-risk upper-gastrointestinal haemorrhage: multicentre validation and prospective evaluation. *Lancet* 2009; 373(9657): 42–47.

4. Forrest JA, Finlayson ND, Shearman DJ. Endoscopy in gastrointestinal bleeding. *Lancet* 1974; 2(7877): 394–397.

Further reading

Barkun AN, Martel M, Toubouti Y, Rahme E, Bardou M. Endoscopic hemostasis in peptic ulcer bleeding for patients with high-risk lesions: a series of meta-analyses. *Gastrointest Endosc* 2009; 69(4): 786–799.

Jalan R, Hayes PC. UK guidelines on the management of variceal bleeding in cirrhotic patients. *Gut* 2000; 46: iii1–iii15.

NICE. Acute Upper Gastrointestinal Bleeding: Management. National Institute for Health and Care Excellence CG141, June 2012.

SIGN. Management of Acute Upper and Lower Gastrointestinal Bleeding. Scottish Intercollegiate Guidelines Network, 2008.

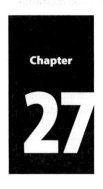
Haematuria

Duncan Whitehead

Introduction

Detection of blood in the urine always requires some consideration as to how it got there. Blood can enter the urine at any point from glomerulus to urethral meatus. The concentration of blood determines whether it is visible or invisible.

Scenario 27.1

Mr GN is an 81-year-old man, referred to the acute medical take with 'SOB uncertain cause'; the history is of 4 weeks of feeling unwell with a reduced appetite and lethargy, and he reports some epistaxis. He has recently developed a non-productive cough and shortness of breath on exertion; he was previously fit and fully independent. BP = 175/92 and his CXR demonstrates some bilateral patches of consolidation; his blood tests show WCC 10×10^9, CRP of 56 mg/L and a creatinine of 350 μmol/L. He has a creatinine from 5 months earlier of 112 μmol/L. Urine dipstick reveal blood +++ and protein +++.

There are a number of features in this history which suggest this man has more than a community-acquired pneumonia with associated AKI, although this should be the first diagnosis in the differential diagnosis. It is essential at this point not to start antibiotics and fluids and consider the 'job done'. The whole scenario needs consideration and a full differential needs formulating and investigating appropriately. He has an ANCA-positive vasculitis with pulmonary and renal involvement; delay or completely missing this diagnosis will result in very poor outcome.

Anatomy of the urinary tract

The anatomy of the urinary tract is shown in Figure 27.1.

Common causes of haematuria

There is always an explanation for haematuria; the common causes are:

- Transient haematuria is commonly a benign finding; causes include contamination from menstruation or minor trauma
- Urinary tract infections (UTI) are the commonest pathological cause
- Renal or bladder calculi
- Tumour within the urinary tract (higher probability with visible haematuria)
- Trauma
- Glomerulonephritis
- Thin basement membrane disease (benign inherited abnormality in type IV collagen)
- Endocarditis
- Haematuria can result from haemolysis.

Anticoagulants will increase the degree of haematuria but are not a cause.

Clinical assessment

History

Enquire regarding:

- Symptoms of a UTI: dysuria, frequency, urgency
- Abdominal pain of renal colic
- Recent infection suggestive of post-infectious glomerulonephritis
- Recent abdominal/pelvic trauma
- Recent intense exercise
- Foreign travel, e.g. schistosomiasis

Acute Medicine, ed. Stephen Haydock, Duncan Whitehead and Zoë Fritz. Published by Cambridge University Press. © Cambridge University Press 2015.

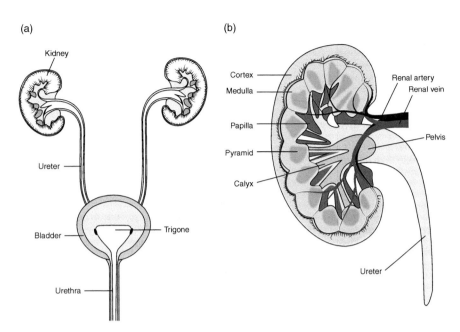

(a)

Kidney

Ureter

Bladder

Trigone

Urethra

(b)

Cortex

Medulla

Papilla

Pyramid

Calyx

Renal artery
Renal vein

Pelvis

Ureter

Figure 27.1 Basic anatomy of the urinary system. (A) Gross anatomy of the renal tract. (B) Anatomy of the kidney. (C) Microscopic structure of glomerulus, nephron and collecting duct.

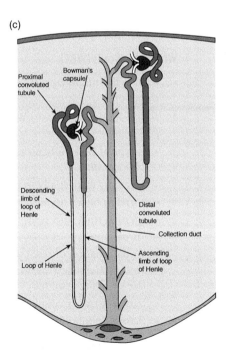

(c)

Proximal convoluted tubule

Bowman's capsule

Descending limb of loop of Henle

Distal convoluted tubule

Collection duct

Loop of Henle

Ascending limb of loop of Henle

- Occupational exposure, e.g. benzenes, arylamines in rubber and plastics industry (now banned due to risk of bladder cancer)
- Past history of hypertension
- Drug history, e.g. sulphonamides, cyclophosphamide
- Smoking history: increases risk of bladder cancer four-fold
- Unexplained weight loss.

Examination

A full examination is indicated; the key features to examine for are:

- Temperature
- Blood pressure
- Heart rate
- Oxygen saturations
- Respiratory rate
- Abdominal examination:
  - palpate the bladder for tenderness and urinary retention
  - ballot the kidneys; considering renal cell carcinoma and polycystic kidneys
- Per rectum examination:
  - rectal masses with possible anterior invasion
  - prostate gland in males: tenderness (prostatitis), masses and size
- Respiratory system; crepitations consistent with pulmonary haemorrhage, pleural effusions from fluid overload
- Cardiac auscultation; endocarditis, AF with fast ventricular response
- Finger nails for splinter haemorrhages and nail bed infarcts; vasculitis, endocarditis
- Eyes including fundoscopy; Roth spots, uveitis
- Skin rashes; purpuric rash of vasculitis
- Joints; arthritis and synovitis
- Neurological assessment; mononeuritis multiplex, cerebral vasculitis

Investigation of the urine in haematuria

Dipstick

- *Nitrites*: some bacteria such as *E. coli* reduce nitrates into nitrites not all pathogenic bacteria produce nitrites.
- *Leucocyte esterase* indicates the presence of white cells in the urine suggesting UTI, or another cause, interstitial nephritis for one.

In a symptomatic patient a negative dipstick for nitrites and leucocytes does not exclude UTI. Nor do positive results when asymptomatic confirm a UTI.

- *Haemoglobin*, positive if myoglobin, erythrocytes or haemoglobin present.
- *Protein*: most strips are more sensitive to albumin than other proteins, and generally do not show positive with isolated BJP in the urine.

- *Glucose*: proximal tubular cells reabsorb glucose, so glucosuria only occurs if the serum glucose level is above 10 mmol/L, the '*renal glucose threshold*'. When renal tubules are not functioning normally, renal glucosuria can occur with normal serum glucose.
- *pH*: normal urinary pH range is 4.5–8.0. The presence of an acidosis should result in renal compensation, acidifying the urine; a urinary pH ≥5.5 with an acidosis would be abnormal and suggests renal tubular acidosis type 1 or 2.

Urinary tract infections are the commonest pathological cause of haematuria or proteinuria on dipstick testing; their presence should trigger mid-stream urine (MSU) analysis with microscopy, culture and sensitivity (MC&S). If specific requests are made, fresh urine can give further diagnostic information.

The 'piss-prophets' of the eighteenth and nineteenth centuries knew urine held key diagnostic information; we should not forget this wisdom!

Microscopy

White blood cells (WBC)

- $>10^4$ WBC/mL is suggestive of a urinary tract infection.
- If the culture is negative this is termed *sterile pyuria*; causes include:
  - atypical UTI, difficult to culture, e.g. *TB, Chlamydia*
  - recently or partially treated UTI
  - foreign body; ureteric stent, urethral catheter
  - genital tract infection
  - prostatitis
  - inflammation of renal parenchyma as in acute interstitial nephritis, urinary eosinophils may be seen if stained for
  - urinary tract malignancy
  - sample contamination.

Red blood cells (RBC)

- Normally ≤5 RBC/high power field (HPF) on microscopy.
- Dipstick positive haematuria with ≤5 RBC/HPF on microscopy suggests myoglobin or haem is present, so rhabdomyolysis and haemolysis need consideration.

- Dysmorphic urinary red cells result from erythrocytes entering Bowman's capsule and passing through the renal tubules; the osmotic pressures cause the crenated or dysmorphic appearance.
- Non-dysmorphic red cells most commonly enter the urine distal to the nephron unit.

Casts

- Casts form within the tubules giving the classic vermiform shape; they are bound together by Tamm–Horsfall protein, secreted from the loop of Henle.
- *Red cell casts* typically indicate a glomerulonephritis but occasionally arise in interstitial nephritis and ATN.
- *White cell casts* can occur in pyelonephritis and active interstitial nephritis.
- *Fractured casts* from Bence Jones protein aggregation in myeloma cast nephropathy are seen on renal biopsy within the tubules; microscopy can reveal these as waxy or granular casts with associated reactive cells.

The absence of dysmorphic red cells or urinary casts does not exclude glomerular pathology, nor do these findings clarify the type of glomerulonephritis present.

Culture

- The gold standard technique to obtaining urine for culture is suprapubic aspiration; this is rarely done unless a suprapubic catheter is being inserted.
- MSU is an acceptable alternative but can be contaminated by urethral bacteria.
- $\geq 10^5$ cfu/mL of a single organism is defined as a positive culture.
- In symptomatic females a culture result is considered positive with as few as $\geq 10^2$ cfu/mL; early infection can be present with $<10^5$ cfu/mL in males.
- Symptoms and signs of UTI need correlation with the result, and include:
  - dysuria
  - frequency
  - urgency
  - polyuria
  - suprapubic or loin tenderness
  - haematuria
  - fever
  - rigors

- other signs of the systemic inflammatory response syndrome (SIRS).
- Asymptomatic bacteriuria is common; present in ≈17% of women over 75 years old, it is a near universal finding with long-term catheters.
- Harm can result from treating asymptomatic bacteriuria, so restrict treatment to those who are symptomatic.
- Symptomatic catheterized individuals should be treated with 7 to 14 days of antibiotics, and there is evidence for an *early catheter change while on antibiotics.*

UTIs cause ≈40% of hospital-acquired infections.

Sensitivities

- When urine culture is positive, antibiotic sensitivities will be released; these should guide antibiotic choice, alongside local antibiotic prescribing policy

If UTI is excluded or the clinical picture is suspicious for another cause of haematuria then further evaluation is required.

Cytology

- Lacks sensitivity and specificity for low-grade urinary tract malignancies so is not an investigation of exclusion.
- Adjunctive test to USS and cystoscopy.
- It has a place in monitoring of high-grade urinary tract tumours.

Blood tests

Glomerulonephritis screening, blood tests as AKI and consider additional tests depending on the clinical scenario:

- anti-neutrophil cytoplasmic antibodies (ANCA-associated vasculitis)
- anti-glomerular basement membrane antibodies (anti-GBM disease)
- anti-nuclear antibodies (ANA) and double-stranded DNA (positive in SLE)
- rheumatoid factor (rheumatoid-associated vasculitis can affect kidneys, also typically positive in cryoglobulinaemia)
- cryoglobulins (rare but important cause of rapidly progressive glomerulonephritis)

- complement: C3 and C4 (low levels in lupus nephritis and endocarditis associated glomerulonephritis)
- hepatitis B and C (associated with several glomerulonephritides)
- anti-streptolysin O titre (raised in post streptococcus glomerulonephritis)
- Immunoglobulins (raised IgA in 50% of patients with IgA nephropathy).

Additional tests to consider:

- Haemolysis screen
  - blood film
  - lactate dehydrogenase
  - haptoglobin
- CK
- Prostate specific antigen (PSA).

Nephrological haematuria

Glomeruli are specially adapted capillary bundles with a triple layered (endothelial cells, basement membrane and podocyte foot processes) permeable barrier between the capillary lumen and the Bowman's capsule. Disruption of this barrier results in blood and/or protein crossing from the bloodstream into the urine, as seen in glomerulonephritis.

Several features should make the physician question whether haematuria is from a glomerular pathology. Assessment for glomerular causes requires the following steps:

History and examination

- Systemic symptoms of autoimmune condition, e.g. vasculitic rash, haemoptysis, epistaxis, sinusitis, arthritis.
- Hypertension is frequently present with acute or chronic glomerulonephritis.
- No obvious cause for AKI.

Urine analysis

Quantifying proteinuria

A urinary protein:creatinine ratio should be performed if the dipstick indicates proteinuria; this gives a rapid quantification of proteinuria:

- 50 mg/mmol ($\approx$0.5 g/24 hours), significantly raised
- >100 mg/mmol ($\approx$1.0 g/24 hours), suggests glomerular disease

- >300 mg/mmol ($\approx$3 g/24 hours) is nephrotic range proteinuria requiring a nephrology referral.

Proteinuria of renal origin occurs from:

1. Glomerular pathology
2. Reduced tubular reabsorption of protein.

Normally $\leq$1 g/24 hours of small protein molecules pass through the glomerular membrane and are reabsorbed in the tubules. Damage to the tubules can reduce this reabsorption of protein, for example in acute interstitial nephritis, and may result in proteinuria up to $\approx$1 g/24 hours.

3. Excessive production of abnormal proteins (*overflow proteinuria*).

Myeloma producing a large quantity of (small) free light chain proteins can overwhelm tubular protein reabsorption overflowing into the urine as BJP.

Microscopy (fresh urine)

- Red cell casts or dysmorphic erythrocytes are consistent with glomerulonephritis.

Blood tests

- Progressively rising creatinine over days (see 'AKI', Chapter 6)
- Raised CRP without obvious infection
- Autoantibodies present
- Reduced complement levels
- Hepatitis B or C positive; association with several types of glomerulonephritis.

Urine output

- Oliguria despite euvolaemic without urinary obstruction (see 'AKI', Chapter 6).

Ultrasound

- Echobright or normal appearance is compatible with an active glomerulonephritis.

Nephrology referral

A glomerulonephritis should be suspected on clinical grounds; definitive diagnosis requires a renal biopsy for histology. Urgent nephrology referral is indicated when a glomerulonephritis is suspected and renal function is worsening as this is consistent with a rapidly progressive glomerulonephritis (RPGN).

Early diagnosis of RPGN enables prompt intervention and gives the best renal and patient outcome, illustrated clearly in anti-GBM disease. Where diagnosis is delayed until renal replacement therapy is required or creatinine is >600 µmol/L, the kidneys are almost never salvageable. If the patient is dialysis free with a creatinine <600 µmol/L when plasma exchange is initiated there is an ≈80% dialysis-free survival rate.

When concerned do not delay referral, waiting for an ultrasound or autoimmune screen. High quality referrals include:

- History
- Patient's normal level
- Medications
- Examination findings
- Observations
- Fluid input and output
- Urine dipstick result
- Proteinuria quantification
- Creatinine results and other blood results currently available
- Ultrasound result if performed
- Current differential diagnosis for AKI.

Urological haematuria

Indications for rapid urological assessment for haematuria are suspected malignancy and the prevention of complications from haematuria:

- Visible (macroscopic) haematuria:
  - dark 'claret' haematuria or visible clots require admission and bladder irrigation with a three-way catheter to avoid clot retention.

- *Persistent invisible (microscopic) haematuria* with risk factors for urinary tract malignancy:
  - age >40
  - male
  - smoking history
  - prior exposure to carcinogens; cyclophosphamide, benzenes, aromatic amines
  - previous pelvic radiation
  - irritative urinary tract symptoms; urgency, frequency or dysuria
  - history of urological pathology or treatment.

These patients should have outpatient referral for investigation with USS KUB and flexible cystoscopy.

Other indications for urology assessment include:

- renal cell carcinoma or bladder tumour suggested on imaging
- suspicion of prostate mass on PR examination.

Further reading

Joint Consensus Statement on the Initial Assessment of Haematuria Prepared on behalf of the Renal Association and British Association of Urological Surgeons (2008). Available to download at www.baus.org.uk/AboutBAUS/publications/haematuria-guidelines.

Management of suspected bacterial urinary tract infection in adults. SIGN guideline 88 (2012). Available to download at www.sign.ac.uk/pdf/sign88.pdf.

Chapter 28

Haemoptysis

Marko Nikolić and Jonathan Fuld

Introduction

Haemoptysis stems from the Greek words haima ('blood') and ptysis ('spitting') and thus refers to the expectoration of blood. For centuries, haemoptysis was considered pathognomonic of pulmonary tuberculosis; more latterly smoking has made lung cancer the diagnosis of exclusion.

Causes

Common >60% [1]

- Bronchiectasis
- Chronic bronchitis
- Acute bronchitis
- Lung cancer

Less common ~30%

- Pneumonia
- Pulmonary embolism
- Tuberculosis
- Interstitial lung disease
- Drugs (e.g. anticoagulants, aspirin)
- Iatrogenic (e.g. bronchoscopy, percutaneous lung biopsy, radiotherapy)
- Haematological (e.g. coagulopathies, abnormal platelet function)

Rare <10%

- Goodpasture's syndrome
- Vasculitides (e.g. Wegener's granulomatosis)
- Arteriovenous malformations or bronchial artery malformations
- Foreign body inhalation
- Chronic congestive heart failure
- Mitral stenosis

Non-pulmonary bleeding

- Oropharynx, e.g. gingival disease
- Gastro-oesophageal reflux disease

Idiopathic

> **Scenario 28.1**
>
> *A 60-year-old male patient is referred to the medical assessment unit by the emergency department with a 2-day history of coughing up sputum and blood. The sister-in-charge asks you what investigations are required and whether you are planning to admit the patient.*

This is a common referral to the on-call medical team and requires exclusion of serious underlying pathology, though not necessarily as an inpatient.

History

Information from the history is vital for tailoring the management of the patient presenting with haemoptysis, though is often insufficient to make the diagnosis or identify the cause [2].

It is important to confirm that the source of the bleeding is from the lungs.

- Any bleeding from the nose or pharynx?
- Any dental problems?
- Any gastro-oesophageal reflux?
- Any vomiting?
- Is the blood mixed with the sputum? (If yes, then this is clearly haemoptysis.)

Detailed questions about the sputum will help differential diagnosis.

- Frothy or pink suggests heart failure.

Acute Medicine, ed. Stephen Haydock, Duncan Whitehead and Zoë Fritz. Published by Cambridge University Press. © Cambridge University Press 2015.

- Purulent or rusty-coloured suggests a bacterial infection.
- White sputum with blood streaks is more likely to indicate tumour [2].

Asking about the frequency of episodes will help differential diagnosis.

- Are the episodes recurrent? (Recurrent bleeding suggests malignancy, particularly if it continues for more than a few days [2].)

Infection is a very common cause.

- Any infective symptoms? Any fevers? Any yellow/green-coloured sputum?

Establish the severity of anaemia.

- Check for symptomatic anaemia: chest pain or dyspnoea?

Ask about past medical history and drug history.

- Any known bleeding tendencies?
- Any medications which increase the bleeding tendency?

Identify any clues that there may be an undiagnosed malignancy.

- Ask about smoking status, weight loss, back pain.

Venous thromboembolism is a potentially life-threatening cause of haemoptysis.

- Ask about major risk factors of venous thromboembolism (VTE):
  - reduced mobility
  - recent surgery
  - pregnancy
  - malignancy
  - previous VTE.

Establish whether there has been exposure to tuberculosis.

- Ask about travel history.

Ask about anything else unusual.

- Any foreign body inhalation?

Examination

The principle of the clinical examination is to determine an appropriate differential diagnosis.

On inspection

- Any finger clubbing? Respiratory causes of clubbing associated with haemoptysis include:
  - bronchial carcinoma
  - bronchiectasis.
- Are there signs of significant anaemia:
  - subconjunctival pallor
  - raised respiratory rate
  - central or peripheral cyanosis.
- Any leg swelling:
  - subconjunctival pallor
  - raised respiratory rate
  - central or peripheral cyanosis.
- Sputum pot:
  - blood mixed with sputum confirms the lung as the bleeding source.

On palpation

- Lymphadenopathy suggests malignancy.

On percussion

- Stony dull percussion note suggests pleural effusion.

On auscultation

- Localized, coarse inspiratory crackles suggest infection or bronchiectasis.
- Fixed wheeze suggests endobronchial tumour until proven otherwise.
- Fine inspiratory crackles suggest interstitial lung disease.
- Absent breath sounds suggest pleural effusion.

Basic investigations

Request the following at time of presentation (regardless of the degree of haemoptysis).

Blood tests

- FBC, U&E, creatinine, LFTs.
- Clotting screen, and consider group and save. Act swiftly on any significant clotting abnormalities or anaemia (Hb <8 or Hb <10 with symptoms).

Imaging

- CXR. Any obvious abnormalities: Consolidation? Masses?

Other

- ECG. Sinus tachycardia is the commonest ECG change in pulmonary embolism. The classic changes of $S_1Q_3T_3$ are rare.
- Sputum inspection and culture (as described above).
- Urine analysis. Blood and protein in the urine could indicate pulmonary-renal syndrome.
- *Arterial blood gas* if SpO_2 abnormal. Hypoxia can be associated with various causes of haemoptysis and needs to be corrected. *The cause of death in patients with massive haemoptysis is usually asphyxiation, not exsanguination* [3].

Specialist investigations

The following may not be required on the day of presentation. Nevertheless, it is important to consider these specialist investigations as a junior doctor because there are certain requirements for them to be done safely, e.g. adequate renal function for CTPA, normal clotting for bronchial biopsy.

Contrast CT scanning now sits at the cornerstone of investigation of patients with haemoptysis, and should include arterial phase imaging if pulmonary embolus is suspected as a possible cause.

CT chest

- *Benefits*: diagnosis of bronchiectasis, bronchogenic carcinoma and aspergilloma.
- *Cautions*: radiation.

CT pulmonary angiogram

- *Benefits*: gold standard for the diagnosis of pulmonary embolism.
- *Cautions*: radiation.

If pulmonary embolism is suspected in a patient with haemoptysis, then a V/Q scan should not be performed as lung cancers can also cause a V/Q abnormality and may therefore be missed.

Bronchoscopy

- *Benefits*: visualizes the airways and localizes the site of bleeding; useful for evaluating central bronchial lesions by biopsy, also allowing the local infusion of a vasoconstricting drug (adrenaline) or catheter insertion for tamponade (see massive haemoptysis) to control the bleeding.

- *Cautions*: any clotting abnormalities need to be corrected.

Bronchial artery angiogram

- *Benefits*: required to determine the optimal approach for bronchial artery embolization.
- *Cautions*: radiation.

Specialized blood tests

- ANCA, anti-GBM, ANA.

Management

Minor haemoptysis

- Blood streaking of the sputum or more obvious haemoptysis with normal radiograph.
- Significant radiological changes are associated with the most serious causes of haemoptysis. A normal chest X-ray will reduce the probability of cancer or pulmonary embolism and suggests that the bleeding source lies in the tracheobronchial tree rather than in the pulmonary parenchyma [4]. The overall incidence of cancer in this set of patients is only 3% [2] and it is likely that these tumours are surgically resectable.
- We therefore need to select the patient group which requires *further investigations* (CT chest in the first instance and bronchoscopy for cases where the CT is inconclusive). The following criteria favour malignancy [1]:
  - *age* over 40 years
  - current *smokers*
  - haemoptysis lasting *more than one week.*
- In the absence of these factors, the incidence is only 0.13% [1].
- Irrespective of these criteria, *all* patients with haemoptysis and a normal chest radiograph can be managed as *outpatients, usually via a 2-week cancer referral to respiratory medicine.*
- On discharge, have a low threshold for prescribing a course of oral antibiotics.
- *Bronchoscopy* can be considered as the first-line investigation if there is doubt that the reported bleeding was indeed haemoptysis.
- *CT chest* and *bronchoscopy* can supplement each other: bronchoscopy cannot detect peripheral lesions and CT may miss endobronchial tumours or may misattribute small opacities to other causes [5].

- Consider stopping *anticoagulants* depending on the importance of the indication.

Major haemoptysis

Life-threatening

Life-threatening haemoptysis is defined by any one of the following criteria:

- >500 mL in 24 h [7]
- Abnormal gas exchange/airway obstruction
- Haemodynamic instability.

Immediate management

- *Immediate resuscitation* with intravenous fluids (large bore intravenous access) and/or blood products and oxygen therapy.
- Referral to *intensive care* and *specialist advice*, including from interventional respiratory physicians or cardiothoracic surgeons. This might involve isolation of the healthy lung by intubating the contralateral main bronchus.

Specialist management

- Consider oral *tranexamic acid* (500 mg tds, not in severe renal failure).
- Early *bronchoscopy* (rigid is preferable) to localize bleeding and insert Fogarty catheter for balloon tamponade.
- *Bronchial artery embolization*.
- *Surgical resection* of bleeding lobe (if all other measures fail).

The commonest causes

1. Malignancy
2. Bronchiectasis
3. Aspergilloma
4. Tuberculosis when a major vessel has been invaded or damaged

Mortality has been reported to be up to 85% [8] and in view of this an early palliative approach may be appropriate.

Non-life-threatening

- *CT chest with contrast* is required to rule out pulmonary embolism and rare causes such as arteriovenous malformations. CT scanning aids

planning of bronchial artery embolization and should be performed urgently.

- *Angiographic embolization* should be considered for all patients with an identified focus of bleeding (e.g. from tumour, bronchiectasis).
- Conservative medical resuscitation is likely to be as effective as urgent *bronchoscopy/surgery* [9], but this obviously depends on the individual patient.
- Consider early referral to intensive care, as *endotracheal intubation* allows aspiration to clear the airways of clots.
- For lesser degrees of bleeding, airway clearance can be encouraged by *postural drainage* and *bronchodilators*.
- A *chest radiograph* may help to identify the source of bleeding.
- *Bronchoscopy* is required to localize the bleeding source and possibly identify the cause. Only 30–50% of bronchoscopies find a cause [2].
  - There is usually time for the procedure to be done electively and some studies have shown that the likelihood of identifying the source of bleeding and the overall clinical outcome do not differ if delayed by up to 48 hours [10].
- Correct any coagulopathy and arterial oxygenation and consider any underlying causes, e.g. leukaemias, Goodpasture's syndrome.
- Stop any anticoagulants and consider reversal depending on the importance of the indication.

Key points

- Although infection is the commonest cause, lung cancer must not be missed.
- In up to one-third of patients, no cause is identified. This has a good prognosis.
- Patients with haemoptysis and a normal chest radiograph can be managed as outpatients by the respiratory team.
- Patients with haemoptysis and an abnormal chest radiograph should have an urgent (within 2 weeks) CT chest with contrast.
- CTPA, not V/Q, is the test of choice to exclude pulmonary embolism in a patient with haemoptysis.
- Major haemoptysis warrants consideration of bronchial artery embolization if a bleeding source is evident.

References

1. Tsoumakidou M, Chrysofakis G, Tsiligianni I, Maltezakis G, Siafakas NM, Tzanakis N. A prospective analysis of 184 hemoptysis cases: diagnostic impact of chest X-ray, computed tomography, bronchoscopy. *Respiration; International Review of Thoracic Diseases* 2006; 73: 808–814.

2. John Gibson DMG, Costabel U, Sterk P, Corrin B. *Respiratory Medicine*, 3rd edn. Saunders; 2003.

3. Marshall TJ, Jackson JE. Vascular intervention in the thorax: bronchial artery embolization for haemoptysis. *European Radiology* 1997; 7: 1221–1227.

4. Israel RH, Poe RH. Hemoptysis. *Clinics in Chest Medicine* 1987; 8: 197–205.

5. White CS, Romney BM, Mason AC, Austin JH, Miller BH, Protopapas Z. Primary carcinoma of the lung overlooked at CT: analysis of findings in 14 patients. *Radiology* 1996; 199: 109–115.

6. Naidich DP, Funt S, Ettenger NA, Arranda C. Hemoptysis: CT-bronchoscopic correlations in 58 cases. *Radiology* 1990; 177: 357–362.

7. Thompson AB, Teschler H, Rennard SI. Pathogenesis, evaluation, and therapy for massive hemoptysis. *Clinics in Chest Medicine* 1992; 13: 69–82.

8. Santiago S, Tobias J, Williams AJ. A reappraisal of the causes of hemoptysis. *Archives of Internal Medicine* 1991; 151: 2449–2451.

9. Corey R, Hla KM. Major and massive hemoptysis: reassessment of conservative management. *American Journal of the Medical Sciences* 1987; 294: 301–309.

10. Gong H, Jr, Salvatierra C. Clinical efficacy of early and delayed fiberoptic bronchoscopy in patients with hemoptysis. *American Review of Respiratory Disease* 1981; 124: 221–225.

Head injury

Cliff Mann

Introduction

Head injuries requiring admission to hospital have an annual incidence in the UK of almost 300/100 000 population, with a male to female ratio in excess of 3:1. In patients under 65, road traffic accidents account for more than half of admissions whilst falls are the predominate cause in older patients. NICE guidance in this area was published in 2007 and is due for updating at the time of writing. Physicians need an understanding of head injury as they encounter them in the elderly falls patient presenting on the acute medical take and sadly, though hopefully rarely, they can be sustained by our patients in the ward environment.

> **Scenario 29.1**
>
> *A 70-year-old man is referred by his GP. He has a history of falls and has fallen in his garden and was unable to mobilize. He has sustained an injury to his face. Initially alert, his GCS score on arrival on the MAU has fallen to 12/15.*

The physician is frequently involved in the care of patients who have fallen and sustained a head injury. We need to be able to decide on the urgency for CT scanning, frequency of nursing observation and when to contact neurosurgery.

Clinical assessment

Basic principles

Use the ABCDE approach. Always look for other major injuries resulting in hypotension and/or hypoxia; these must be addressed first since either results in diminished cerebral function or significantly increases the morbidity and mortality of any brain injury. Ensure cervical spine immobilization until a full risk assessment has been completed:

- GCS score <15
- neck pain or tenderness
- focal neurology
- paraesthesia of extremities
- other suspicion of cervical spine injury.

Always attempt to assess neurological function (although clearly this should not delay life-saving treatments) before the patient is intubated because anaesthetic drugs will obtund or mask neurological responses to stimuli (see Chapter 62 for indications for intubation). The following should be recorded:

- GCS score
- pupillary responses
- evidence of lateralizing signs
- decorticate and decerebrate posturing.

Determination of severity

See Table 29.1. (The derivation of the GCS score is given in Chapter 62.)

A. Functional status

- Patients with a GCS score of 8 or less are often referred to as comatose.
- Patients who are able to localize a painful stimulus are *not* comatose.

B. Anatomical description (as determined by CT imaging)

(a) Sites of haemorrhage:
- extradural
- subdural

Acute Medicine, ed. Stephen Haydock, Duncan Whitehead and Zoë Fritz. Published by Cambridge University Press. © Cambridge University Press 2015.

Table 29.1 In assessing the GCS, record the *best* response to verbal and physical stimuli. Record individual components and total score

Severity	GCS	Loss of consciousness	Post-traumatic amnesia
Mild	13 or greater	<30 minutes	<1 day
Moderate	9–12	<24 hours	<1 week
Severe	8 or less	>24 hours	>1 week

- subarachnoid
- intracerebral.

(b) Non-haemorrhagic signs of injury:
- contusions on side of impact (coup) or opposite side (contrecoup)
- diffuse axonal injury:
  - shear forces acting on brain tissues of slightly different density, most evident at the grey and white matter interface
  - signs are absent or subtle on both CT and MRI despite significant damage and is inferred on the basis of micro-haemorrhages within the cerebral cortex or corpus callosum
- midline shift.

(c) Raised intracranial pressure:
- decreased size of ventricles or basal cisterns
- evidence of herniation.

CT imaging

This is the definitive investigation in all patients with a serious head injury. NICE (2007) guidance recommends urgent CT scanning for two groups.

Group 1

Any one of the following:
- GCS score <15 when assessed on arrival
- Evidence of skull fracture
- Post-traumatic seizure
- Focal neurological signs
- Vomited twice or more
- Retrograde amnesia for >30 min before impact.

Group 2

Anterograde amnesia *or* any loss of consciousness *plus*:
- age >65
- known coagulopathy/anticoagulation
- dangerous mechanism.

Ten per cent of patients with significant head injuries have a cervical spine injury; CT scans of the cervical spine should be performed as a matter of routine in these patients.

Sensitivity

CT is very sensitive for the detection of:
- acute haemorrhage
- intracranial air
- foreign bodies.

CT is less sensitive for other important pathologies:
- diffuse axonal injury
- posterior fossa lesions
- skull fractures in the plane of the scan.

The following early CT scan findings correlate with poorer outcome:
- subarachnoid haemorrhage in the basal cisterns
- midline shift determined at level of foramen of Munro
- compression or absence of the basal cisterns evaluated at level of midbrain.

MR imaging

- Suspected cervical spinal lesions (including suspected dissection).
- Altered consciousness/mentation that cannot be explained by CT findings.

Criteria for admission

- Significant new abnormality on imaging
- GCS remains <15
- Delay in CT imaging although indicated
- Persistent vomiting, severe headaches
- C spine lesion
- Meningism

- CSF leak
- Other concerns, e.g. alcohol, drug intoxication

Patients with head injury should be admitted under the care of a team led by a consultant with higher specialist training in management of patients with head injuries. Patient with multiple injuries should be admitted under the team best able to manage the most severe problem.

Patients may be discharged home if none of the above conditions apply and there is appropriate home support. They should be provided with verbal and written head injury advice (all trust emergency departments have a *'head injury card'*) that makes them aware of warning signs and how to seek help if they develop. Patients should also have advice regarding post-concussion syndrome.

Recommended nursing observation

For those patients requiring admission, nursing staff should record the GCS, heart rate, temperature, blood pressure, respiration rate and oxygen saturations:

- half-hourly observations until GCS = 15 then
- half-hourly for 2 hours
- 1-hourly for 4 hours
- then 2-hourly.

Medical staff should be advised if:

- Patient becomes agitated or develops abnormal behaviour
- GCS falls by
  - >1 point drop for more than 30 minutes (especially motor)
  - 2 points in motor response
  - a drop of 3 or more points in the eye-opening or verbal response
- New or evolving neurological symptoms or signs
- Severe or worsening headache
- Persistent vomiting.

Management

Primary injuries

These occur at the moment of impact due to mechanical forces of acceleration, and deceleration (closed injuries) or penetration (open injuries) (Figure 29.1).

Extradural haemorrhage

- Bleeding from an intracranial but extracerebral artery commonly due to direct blow to the head,

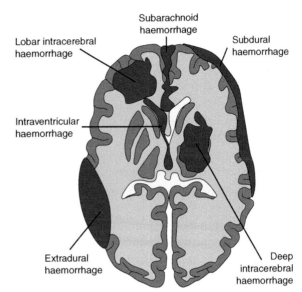

Figure 29.1 Location of different types of intracranial haemorrhage.

especially *middle cerebral artery* overlying the squamous temporal bone which is the thinnest and weakest area of the skull.

- Typically few seconds loss of consciousness following the transient neurological dysfunction of initial blow or impact before regaining consciousness.
- Subsequent loss of consciousness due to mass effect of continuing haemorrhage.
- Prompt neurosurgical evacuation of haematoma is associated with good outcomes and full recovery is not unusual. Recommended for:

  - volume >30 mL
  - midline shift >5 mm
  - focal deficits.

Subdural haemorrhage

- Tear of the vessels (usually venous) lying between brain and the dura mater, and bleeding is usually associated with a contusional injury to the brain which determines the initial presentation and potential for recovery.
- Patients can present days or weeks after a head injury, with cognitive changes, subtle motor deficits, persistent headache or seizure, whereas others are comatose from the moment of impact.

- Haematoma evacuation is recommended regardless of the patient's GCS score in cases of *acute* subdural haematoma with:
  - thickness >10 mm
  - midline shift >5 mm
  - smaller bleeds if GCS has fallen by 2 or more points since time of injury and/or pupillary abnormality.
- Mortality depends on age, associated parenchymal injury and GCS prior to surgery:
  - patients over 40 have a substantially higher mortality
  - majority of those requiring surgical intervention do not achieve a full recovery.
- Assess blood volume by the ABC/2 formula: Where A = largest cross-sectional diameter, B = largest diameter 90° to A on the same slice, C = approximate number of 10 mm slices on which the ICH is seen and halve to approximate volume of an ellipsoid.

Traumatic subarachnoid haemorrhage

- Commonest intracranial haemorrhage following trauma and found in over one-third of patients with a severe head injury.
- Neither surgery nor nimodipine is of value.
- Mortality from any head injury doubles in the presence of traumatic subarachnoid haemorrhage.

Intracerebral haemorrhage

- Result of mechanical deformation of the brain with consequent disruption of small cortical vessels.

Secondary injuries

Primary injury causes the brain to become uniquely susceptible to secondary internal insults due to:

- hypoxia
- hypoperfusion
- hypoglycaemia
- pyrexia
- damage to the blood–brain barrier
- neurotransmitter release

  resulting in:
- oedema
- secondary haemorrhage

- raised intracranial pressure which if not reversed can result in herniation of the temporal lobes or brainstem leading to death.

Forty per cent of patients suffer further deterioration after admission to hospital due to secondary injury [1]. Therapeutic interventions are targeted at avoiding, ameliorating and reversing secondary injuries.

Contacting the neurosurgical team

The neurosurgical unit should be contacted if imaging reveals a structural abnormality.

Factors that favour surgical removal of intracerebral haematoma include:

- superficial haemorrhage
- clot volume between 20 and 80 mL
- relatively young
- haemorrhage causing midline shift/raised intracranial pressure (ICP)
- cerebellar haematomas >3 cm or causing hydrocephalus.

Factors mitigating against surgical interventions include:

- large haemorrhage in a moribund patient (GCS <5)
- orientated patient with a small haematoma (<2 cm).

Surgical intervention may also be indicated for treatment of depressed skull fractures. Otherwise discuss with neurosurgery if:

- persisting GCS ≤8 after resuscitation
- unexplained confusion >4 hours
- deterioration in GCS after admission (especially motor response)
- progressive focal neurology
- seizure without full recovery
- penetrating injury
- CSF leak.

For transfer to tertiary centre, refer to local guidelines. The patient should be first adequately resuscitated and stabilized and accompanied by a doctor with appropriate training and experience and an adequately trained assistant. In particular they should be *capable of managing the airway* should it become compromised and *treating seizures* complicating the injury.

Conservative management

It is essential to avoid both hypotension and elevation of ICP (Figure 29.2).

> CPP = MAP – ICP
>
> *where:*
>
> CPP (cerebral perfusion pressure)
> MAP (mean arterial pressure)
> ICP (intracranial pressure)
>
> It is essential to avoid both hypotension and elevation of ICP

Figure 29.2 Blood flow in the injured brain is inversely proportional to intracranial pressure.

Reducing haemorrhage volume

It is essential to reverse anticoagulation even before results of coagulation tests are available in patients on warfarin therapy. Prothrombin protein complex should be used. The CRASH 3 trial is currently under way to examine the role of tranexamic acid in patients with traumatic brain injury.

Reducing intracranial pressure

ICP is the key outcome predictor and rises exponentially with increases in intracranial volume beyond 150 mL. Before ICP rises, CSF and venous blood are displaced out of the cranium to accommodate the mass lesion resulting in worsening headache and vomiting. Aim to reduce ICP by:

- nursing with 15 degrees head-up tilt
- avoiding neck constrictions or obstruction to venous return from head
- ventilation setting to keep PCO_2 low normal and prevent vasodilatation and hypotension reducing intracranial blood flow.

Where signs of raised intracranial pressure are present and neurosurgery is not immediately feasible, measures aimed at temporizing the situation can be life-saving.

Hypertonic solutions (mannitol or saline) osmotically draw intracellular water into the circulation with a consequent reduction in brain cell mass. Although the mass reduction is slight, the exponential relationship of ICP to intracranial volume gives a significant albeit temporary benefit.

Maintaining cerebral perfusion pressure

Failure to adequately perfuse the damaged brain will cause worsening hypoxia, cell death and oedema. Cerebral auto-regulation is lost in injured brain, rendering it susceptible to hypotension with even brief

periods associated with significant rise in morbidity and mortality.

All brain tissue is uniquely susceptible to hypoxia and even brief periods of hypoxia are associated with worse functional outcomes.

- Patients should always be treated with supplemental oxygen at high concentration.

Reducing cerebral metabolic requirements

Seizures are common with severe brain injury and must be avoided. Aetiological factors include:

- Increased metabolic requirements.
- Uncontrolled chaotic release of neurotoxic transmitters.

Provide *seizure prophylaxis* for all patients with *severe* head injury and continue for 7 days. Routinely use paracetamol to prevent increased metabolic demand of pyrexia.

Consequence of treatment failure

Failure to control rises in intracranial pressure results in various parts of the brain becoming squeezed into small potential spaces and the physical and functional consequences of brain herniation (Figure 29.3). The two commonest syndromes are:

1. *Herniation of the incus of the temporal lobe* through the tentorium cerebri causing compression of the oculomotor nerve and resulting in fixed dilation of the ipsilateral pupil ('surgical III nerve palsy').
2. *Herniation of the cerebellar tonsils* through the foramen magnum causing brainstem compression and resulting physiological changes of 'coning' characterized by Cushing's triad of:

   - rising blood pressure
   - bradycardia
   - periodic respiration.

There are two other classic signs of cortical and cerebral failure referred to respectively as decorticate and decerebrate posturing.

- In both, the legs are extended, adducted and internally rotated (as in spasticity).
- In decorticate posturing the arms are flexed.
- In decerebrate posturing, the arms are extended.
- Both are grave signs with decerebrate posturing associated with the poorest outcomes.

In intracranial haemorrhage the mass effects are usually (though not exclusively) unilateral and there

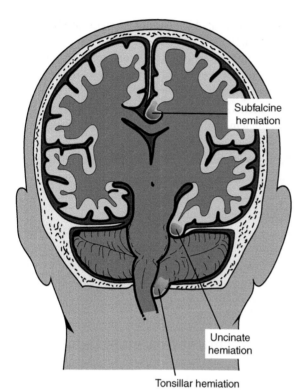

Subfalcine hemiation

Uncinate hemiation

Tonsillar hemiation

Figure 29.3 Cerebral herniation due to uncontrolled elevation of intracranial pressure.

- locked in syndrome (rare)
  - damage to brainstem
  - fully conscious and aware but unable to communicate
- secondary epilepsy
- secondary hydrocephalus
- cranial nerve palsies
- language and communication problems
- impaired cognition
- behavioural problems often related to impulsivity
- impaired sensorium
- emotional and psychiatric problems
- degenerative brain disease.

Patients and their families will require counselling with regard to the potential problems prior to discharge. Patients may require the ongoing support of a multidisciplinary therapy team specializing in neurorehabilitation.

may be significant lateralization of the physical signs with posture and pupil normal on one side but abnormal on the other, suggesting a contralateral space-occupying haemorrhage. This mandates immediate CT and probable neurosurgical intervention.

Prognosis

The outcome of coma following trauma is significantly better than that due to hypoxic and ischaemic brain injury. Of those presenting with a GCS of 8 or less, 35% can be expected to have made a good recovery at one month. Patients with a GCS of 3 have mortality approaching 75% *but* at least 10% will have functionally good outcomes [2].

Complications of severe head injury

Patients who survive a severe injury may go on to develop

- persistent vegetative state
- minimally conscious state
  - markedly altered consciousness with some awareness of environment

Concussion

Patients with less severe injuries may also suffer significant morbidity due to the pathophysiological processes of secondary brain injury previously discussed. These can be protracted and characterized by:

- headaches
- nausea
- cognitive impairment
- irritability
- impaired balance.

Patients with head injuries have a greater risk from subsequent injury and it is important to counsel patients with regard to minimizing this risk. Whilst most patients with concussion recover fully within 3–5 days, the greatest period of risk from a further concussion is for a further 10 days. For this reason any patient who has sustained a concussion severe enough to cause even a brief loss of consciousness should be advised to avoid contact sport for 10 days after complete recovery. Specific advice should be given for particular sports, e.g. horse racing.

References

1. Narayan RK, Michel ME, Ansell B, et al. Clinical trials in head injury. *J Neurotrauma* 2002; 19(5): 503–557.

2. MRC CRASH Trial Collaborators. Predicting outcome after traumatic brain injury: practical prognostic models based on large cohort of international patients. *BMJ* 2008; 336: 425.

Further reading

Advanced Trauma Life Support for Doctors: ATLS Student Manual (2012) American College of Surgeons.

Brain Trauma Foundation, American Association of Neurological Surgeons, Congress of Neurological surgeons, et al. Guidelines for the management of severe traumatic brain injury. Introduction. *J Neurotrauma* 2007; 24 (Suppl 1): S1.

CG56 Head Injury: NICE guideline 2007. Available to download at www.nice.org.uk/nicemedia/live/11836/36257/36257.pdf.

Lingsma HF, Roozenbeek B, Steyerberg EW et al. Early prognosis in traumatic brain injury; from prophecies to predictions. *Lancet Neurol* 2010; 9: 543.

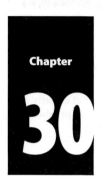

Chapter

30

Headache

Stephen Haydock

Introduction

Headaches account for ≈5% of emergency department attendances and ≈3% of emergency referrals/admissions to the acute medical take. Patients seek help for headache either because it is sudden and severe (thunderclap headache) or because it fails to improve with time. It is accepted convention to divide headaches into:

- *Primary*: no underlying causative medical condition (90% of cases seen in ED):
  - tension type headache
  - migraine
  - cluster headache
  - trigeminal neuralgia
  - atypical facial pain
  - benign paroxysmal.
- *Secondary*: identifiable medical problem:
  - intracranial haemorrhage
  - raised intracranial pressure
  - infective
  - inflammatory
  - post-herpetic
  - referred.

Approach to management should be:

- *Recognition of primary headache syndromes* to avoid unnecessary investigation, provide reassurance and appropriate symptomatic relief:
  - migraine
  - cluster headaches
  - tension headache
  - analgesic headache.
- Identification of those patients presenting with a life-threatening or potentially disabling secondary

headache to permit prompt investigation and management:

- thunderclap headache
- temporal arteritis
- idiopathic intracranial hypertension
- CNS infections (see Chapter 23).

The pathophysiology of headache remains poorly understood. Pain receptors are not present in the brain but are found in the scalp, large intracranial vessels and dura mater. Nociceptive impulses are elicited from these structures as a result of distension, stretch and inflammation. Impulses pass along the trigeminal nerve, first to third cervical nerves, facial nerve and glossopharyngeal and vagus nerves. Pain can therefore also arise by compression, traction or inflammation of these nerves and muscles that they receive afferents from.

History

This is essential to making the diagnosis as most patients will have a normal examination and subsequent investigations.

- Time of onset of acute presenting episode
- Time from onset to maximum severity:
  - instantaneous
  - a few minutes
  - longer
- If recurrent:
  - age at first onset
  - frequency
  - duration
  - severity
  - response to previous treatments

Acute Medicine, ed. Stephen Haydock, Duncan Whitehead and Zoë Fritz. Published by Cambridge University Press.
© Cambridge University Press 2015.

- Associated prodrome; visual, sensory or motor auras
- Quality, severity, location and radiation
- Fluctuations/variation of headache with movement or postural change
- Precipitating, aggravating and relieving factors
- Previous or family history of migraine
- History of recent head trauma
- Visual symptoms including photophobia
- Headache-specific associated symptoms, e.g. jaw claudication in temporal arteritis
- General health/systemic enquiry
- Relationship to menstrual cycle or exogenous hormones, e.g. HRT and OCP

'Red flags' in history

- Sudden onset of excruciating pain (worst ever) that has onset in seconds or a few minutes
- First ever episode and never had anything like this previously
- Headache associated with syncope
- Severe, progressive headache if over 50 years of age
- Immunosuppression including HIV
- History/suspicion of malignancy
- Family history of subarachnoid haemorrhage
- Headache predominantly in the occipital region
- Anticoagulant therapy
- Sudden visual loss, tender scalp or jaw claudication
- Cluster of patients in winter/camping/holiday home suggestive of carbon monoxide poisoning

Examination

'Red flags' on examination

- Reduced conscious level
- Fever
- Meningeal irritation
- Abnormal neurological signs
- Evidence of cranial trauma
- Papilloedema
- Tender temporal arteries
- Petechial rash

Investigation

Blood tests

- FBC
- CRP

- ESR
- Clotting
- Electrolytes
- Liver function tests
- Carboxyhaemoglobin if suspect carbon monoxide poisoning

Radiology

- Non-contrast CT for those patients with high risk features at presentation listed above consistent with an intracranial mass or haemorrhage.

Lumbar puncture

- First choice if infective cause suspected. It is prudent to proceed to LP only after CT imaging in those patients where there is evidence of raised intracranial pressure as suggested by:
  - papilloedema
  - focal neurological deficits
  - reduced conscious level.

Common primary headache syndromes

Scenario 30.1

A local GP calls you for advice. A 19-year-old girl is in his surgery; she has developed a severe right-sided throbbing headache while at work. This was preceded by bright flashing lights in the lateral right visual field and subsequent numbness of the left arm. The headache developed in severity over 15 minutes. There is no longer any neurological deficit on examination. The GP thinks this might be migraine but is worried he is missing a subarachnoid haemorrhage (apparently he has been 'caught out' once before).

Migraine

The history above is certainly suggestive of classic migraine with aura. Further confirmation should be obtained by clarifying:

- headache is worse on moving and relieved by rest
- associated with nausea and vomiting
- patient wants to lie in a darkened room and describes photophobia
- previous episode
- normal examination with no neck stiffness
- no 'red flag' features.

Subject to the answers to these questions the patient can be considered to have classical migraine.

- *Neuroimaging is not indicated* for patients with a clear history of migraine without history or examination red flags who meet International Headache Society (IHS) diagnostic criteria (see below).
- *Migraine is a clinical diagnosis.* Patients who present with recurrent episodes of severe and disabling headache associated with nausea and light sensitivity and who have a normal neurological examination should be considered to have migraine.

The IHS indicate that a diagnosis of *migraine without aura* is suggested by at least five episodes of:

- Headache lasting 4–72 hours without treatment or if treatment unsuccessful.
- Two or more of:
  - unilateral
  - pulsating
  - moderate or severe intensity
  - worsened by routine physical activity.
- Headache associated with one or more of the following symptoms:
  - nausea
  - vomiting
  - photophobia
  - phonophobia.
- History and examination do not suggest an alternative diagnosis.

A diagnosis of *migraine with aura* is suggested by at least two attacks in which:

- A headache characteristic of migraine (as above) develops during the aura or within 60 minutes of its onset.
- The aura is fully reversible and characterized by:
  - positive and/or negative visual features
  - positive and negative sensory symptoms
  - dysphasia.
- At least one of the following is seen:
  - homonymous visual symptoms
  - unilateral sensory symptoms
  - at least one aura symptom developing gradually over 5 minutes or more and/or different aura symptoms occurring in succession over 5 minutes or more
  - each symptom lasts more than 5 minutes and less than 60 minutes.

Specific migraine variants are described according to the associated neurological deficit seen:

- hemiplegic
- basilar
- ophthalmoplegic.

Management

First line

- Paracetamol 1 g orally for mild to moderate migraine
- Aspirin 900 mg orally for all severities
- Ibuprofen 400 mg orally for all severities
- Metoclopramide 20 mg orally or domperidone 30 mg rectally for nausea and vomiting and to aid gastric emptying

Second line

- Oral sumatriptan 50–100 mg
- Stronger oral NSAIDs such as naproxen 250–500 mg
- Intranasal zolmitriptan if vomiting
- Severe resistant migraine may be treated with 6 mg sumatriptan subcutaneous injection

Prophylaxis

Not all patients with migraine will require prophylaxis, depending on frequency, severity and response to acute treatments, and this rarely needs to be initiated in the acute setting. Commonly prescribed agents are:

- beta-blockers, e.g. atenolol 25–100 mg
- tricyclic antidepressants, e.g. amitriptyline 10–150 mg daily
- sodium valproate 250–1500 mg daily
- topiramate 50–100 mg daily
- gabapentin 300–3600 mg daily
- calcium channel blockers.

> **Scenario 30.2**
>
> *You are asked to see a 30-year-old man in the early hours of the morning. He has been driven to the ED by his wife due to a 10/10 right-sided retro-orbital head-ache that developed over a few minutes after going to bed. He remains in extreme pain despite a range of opi-oid analgesics. Similar headaches have occurred in the early hours over the last 3 nights lasting up to 45 minutes. This attack is even more severe and has not settled like the others. He is clearly very distressed and says the pain is unbearable.*

Cluster headache

Cluster headaches affect 1/1000 of the population, especially young male (male: female 6:1) smokers and may be precipitated by a head injury.

Characteristics

- Intense unilateral pain especially around eye.
- Lasting 15–180 minutes with rapid onset and cessation.
- Typically in clusters over several weeks.
- Often similar time of day.
- Significant motor restlessness.
- Up to 20% have classical symptoms that occur *persistently without clustering.*
- 97% have autonomic features:
  - ipsilateral conjunctival injection
  - lacrimation
  - sweating
  - rhinorrhoea
  - partial Horner's syndrome.

Management

Acute

- Sumatriptan 6 mg SC is usually effective in 15 minutes.
- Nasal zolmitriptan if needle phobic.
- High flow oxygen.
- Lidocaine nasal drops 4–10% (may work by blocking the sphenopalatine ganglion that lies only a few millimetres below the nasal mucosa above and behind the middle turbinate bone).

Prophylaxis

- Prednisolone 80 mg for 7 days and then rapidly taper dose (usually rapidly effective and stop if fails to prevent attacks within 48 hours).
- Verapamil useful for long-term prevention.

  All patients in whom the diagnosis is made or suspected should have neurology follow-up.

Tension type headache

This is the commonest and unfortunately least well studied and understood (*would you want to make this your life's work!*) of the primary headache syndromes. It is classically:

- Mild to moderate intensity
- Bilateral

- Not throbbing
- Described as '*head fullness*' or '*tight band*' (may place hands either side of temples to illustrate pressure)
- Tenderness of head and neck muscles (demonstrated on examination by pressing with rotatory movements of fingers)
- Precipitated by recent stress
- Worse at the end of the day
- Normal investigations
- No red flag symptoms/signs.

Management

In the acute setting it is best managed by reassurance and simple analgesics such as paracetamol, aspirin or ibuprofen. In the longer term non-pharmacological treatments including cognitive training and physiotherapy can be useful and have some evidence to support their use. Exercise and weight loss should also be advised as this can help improve chronic symptoms.

Analgesic headache

These are chronic daily headaches related to analgesic overuse for a primary headache syndrome, frequently a tension type-headache or migraine syndrome, particularly associated with:

- codeine especially compound preparations, e.g. co-codamol
- tryptans
- ergot alkaloids.

  It generally develops after 10–15 days of repeated use but sometimes earlier.

Management

- *Abrupt withdrawal of analgesia!*
- Full explanation of the basis of the condition including likely initial increase in severity on stopping analgesics.
- Short-term use of naproxen 250 mg tds can be helpful in managing the withdrawal headache.
- Appropriate prophylaxis of underlying headache syndrome if appropriate.
- Consider possibility of drug dependence issues.

Secondary headaches

Thunderclap headache

A thunderclap headache is of sudden onset reaching maximum intensity within 5 minutes of onset and lasting for more than one hour.

Principal causes of thunderclap headache

- Subarachnoid haemorrhage
- Cerebral venous sinus thrombosis
- Cervical artery dissection
- Coital headache
- Spontaneous intracranial hypotension
- Stroke (both ischaemic and haemorrhagic)
- Pituitary apoplexy
- Reversible cerebral vasoconstriction syndrome

Scenario 30.3

A 35-year-old woman with a history of migraine develops a sudden onset of very severe headache associated with vomiting and transient loss of consciousness. She is brought to the emergency department as her husband feels she is confused. On examination she is clearly unwell with headache, photophobia and neck stiffness.

Despite the history of migraine, this woman has a classical history of subarachnoid haemorrhage and this clearly requires urgent investigation.

Subarachnoid haemorrhage

Most are due to ruptured saccular aneurysms of the arteries of the circle of Willis (80%) (present in 5% of the adult population). It has a lifelong incidence of about 10 per 100 000 of the population. The mean age of onset is 55 years (40–60 years).

Important risk factors are:

- systemic hypertension
- smoking
- moderate to heavy alcohol consumption
- previous family history:
  - first degree relatives have three- to five-fold increased risk
- rare genetic syndromes:
  - autosomal dominant polycystic kidney disease
  - Ehlers–Danlos syndrome
  - glucocorticoid remediable aldosteronism
- sympathomimetic drugs including cocaine.

Antithrombotic/anticoagulant drugs do not increase the risk but do increase the severity of a bleed.

Classical presenting features

- Sudden onset of severe headache ('worst ever', 'hit with hammer') either bilateral or lateralized
- Often on physical exertion
- Transient loss of consciousness
- Nausea and vomiting
- Seizure
- Neck stiffness
- Previous history of sudden severe '*sentinel headache*' in preceding 3 weeks although the significance and validity of the concept of sentinel headache has been challenged

All patients presenting with a sudden, severe onset of headache should be investigated for subarachnoid haemorrhage by CT imaging followed by lumbar puncture (after 12 hours from the onset of symptoms).

CT scanning in subarachnoid haemorrhage

Greater than 92% sensitivity for CT imaging within 24 hours is quoted; sensitivity falls off with time. Most patients seen by on-take medical teams are a selected group where the diagnosis is not obvious and the only presenting feature is headache. *The sensitivity of CT scanning in this group may be half that quoted* and in part dependent on the expertise of the individual radiologist reviewing the scan. A negative scan early after onset of headache *cannot entirely exclude a bleed* on its own.

CT angiography is used to identify the aneurysm/ bleeding source after diagnosis and can also be useful if the patient presents late (>14 days) when normal CT imaging and LP are unlikely to be helpful.

Lumbar puncture

Lumbar puncture should always be performed (if the CT scan is negative), after 12 hours from the onset of headache and *ideally by someone experienced* to reduce the risk of a traumatic tap and consequent diagnostic uncertainty. The following are seen:

- elevated opening pressure
- elevated red cell count
- xanthochromia.

It is customary to take sequential samples to check for a traumatic tap, although a subarachnoid haemorrhage can only be excluded if the final sample is clear of red cells.

Xanthochromia forms within 2 hours of onset of a bleed and can persist in excess of 2 weeks. It occurs from haemoglobin degradation, and is seen in centrifuged samples of the CSF. It is customary to wait 12 hours after headache onset before sampling the CSF for its presence. It appears yellow or pink to the eye; this is assessed by comparing the CSF sample with a clear water specimen held against a white card under bright illumination. False positive tests for xanthochromia can occur with:

- hyperbilirubinaemia
- high CSF protein
- very traumatic taps (>100 000 red cells per microlitre)
- samples that are not protected from light.

False negatives occur in small bleeds where the level of xanthochromia is below that which can be detected by the naked eye. For this reason it is now customary in the UK for the laboratory to perform spectrophotometry on the submitted sample. Oxyhaemoglobin undergoes a degradation initially to methaemaglobin and then to bilirubin. Analysis should be performed on the sample with least blood present and protected from light on its journey to the laboratory.

Management

Half of those affected will die and one-third of survivors are severely disabled and dependent.

Complications include:

- rebleeding
- vasospasm and delayed cerebral ischaemia/ infarction
- hydrocephalus
- raised intracranial pressure
- seizures
- hyponatraemia due to cerebral salt wasting
- cardiac abnormalities due to associated catecholamine release, especially with severe bleeds:
  - abnormal ECG, rhythm disturbances
  - troponin elevation
- hypothalamic dysfunction and pituitary insufficiency.

The case should be discussed with the neurosurgical team as soon as the diagnosis is confirmed. Prior to transfer the medical team should:

- ensure patient nursed in quiet surroundings avoiding bright light
- restrict to bed
- nurse at 30°
- frequently assess neurological status
- insert IV line and administer at least 3 litres of fluid per day
- commence nimodipine 60 mg PO 4-hourly to reduce vasospasm (continue for 3 weeks)
- TED (anti-embolism) stockings
- treat pain with paracetamol, or if insufficient regular codeine
- avoid treating hypertension unless causing organ damage as this will reduce cerebral perfusion pressure.

Spontaneous arterial dissection

Spontaneous arterial dissection is an uncommon cause of stroke (2%) but a common (25%) cause of stroke in younger people. There is loss of vessel wall integrity of the vertebral or carotid arteries. This allows blood to track between the layers of wall causing an intra-mural haematoma resulting in neurological signs due to luminal compression reducing blood flow and embolization of material from the dissection site. It is usually associated with extremes of neck movement and has been described with:

- exercise/yoga
- shampooing at the hairdressers
- whiplash/neck trauma
- decorating a ceiling.

It can occur spontaneously in genetic conditions where there is an underlying vessel weakness:

- Marfan's syndrome
- Ehlers–Danlos syndrome
- osteogenesis imperfecta type 1
- polycystic kidney disease
- fibromuscular dysplasia
- pseudoxanthoma elasticum.

Clinical features

- Patients develop head and neck pain.
- The pain is constant, severe and often ipsilateral to the dissected artery.

Carotid

- >50% of patients with a carotid dissection will have an associated stroke in the carotid territory; this can be delayed by hours or days.
- Painful Horner's syndrome.
- Amaurosis fugax.
- Resulting neurological deficit depends on available collateral circulation from the circle of Willis (usually good in young patients).
- Transient ischaemia or irreversible cerebral infarction can result from embolization from the site of dissection. This explains why the neurological manifestations of the dissection can evolve some time after the onset of headache.

Vertebral

- Severe occipital headache and posterior nuchal pain following a head or neck injury.

- Subsequently develops focal neurological signs attributable to ischaemia of the *brainstem or cerebellum*, these may not appear until after a latent period, lasting as long as 3 days, although delays of weeks and even years have been reported.
- Many patients present only at the onset of neurological symptoms.
- When neurological dysfunction does occur, patients most commonly report symptoms attributable to lateral medullary dysfunction (i.e. Wallenberg syndrome).

Currently diagnosis is by magnetic resonance imaging (detect vessel wall abnormalities) with angiography (detect flow abnormalities) (MRI/MRA).

Management

Refer to neurology or stroke team according to local policy.

- *Anticoagulants and antiplatelet agents* are the drugs of choice to prevent thromboembolic disorders:
  - trials are ongoing
  - heparin then warfarin probably more effective but risk of increasing size of haematoma.
- More potent agents (e.g. intra-arterial thrombolytics) have been used in selected cases.
- Stenting and surgery when medical therapy fails or contraindicated.

Prognosis

Is generally good but key is early diagnosis and treatment, before deficit develops. The diagnosis should be suspected when headache occurs in the context of a known risk factor.

Stroke

Posterior circulation strokes in particular cause headache. A high degree of clinical suspicion should be maintained in any patient with headache and a history of transient neurology especially in posterior arterial territories.

Coital headache

Pre-orgasmic: occipital headaches of gradually increasing intensity during intercourse, the severity develops correlating with increased arousal. It is usually easily recognized and distinguished as such. *Post-coital headache* may be seen on the acute medical take and will be described in more detail.

Clinical features

- Explosive severe sudden onset of headache at time of orgasm followed by severe generalized throbbing headache.
- Can be associated with stroke.
- Can be difficult to distinguish first event from a subarachnoid haemorrhage as intercourse is well documented in the aetiology of subarachnoid haemorrhage ($\approx$10%).
- Acute arterial dissection can also be precipitated by coitus.
- Peak onset in the 30s.
- More common in men ($\female$1:3$\male$).
- Often history of chronic tension/migrainous headache.
- Not associated with loss of consciousness, meningism or focal neurology.

Its aetiology is not well understood as it is rare *and let's be honest … it isn't going to be easy to do functional imaging studies on this!*

Management

After a first episode a patient should be investigated to exclude a subarachnoid bleed with CT and LP as described above. Subsequent episodes are not investigated unless atypical features arise. If other causes have been excluded then the following management is appropriate:

- Reassurance of the benign nature of the condition
- Likelihood of remission over time
- NSAIDs, beta-blockers and tryptans may be used and can be effective as prophylaxis and/or treatment.

Pituitary apoplexy

- Haemorrhage into or infarction of a previously diagnosed or unknown pituitary adenoma.
- Not necessarily associated with headache.
- Sheehan's syndrome describes this in the context of blood loss and hypovolaemia following childbirth (Harold Leeming Sheehan [1900–1988], formerly Professor of Pathology, University of Liverpool).
- Results in acute or chronic onset hypopituitarism.
- Initial diagnosis is by CT but if high clinical suspicion MRI is required as CT is not always diagnostic.

Spontaneous intracranial hypotension

- Sudden onset severe headache due to CSF leak.
- Classically worsens with upright posture.
- Often revealed during investigation of suspected subarachnoid haemorrhage:
  - normal CSF constituents
  - low or unrecordable CSF opening pressure.
- Characteristic appearance on MRI is often diagnostic.

Reversible cerebral vasoconstriction syndrome

- Severe headache of sudden onset due to cerebral arterial vasospasm in the absence of an identifiable precipitating agent.
- May produce focal neurological deficits.
- May be repeated attacks that resolve spontaneously.
- Responds to calcium channel blockers such as nimodipine.

Scenario 30.4

A 30-year-old woman is referred by the ED with a severe sudden onset headache. She has no previous medical history. Her only medication is the combined oral contraceptive pill. On arrival she is slightly drowsy and has nausea and vomiting; the headache is worse lying flat. There are no focal neurological signs. A CT scan and LP are unremarkable.

This patient presents with a history suggestive of a subarachnoid haemorrhage but this has been effectively excluded. The nausea, vomiting and drowsiness merit further investigation. This presentation in a woman on the OCP (when subarachnoid haemorrhage excluded) is suggestive of a cortical venous sinus thrombosis. The headache is more commonly of subacute onset and often worse in the recumbent position.

Cerebral venous thrombosis

Predisposing factors

- Female sex
- Infection, e.g. sinusitis
- Neurosurgery or head trauma
- Hypercoagulability
- Post lumbar puncture or CSF shunt insertion
- Drugs:

- OCP, steroids, epsicapron, tamoxifen, erythropoietin
- Pregnancy/postpartum
- Nephrotic syndrome
- Sickle cell disease
- Collagen vascular disease

Clinical features

- Headache may be thunderclap or slower onset
- Nausea and vomiting
- Variable reduction of conscious level from normal to coma
- Seizures
- Focal neurological deficits
- Cranial nerve palsies

Diagnosis

- Bloods to exclude sepsis, polycythaemia, TTP.
- D-dimer elevated (97% sensitive) and *diagnosis unlikely if negative*.
- Initial CT imaging may identify infarction not corresponding to an arterial territory but is most useful in excluding an alternative pathology. *It is usually (90%) abnormal if there is a focal neurological deficit.*
- Elevated CSF opening pressure.
- The definitive investigation is MRI/magnetic resonance venography.

Management

- As for arterial stroke.
- Discuss with neurological/stroke colleagues.
- Anticoagulants are indicated but remain controversial.

Idiopathic intracranial hypertension (IIH)

Idiopathic intracranial hypertension (formerly benign intracranial hypertension) is a condition that predominantly affects obese women of childbearing age and is of unknown aetiology (may be related to venous hypertension). Most patients are overweight at the time of diagnosis. They are frequently referred by the eye clinic when papilloedema has been recognized.

Clinical features

Raised intracranial pressure results in:

- non-specific, pressure-type headache which is worse on lying down

- diplopia due to VI nerve palsies
- pulsatile tinnitus.

Papilloedema results in:

- progressive loss of peripheral vision in one or both eyes
- orthostatic visual disturbances
- blurring of vision
- sudden visual loss.

Visual function tests are critical in diagnosing and monitoring patients with IIH. Such tests include the following:

- ophthalmoscopy
- visual field assessment
- ocular motility examination.

Investigation

Blood tests

- FBC
- ESR
- Serum iron and iron-binding capacity
- ANA
- Lyme screening test

Radiology

- MRI of the brain with gadolinium enhancement (probably the study of choice)
- Magnetic resonance venography
- CT of the brain

Lumbar puncture

Once a mass lesion has been excluded; diagnosis is made by identifying raised CSF opening pressure (>25 cm in the lateral decubitus position).

Management

The goal is to preserve optic nerve function while managing increased ICP. Therapy may include the following:

- *Repeated* lumbar puncture is no longer recommended.
- 10–15% weight loss is the only definitive treatment.
- Pharmacotherapy includes:
  - acetazolamide (the most effective agent for lowering ICP) and furosemide
  - primary headache prophylaxis with amitriptyline, propranolol, or other commonly prescribed migraine prophylaxis

agents such as topiramate (added benefit of weight loss)
  - corticosteroids.

Surgery is indicated for deteriorating visual function:

- cerebrospinal fluid diversion (i.e. via a lumboperitoneal or ventriculoperitoneal shunt)
- intracranial venous sinus stenting.

> ### Scenario 30.5
>
> *A 72-year-old woman is referred by the ED with a one-day history of generalized headache of sudden onset. She has some blurring of vision in the right eye. She also complains of general fatigue and weight loss. Examination is otherwise unremarkable. ESR is 40 mm/h, CRP is raised at 35. She has a mild anaemia, elevated platelet count and abnormal LFTs with a raised ALP. A CT head scan shows no abnormality. The emergency department wish to discharge her for follow-up in the outpatients clinic.*

Temporal arteritis

The clinical suspicion here is of temporal arteritis. The ESR is not markedly elevated, the normal range for a woman of this age is <41. However, a normal ESR does not exclude the diagnosis. Other clinical features and lab results are suggestive of the diagnosis. This woman requires treatment with corticosteroid and outpatient temporal artery biopsy.

Temporal arteritis (giant cell arteritis) is a relatively common systemic vascular disorder with a predilection for superficial arteries. Histologically it is characterized by transmural inflammation of the vessel with patchy inflammatory cell infiltration. It is important to recognize this condition; failure to make the diagnosis can result in permanent loss of vision. Inflammatory thickening of the wall results in distal ischaemia of those arteries that are particularly involved, namely the temporal (causing headache) and the ophthalmic, posterior ciliary and retinal arteries. Ten per cent of patients with temporal arteritis also meet the diagnostic criteria for polymyalgia rheumatica (PMR) and vice versa.

Epidemiology

- Onset after 50 years (mean age 72 years)
- More common in women (×2–3)
- Incidence 2/10 000 over 50 years
- More common in white northern Europeans

Clinical features

Most common presenting feature is headache (70%).

- Typically sudden onset and bitemporal
- Can be non-specific; slower onset and more diffuse
- Associated with scalp tenderness noticed by patient

  Systemic features include:
- fever, fatigue, malaise and weight loss
- symptoms of PMR.

  Neurological manifestations include:
- permanent visual loss:
  - (unilateral or bilateral)
  - can be sudden and painless
  - may be preceded by transient subtle defects
- TIAs
- strokes
- jaw claudication (maxillary artery involvement).

  Examination may reveal:
- tender, warm, thickened palpable non-pulsatile arteries of head and face (especially temporal arteries)
- areas of scalp necrosis.

  Fundoscopy may be normal or show evidence of venous dilatation and/or arterial occlusion.

Investigation

- Most patients will have an ESR >80 mm/h but 20% can have a normal or low ESR.
- Remember for male ESR is <half age; for female is <half age + 5 mm/h.
- *CRP is more sensitive and does not vary with age or sex; it may be elevated even when the ESR is normal.*
- Leucocytosis, anaemia and thrombocytosis are common.
- Abnormal LFTs, especially elevated ALP, are common.

Note

The 1990 American College of Rheumatology criteria suggest that three of the following five findings are suggestive (93.5% sensitivity and 91.2% specificity):

1. Age of onset greater than 50 years
2. New-onset headache or localized head pain
3. Temporal artery tenderness to palpation or reduced pulsation
4. Erythrocyte sedimentation rate (ESR) greater than 50 mm/h
5. Abnormal arterial biopsy (necrotizing vasculitis with granulomatous proliferation and infiltration).

Those patients for whom the diagnosis is suspected require treatment with corticosteroids and temporal artery biopsy. This should be:

- performed within 1 week (useful up to 3–4 weeks)
- multiple biopsies as patchy disease.

There is interest in using colour duplex sonography. The presence of a halo sign around the artery is specific but not sensitive but may be useful as a screening test to reduce need for biopsy.

Treatment

- Oral prednisolone 60 mg/day.
- Improvement is usually expected within 72 hours.
- Will require long-term steroid treatment.

Further reading

British Association for the Study of Headache. BASH guidelines: www.bash.org.uk/guidelines/.

Van Gijn J, Kerr RS, Rinkel GJ. Seminar. Subarachnoid haemorrhage. *Lancet* 2007; 369: 306–318.

Chapter 31

Hoarseness and stridor

Marko Nikolić and Jonathan Fuld

Scenario 31.1

A 65-year-old woman presents to the medical assessment unit with a one-week history of worsening shortness of breath associated with a hoarse voice and stridor. She does not have any relevant past medical history. She is a current and lifelong smoker. How are you going to manage this patient?

Hoarseness and stridor are quite different symptoms which can present simultaneously.

Hoarseness is an 'abnormality of voiced sounds due to disorganized movement of the vocal cords' [1]. Nearly one-third of the population have impaired voice production at some point in their lives [2]. The words hoarseness and *dysphonia* are sometimes substituted for one other, but have subtly different meanings: hoarseness is a symptom of altered voice quality, whereas dysphonia is a diagnosis.

Dysphonia is generally defined as 'an alteration in voice production that impairs social and professional communication' [3].

Stridor is a loud, harsh, high-pitched sound produced by turbulent airflow through a partially obstructed airway at the level of the main airway or larynx. It has a lower pitch than wheezing [1]. It is loudest in inspiration because:

- the obstruction usually occurs in the extrathoracic trachea and is thus independent of any intrathoracic pressure change
- the obstruction is usually immobile [1].

Inspirational stridor is most common and is caused by obstruction at, or above, the level of the cords.

Biphasic stridor (inspirational and expirational) is caused by obstruction in the subglottis or trachea.

Causes of hoarseness

- *Laryngitis* – infection, inflammation (vocal abuse, reflux, allergic), hypothyroidism [4].
- *Vocal cord polyps/nodules/granulomas/cysts.*
  - Any damage to the vocal cords will produce hoarseness.
- *Laryngeal tumours* (papilloma, squamous cell cancer).
- *Vocal cord paralysis* due to recurrent laryngeal nerve damage, e.g. lung cancer, stroke or myasthenia gravis.
  - If the left cord is paralysed, the possibility of a bronchial neoplasm invading the left recurrent laryngeal nerve at the level of the hilum has to be considered (Figure 31.1).
  - Note that the right recurrent laryngeal nerve is shorter and does not extend into the chest.
- Drugs [3]:
  - ACE inhibitor (by causing cough)
  - inhaled corticosteroids (myopathic weakness of the adductor muscles of the vocal cords, fungal laryngitis, mucosal irritation)
  - warfarin (vocal fold haematoma)
  - antihistamines, diuretics, anticholinergics (drying effect on mucosa).

Causes of stridor

- *Laryngeal pathology*, e.g. inflammation or a foreign body
- *Endobronchial tumour* (Figure 31.1)
- *Goitre*
- *Infective laryngitis* (in children)

Acute Medicine, ed. Stephen Haydock, Duncan Whitehead and Zoë Fritz. Published by Cambridge University Press.
© Cambridge University Press 2015.

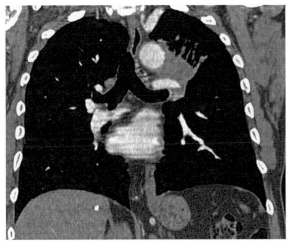

Figure 31.1 CT chest image showing a left-sided lung cancer (histologically proven) invading the left recurrent laryngeal nerve in a patient who presented with hoarseness (provided by Nick Screaton, Cambridge University Hospitals NHS Foundation Trust).

History

Consider input from relatives when diagnosing hoarseness, as some data suggests that *hoarseness may not be recognized by the patient* [5]. Patients with cognitive impairment or severe emotional burden may be unaware or unable to recognize and report on their own hoarseness [6].

- Take a collateral history.

Duration of hoarseness will affect management.

- How long has your voice been hoarse?

Ask about specific symptoms which might help to identify the cause in brackets.

- *Acid reflux?* (gastro-oesophageal reflux (GORD))
- *Halitosis?* (oropharyngeal candidiasis)
- *Unintentional weight loss?* (metastatic disease)
- *Does your voice deteriorate or fatigue with use? Have you noticed any other neurological symptoms?* (myasthenia gravis)
- *Any foreign body inhalation?*

Try to determine the severity of stridor.

- *Any history of colour change (cyanosis), respiratory effort and apnoea?*
- *Is it positional?*

Surgical procedures involving the neck or affecting the recurrent laryngeal nerve (e.g. cardiac surgery, oesophagectomy), recent endotracheal intubation (especially prolonged) and radiation treatment to the neck can cause hoarseness.

- *Any recent surgical procedures?*
- *Any recent radiation treatment to the neck?*

The level of suspicion of a neoplastic cause is increased if the patient is a heavy *alcohol* drinker or heavy *smoker* and is aged over *50 years*.

- *Ask about smoking and alcohol history.*
- The chewing of tobacco (called Gutkha in India) or the chewing of Paan Masala or Betel should also increase the level of suspicion (NICE guidelines, CG27 [7]).

  Vocal overuse is a common aetiological factor.
- *Ask about occupation.* Singers, performers and teachers are at an increased risk.

Various *drugs* can cause hoarseness (see 'Causes of hoarseness' above).

- *Take a drug history (including inhalers).*

What clues can be found on examination?

Perform a full examination, specifically looking for signs which may coexist with stridor or hoarseness.

On inspection

- The severity of stridor can be determined by monitoring the *respiratory rate*, *respiratory effort* and any signs of peripheral or central *cyanosis*.
- *Bovine cough* refers to the non-explosive cough of a patient unable to close his or her glottis.
- *Horner's syndrome* (ptosis, miosis, anhidrosis) suggests an endobronchial tumour causing stridor and hoarseness by involving the recurrent laryngeal nerve.

On palpation

- *Lymphadenopathy* is commonly associated with lung cancer.
- *Thyroid enlargement*:
  - a thyroid swelling and unexplained hoarseness is an indication for urgent referral.
- *Soft tissue masses* of face, neck or chest:
  - benign or malignant tumours can externally compress the airway.
- *Tracheal deviation*:
  - lung cancers can cause tracheal deviation either away from or towards the side of the lesion.

On percussion

- Stony dull percussion note suggests *pleural effusion* which might be malignant.

On auscultation

- It may be difficult to distinguish *stridor* from the inspiratory *wheezing* sounds in a patient with asthma and in this situation the possibility of a tumour in the trachea or around the main carina should be considered.
- *Fixed monophonic wheeze* is a sound which is usually constant in pitch and occurs at a fixed point in the respiratory cycle [1]. It is associated with a fixed obstruction in a large airway, typically due to a bronchial tumour. This is in contrast to *expiratory polyphonic wheeze*, which is a complex multi-pitched sound, with each tone starting at around the same time in expiration [1]. It characteristically occurs late in expiration and is thought to be due to dynamic airway compression, often associated with emphysema [1].

Basic investigations

The following should all be done at assessment for both hoarseness and stridor.

Blood tests

- *Routine bloods*, including liver function tests and Ca^{2+}
- Thyroid function tests in patients with a thyroid swelling

Imaging

- Chest X-ray (CXR)
  - Any obvious abnormalities: Consolidation? Masses?

Other

- Arterial blood gas if SpO_2 abnormal on air
  - Stridor can be associated with marked hypoxia (PaO_2 <8 kPa) as well as hypercapnia ($PaCO_2$ >6 kPa) in life-threatening cases.

Specialist investigations

In contrast to the above basic investigations, it may not be necessary to carry out the following investigations on the day of presentation as far as hoarseness is concerned. Stridor, however, requires immediate attention and urgent investigations need to be considered.

Hoarseness

Bronchoscopy/laryngoscopy (first line)

- *Benefits*: visualizes the airways, useful in evaluating lesions by biopsy.
- *Cautions*: any clotting abnormalities need to be corrected.

Indicated as first-line investigation when hoarseness fails to resolve within 3 months, or irrespective of duration if a serious underlying cause is suspected [3].

CT chest or neck/MRI neck (second line)

- *Benefits*: diagnosis and staging of lung cancer, mediastinal and neck masses.
- *Cautions*: radiation (CT chest gives approximately 7 mS exposure or equivalent of 70 plain chest radiographs, CT neck approximately 4 mS), metal implants/claustrophobia (MRI).

CT or MRI imaging of a patient with hoarseness should not take place before visualizing the larynx [3] as the bronchoscopy findings determine which imaging modality is appropriate.

pH probe

- *Benefits*: diagnosis of GORD.

Stridor

CT chest ± neck (an essential and urgent investigation)

- *Benefits*: diagnosis and staging of lung cancer, mediastinal and neck masses; identification of lung area to be biopsied either during bronchoscopy or a CT-guided procedure.
- *Cautions*: radiation.

Bronchoscopy

- *Benefits*: visualizes the airways, useful in evaluating central bronchial lesions by biopsy.
- *Cautions*: any clotting abnormalities need to be corrected.

MRI neck

- *Benefits*: may be helpful in demarcating lesions of the upper airway and vascular anomalies.
- *Cautions*: metal implants/claustrophobia.

Lung function testing

- *Benefits*: differentiates restrictive and obstructive lung processes and defines the location of the obstruction (upper or lower airways).
- *Cautions*: poor technique can sometimes give false results.

Management

Hoarseness

- Hoarseness is usually a benign symptom of voice overuse or the result of laryngitis. The commonest cause of community-acquired hoarseness is viral and symptoms caused by viral laryngitis usually last 1–3 weeks. *Hoarseness that persists for more than 3 weeks* must be assumed to be laryngeal carcinoma until proven otherwise, and requires an urgent referral for CXR (particularly in smokers older than 50 years of age and heavy drinkers [3]).
  - Positive finding requires urgent referral to the *respiratory team*.
  - Negative finding requires urgent referral to *ENT* [4].
- 'Urgent' means that the patient needs to be seen within the national target for urgent referrals, currently 2 weeks.
- The use of a *spacer* does *not* appear to help with hoarseness associated with inhaled corticosteroid use [8].
- *Anti-reflux medications* should *not* be prescribed for patients with hoarseness without any signs or symptoms of gastro-oesophageal reflux [3], but should be used if there are signs of chronic laryngitis.
- *Oral corticosteroids* should not be routinely prescribed to treat hoarseness as clinical trials have not shown any benefit and there are significant side effects.
- *Antibiotics* should not be routinely prescribed based on systematic reviews and randomized controlled trials [3]. This is because in most patients hoarseness is caused by acute laryngitis or a viral upper respiratory tract infection, not bacterial infections.
- *Surgery* may become appropriate with suspected malignancy.

Stridor

- NICE guidelines (CG27) [7] state that *immediate* referral should be considered for a patient presenting with stridor.
  - Involve specialist team as appropriate: respiratory team or ENT team.
- Involve and recognize the need for *anaesthetic team* promptly in event of significant airway compromise. This is obviously a priority over identifying the cause of the airway obstruction.
- Patients with moderate to severe stridor should be given *nothing by mouth* in preparation for possible intubation, bronchoscopy or tracheostomy.
- Management should be tailored to the *specific cause of stridor*:
  - initiate appropriate antimicrobial therapy if infective cause is suspected.
- The use of a *helium-oxygen* (heliox) mixture in patients with critical airway obstruction is rare nowadays. Heliox does not resolve the obstruction, but decreases airway resistance, giving more time for other treatments to be initiated and to have an effect [9].

Key points

- Suspicion of a serious underlying cause of hoarseness is warranted if there is a history of tobacco or alcohol use or unexplained weight loss.
- Hoarseness that persists for more than *3 weeks* must be considered to be laryngeal carcinoma until proven otherwise.
- Inhaled corticosteroids can cause hoarseness by causing vocal cord paralysis, fungal laryngitis or mucosal irritation.
- CT or MRI imaging of a patient with hoarseness should not take place prior to visualizing the larynx.
- In a patient with stridor, refer immediately to the anaesthetic team in the event of significant airway compromise.

References

1. Gibson J, Geddes D, Costabel U, Sterk P, Corrin B. *Respiratory Medicine*, 3rd edn. Saunders; 2003.
2. Roy N, Merrill RM, Gray SD, Smith EM. Voice disorders in the general population: prevalence, risk

factors, and occupational impact. *The Laryngoscope* 2005; 115: 1988–1995.

3. Schwartz SR, Cohen SM, Dailey SH, et al. Clinical practice guideline: hoarseness (dysphonia). *Otolaryngology – head and neck surgery: official journal of American Academy of Otolaryngology-Head and Neck Surgery* 2009; 141: S1–S31.

4. Rosen CA, Anderson D, Murry T. Evaluating hoarseness: keeping your patient's voice healthy. *American Family Physician* 1998; 57: 2775–2782.

5. Brouha XD, Tromp DM, de Leeuw JR, Hordijk GJ, Winnubst JA. Laryngeal cancer patients: analysis of patient delay at different tumor stages. *Head and Neck* 2005; 27: 289–295.

6. Sneeuw KC, Sprangers MA, Aaronson NK. The role of health care providers and significant others in evaluating the quality of life of patients with chronic disease. *Journal of Clinical Epidemiology* 2002; 55: 1130–1143.

7. *CG27: Referral for Suspected Cancer*. National Institute for Health and Care Excellence Guidelines, June 2005.

8. The use of inhaled corticosteroids in adults with asthma. *Drug and Therapeutics Bulletin* 2000; 38: 5–8.

9. Fu A, Kopec A, Markham M. Heliox in upper airway obstruction. *Official Journal of the Canadian Association of Critical Care Nurses/CACCN* 1999; 10: 12–13; quiz 14–15.

Hypothermia

Mohamed Yousuf

Introduction

Hypothermia is associated with significant morbidity and mortality, being responsible for an estimated 300 deaths per year in the UK. It is defined as a core body temperature below 35°C measured using a rectal thermometer.

Scenario 32.1

An 80-year-old woman is brought into the ED on a cold winter's day. She was found after the weekend on the floor of her bedroom by her carers. She has not been seen for 2 days and the house was unheated. She has a history of hypothyroidism and vertigo for which she takes thyroxine and prochlorperazine, respectively. On arrival she is drowsy, bradycardic and hypothermic with a rectal temperature of 32°C.

Causes

Homoeothermic (warm-blooded) animals maintain their body temperature despite marked fluctuations in the external temperature. Most heat in the body is generated by metabolic processes in the major organs and skeletal muscle contraction. It is lost by convection, radiation, conduction and evaporation through the skin and lungs. Thermoregulation is a complex balance between heat production and loss, principally controlled by the hypothalamus. Hypothermia develops when loss exceeds production. Cold exposure results in a series of reflex mechanisms, most importantly cutaneous vasoconstriction and shivering.

High risk groups for developing hypothermia include:

- elderly (and children)
- homeless
- malnourished
- substance abusers
- patients with co-morbid chronic psychiatric and medical conditions.

Though accidental hypothermia is a more common presentation, we are not infrequently starting to see hypothermia in elderly frail patients living alone, where the underlying causes are a lack of bodily reserve to generate heat due to malnourishment, sepsis and a reduced awareness of the external environment.

Many medical conditions can result in hypothermia:

- Major trauma
- Skin conditions such as burns, psoriasis
- Hypothyroidism
- Hypoadrenalism
- Neuromuscular disease
- Thiamine deficiency
- Hypoglycaemia
- Central lesions affecting the hypothalamus including strokes and subarachnoid haemorrhages.

Drugs contributing to hypothermia

(a) Direct impairment of thermoregulatory mechanisms

- Anxiolytics
- Antidepressants
- Antipsychotics (including prochlorperazine)
- Opioids

(b) Impair judgement of external environment

- Ethanol

Acute Medicine, ed. Stephen Haydock, Duncan Whitehead and Zoë Fritz. Published by Cambridge University Press.
© Cambridge University Press 2015.

(c) Impair mechanisms that compensate for low external temperatures

- Oral hypoglycaemics
- Beta-blockers
- Alpha-adrenergic agonists (e.g. clonidine)

Clinical assessment

If the symptoms are inconsistent with the severity of hypothermia, it should raise suspicions of other coexisting pathologies.

Mild hypothermia (32–35°C)

- Tachypnoea, tachycardia, ataxia, dysarthria, impaired judgement, and shivering.

Moderate hypothermia (28–32°C)

- Proportionate reductions in pulse rate and cardiac output, hypoventilation, CNS depression, hyporeflexia, loss of shivering. Cardiac arrhythmias (AF, bradycardia, junctional rhythm) may develop.

Severe hypothermia (less than 28°C)

- Pulmonary oedema, oliguria, areflexia, coma, hypotension, bradycardia, ventricular arrhythmias (including ventricular fibrillation) and asystole.

Always carry out a general survey looking for injuries and trauma. Clues such as a thyroidectomy scar, smell of alcohol, etc., could point towards the aetiology of the hypothermia.

In addition, patients commonly develop the following conditions.

Dehydration

Careful attention needs to be paid to fluid balance, especially in the elderly with multiple co-morbidities. They are also more prone to complications from fluid overload during intravenous rehydration.

Dehydration results from:

- Reflex peripheral vasoconstriction causing a transient increase in central vascular volume and resulting 'cold diuresis'.
- In later stages fluid shifts from intravascular to extravascular space.
- If uncorrected it progresses to acute kidney injury.

Haemorrhage

Moderate and severe hypothermia predisposes to bleeding and haemorrhage due to inhibition of clotting factors.

Sepsis

Always consider as it carries a significant mortality in hypothermia.

Investigations

- Full blood count
- Urea and electrolytes
- Blood glucose
- Liver function tests
- Creatine kinase (risk of rhabdomyolysis)
- Lactate
- CRP (high value may suggest occult sepsis)
- Clotting screen
- Amylase (exclude hypothermia-induced acute pancreatitis)
- Toxicology screen (if drug abuse suspected)
- ECG
- Plain chest radiograph

Care should be taken when interpreting the laboratory values for clotting screen and blood gases as these could be spuriously normal. Use uncorrected values when interpreting blood gas values and be aware that the patient could still have a coagulopathy despite lab values being normal.

Insulin is ineffective at low temperature so patients are frequently hyperglycaemic on admission. They may become hypoglycaemic as temperature rises. Consider diabetic hyperglycaemic state if blood glucose does not fall on warming. Ensure frequent monitoring of blood glucose.

ECG changes in severe hypothermia are common due to cardiac irritability:

- Baseline shivering artefact (has been misinterpreted as VF!).
- AF with slow ventricular response.
- VF and VT.
- The PR, RR and QT intervals are prolonged and there may be elevation of the 'J' point (Osborn or J waves). These changes can be misinterpreted as cardiac ischaemia (see Figure 32.1).
- *Avoid rough handling of patients* as this increases risk of inducing an arrhythmia.

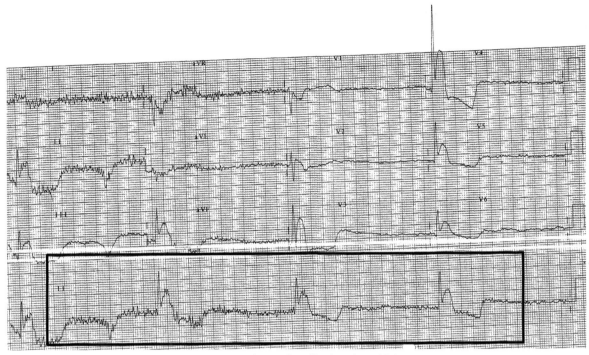

Figure 32.1 ECG in hypothermia illustrating shivering artefact, profound bradycardia and Osborn waves.

Chest radiograph may show:

- aspiration pneumonia
- consolidation
- pulmonary oedema.

Management

Resuscitation

Airway/breathing

Consider endotracheal intubation if low GCS, unable to protect airway and/or respiratory distress. It aids in clearing respiratory secretions and allows delivery of warm oxygen.

- Reduced GCS is *uncommon* in mild hypothermia and if present may indicate associated CNS pathology (stroke, haemorrhage, infection) or drugs.
- Tachypnoea is unusual in moderate and severe hypothermia; if present it may indicate diabetic ketoacidosis or lactic acidosis.

Circulation

Palpation of peripheral pulses may be difficult due to peripheral vasoconstriction, dehydration and bradycardia. Check the carotid pulse for up to 60 seconds. Dopplers or bedside echocardiogram are useful where available.

- Tachycardia is unusual in moderate and severe hypothermia.
- If present think sepsis, fluid loss/haemorrhage or overdose.

Obtain IV access and start replacing fluids using crystalloids.

- Large fluid volumes may be needed to achieve euvolaemia.
- Large fluid shifts occur during rewarming.
- Blood pressure can drop with warming due to peripheral vasodilatation.
- Fluid may shift from the extravascular space to the intravascular space which along with aggressive fluid resuscitation can lead to pulmonary oedema (may need monitoring of central pressure).
- Urinary catheterization will be required.

Cardiorespiratory arrest

After checking for signs of life, follow the appropriate ALS algorithm. Continue resuscitation indefinitely until the temperature is 32–35°C.

Ventricular arrhythmias and asystole are refractory to conventional treatments in this setting. Treatment is focused on aggressive rewarming and use of vasopressors.

Rewarming

Passive external rewarming can be used to treat mild hypothermia in those who are well with sufficient reserve to generate heat by shivering.

- Remove patient from cold environment to a warm room.
- Cover with blankets to prevent further heat loss.
- Rate of rewarming by this method is 0.5–2°C per hour.

Active external rewarming is used in moderate to severe hypothermia and in those with mild hypothermia who fail to rewarm adequately by the above measures.

- Warm blankets, heat pads, warm bath or warm air blown over the skin surface area.
- Take care to prevent body surface burns.

Significant fluid shifts may have occurred in patients who have been hypothermic for some time. These patients have lost their reserve to generate heat and can take longer to warm up despite adequate rewarming techniques.

Active internal rewarming is employed in more severe cases:

- Warmed crystalloid infusion (40–42°C)
- Warmed humidified oxygen
- Irrigation of body cavities (pleural irrigation, peritoneal irrigation, colonic lavage, gastric lavage) using warmed crystalloid
- Extracorporeal blood (haemodialysis, continuous arteriovenous rewarming, and cardiopulmonary bypass)
- Expected rate of rewarming is 2°C per hour.

Failure to rewarm despite these measures should prompt a search for other causes:

- Infection
- Hypoglycaemia
- Adrenal insufficiency
- Hypothyroidism.

Core temperature 'after-drop' is a risk of active external rewarming and can cause arrhythmias during the rewarming when the extremities and trunk are warmed simultaneously. Cold acidotic blood from the peripheries moves to the centre, thereby lowering the core body temperature and inducing arrhythmias. The risk may be reduced by warming the trunk before warming the peripheries.

Co-morbidities

Sepsis can present with hypothermia. Mortality may be high in such patients and they are slower to rewarm. Empirical antibiotics should be started if

- there is an obvious source of infection
- patients fail to raise their core body temperature despite adequate measures
- patients are elderly.

Adrenal insufficiency: If there is failure to rewarm despite adequate measures and there are other features that suggest adrenal insufficiency, consider treating with dexamethasone 4 mg IV or hydrocortisone 100 mg IV.

Trauma: always assess for co-morbid trauma and in particular fractures. Rule out spinal injury in patients with absent reflexes and paralysis before attributing to hypothermia.

Further reading

Brown DJ, Brugger H, Boyd J, Paal P. Accidental hypothermia. *N Engl J Med* 2012; 367:1930–1938.

Headdon WG, Wilson PM, Dalton HR. The management of accidental hypothermia. *BMJ* 2009; 338:b2085.

Mulcahy AR, Watts MR. *Accidental Hypothermia: An Evidence-Based Approach.* Emergency Medicine Practice EBMedicine.net; 2009.

Chapter

33

Immobility

Matthew R. Hayman, Cally Williamson and Stephen Haydock

Introduction

Immobility was one of the original *'geriatric giants'* (the others being *instability, incontinence* and *impaired intellect*) described by Professor Bernard Isaacs [1], one of the founding fathers of geriatric medicine in the UK: *'If examined closely enough all common problems with older people relate to one or more giants'.*

Immobility is a common reason for requesting hospital admission, as the primary reason for referral or as a component of the *frailty syndrome*. In order to be supported in the community the elderly often require a certain level of mobility. If they fall below this level, the existing family and social support package may become inadequate to safely maintain them at home or in residential care. Unfortunately, it is often not possible to provide the extra support needed in the community within a time frame that can ensure their continued safety, and an acute admission results.

Ambulation is a complex process; dependent upon many sensory neuronal inputs, accurate central computation of these inputs, and then appropriately coordinated neuronal outputs to initiate multiple coordinated muscular contractions. Good function of the sensorium, brain and neuronal conduction, along with muscular and joint function, is essential for safe, stable ambulation. It is not surprising that the frail elderly frequently develop gait and balance problems at times of even minor added psychological or physical stress. As a syndrome there are multiple diagnoses that can lead to this 'final common pathway' of immobility ranging from the relatively simple and potentially curable to those heralding the final days of life.

The approach of the acute physician to immobility should be to recognize the syndrome as *potentially life-threatening and rewardingly complex*. A complete and thorough assessment, often involving members of the multidisciplinary team, is usually required to uncover the one or more diagnoses present, thus enabling the formulation of an appropriate management plan. *If you don't look carefully you won't find out what is wrong. If you don't know what is wrong, you will not be able to fix it!*

Sometimes the cause is straightforward...

Scenario 33.1

Mrs EG is an 82-year-old woman with known osteo-arthritis and mild IHD. She is admitted to the MAU having been found 'off legs' in her bath by her carer. She has longstanding dysphasia following a stroke. CK is 9000 IU/L and renal function mildly impaired. There is bilateral buttock and abdominal bruising. Following initial assessment she is inappropriately treated for a UTI on the basis of a urine dip (Blood ++, Protein +).

When time is taken to elicit a full history from this patient with dysphasia it transpires that the bath seat she uses due to her arthritis collapsed beneath her and she was unable to get out of her steep-sided bath. Her 'piper alarm' wrist band was carefully removed and placed out of reach prior to her entering the bath.

...and sometimes it isn't...

Scenario 33.2

Mr AS, a 69-year-old man, is referred to the MAU on Friday afternoon complaining of general lethargy and unsteadiness. Examination (including CNS) is unremarkable. His investigations show a mild normochromic and normocytic anaemia and hyponatraemia (sodium = 120 mmol/L). He is fluid restricted and paired osmolalities sent. On Monday the ward nurse comments that Mr AS has developed a sacral pressure sore, having not been out of bed all weekend. Repeat neurological examination reveals a sensory level at T12

Acute Medicine, ed. Stephen Haydock, Duncan Whitehead and Zoë Fritz. Published by Cambridge University Press. © Cambridge University Press 2015.

and reduced lower limb power and sphincter dysfunction. MR of the whole spine reveals spinal cord compression at T12 which is subsequently found to be due to a plasmacytoma.

Common causes of immobility

Musculoskeletal

- Arthritides
- Osteoporosis
- Fractures (hip/femur)
- Podiatric
- Other (Paget's)

Neurological

- Impaired cognition
- Stroke
- Parkinson's disease
- Cerebellar dysfunction
- Neuropathies
- Visual impairment

Cardiovascular

- Congestive cardiac failure (limiting breathlessness)
- Ischaemic heart disease (frequent angina)
- Peripheral vascular disease (claudication pain)

Respiratory

- Chronic obstructive pulmonary disease
- Interstitial lung disease

Psychological

- Depression
- Anxiety including fear of falling
- Social isolation

Medication

- Parkinsonian drugs
- Sedation
- Hypotensives
- Drugs causing blurred vision

Environmental

- 'Enforced immobility' due to physical, chemical or treatment restraints in hospital or care home and associated deconditioning

Pain

- Acute
- Chronic

In fact immobility can result from any significant systemic illness.

Causes of immobility not to be missed

While many serious medical conditions can lead to immobility there are some that the acute physician should always consider when there has been a *sudden or rapidly progressive* loss of mobility:

- spinal cord compression
- Guillain–Barré syndrome
- septic arthritis
- undisplaced fracture of the neck of femur/pubic ramus/acetabulum
- stroke
- new medications (antipsychotics, anticholinergics, antihypertensives, etc.).

Clearly this is not an exhaustive list and the more open-minded regarding the cause or causes one can be, the less likely it is that important, treatable causes of immobility will be missed.

Clinical assessment of immobility – the multidisciplinary team

The clinical assessment of frail older people can be difficult due to communication and cognitive problems. Information should be sought from carers, family members, close friends and the general practitioner where possible.

The best approach to assessment of the frail patient is a multidisciplinary team (MDT) one; incorporating a comprehensive geriatric review to identify the medical, psychological, social and functional impediments for the patient. The subsequent management involves coordination of the MDT to provide an integrated treatment that addresses all identified reversible issues to *optimize the function and health of the patient.*

Clear communication and close team working between medical, nursing and therapy staff ensures that the patient is treated and discharged in a timely manner, as safely as possible to the appropriate setting.

Composition of the multidisciplinary team

- Medical staff
- Nursing staff

- Physiotherapist
- Geriatric nurse specialist
- Occupational therapist
- Social worker
- Pharmacist (medicines reconciliation)

Supported by

- District nurse and community matron
- Psychiatric liaison, mental health and community psychiatric nurse
- Specialist nurses; learning difficulties team, tissue viability
- Speech and language therapist
- Adult safeguarding team
- Palliative care/end of life team

The patient (and their family) must remain central and fully involved with this process. The success of the multidisciplinary team approach depends upon clear, regular communication with interactive meetings where all parties are able to contribute equally.

If the patient is considered safe to manage at home, but requires increased support, nursing staff and therapists can identify the need and engage the community MDT or alternative services and charities. If further rehabilitation is necessary, therapists create a rehabilitative treatment plan with specific goals with continuous monitoring of progress. If goals cannot be met, the team works together to establish adaptive strategies to achieve the maximal independence for the patient. Should these approaches also fail to enable safe discharge home then social workers will need to start the process of identifying alternative housing or placement.

Emergency therapy in the acute care setting

- As acute medicine emerged as a distinct clinical specialty, therapists started to explore how their expertise could be better utilized in the acute setting. Therapy had been traditionally rehabilitation based, with less emphasis on assessment, and limited to normal working hours.
- During the 1990s the physiotherapy and occupational therapy professions were increasingly involved in delivering NHS targets with regard to reducing length of stay, inpatient costs and health promotion, necessitating

increased out-of-hours provision. Early trials were conducted using therapy teams to facilitate discharges from the ED and MAU; reducing unnecessary admissions and length of stay without adversely affecting the quality of care or patient experience [2].
- A 2005 study sought to examine the benefits of consistent access to the geriatric care pathway for patients aged over 70 years. The resulting 'Older Persons Assessment and Liaison' (OPAL) Team consisted of an elderly care specialist nurse, physiotherapist and geriatrician. Collaboratively, the nurse and physiotherapist identified moderate-high clinical risk patients using a Comprehensive Geriatric Assessment and discussed these with the team geriatrician. Bed occupancy was reduced and 'OPAL' became nationally recognized as an excellent model of interdisciplinary care [3] and was emulated in many acute trusts in the UK.
- The acute care therapist requires a good understanding of how both acute and chronic disease processes can impact adversely on the functional status of a patient and hence their ability to cope in their usual living environment.
- Occupational therapists and physiotherapists have complementary specialist skill sets that make them ideal professions to work closely together, providing elements of care which combine to maximize the patient's overall function and facilitate their discharge to a suitable location.

Occupational therapists' skills

- Assessing previous and current cognitive ability; distinguishing 'new confusion' from the patient's usual level of cognitive function. They may discuss with the community psychiatric nurse, community social worker, family or carer.
- Assessment of functional status in relation to their home environment, and advising on environmental modifications to assist the patient's independence, potentially completing a visit to the patient's home, with or without the patient accompanying.
- They are crucial in coordinating complex discharge plans, often liaising with the patient, their family, friends and the wider MDT and charities.

Physiotherapists' acute care skills

- Musculoskeletal, cardiorespiratory and neurological assessments and physical treatments, enabling them to initiate and plan the required rehabilitation for a given individual.
- Implementation of a range of acute respiratory interventions and frequently link with the respiratory early supported discharge schemes; usually focused towards COPD patients.

History

Take a *detailed history of the presenting problem*, in particular:

- Duration of mobility problems and current functional status.
- Nature of decline: acute or gradual.
- Patient's understanding of the problem; what is limiting mobility, e.g. pain, confidence, weakness, stiffness, dizziness.
- Ask specifically about pain *(it is never acceptable to document that a patient is in pain on admission and then do nothing about it until the post take ward round!)*.
- What are the patient's goals: getting to toilet, getting to shops, etc.

Medication history

Pay particular attention to medications that can cause postural symptoms or sensory/neurological impairment:

- Current medication
- Recent changes
- Over-the-counter medications
- Enquire as to whether patient self-administers or is supervised; care staff, Dossette box.

Nutritional history

- What does the patient eat during the day?
- Who provides these meals, who does the patient's shopping?
- How has decline in mobility impacted on nutrition and hydration; is the patient able to make hot drinks, etc.?

Mental health and psychological well-being

- Is there evidence of cognitive impairment (assess formally)?
- Ask regarding symptoms of anxiety or depression.

- Is the patient socially isolated; who visits? Family, carers, friends?
- Access to day care facilities.
- What are the patient's '*hopes and fears*' for the present and future?

Continence

- Urinary continence
- Faecal continence
- How has this changed recently, in particular in relation to decline in mobility?

Examination

Carry out as full a system examination as is possible. Pay particular attention to:

- *Skin integrity* and document evidence of impending or existing pressure damage
- *Combined musculoskeletal assessment*: muscle tone and strength, joint range of movement, foot deformities and skin lesions
- *Neurological assessment*: focal weakness and deficit, peripheral neuropathy
- *Cognitive assessment*: using a validated tool, e.g. MMSE.

Always enlist the help and expertise of nursing and therapy staff to ensure that these aspects of an examination are accurately performed and recorded. Immobility is impossible to diagnose without an attempt to assess mobility (bed mobility, ability to transfer, standing or sitting balance, gait and the presence or absence of pain on movement) and *doctors are notoriously poor at these assessments*.

Following the assessment and taking into account the associated assessments by therapists and other members of the multidisciplinary team a *problem list* should be generated. This should list any issue (*not just medical*) that requires attention by members of the team. This should include a consideration of the:

- medical problems
- nutritional problems
- functional problems
- psychological problems
- social implications
- proposed intervention target.

Complications of immobility

Even short periods of immobility are associated with deterioration in almost all organ systems. It should be the primary goal to actively intervene to restore mobility as soon as possible following admission to hospital.

Skin

- Pressure ulcers (see Box 33.1)

Musculoskeletal

- Muscular deconditioning
- Muscle atrophy
- Rhabdomyolysis
- Contractures
- Loss of bone density

Muscular deconditioning begins *after only 24 hours of immobility* and progresses at a rate of 1–3% per day, meaning that there can be 50% muscle loss in 2 months. Similarly bone mineral loss is progressive with vertebral loss estimated at 1% per week.

Cardiovascular

- Cardiovascular deconditioning
- Orthostatic hypotension
- Venous thromboembolic disease

Respiratory

- Decreased ventilation
- Atelectasis
- Aspiration pneumonia

Gastrointestinal

- Anorexia
- Constipation
- Faecal impaction
- Faecal incontinence

Genitourinary

- Urinary tract infection
- Urinary retention
- Urinary incontinence
- Bladder calculi

Metabolic

- Decreased plasma volume
- Negative nitrogen balance
- Impaired glucose tolerance
- Decreased PTH, raised serum calcium
- Raised renin/aldosterone

- Altered growth hormone, androgen secretion and circadian rhythm

Psychological

- Sensory deprivation
- Delirium
- Depression

Box 33.1 Pressure ulcers: classification, prevention and treatment

Classification

Pressure ulcers are graded 1–4 according to the European Ulcer Advisory Panel Classification System:

- *Grade 1*: Non-blanchable erythema of intact skin
- *Grade 2*: Partial thickness skin loss involving epidermis, dermis or both
- *Grade 3*: Full thickness skin loss involving damage and necrosis of subcutaneous tissues that may extend to but not through underlying fascia
- *Grade 4*: Extensive destruction, necrosis or damage to muscle, bone or supporting structures (with/without full thickness skin loss)

Prevention

- Regular assessment and documentation of risk using recognized risk assessment, e.g. 'Waterlow Pressure Area Risk Assessment'
- Encourage early mobilization
- Positioning and repositioning interventions and minimize pressure on bony prominences
- Provide nutritional support according to nutritional assessment with a recognized tool, e.g. MUST score (see Chapter 67)
- Use of pressure-relieving devices, e.g. foam mattresses, air mattresses

Treatment

- Document depth, area and EPUAP grade (development of grade 2–4 ulcers should be reported as a local clinical incident)
- Manage by modern dressing to encourage wound healing
- Consider antimicrobial therapy if signs of local or systemic infection
- Consider surgical referral if conservative management unsuccessful, taking the level of anaesthetic and surgical risk into account

Management

- Identify the possible cause(s) of immobility and reverse all of these, that it is possible to, by appropriate medical interventions and input from therapists.
- Maintain an adequate fluid intake to reduce the likelihood of: postural hypotension, rhabdomyolysis, thickened respiratory secretions, constipation, venous thromboembolism.
- Ensuring adequate nutritional support; high protein and high calories, possibly with supplemental vitamin D, C and B complex.
- Scrupulous medical, nursing and therapy care aimed at avoiding the complications of immobility: loss of muscle bulk and bone density, development of contractures and pressure damage to skin.
- Regular formal MDT meetings to update all team members on progress, highlight the issues still to be addressed, and consider opportunities for further improvement (titration of pain relief, splinting, changes to medications).
- *Rapid investigation and response to unexpected deteriorations* that might indicate a progressive neurological conditions (Guillain–Barré, cord compression) or acute rheumatological/vasculitic conditions (PMR, temporal arteritis, gout/ pseudogout, non-displaced hip fractures).

Rehabilitation

- The aim of treatment must always be kept at the forefront of the mind when rehabilitating the immobile patient: *to return the patient to their normal level of function as rapidly as possible.* When this is not possible the aim is to minimize the acquired deterioration in function as much as possible (e.g. post stroke, fracture, etc.).
- Optimal rehabilitation requires prompt and full diagnosis, followed by appropriate therapy interventions aimed at maintaining and increasing mobility *as soon as possible.*
- There is no firm point at which '*acute treatment*' ends and '*rehabilitation*' begins, as rehabilitation can and often should commence and proceed while any acute problems are being treated.
- Rehabilitation commonly involves early goal setting and frequent reviews of progress and involves multidisciplinary teams; doctors may be involved as supporting members of the team with the lead being taken by nursing and therapy staff.
- The venue for rehabilitation can be any setting from the acute hospital ward to the patient's own home. It is often most effective when performed in a location as similar to the patient's normal environment as possible, so ideally in their home.

In the UK there are a variety of local systems in place for assessment, rehabilitation and delivery of care:

Rapid response teams can be based within the ED or the community; they consist of therapists and nursing staff with the skills to assess the individual struggling and at a crisis point. They may facilitate patients returning to or remaining in their own home with additional support (care or therapy input) or can refer on to a community hospital. They reduce inappropriate admissions to the acute Trust of patients with minimal new medical needs.

Day hospital: the geriatric day hospital developed in the UK in the 1950s and 1960s has traditionally focused on rehabilitation needs with ready access to occupational and physiotherapy services. They also provide comprehensive geriatric medical input through specialty clinic services, e.g. falls, Parkinson's disease, leg ulcers, memory and incontinence services.

These clinics are supported by on-site therapy and nursing staff with the appropriate expertise to provide a 'one stop shop' approach. They can also provide an alternative route to urgent assessment to that of the emergency department and have access to a range of laboratory and radiological investigations.

Hospital at home: provides short-term acute medical care (several days) within the homes of patients (including residential and nursing homes) when they have ongoing medical and therapy needs that can be delivered outside of the acute Trust, e.g. IV antibiotics, nebulizers for COPD treatment, anticoagulant titration post PE, physiotherapy and occupational therapy needs. Patients may remain under the care of a hospital consultant and be managed on a '*virtual ward*'.

Community hospitals aim to provide a range of services as close to the homes of the local population as possible. They are most commonly located in rural communities, where there are considerable distances to the closest acute hospital, making travelling onerous for patients and their visitors. The services provided vary but usually include a combination of inpatient facilities providing respite, step-down care from the acute trust and rehabilitation, together with outpatient therapy, medical clinics and procedures, e.g. IV therapies, transfusions and endoscopy.

Step-up/step-down facilities: ward-based facility providing therapy input for patients admitted from the community (step up) or from the acute Trust (step down). Patients are medically stable, but require ongoing therapy to improve mobility and independence, before returning to independent living in their own home. May have a degree of specialization such as stroke step-down beds; these can be on the site of the acute Trust or be part of a community hospital.

Respite care: sometimes referred to as a 'short break service', it aims to provide the carers with an essential break to recuperate from the physical and emotional fatigue of the caring role. Without such breaks the carers might be unable to continue to manage the patient at home. This can be for a few hours, overnight or for several days and provided at the patient's home or in an alternative residential setting, usually either a care home or community hospital.

Despite appropriate medical and therapy input, many elderly patients are unable to return to independent living in their own home. Long-term care ranges from sheltered housing, extra care housing to residential and nursing home placements. An estimated 468 000 places were provided in 2006 for nursing, residential and long-stay hospital care in the UK. This was provided by the NHS, local authorities and the private and voluntary sector (including 12 208 registered care homes).

Conclusion

Immobility is frequently a multifactorial presentation, often in an elderly patient, which can be caused by problems with almost any of the body's organs or systems. It is important to note that pain is a common pathway by which many disorders present with immobility and its treatment is a vital part not only of good patient care but also of the diagnostic process (*once out of pain a patient may well show more localizing signs or provide vital clues to the diagnosis*).

A critical part of the treatment of patients presenting with immobility is the early involvement of the multidisciplinary team, who can provide skills that acute physicians lack and are likely to play a vital role in the ongoing treatment and rehabilitation of such patients. Many causes of immobility are treatable and at least partially reversible. Given the severe complications that can arise from extended periods of immobility, rapid diagnosis and treatment with early therapy to ensure optimal rehabilitation are essential.

References

1. Isaacs B (1981) Ageing and the doctor. In: Hobman D (ed.) *The Impact of Ageing*. London: Croom Helm.

2. Hardy C, Whitwell D, Sarsfield B, Maimaris C (2001) Admission avoidance and early discharge of acute hospital admissions: an accident and emergency based scheme. *Emergency Medicine Journal* 18(6): 435–440.

3. Harari D, Martin FC, Buttery A, O'Neill S, Hopper A (2007) The older person's assessment and liaison team 'OPAL': evaluation of comprehensive geriatric assessment in acute medical inpatients. *Age and Ageing* 36: 670–675.

Further reading

Gosney M, Harper A, Conroy S (eds.) (2012) *Oxford Desk Reference: Geriatric Medicine*. Oxford: Oxford University Press.

Jiricka MK (2008) Activity tolerance and fatigue pathophysiology: concepts of altered health states. In: Porth CM (ed.) *Essentials of Pathophysiology: Concepts of Altered Health States*. Philadelphia, PA: Lippincott Williams & Wilkins.

Mearns N, Millar A, Murray F, Fraser S (2008) Developing occupational therapy best practice guidelines for acute medical services. *Acute Medicine* 7(2): 97–100.

NICE Guidelines (2005) The Prevention and Treatment of Pressure Ulcers. NICE Clinical Guideline 29. Available to download at www.nice.org.uk/nicemedia/live/10972/29887/29887.pdf.

NICE Guidelines (2013) Falls: Assessment and Prevention of Falls in Older People. NICE Clinical Guideline 121, Issued June 2013. Available to download at www.nice.org.uk/nicemedia/live/14181/64166/64166.pdf.

Incidental findings

Stephen Haydock

Introduction

Incidental findings describe apparently asymptomatic and unexpected findings on either examination or investigation that may or may not require further investigation depending on the particular finding and the clinical situation in which it was discovered. They are commonly referred to amongst physicians by the generic term '*incidentalomas*'. Such discoveries are increasingly common due to:

- Large number of 'routine' blood, urine, cardiological and radiological investigations performed on patients in primary and secondary care
- Improved availability and resolution of CT and MRI imaging modalities to identify lesions below resolution of older scanners
- Availability of private CT scan 'health checks' detecting abnormalities in otherwise healthy individuals
- Screening and study investigations performed on subjects as part of academic or pharmaceutical research studies
- Increased life expectancy and imaging of increasingly elderly patients with an increased burden of occult disease.

Incidental abnormalities

These may be detected on:

Physical examination

- *Hypertension* including hypertensive retinopathy noted on ophthalmoscopic examination
- Organomegaly
- Lymphadenopathy
- Skin lesions

Blood and urinalysis

- Anaemia
- Thrombocytopenia
- Abnormal clotting
- Serum electrolyte abnormalities, e.g. hypo- and hyperkalaemia
- Hyper- and hypocalcaemia
- Proteinuria
- Non-visible haematuria

ECG/ECHO

- LV hypertrophy
- Disorders of cardiac conduction
- *Pulmonary hypertension*

Radiology

- Mass lesions on plain chest radiograph
- Abdominal masses on CT or MRI, e.g. *incidental adrenal masses*
- Intracranial masses on CT or MRI, e.g. *incidental pituitary masses*

Most commonly, problems arise from unexpected findings on radiological imaging. The likelihood of detecting such an abnormality increases with increasing age. A review of 1426 imaging studies performed for research purposes [1] used the definition of an incidental finding as 'an observation noted in the dictated radiology report not directly related to the aims of the study' and excluded comments regarding old injuries, non-pathological anatomical variants or normal line or pacemaker insertions. The following rates of incidental findings were reported for subjects with a mean age of 58 years (range 3–97 years):

Acute Medicine, ed. Stephen Haydock, Duncan Whitehead and Zoë Fritz. Published by Cambridge University Press. © Cambridge University Press 2015.

- MR head — 43%
- MR (all other) — 20%
- CT scans of abdomen and pelvis — 61%
- CT scans of thorax — 55%
- CT scan (all other) — 25%
- ultrasounds scans — 9%
- nuclear medicine scans — 4%
- plain radiology — 39%

Therefore 567 of the 1426 research imaging studies reported incidental findings comprising 40% of subjects imaged. Other studies have reported similar incidences for these imaging modalities and noted the highest incidence for CT imaging of abdomen and pelvis. Of the 567 individuals identified above:

- Only 35 (6.2%) subjects had an abnormality that required further clinical action.
- Of these, 6 individuals derived clear benefit from the discovery and subsequent investigation (potentially life-threatening infections and tumours).
- However, 3 patients had additional unnecessary medical burden having undergone surgery for essentially benign disease not likely to impact on morbidity and mortality.

In general, most findings can be managed on an outpatient basis. Few incidental findings are likely to be life-threatening. It is important that the finding is explained to the patient in such a way that undue anxiety does not result. It is important to ensure that an appropriate investigation plan is in place if indicated, involving follow-up by either the patient's general practitioner or the appropriate specialty team. The subsequent investigation and follow-up should be carefully judged to avoid an unnecessary burden of anxiety and morbidity on the patient and their family. Particular issues arise in relation to unexpected masses and nodules that might indicate an underlying neoplasm.

Incidental pituitary tumours

Post-mortem studies give a prevalence of about 10% and incidental findings of tumours on cranial imaging are therefore not uncommon. Ninety per cent of intrasellar tumours are adenomas, the remainder are Rathke's cleft cysts, craniopharyngiomas, metastases, chordomas or meningiomas. Incidental pituitary adenomas are classified according to size:

Macroadenomas

- >1 cm in diameter

- 2% of adenomas
- May cause symptoms due to mass effect, e.g. headache, visual loss (classically bitemporal hemianopia) due to optic chiasm compression
- May cause pituitary insufficiency due to compression of remainder of gland
- 20% may be autonomously secreting

Microadenomas

- <1 cm
- 98% of adenomas
- Do not produce symptoms due to mass effects
- Do not cause pituitary insufficiency
- 50% may be autonomously secreting

The markedly greater prevalence of microadenomas suggests that transformation from a micro- to a macroadenoma is a fairly rare event.

The anterior pituitary contains the following cell lines:

- corticotrophs secreting adrenococorticotrophic hormone (ACTH)
- thyrotrophs secreting TSH
- gonadotrophs secreting luteinizing hormone and follicle stimulating hormone
- growth hormone secreting cells.

In practice hypersecretion from a pituitary incidentaloma usually results in overproduction of growth hormone or more commonly prolactin (rarely ACTH and almost never TSH). Reassuringly, though, most are non-functioning.

Investigation

Incidental microadenoma

- Exclude hyperprolactinaemia by measuring serum prolactin.
- Exclude growth hormone secretion by measuring insulin-like growth factor-1 (IGF-1).
- Exclude Cushing's if clinical suspicion by 1 mg dexamethasone suppression test.
- Exclude TSH secretion by measurement; although TSH secretion is extremely rare, measurement is simple and inexpensive.

Incidental macroadenoma

- Need to exclude hypersecretion and hyposecretion due to mass effect.

- Measure TSH, thyroxine, cortisol, prolactin and IGF-1, testosterone 9 am sample (male), menstrual history (female).
- 1 mg dexamethasone suppression test if features of Cushing's present.
- Short Synacthen test if features of Cushing's absent.
- Note that prolactin may be elevated due to mass effect as dopamine is *prolactin release inhibitory factor*.
- Need formal assessment of visual fields.

Management

- Incidental pituitary tumours should be discussed with the endocrine team.
- Both micro- and macroadenomas may increase in size, remain stable or reduce in size.
- If no evidence of hypo- or hyperfunction and not threatening visual loss then follow up with MRI at regular intervals.
  - Macroadenomas at 6 months then annually for 5 years (minimum).
  - Microadenomas annually for up to 3 years (consider repeating prolactin measurements at 12 months).
- In addition, non-functioning macroadenomas need monitoring of visual fields. The decision to excise relates to risk to vision; those that threaten vision are removed via a trans-sphenoidal approach.
- Surgery is indicated for secretory tumours not responding to medical therapy.

Incidental adrenal tumours

Functional anatomy of adrenal gland

The adrenal glands lie above the kidneys and are about 7–10 g in weight. They are divided anatomically and functionally into an outer cortex composed of three layers, from outer to inner:

- zona **g**lomerulosa producing aldosterone (*Conn's syndrome*)
- zona **f**asciculata producing glucocorticoids (*Cushing's syndrome*)
- zona **r**eticularis producing androgens (*congenital adrenal hyperplasia*).
  Think GFR!

And an inner:

- medulla producing catecholamines (*phaeochromocytoma*).

Aetiology

It is increasingly common to identify incidental adrenal mass lesions on abdominal and chest imaging with CT or MRI. Using current imaging modalities these are detected at a rate of 4–5% of scans performed. The incidence increases with increasing age from 0.2% of scans in 20- to 29-year-olds to 7% of patients over the age of 70. This is consistent with a reported post-mortem prevalence of adrenal tumours of between 1% and 9%. Incidental adrenal tumours may be functional (hormone secreting) or non-functional. They may be benign or malignant. The *majority are non-functional benign adenomas.*

It is difficult to be precise regarding the actual aetiologies as studies vary widely depending on precise entry criteria and population studied. For example the incidence of phaeochromocytoma is quoted as between 0.3% and 9% of adrenal incidentalomas. There is similar variation in the quoted risk of malignancy. Common causes of an incidental adrenal mass to be considered include:

- benign non-functional adenoma (the majority)
- cortisol secreting adenoma
- phaeochromocytoma
- myolipoma
- haematoma
- aldosterone secreting adenoma
- adrenocortical carcinoma
- metastatic carcinoma
- congenital adrenal hyperplasia.

Many other rarer causes including other benign tumours and granulomatous disease may occur.

When faced with an adrenal incidentaloma ask two questions:

1. Is it likely to be malignant?
2. Is it likely to be functional?

Incidental malignant adrenal tumours

Malignancy is uncommon and certainly below 5% of incidental tumours. Some studies quote much lower figures. The adrenal is a common site of metastases and a mass may represent a metastatic deposit in a patient not known to have a primary malignancy. It can be difficult to decide if a lesion is malignant. The risk of malignancy increases if:

- large size >4 cm
- irregular in outline
- non-homogeneous
- high attenuation on pre-contrast CT scan (low attenuation suggests high fat content and therefore myolipoma or lipid-rich benign adenoma).

Functional adenomas

Although functional adrenal adenomas may give rise to the characteristic syndromes associated with excess secretion, there is a wide range in the level of secretion and patients may be entirely asymptomatic or have very mild disease. In the absence of clinical manifestations of hypersecretion, the interpretation of tests for hypersecretion is difficult. In the absence of any clinical clues:

Hypercortisolism

- 24-hour urinary free cortisol
- 1 mg overnight dexamethasone suppression test

Hyperaldosteronism

- Plasma renin:aldosterone ratio >20–40

Phaeochromocytoma

- 24-hour urinary metanephrines and catecholamines

Management

There is still disagreement regarding the best approach. There is clearly a balance to be struck between managing risk and avoiding unnecessary anxiety to the patient. Patients should be referred for advice, counselling and investigation by an endocrinologist with an interest in adrenal disease.

- There is general agreement that tumours greater than 4 cm in diameter are best surgically resected unless there is very strong evidence to suggest that they are benign or co-morbidities limit surgical options.
- For others, traditional follow-up has included repeat endocrine testing (annually) combined with one to three interval CT scans. Such an approach has been challenged on grounds of:
    - cost of testing
    - radiation exposure

in the context of:

- low risk of conversion to hyperfunction
- low risk of malignant transformation.

As a *minimum* one follow-up scan at 6 months is required.

Incidental pulmonary hypertension

Pulmonary hypertension is defined as a mean pulmonary artery pressure at catheterization of 25 mmHg or greater. It is rare in the general population but is found at much higher frequency in some patient groups:

- systemic sclerosis
- portal hypertension
- HIV
- congenital heart disease
- following pulmonary emboli.

WHO classification

Group 1 Idiopathic, inherited, disorders of small arterioles, e.g. connective tissue disease

Group 2 Secondary to diseases of left side of heart, e.g. systolic dysfunction

Group 3 Secondary to hypoxaemia/lung disease

Group 4 Secondary to chronic thromboembolic disease

Group 5 Unclear or multifactorial mechanisms

In patients in whom pulmonary hypertension is found as an incidental feature on examination or imaging, the clinical approach should be aimed at assessing for any related signs, symptoms or sequelae.

History

- Progressive breathlessness
- Exertional syncope/presyncope
- Angina due to increased oxygen demand of hypertrophied right ventricle
- Eventually oedema and ascites due to right heart failure

Examination

- Signs of underlying condition, e.g. systemic sclerosis
- Atrial flutter
- Loud pulmonary component of second heart sound

- Tricuspid regurgitation
- Elevated JVP, ascites and oedema
- 6-minute walk test to assess severity (and subsequent response to therapy)

Investigation

Blood tests:

- if suggestive of an underlying cause, e.g. HIV, autoimmune screen
- BNP and N-terminal BNP as markers of disease severity and prognosis.

    ECG may show evidence of right heart strain.

    CXR may show prominent pulmonary arteries, cardiomegaly.

    Lung function testing with gas transfer coefficient may show reduced gas transfer.

    Echocardiography: pulmonary hypertension may be detected on echocardiography performed to assess left ventricular systolic function. It is characterized by:

- elevated systolic pulmonary artery pressure
- dilated right atrium and/or ventricle
- right ventricular hypertrophy
- impaired right ventricular function
- pulmonary artery enlargement
- abnormal motion of interventricular septum.

    More specialized investigations include:

- isotope perfusion lung scanning
- HRCT (high resolution CT) and CTPA
- MRI and MRI pulmonary angiography
- right heart catheterization.

Management

Pulmonary hypertension is an unusual condition and severe disease requires specialized management provided through a series of national centres. Specific treatment modalities depend upon the underlying aetiology.

General

- Diuretic therapy to reduce oedema, but can reduce cardiac output due to reduction in preload and cause electrolyte imbalance
- Long-term oxygen therapy to maintain oxygen saturations >90% at rest and ideally during sleep and exercise
- Digoxin therapy to improve cardiac output and for rate control

- Exercise training
- Anticoagulation with warfarin is clearly of benefit in pulmonary hypertension secondary to thromboembolic disease but may be beneficial with other aetiologies due to the increased risk of thromboembolism and marked deterioration that could result

More advanced and specific drug therapies should be administered to specific patient groups by specialists at regional centres. Patients undergo cardiac catheterization studies and tests of vasoreactivity to assess likely drug responsiveness. Options include:

- calcium channel blockers, e.g. diltiazem, nifedipine and amlodipine
- prostanoids, e.g. iloprost, epoprostenol, treprostinil
- endothelin ET-1 antagonists, e.g. bosentan, ambrisentan, macitentan
- phosphodiesterase PDE5 antagonists, e.g. sildenafil, tadalafil, vardenafil.

    Surgical therapies include:

- thromboendarterectomy for severe chronic thromboembolic pulmonary hypertension (<5% operative mortality)
- creation of a right to left shunt considered in adults with severe refractory disease with recurrent syncope or as a bridge to transplantation
- bilateral lung or heart lung transplantation.

Hypertensive urgencies and emergencies

> **Scenario 34.1**
>
> *You are contacted by the ophthalmology registrar who has seen a 55-year-old patient in clinic. On fundoscopy he has exudates, fundal haemorrhages and papilloedema. The registrar has checked his BP and recorded a reading of 220/120. The patient denies any symptoms. He has admitted that he was on treatment for hypertension 'some years ago' but has stopped taking his medication 2–3 years ago.*

When managing patients with severe hypertension it is important to recognize the harm that can result from overly aggressive blood pressure reduction. True hypertensive emergencies are rare and most patients can be managed with oral therapy in an ambulatory setting.

It is common for patients to be referred to the on-take medical team due to significant hypertension. This often occurs in patients with known hypertension who attend their GP and are found to have markedly elevated blood pressures, commonly due to compliance issues. Less commonly it is discovered during a routine health check or following an ophthalmic review involving fundoscopy. The vast majority of the patients will fall into the category of the *hypertensive urgency* whilst very few will constitute a true *hypertensive emergency*.

Hypertensive urgency: severely elevated blood pressure (generally systolic >180, or diastolic>120 mmHg) *without* symptoms and signs of acute end organ damage. Such patients can be managed as an outpatient with oral therapy.

Hypertensive emergency: severely elevated blood pressure (generally systolic >180, or diastolic >120 mmHg) *with* symptoms and signs of acute end organ damage. Such patients require admission and consideration of parenteral therapy.

'*Acute end organ damage*':

- *Cerebral*: encephalopathy, intracerebral haemorrhage
- *Cardiac*: acute coronary syndrome, acute pulmonary oedema
- *Kidney*: acute kidney injury
- *Pregnancy*: pre-eclampsia and eclampsia

The symptoms at presentation of 108 patients who met criteria of hypertensive emergency were reviewed by Zampaglione and co-workers in 1996 [2]. For this group of patients the mean systolic and diastolic BP at presentation were 210 ± 32 mmHg and 130 ± 15 mmHg, respectively:

- Chest pain   27%
- Breathlessness   22%
- Neurological deficit 21%
- Headache   3%
- Epistaxis   0%

In those patients in the same study presenting with hypertensive urgency, 22% complained of headache and 17% of epistaxis at presentation.

History

As part of a full history with systems enquiry ask specifically:

- Does the patient have a current diagnosis of hypertension? If not, how was it detected prior to this visit?

- Has blood pressure control been good, who monitors it, how frequently?
- Has compliance been good? (accepting that patients may not be entirely honest about this!)
- What is the current BP treatment regime, what drugs have been used previously, why were they discontinued?
- What investigations have been performed previously to look at possible aetiology and end organ damage
- What other prescribed and OTC medications taken?
- Ask specifically regarding recreational drug use, e.g. cocaine, amphetamines, phencyclidine.
- Family history of hypertension?
- Alcohol intake?
- Past history of pregnancy-related hypertension?
- Other cardiovascular risk factors?

Examination

- Measure the blood pressure carefully with the patient seated for 5 minutes, relaxed, not talking and with the blood pressure cuff supported at the level of the heart.
- Measure the blood pressure in both arms.
- Ensure that the cuff size is appropriate (you shouldn't be struggling to keep it in place). The bladder of the BP cuff should fit around 80% of the arm and no more than 100%. The average arm diameter is increasing in the UK! Consequently standard ward cuffs are often too small and this will result in an overestimation of the BP.

*Further information on the correct procedures for BP measurement (and all things 'hypertension') is available on the British Hypertension Society website (*www.bhsoc.org/*).*

- Perform a full systems examination, in particular looking for end organ damage.
  - *CNS*: evidence of hypertensive encephalopathy with reduced conscious level, nausea, vomiting, and seizures. Lateralizing signs are rare in absence of associated CVE.
  - *Cardiovascular*: gallop rhythm, renal bruits (renovascular disease), murmurs.
  - *Respiratory*: crackles of pulmonary oedema.
  - *Fundoscopy*: see below.

Classification of hypertensive retinopathy

Grade 1: Mild arteriolar narrowing (vein: artery diameter should be 1.1:1)
Increased light reflex (copper or silver wiring)
Variation in vessel calibre

Grade 2: Moderate arteriolar narrowing
AV nipping

Grade 3: Severe arteriolar narrowing
Haemorrhages, cotton wool spots, hard exudates

Grade 4: Grade 3 changes plus papilloedema

Grade 2 changes occur with longstanding significant hypertension. *Grade 3 and 4 changes are related to development/presence of significant end organ damage.*

Investigation

For end organ damage

- Full blood count
- Urea and electrolytes
- Consider troponin measurement
- Urinalysis for proteinuria
- ECG: LV hypertrophy or ischaemia
- CXR: dissection and pulmonary oedema

Cardiovascular risk profile

- Blood glucose
- Fasting lipid profile

Aetiology (consider)

- Renin:aldosterone ratio (primary hyperaldosteronism)
- 24-hour metanephrine collection (phaeochromocytoma)
- 24-hour urinary free cortisol (Cushing's syndrome)
- MRA/CT angiogram/Doppler USS to exclude renal artery stenosis

Other investigations will be indicated for patients presenting with a hypertensive emergency depending on symptomatic manifestations (e.g. CT head for encephalopathy or urgent aortogram if dissection suspected).

Management

Hypertensive urgency

- More harm can be done by too rapid reduction of blood pressure than no treatment, especially in the elderly.
- Aim to reduce blood pressure over 1–2 days and then normalize blood pressure over following weeks.
- The greater the likely chronicity of the rise, the slower the reduction.
- Those *already on medication*:
  - can increase dose of existing medication or add another agent
  - keep on current regime and observe if suspect compliance issues
  - institute frequent external monitoring to reinforce compliance.
- For those not on medication:
  - start oral therapy with a calcium channel blocker, e.g. amlodipine 5 mg od or a highly selective beta-blocker, e.g. bisoprolol 2.5–5mg od
  - most patients will require two agents to reach target BP
  - ACE inhibitors and angiotensin-II antagonists are best avoided in this situation as some patients can be very sensitive with rapid and marked BP reductions.

Hypertensive emergency

In practice with modern management in the UK *such situations are now extremely rare*. Blood pressure reduction with an intravenous agent should occur only within an HDU or ITU setting *with dynamic invasive arterial pressure monitoring*:

- Goal is to reduce BP by no more than 25% over 2–6 hours and aiming for diastolic of 105 mmHg.
- More rapid reductions can precipitate myocardial and cerebral ischaemia.
- Preferred agents depend on the *specific circumstances of target organ damage* but labetalol and sodium nitroprusside are commonly used.

Sodium nitroprusside

- Potent vasodilator with immediate onset of action and short duration of 1–2 minutes.
- Adverse effects include nausea, vomiting, sweating and muscle twitching.
- Decomposes on exposure to light to give toxic thiocyanates and cyanide so *giving set must be protected from light exposure* and long infusions avoided.

Labetalol

- Combined alpha- and beta-blocker with 5–10 minute onset of action and duration of 3–6 hours.
- Adverse effects include vomiting and scalp tingling and can precipitate bronchoconstriction and heart block.

Once the patient has an immediate, safe management plan and treatment is implemented it is highly appropriate to hand over their care to a hypertensive specialist. In most hospitals this would be a nephrologist or cardiologist; if the patient presents in working hours they may be available from the outset.

References

1. Orme NM, Fletcher JG, Siddiki HA, Harmsen WS, O'Byrne MM, Port JD, Tremaine WJ, Pitot HC, McFarland EG, Robinson ME, Koenig BA, King BF, Wolf SM. Incidental findings in imaging research: evaluating incidence, benefit, and burden. *Archives of Internal Medicine* 2010; 170(17): 1525.

2. Zampaglione B, Pascale C, Marchisio M, Cavallo-Perin P. Hypertensive urgencies and emergencies. Prevalence and clinical presentation. *Hypertension* 1996; 27: 144–147.

Further reading

Bevan JS. Pituitary incidentaloma. *Clinical Medicine* 2013; 13: 296–298.

Kiely DG, Elliot CA, Sabroe I, Condliffe R. Pulmonary hypertension: diagnosis and management. *BMJ* 2013; 346: f2028. Available online at www.bmj.com/content/346/bmj.f2028.

US Department of Health and Human Services. The Seventh Report of the Joint National Committee on Prevention, Detection, Evaluation and Treatment of High Blood Pressure. Available to download at www.nhlbi.nih.gov/guidelines/hypertension/jnc7full.pdf.

Williams B, Poulter NR, Brown MJ, Davis M, McInnes GT, Potter JF, Sever PS, Thom SM. British Hypertension Society guidelines for hypertension management (BHS-IV). *BMJ* 2004; 328:634–640. Available to download at www.bhsoc.org/files/1913/3517/8212/Summary_Guidelines_2004.pdf.

Young (Jr) WF. The incidentally discovered adrenal mass. *New England Journal of Medicine* 2007; 356:601–610.

Involuntary movements

Mark Fish

Scenario 35.1

You are called urgently to the emergency department to review an 18-year-old girl whose eyes are deviated upwards and head pointed back. Two days ago she had visited her GP and had been treated for acute vertigo.

Introduction

When meeting a patient with involuntary movements a 'spot diagnosis' may be possible such as in the above case of oculogyric crisis. Probing the patient revealed that the patient had received an injection of prochlorperazine from her GP. The history is key to illuminating the cause of a movement disorder.

It is useful to note the following features which will either confirm initial impressions or help you to make a diagnosis if the classification of the movement(s) or cause is not immediately clear.

History

Onset and progression

The timing of onset and tempo of progression is a crucial aspect of the neurological history.

- Is the problem progressive?
- How quickly is it getting worse?
- Has it been gradually developing over years (most often due to degenerative disease) or weeks to months (possibly tumour)?
- Did it come on suddenly (always think cerebrovascular event)?
- Was onset early in life (could be developmental if progressive)?
- Has the problem now stopped getting worse (suggesting previous cerebral insult)?

Exposures

This is important to consider in all cases as reversible causes of involuntary movements are easy to miss when they mimic organic brain disease. Drug-induced causes are the most important causes to identify. Always ask about exposure to:

- psychiatric drugs
- antiemetics
- vestibular sedatives
- illicit drugs and 'novel psychoactive substances' (see Chapter 8).

Timing and triggers

- When does the movement occur? (e.g. during the morning, or at night)
- What triggers or aggravates it? (e.g. doing nothing, particular actions, stress)

Aggravation by stress does not necessarily indicate a psychological cause; for instance the following are all aggravated when patients are psychologically distressed:

- tremor of Parkinson's disease
- tics in Tourette's syndrome
- chorea in Huntington's disease.

Examination

Associated symptoms and signs

- Is there evidence of a systemic disorder (e.g. thyrotoxicosis, liver disease: think Wilson disease, or lupus) which could be the cause?

Acute Medicine, ed. Stephen Haydock, Duncan Whitehead and Zoë Fritz. Published by Cambridge University Press. © Cambridge University Press 2015.

- Are there associated neuropsychiatric or cognitive symptoms which are commonly associated with movement disorder?
- Is there evidence of delirium or frank dementia?

Neurological localization

- Which part of the body is affected?
- Is the movement generalized or focal?
- Is only one half of the body affected (suggesting contralateral hemispheric involvement)?
- Are there other localizing neurological signs (e.g. upper motor neurone signs to suggest CNS involvement, extrapyramidal signs seen when the basal ganglia are affected)?

Classification of the involuntary movement

- Most involuntary movements will fit into one of the phenotypes described below.
- Try not to jump too quickly to diagnosis, although some of the presentations are almost synonymous with diagnoses.
- If the classification of the movement is not obvious do not worry, describe what you see, which part of the body is affected and note the features above which will give you important diagnostic clues.

Tremor

Tremor is a shaking of all or part of the body; a rhythmic oscillation superimposed on normal movements or postures, most often the upper limbs but sometimes affecting other parts of the body such as head, face or legs.

Causes to consider

Rigor: occurs in an acutely systemically unwell patient with paroxysms of coarse shaking affecting the whole body. This is not uncommonly confused with seizures which can also occur in the systemically unwell – retention of some awareness and ability to communicate is a key feature that will distinguish a rigor from a generalized seizure when all limbs are involved.

Spasms: these tend to occur in patients who have a known disorder affecting the central nervous system (CNS), for instance a history of stroke, multiple sclerosis or spinal injury. Typically either an awkward movement or pain will trigger a violent shaking and/or severe increase in stiffness in a limb with a background

high tone (and other upper motor neurone signs). This rarely causes a diagnostic conundrum because patients usually have established chronic disease. Manage acutely by treating pain and aggravating factors such as infection. In the medium term specialist physiotherapy input is valuable; anti-spasmodics such as baclofen can be useful.

Where spasms occur de novo they need investigating:

- Consider tetanus: is there a history of penetrating injury?
- Check calcium/parathyroid hormone (consider hypocalcaemic tetany).
- Image brain and spinal cord above the level of the symptoms to exclude possibilities such as space-occupying lesion (SOL), myelopathy or demyelination.

Asterixis: a tremor elicited on examination. When patients hold their hands outstretched with wrists extended, there is a characteristic periodic sudden flexion at the wrists. This sign usually leads to consideration of hepatic encephalopathy (check serum ammonium, there are not always signs of chronic liver disease); however, many forms of metabolic disturbance can cause this sign.

Physiological tremor: is by definition normal. It is a fine tremor, barely perceptible, which can be made more prominent by maintenance of posture such as outstretching arms, and reduced by loading with weight. Physiological tremor may come to clinical attention when it becomes enhanced by strong emotion, exercise, fatigue, beta-agonist/stimulant excess (typically caffeine) or alcohol withdrawal. Endocrinopathies are the main pathological causes to consider with a new presentation of enhanced physiological tremor, so exclude:

- hypoglycaemia
- thyrotoxicosis
- corticosteroid or catecholamine excess.

Essential tremor (ET): characteristically worse with action. Usually one side is worse affected. There is often a family history (autosomal dominant inheritance) and patients may have noticed that it is relieved by alcohol. Typically patients will describe difficulty with actions such as carrying a drink. The best way to demonstrate ET is to ask the patient to pour water from cup to cup, when the large amplitude tremor will often cause spillage or cups will be held very close together, clattering. ET was formerly known as 'benign' ET. This was a misnomer; ET is progressive, may be socially embarrassing and is often disabling. Nevertheless patients are usually relieved to hear that they haven't got Parkinson's disease (PD). Response to treatment is variable; first-line management is with propranolol.

Focal seizures: may occur in full consciousness (simple partial seizures) when they are often not recognized as such. Seizure should be considered as a possible cause of involuntary abnormal tone, posturing or shaking if they spread anatomically over seconds. Imaging of the brain is first-line urgent investigation with de-novo presentation of simple partial seizures to exclude SOL or more acute focal lesions such as infarct or haemorrhage. When presentation is acute or subacute probe for features of encephalopathy (e.g. cognitive compromise, confusion or behavioural disturbance), headache or pyrexial illness, in which case encephalitis would need to be excluded with lumbar puncture after brain imaging.

Parkinsonion tremor: predominantly a rest tremor in contrast to ET.

- Ask the patient if they have a tremor when they are relaxing (difficult to achieve in medical consultation), for instance watching the television.
- In the early stages of PD it is unilateral, and may be quite subtle.
- The patient may be aware of clumsiness or slowness in the affected limb.
- There is often a history of musculoskeletal problems such as frozen shoulder on the same side.
- Typically exaggerated by psychological distress, or emerges when walking.
- There may be an associated action tremor in patients with PD (and subtle extrapyramidal signs in ET), so the distinction with ET is not always straightforward.

Look for other signs of parkinsonism worse on the same side:

- Bradykinesia (increasing slowness *and* decreasing amplitude of repetitive movement, e.g. ask the patient to open and close their hands repeatedly).
- Cog-wheel rigidity, best assessed with a gentle passive alternating flexion/extension at the wrist.
- Postural instability is another cardinal feature, also look for reduced facial expression and an ipsilateral reduction in arm swing.

Patients with suspected PD *should be referred to a specialist service.*

Drug-induced parkinsonism: symptoms and signs can look like PD.

- Pronounced asymmetry does not rule out drug-triggered parkinsonism although it increases suspicion for subclinical disease precipitated by dopamine receptor blockade.
- Most cases occur early (within days) after initial exposure, though delayed presentation is not uncommon.
- The risk is less with the atypical neuroleptics than with first generation antipsychotics.
- Metoclopramide and prochlorperazine are dopamine antagonists that are still used commonly as antiemetics and vestibular sedatives.
- Treatment (and confirmation of diagnosis) is by withdrawal of causative drug.
- Symptoms may take 3 months or longer to settle.

Dystonic tremor: if a patient with a seeming ET has coexistent dystonia (typically cervical dystonia with sustained abnormal head posturing), they may have a dystonic tremor. Dystonic tremor tends to be more irregular and jerky than other types of tremor. It may respond to an anticholinergic or clonazepam.

Cerebellar tremor: may be accompanied by other signs of cerebellar dysfunction:

- gait ataxia
- dysarthria
- nystagmus
- other signs of brainstem involvement.

The most important distinguishing feature of a cerebellar tremor can be brought out by finger–nose pointing; ask the patient to touch their nose (or chin if they have a severe tremor) and then to touch the proffered finger tip of the examiner at arm's length from the patient. The amplitude of the tremor increases towards target and frequently they will miss the target ('past-pointing'). This is called an intention tremor.

Head tremor: can occur as part of ET, cervical dystonia and due to cerebellar disease. Ancillary features (which may be obvious or may need to be sought) will usually make the diagnosis.

A comparison of the common causes of tremor is given in Table 35.1.

Abnormal facial movements

Myokymia (eyelid and facial): is a fine flickering of the eyelid that is a benign phenomenon and is usually self-limiting; aggravating factors are similar to physiological

Table 35.1 Comparison of common causes of tremor

	Tremor present upon:		
	Rest	Maintenance of posture	Action
Physiological	–	✓✓	– Reduces with loading
Cerebellar	Rarely	✓	✓✓ Worse towards target
Essential	–	✓	✓✓✓ Present through whole movement
Parkinsonian	✓✓ Can support diagnosis but variable	Variable	Variable Typically more pronounced when walking

tremor. This doesn't cause the eyelids to close tight unlike blepharospasm. However, if rippling of the muscles is more widespread than the eyelids involving more of the face (facial myokymia), brainstem pathology needs to be excluded with MR imaging.

Blepharospasm: involves involuntarily scrunching up of the eyes, repeatedly in bursts. Usually this is bilateral (unlike hemifacial spasm). If symptoms are persistent and troubling the patient should be referred to the neurology service for consideration of botulinum toxin (bo-tox) injections, which can be a very effective treatment.

Hemifacial spasm: looks similar to blepharospasm but is usually unilateral and in addition to eye closure the lower face is affected, typically the corner of the mouth being pulled up and out at the same time as eyelid closure. Treatment is also with bo-tox and is usually effective. Patients should be imaged to exclude an SOL.

Abnormal lip and tongue movements

Automatisms: semi-coordinated, repetitive motor activities that are associated with altered awareness, occurring in the context of seizure. They typically involve the mouth or hands. Typically patients are seen to fumble, pick, chew or lip-smack but more elaborate actions can occur. They are usually indicative of complex partial seizures secondary to temporal lobe epilepsy.

Tardive dyskinesia: may first manifest with abnormal movement of the lips and tongue and is a consequence of prolonged exposure to dopamine receptor blockade (usually neuroleptics).

NMDA receptor antibody-mediated encephalopathy: consider when unusual involuntary movements, particularly of the face, are associated with subacute onset of psychosis or encephalopathy. It is a form of autoimmune encephalitis which may respond to immune therapy. There may be underlying malignancy. The full range of movement disorders can occur in this condition.

Chorea and related hyperkinetic movement disorders

The different hyperkinetic movement disorders can be tricky to distinguish; however, the causes to consider overlap to a large degree so initial identification of hyperkinetic (too much movement) disorder is a useful start!

Choreic movements: involuntary, irregular and abrupt movements. Patients have a 'fidgety' appearance. Huntington's disease is an autosomal dominant (ask about family history) neurodegenerative disorder which causes cognitive impairment and psychiatric symptoms as well as a variety of abnormal movements including chorea. There are a number of inherited disorders that cause a similar picture.

Simple motor tics: can appear similar to chorea but tend to be more repetitive. Complex tics involve more elaborate movements or gestures (e.g. touching, squatting, gesticulating) that may seem semi-purposeful. Vocal tics can be simple such as coughing or grunting or involve vocalizations such as swearing (coprolalia). Tics are associated with prior urge and subsequent relief and are temporarily suppressible with an effort of will. Gilles de la Tourette's syndrome (GTS) may be diagnosed when there are multiple tic types, onset is in childhood and there is chronicity. Obsessive

Table 35.2 Important drug-induced movement disorders

	Tremor	Parkinsonism	Chorea and other hyperkinetic movements	Dystonia
Dopamine blockers (antipsychotics and antiemetics)	✓	✓		
Dopamine enhancers (levodopa and agonists)			✓	✓
Stimulants (e.g. amphetamine, methylphenidate)	✓		✓	
Anticonvulsants	✓	✓ In particular sodium valproate	✓	✓
Antidepressants (including SSRIs and tricyclics)			✓	Rarely
Lithium	✓	✓	✓	
Oestrogen			✓	
Calcium channel blockers		✓		

compulsive disorder and attention deficit hyperactivity disorder commonly co-occur with GTS. GTS is an organic brain disorder.

Sterotypies: repetitive movements (e.g. nodding, rocking) which are without purpose and more constant than tics. They often occur in the context of autism, schizophrenia or frontal dementia but can also occur as a consequence of chronic neuroleptic exposure.

Hemiballismus: unilateral, large amplitude, vigorous flinging movement, affecting limb or trunk. When onset is acute the cause is usually a vascular event (haemorrhage or infarct) affecting the basal ganglia, classically the subthalamic nucleus. In the absence of a relevant cerebrovascular accident, other causes to consider (even if unilateral) include SLE, syphilis and drugs.

Myoclonus: shock-like involuntary movement, which can arise due to sudden bursts of activity (or inhibition of tonic activity) in the brain or spinal cord. Myoclonus is a common physiological phenomenon at the point of falling asleep. Hiccups is myoclonus affecting the diaphragm. The presence of myoclonus is often indicative of a degenerative disorder; if progression is very rapid consider prion disease or underlying malignancy. When it occurs in idiopathic generalized epilepsy, it is often an indication that treatment needs to be increased. Generalized myoclonus can be a troubling part of hypoxic ischaemic brain injury. Valproate and clonazepam are moderately effective symptomatic treatments.

Dystonia: sustained or periodic muscle contraction (often there is co-contraction of agonist and antagonist

groups) which often causes abnormal posturing and may be painful. Any part of the body may be affected. Dystonia may be a manifestation of neurodegenerative disease, metabolic disorder such as Wilson's disease, drug triggered or idiopathic. Blepharospasm, cervical dystonia and writer's cramp are all forms of dystonia that respond to botulinum toxin. Dystonia often complicates later stage Parkinson's disease and its treatment.

A subacute onset of dystonic reaction typically causing abnormal posturing of head, jaw opening/closure or abnormal eye position may be drug induced. Oculogyric crisis with involuntary upward deviation of the eyes is well known as a consequence of de-novo neuroleptic exposure. Such reactions can also occur secondary to other drugs such as antidepressants or after dose increment of neuroleptics. Management is withdrawal of the causative drug and use of anticholinergic with or without benzodiazepine.

Causes of subacute hyperkinetic movement disorder to consider

- *Always take a drug history*; as well as the 'obvious' dopaminergic drugs, dopamine depleting drugs, oestrogen and antidepressants can cause subacute onset of movement disorder (Table 35.2).
- *SLE is always a consideration* with fulminant hyperkinetic movement disorder especially chorea. Polycythaemia rubra vera and hyperthyroidism can also cause chorea. HIV can affect all parts of the nervous system and

Table 35.3 Clinical features of neuroleptic malignant syndrome and serotonin syndrome

	Changed mental state	Dysautonomia	Muscle rigidity	Tremor	Myoclonus, hyperreflexia, incoordination	Risk of rhabdomyolysis
Neuroleptic malignant syndrome	✓	✓	✓	✓		✓✓✓
Serotonin syndrome	✓	✓		✓	✓	✓✓

should always at least be considered when there is unexplained neurological disorder. *Where there is rapid progression* of neurological symptoms and deficits, including movement disorder such as chorea or myoclonus, then think about an underlying malignancy causing a paraneoplastic syndrome or prion disease (CJD). A CT scan of the chest, abdomen and pelvis will be the first line of investigation in this instance.

Movement disorder associated with sleep

Nocturnal seizures: may or may not be obvious when observed and the patient may not be aware of them. Seizures arising from the frontal lobes are often nocturnal, can be bizarre, and often have a rapid onset and resolution, without an obvious post-ictal period, which can make diagnosis challenging.

Restless legs syndrome (RLS): creeping sensations in the legs combined with an irresistible urge to move, particularly when trying to get off to sleep. Walking about, rubbing the limb, or succumbing to the urge to move the leg about can provide temporary relief. Excess caffeine, fatigue and heat can be trigger factors. With a first presentation check for iron deficiency, uraemia and pregnancy if relevant. Mainstays of treatment are dopamine agonists, weak opiates such as codeine, or benzodiazepines such as clonazepam.

Periodic limb movement disorder: related condition to RLS that causes repeated clusters of leg movement during sleep lasting 10–90 seconds. This can disturb sleep and cause daytime somnolence. It responds to a similar range of medication to RLS.

REM behavioural sleep disorder manifests as seemingly purposeful behaviour during sleep, literally the acting out of dreams. Sufferers may hit their spouses and shout in their sleep. This is common in patients with Parkinson's disease and related disorders, and

may be a prodromal symptom years in advance of the clinical presentation of the neurodegenerative disorder. This responds well to a small dose (500 μg) of clonazepam nocte.

Movement disorder emergencies

Both '*neuroleptic malignant syndrome*' and the '*serotonin syndrome*' occur soon after exposure to the provocative drug (Table 35.3).

In both these syndromes patients can be critically unwell with:

- pyrexia
- autonomic instability
- delirium.

Neuroleptic malignant syndrome

- Can be associated with all neuroleptics and occurs usually on initiating treatment, on dose escalation or in overdose.
- Parkinsonism, dystonia and rigidity occur.
- Rhabdomyolysis leads to climbing creatine kinase and myoglobinuria with associated risk of acute kidney injury.
- Neuroleptics are withdrawn and treatment is largely supportive with particular attention to fluid balance and cooling.
- Dantrolene is used as a muscle relaxant. It abolishes excitation–contraction coupling in muscle cells.

Serotonin syndrome

- Combination of drugs such as monoamine oxidase inhibitor and selective serotonin reuptake inhibitor (SSRI), triptan and SSRI or multiple stimulant drugs such as amphetamine/cocaine with MDMA push up serotonin levels precipitously.

- There is more agitation and restlessness than in neuroleptic malignant syndrome with more prominent involuntary movements such as myoclonus and tremor. Reflexes are brisk.
- Rhabdomyolysis can also occur as a complication.
- After withdrawal of causative drugs, treatment is supportive.

- Benzodiazepines and beta-blockers are first- and second-line management, respectively.

Further reading

Sawle GV (1999) *Movement Disorders in Clinical Practice.* ISIS Medical Media.

Jaundice

Jane Chalmers and Rudi Matull

Introduction

Jaundice describes yellow pigmentation of the skin and sclera due to deposition of excess circulating bilirubin (>50 μmol/L). Causes of jaundice can be divided into pre-hepatic, hepatic and post-hepatic. It can also be described as acute or chronic. *High levels of bilirubin with signs of sepsis should be considered an emergency.*

Pathophysiology

Pre-hepatic

- Caused by increased turn-over (breakdown) of red blood cells resulting in:
  - increased serum unconjugated bilirubin (water-insoluble)
  - increased urinary uro-bilinogen (water-soluble).
- It can be caused by a range of inherited (glucose-6-phosphate dehydrogenase deficiency, hereditary spherocytosis, sickle cell, thalassaemia) and acquired (haemolytic anaemia) disorders.
- Gilbert's syndrome is found in approximately 5% of the population; it is characterized by reduced conjugation of bilirubin leading to a mild jaundice during fasting or illness.

Hepatic

- Caused by direct damage to the liver cells (necrosis) resulting in defects at different steps in bilirubin metabolism, namely uptake of unconjugated bilirubin, intracellular processing of bilirubin, or excretion of conjugated bilirubin into bile. This results in raised levels of varying degrees of both:
  - serum unconjugated bilirubin
  - serum conjugated bilirubin.
- There are many causes, including:
  - all causes of chronic liver disease – jaundice is a sign of progression or decompensation
  - transient viral infections (CMV/EBV/ hepatitis A/resolving hepatitis B or C)
  - drug-induced liver injury, e.g. co-amoxiclav
  - carcinoma/metastases
  - abscess
  - rare infections, e.g. leptospirosis, or tropical diseases
  - pregnancy (*when jaundice is an emergency*)
  - rare inherited disorders, e.g. Rotor syndrome, Dubin–Johnson syndrome.

Post-hepatic (obstructive jaundice)

- Caused by failure of drainage of the bile through the biliary system resulting in:
  - high levels of conjugated serum bilirubin (having bypassed conjugation to uro-bilinogen in intestine) causing pale stool and dark urine.
- Although usually caused by blockage of the biliary system after the liver, sometimes hepatocellular damage can cause intrahepatic obstruction of bile drainage through swelling or fibrosis of the biliary canaliculi giving a similar picture. Common causes include:
  - gallstones within the common bile duct

Acute Medicine, ed. Stephen Haydock, Duncan Whitehead and Zoë Fritz. Published by Cambridge University Press. © Cambridge University Press 2015.

- carcinoma (cholangiocarcinoma/pancreatic/ gallbladder)
- nodal disease, often metastatic (usually at the porta hepatis)
- primary sclerosing cholangitis
- pancreatitis/pseudocyst
- other bile duct strictures, e.g. post-surgical
- hepatic artery thrombosis (ischaemia)
- tropical diseases, e.g. schistosomiasis.

Scenario 36.1

A 56-year-old man is referred to the medical admissions unit (MAU) with jaundice. He gives a history of his skin and eyes becoming yellow over the past 2 weeks. He rarely sees his GP, has no other past medical history and is on no regular medication. He currently works as a farm labourer.

Discussion

- Jaundice is a common presentation to MAU. In this particular case, the lack of detail within the history of presenting complaint, i.e. presence/ absence of pain, makes further division of causes of the patient's jaundice difficult. The absence of past medical history and the short, 2-week course of illness does not necessarily exclude a chronic liver condition as the cause for jaundice.
- Although common causes for jaundice come to mind, for example alcohol, viruses and biliary stones, it is important to consider rarer causes from the outset, such as toxins, drugs, leptospirosis, hepatitis E or hydatid disease (farm labourer).
- The patient does not sound particularly unwell, but one must contemplate the reason for admission – are there signs of sepsis?
- Investigation of such a patient needs to be done in a systematic manner, asking pertinent questions to organize the information into pre-hepatic, hepatic or post-hepatic causes of jaundice in order to arrange appropriate investigations.
- In particular, it is important to identify those patients in need of urgent medical attention or rapid investigation, such as those presenting with acute sepsis, acute liver failure or those with high risk of a cancer diagnosis.

History

Take a full history of presenting complaint including onset of jaundice and full systematic review.

Important associated symptoms/factors to consider include:
- pain (or nausea)
- obstructive symptoms (pale stool, dark urine, pruritus)
- weight loss/anorexia (loss of appetite)
- recent illness or prodrome
- symptoms of anaemia/abnormal blood count
- signs and symptoms of sepsis (e.g. rigor).

Take a full past medical history including:
- previous episodes of jaundice
- autoimmune disorders
- risk factors for the metabolic syndrome, inflammatory bowel disease or cancer
- pregnancy if female
- any blood product transfusions received, especially overseas.

A full drug history is essential, including:
- any recent changes to medication
- antibiotic use
- over-the-counter medications (including herbal remedies, non-steroidals and supplements)
- any paracetamol use – particularly in excess; even low doses (4–6 g/day), taken over several days (staggered), can be hepatotoxic in malnourished patients (e.g. alcohol use).

Think about a family history of:
- autoimmunity
- congenital disorders
- metabolic problems (e.g. diabetes)
- viruses that could be passed from mother to child (e.g. hepatitis B).

Social history will give significant amounts of information about risk factors for liver disease:
- alcohol history
- history of illicit drug use
- occupation (farming, rodents, exposure to chemicals)
- sexual history
- tattoos
- travel history (e.g. tropical countries).

When taking a history from a patient with liver disease, it must be done with *sensitivity*. Patients can become defensive when asked about their personal habits, in particular regarding alcohol intake or drug use, and inquiring about sexual preference requires privacy which is not easily available in admission units.

In order to obtain accurate information it is important to adopt a non-judgemental attitude, reassuring the patient that these are routine questions. When asking about drugs and alcohol, try to get them to be specific:

- Which alcohol (e.g. 4% or 8% cider)? How much? Every day? 'How often do you drink ≥6 units on a single occasion?', if more than monthly, an alcohol problem becomes more likely. If not a current drinker, previous history of alcohol excess? Sharing needles? Last time they used?

Examination

Initial focus when examining a patient with jaundice is to identify life-threatening problems using an ABCD approach, correcting abnormalities as they are found. It is then important to conduct a *full* examination of the patient as many signs found in other systems may aid diagnosis. The important signs to look for are:

- Evidence of chronic liver disease, i.e. liver cirrhosis possible:
  - spider naevi (>5)
  - palmar erythema
  - gynaecomastia
  - hepato/splenomegaly
  - Dupuytren's
  - clubbing
  - ascites
  - oedema (pulmonary/peripheral)
  - caput medusa
  - parotid enlargement
  - xanthelasma
- Evidence of autoimmunity (e.g. vitiligo)
- Abdominal tenderness
- Evidence of sepsis
- Evidence of IV drug use
- Signs of anaemia
- Nutritional status.

In particular it is important to recognize those patients showing signs of decompensated liver disease (jaundice being one of the relevant indicators of decompensation). These patients require urgent specialist input from the gastroenterology/hepatology team:

- *Ascites*/peripheral oedema
- *Encephalopathy*: flap/confusion/drowsiness/fetor hepaticus (Table 36.1).

Table 36.1 Grading of hepatic encephalopathy

Grade	Clinical features
Grade 1	Changes in behaviour, mood disturbance, sleep pattern alteration, mild confusion
Grade 2	Lethargy, moderate confusion, flap (asterixis)
Grade 3	Marked confusion, drowsy, incoherent speech
Grade 4	Coma

Investigations

A lot of information can be gained from simple investigations. Routine bloods can give a wealth of information separating chronic disease from an acute liver injury, as well as the pathophysiological site of the cause.

FBC:

- Haemolysis/anaemia, low platelets (potential sign of advanced liver disease), raised MCV
- Evidence of infection
- Blood film (e.g. rouleaux in immune-mediated haemolytic anaemia)

U&E:

- Assessment of fluid and electrolyte status (check Mg, PO_4, calcium if nutrition poor)
- Urea (low in cirrhosis or poor nutrition; high may indicate blood loss within upper GI tract)
- Creatinine – used in mortality predictive scores in liver disease (consider hepatorenal syndrome if creatinine remains high after fluid and sepsis management, and no obstruction)

Clotting: coagulopathy is associated with severe liver injury (chronic or acute).

Glucose: hypo- and hyperglycaemia can be seen.

pH and lactate: part of scoring systems to assess severity of liver injury.

Cultures: blood, urine and ascites (spontaneous bacterial peritonitis).

LFT:

Pre-hepatic: isolated rise in bilirubin (conjugated vs. unconjugated)

Hepatic: high ALT out of proportion to ALP

Post-hepatic: high ALP out of proportion to ALT

- Often the abnormalities seen in liver function tests do not follow the pattern described above.
- Some hepatic causes of liver injury give rise to an obstructive picture, e.g. cholestatic liver injury from antibiotic use. This is because swelling of the

hepatocytes causes blockage to the drainage of bile. Conversely, post-hepatic causes of liver injury can give high levels of ALT due to back-pressure causing damage to hepatocytes (e.g. common bile duct stones).

ECG and chest X-ray: to evaluate cardiovascular status and pleural effusion.

Ultrasound is a valuable tool when investigating jaundice and should be performed early, giving information regarding each pathological group of jaundice; in particular:

- Common bile duct diameter (indicating post-hepatic obstruction). The normal diameter of the common bile duct varies with age, ranging up to 8–10mm in the elderly or post-cholecystectomy. Dilatation of the biliary system indicates obstruction. The point at which dilatation occurs indicates the point of pathology, e.g. dilatation of both common bile duct and pancreatic duct is particularly worrying as it may indicate ampullary or pancreatic head malignancy.
- It can show early changes such as fatty infiltration of the liver (seen in non-alcoholic fatty liver disease or with alcoholic liver disease or drug- or virus-induced liver injury) through to cirrhosis, made more convincing by the presence of splenomegaly and ascites.
- It may show lesions within the liver, biliary tract or pancreas.
- It is also useful for assessing patency of vessels via Doppler – looking for portal and hepatic vein thrombosis (Budd–Chiari syndrome).

CT of the abdomen/pelvis if there are concerns about malignancy and in particular to assess disease spread.

Decisions about more specialist investigations:

- MRCP – magnetic resonance cholangio-pancreatography
- ERCP – endoscopic retrograde cholangio-pancreatography
- PTC – percutaneous trans-hepatic cholangiography

should be made by the gastroenterology/hepatology team; therefore it is important *to involve them early*.

MRCP is indicated if more detailed imaging of the bile ducts is required, e.g. to assess hilar strictures or the intrahepatic ducts to decide on how best to achieve drainage.

ERCP is used for both investigation (tissue sampling) and treatment of biliary obstruction (gallstone removal or stent insertion). Decisions about the type of therapy applied during ERCP depend largely on the pathology, e.g. non-resectable cancer requires palliative stenting, as opposed to biliary sphincterotomy and balloon trawl for gallstones.

In patients who are going to undergo invasive procedures it is important to consider clotting and risk of bleeding. Patients who are auto-anticoagulating (e.g. due to liver disease) may need 10 mg of vitamin K IV if INR is ≥1.3 – keeping in mind the risk of thrombosis. For patients on anticoagulation (warfarin and newer agents like dabigatran) or antiplatelet agents such as clopidogrel, advice should be sought from either the haematologists or from the BSG website (www.bsg.org.uk/clinical-guidelines/endoscopy/anticoagulant-antiplatelet-therapy.html).

In the presence of clinically detectable ascites, a diagnostic tap can yield valuable information (see Chapter 3):

- Presence of spontaneous bacterial peritonitis (SBP – normally only seen in patients with liver cirrhosis; definition: >250 neutrophils per mm^3 ascites fluid)
- Serum-ascites-albumin gradient (SAAG; differentiates ascites due to portal hypertension from non-portal hypertension causes; definition for transudate: >11 SAAG)
- Amylase (pancreatic injury)
- Triglycerides (lymphatic injury – chylous ascites; definition: >110 mg/dL = 1.25 mmol/L)
- Cytology.

If SBP is suspected, this is an urgent investigation (*one that should not wait until morning*) and once the sample has been sent, the *results should be chased as a matter of priority* (similar to a CSF sample in suspected meningitis) so that antibiotics can be started without delay.

If the ultrasound does not identify biliary obstruction as the cause for jaundice, then a non-invasive liver screen (NILS) is indicated. This may include the tests shown in Table 36.2.

Finally, in cases of diagnostic uncertainty, a liver biopsy can be helpful, but being an invasive procedure in patients who may have coagulopathy, decisions regarding this should be left to the gastroenterology specialist team.

Table 36.2 Possible components of a non-invasive liver screen

Test	Interpretation
Hepatitis B surface antigen (HBsAg)	Detected in active hepatitis B infection and indicates individual is infectious to others (if positive after 6 months = chronic infection)
Anti-hepatitis C virus antibodies (anti-HCV Ab)	Elevated in acute and chronic hepatitis C infection
Anti-nuclear antibodies (ANA), Anti-mitochondrial antibodies (AMA), Anti-smooth muscle antibodies (SMA) Anti-liver kidney microsomal antibodies (LKMA) Immunoglobulins, IgM and IgG	Autoimmune hepatitis (AIH) and primary biliary cirrhosis (PBC) (IgG raised in AIH, IgM raised in PBC)
Ferritin, transferrin saturation	Elevated ferritin and transferrin saturation >55% suggestive of haemochromatosis
Fasting glucose and fasting lipids	Hyperglycaemia, low HDL and elevated triglycerides define metabolic syndrome (non-alcoholic fatty liver disease)
Aspartate aminotransferase (AST) Alanine aminotransferase (ALT)	AST/ALT ratio more likely seen in non-alcoholic fatty liver disease and alcoholic liver disease
Serum copper and caeruloplasmin (patients <40 years of age)	Elevated copper and reduced caeruloplasmin found in Wilson's disease
Anti-tissue transglutaminase (anti-TTG) antibodies and IgA	Screen for coeliac disease (associated with several liver disorders)
Alpha-1-antitrypsin	Alpha-1-antitrypsin (a rare cause of cirrhosis in adults)
Thyroid stimulating hormone (TSH)	Thyroid dysfunction can result in ALT rises

Decompensated liver disease vs. acute liver failure

Jaundice is a symptom of both *decompensation* of chronic liver disease (CLD) and of *acute liver failure* (ALF). The clues for CLD are found in the history and/or stigmata on clinical examination.

Decompensated liver disease

Decompensation in a patient with chronic liver disease (acute-on-chronic liver failure) is a strong predictor of mortality with 1-year survival dropping from 84% in a patient with 'early' cirrhosis (i.e. Childs–Pugh A) to 42% in a patient with 'advanced' cirrhosis (i.e. Childs–Pugh C) [1,2]. It is indicated by the presence of:

- jaundice
- ascites
- encephalopathy.

It can be caused by a number of different factors, with infection being the most common:

- infection (consider SBP)
- bleeding (consider variceal)
- dehydration (AKI)
- constipation
- drugs (opiates)

- flare or progression of cause of cirrhosis, e.g. hepatitis B, autoimmune hepatitis
- hepatocellular carcinoma – raised alpha-fetoprotein levels
- metabolic derangement
- toxins, e.g. alcohol
- non-compliance with medication
- thrombosis (portal or hepatic veins).

Assessment of these patients through history, examination and investigation is the same as that documented above but can be tailored to the case. Ensure that:

- PR examination is performed to assess for melaena or constipation.

These patients should be identified to the gastroenterology/hepatology specialist team early and management should be guided by them. In the meantime, the best approach is to treat the underlying cause and support the patient as a whole, considering that many patients may require HDU-type attention.

- Treat infection (consider SBP).
- Support and monitor renal function.
- Treat gastrointestinal bleeds (in case of variceal origin, including antibiotics according to local protocol).
- Avoid contributing drugs (e.g. opioids if possible at all) or toxins.

- If encephalopathic, give regular lactulose aiming for bowels to open twice daily.

Renal dysfunction in cirrhotic patients

- Cirrhotic patients tend to have lower creatinine levels (due to lower muscle mass) and some have a lower urine output; therefore these are poor markers of renal function.
- A rise in creatinine of >50% from baseline or of >25 μmol/L in 48 hours is diagnostic for acute kidney injury [3] in cirrhotic patients (this rise may still give them a creatinine within the normal range).
- Ensure the patient is adequately filled.
  - Be aware of potential to worsen ascites, *but not being restricted by it.*
  - Correct intravascular volume depletion as with any other patient (e.g. using Hartmann's solution).
  - Correct electrolyte imbalances, e.g. many patients will have low potassium and magnesium levels.
  - 20% human albumin solution can be added in patients with serum albumin levels <30 g/L (e.g. 100 mL every 6 hours) as well as low dose terlipressin (0.5–1 mg qds), although again, specialist input is advised at this stage.
- Other causes of kidney injury need to be considered such as drugs – stopping diuretics temporarily – and post-renal obstruction (US renal tract).

Acute alcoholic hepatitis

- Is a specific aetiology behind an acute decompensation of chronic alcoholic liver disease (or can be the first presentation of such?). Most patients with alcoholic hepatitis will be cirrhotic.
- It can be precipitated by either chronic high consumption of alcohol or a recent binge.
- It may present as acute decompensation (as described above), as GI bleeding, sepsis or 'just jaundice' (alcohol-related hepatitis has a high mortality).
- Bloods usually show a high bilirubin and INR (coagulopathy) and often low albumin (and platelets). The ALT tends to be only mildly raised,

and if ALT >300 an alternative cause is more likely.
- Mortality can be from 25% in 1 month, but can be more accurately assessed using one of the following predictive scores, which can be found online (www.mdcalc.com/):

1. *Maddrey's coefficient* [4] (discriminant function, DF): requires bilirubin and prothrombin time (PT), as well as lab control PT.
   A value >32 indicates moderate-severe alcoholic hepatitis which carries a poor prognosis. Steroids may reduce mortality in this group of patients in absence of sepsis or GI bleeding.
2. Glasgow alcoholic hepatitis score [5]: requires age, WCC, urea, bilirubin and INR.
   A value >9 indicates a <50% chance of survival at 28 days. This in conjunction with a Maddrey's DF >32 is a strong indicator of poor outcome and consideration of treatment with steroids.

Management of patient with acute alcoholic hepatitis is largely supportive:

- Abstinence from alcohol (supported by withdrawal regime, e.g. CIWA score-guided benzodiazepines).
- Fluid resuscitation and electrolyte corrections (potassium and magnesium; avoid rapid sodium correction) and management of renal failure, if present.
- Management of sepsis and GI bleeding (correct coagulopathy), if present.
- Nutritional support (high dose vitamin replacement plus supplements (Pabrinex); watch for refeeding syndrome).
- Steroids administration should be done under guidance of specialist team.
- Manage encephalopathy to reduce risk of aspiration/injury to self (consider nasogastric (NG) feeding and lactulose).

Ultimately, these patients should be under the care of the gastroenterology/hepatology team who should be informed as soon as they are identified.

Acute liver failure

Assessment

Acute liver failure (ALF) is defined as: 'development of encephalopathy and coagulopathy (INR>1.5) in a patient without pre-existing liver disease'.

- It can be subdivided depending on length of illness, i.e. time from first signs to encephalopathy development:
  - hyperacute (<7 days)
  - acute (<4 weeks)
  - subacute (4–26 weeks)

Hyperacute and acute patients have a better outcome than subacute ALF.

- The most common cause of acute liver failure in the UK is drug-induced (most commonly paracetamol), whereas worldwide acute viral hepatitis is the most common. Other causes include hypoperfusion (ischaemic hepatitis), autoimmune hepatitis, poisoning (e.g. mushroom, 'death cap' amanita) and veno-occlusive disease (including Budd–Chiari syndrome).
- Diagnosis is not always easy as symptoms can be non-specific. Patients may present with jaundice, hepatomegaly and RUQ tenderness, fatigue, anorexia, nausea and later on with ascites. It is vital to recognize early signs of encephalopathy (see time line above) and complete the full history, examination and investigations as described above. As well as encephalopathy and coagulopathy patients may also develop other complications:
  - acute kidney injury
  - metabolic derangement (acidosis, dysglycaemia, hyperlactataemia)
  - haemodynamic compromise (vasodilatation)
  - pulmonary complications (frequent infection/oedema).
- When looking at blood tests, one would expect the aminotransferases to be particularly raised. Tracking the ALT, however, is not the best way to monitor 'liver failure' progression as a fall in ALT may represent recovery, but may also represent hepatocyte death (no cells left to release the enzyme). Therefore it is important to monitor bilirubin and INR closely as these reflect 'true' liver cell function and are better markers of prognosis. Because INR is such an important prognostic marker, including transplant criteria, the use of fresh frozen plasma (FFP) is discouraged unless discussed with the tertiary liver centre.
- Patients with acute liver failure have a 30–50% chance of having concurrent acute kidney injury (often depending on underlying aetiology), so renal function must be closely monitored and organ support (i.e. renal replacement therapy) considered if required.
- Following blood tests (including full non-invasive liver screen plus paracetamol levels), ultrasound of the liver (+/– kidney) plus Doppler flow assessment of hepatic and portal veins is the preferred imaging technique as it negates the need for intravenous contrast in patients with vulnerable renal function.
- Chest X-ray is important to exclude pulmonary oedema, infection or effusions.
- If the aetiology remains uncertain, liver biopsy can be considered, though this tends to require a trans-jugular approach in view of pronounced coagulopathy (and low platelets) and the histology may well be 'non-specific'.

Management

- Once a patient has been identified as having acute liver failure they should be considered for early discussion +/– transfer to a liver centre with transplant capabilities.
- Patients with mild encephalopathy (grade 1) could potentially be managed on a gastroenterology-specialty ward but would require regular reviews and should be considered for transfer to HDU/ITU if critical-care parameters change.
- Management is largely supportive (there are a few specific treatments, e.g. N-acetyl-cysteine for paracetamol overdose). If toxins are implicated, the local toxicology centre should be consulted early on (even out-of-hours).
- Fluid resuscitate (be careful not to over-hydrate as may worsen cerebral oedema – consider CVP monitoring).
- Correct metabolic abnormalities (hypokalaemia, hypomagnesaemia, hypophosphataemia, dysglycaemia).
- Monitor for early signs of sepsis and treat accordingly (no evidence for prophylactic antibiotics).
- Nutritional support (enteral preferably).
- Avoid sedation or opioids where possible, to enable monitoring of encephalopathy grade.
- N-acetyl-cysteine: Give if *any concern* about paracetamol consumption.
- Prophylactic antacids (e.g. proton pump inhibitors) may be considered to reduce the risk of spontaneous GI bleeding.

- Patients with higher grades of encephalopathy should be managed in a liver centre ITU where intracranial pressure monitoring can be performed. Management strategies such as endotracheal intubation, nursing at a 30-degree tilt, CVP and CO_2 monitoring can be done in the interim.

Liver transplantation

Decisions around suitability for liver transplant are made using prognostic scores [6]; i.e. where the likelihood of death is higher than the risk of emergency transplantation. Patients with ALF deemed suitable for transplant are automatically put at the top of the transplant list. The King's College criteria are the most commonly used prognostic scoring system. The system is made up of two separate scores (assessed after initial fluid resuscitation).

For paracetamol-related ALF:

pH <7.30 *or*

Grade 3–4 encephalopathy *plus* PT >100 s *and* creatinine <300 µmol/L.

For non-paracetamol-related ALF:

PT >100 s *or*

Any three of:

(a) Age <10 or >40 years

(b) Unfavourable disease (viral, drug, Wilson's)

(c) Jaundice >7 days

(d) PT >50 s

(e) Bilirubin >300 µmol/L

Patients who meet King's College criteria should be immediately considered for liver transplantation listing; i.e. if out of hours, the referral to the tertiary liver unit may need to be done by bypassing the local gastroenterology team and through discussion directly with the regional liver transplantation unit.

Scenario 36.1 continued

Detailed history revealed that the patient usually consumed around 4 pints of 8% cider a night; however, in the last week this amount had doubled due to stress relating to his work. He had no other risk factors for liver disease, his examination was normal except for jaundice and NILS and US abdomen were unremarkable. He was diagnosed with alcoholic hepatitis with a Maddrey's coefficient of 34 and a Glasgow score of 9. He was treated with oral prednisolone and was monitored over the following week. He was discharged once his bilirubin consistently dropped, without INR rise, and is due to be reviewed in the gastro/hepatology clinic in the next 2 months.

- Throughout this process it is important to keep the patient informed of the diagnosis, i.e. unequivocally linking the severe illness to the alcohol consumption, and management plan which tends to include cirrhosis work-up. This includes giving information about prognosis and likely follow-up. It can be helpful to involve specialist nurses to allow for more time and reinforcement.

- When dealing with patients with a history of alcoholism or substance abuse, it is important, once the acute phase of illness has been managed, to engage the patient in discussion about their lifestyle choices and the impact these have on their health, both acutely and chronically. The first acute presentation may well be the wake-up call these patients need, so this opportunity to offer health promotion advice should not be missed ('opportunistic moment') – whether it is alcohol cessation or advice about needle-sharing. An in-hospital alcohol (and drug) liaison team has been shown to be patient-centred and cost-effective (reduced readmissions) and can be the link to the support services in the community.

- In patients with chronic liver disease due to alcohol it is important to document these discussions in the notes, as most liver centres will require patients to have been abstinent from alcohol for >3–6 months in order to be considered for transplantation.

References

1. Child CG, Turcotte JG. Surgery and portal hypertension. In: *The Liver and Portal Hypertension*. Philadelphia and London: WB Saunders; 1964: 50–64.

2. Pugh RN, Murray-Lyon IM, Dawson JL, et al. Transection of the oesophagus for bleeding oesophageal varices. *British Journal of Surgery* 1973; 60(8).

3. Wong F, Nadim MK, Kellum JA, et al. Working party proposal for a revised classification system of renal dysfunction in patients with cirrhosis. *Gut* 2011; 60: 702–709.

4. Maddrey WC, Boitnott JK, Bedine MS, et al. Corticosteroid therapy of alcoholic hepatitis. *Gastroenterology* 1978; 75(2): 193–199.

5. Forrest EH, Evans CD, Stewart S, et al. Analysis of factors predictive of mortality in alcoholic hepatitis and derivation and validation of the Glasgow alcoholic hepatitis score. *Gut* 2005; 54(8):1174–1179.

6. Bailey B, Amre DK, Gaudreault P. Fulminant hepatic failure secondary to acetaminophen poisoning: a systematic review and meta-analysis of prognostic criteria determining the need for liver transplantation. *Critical Care Medicine* 2003; 31(1): 299–305.

Further reading

EASL clinical practical guidelines: management of alcoholic liver disease. *European Association for the Study of Liver. Journal of Hepatology* 2012; 57(2): 399.

Polson J, Lee WM. AASLD Position Paper: The management of acute liver failure. *Hepatology* 2005; 41(5).

Chapter 37

The swollen joint

Catherine Laversuch

Introduction

Joints can be subdivided into fibrous, cartilaginous and synovial. The fibrous skull sutures and the fibro-cartilaginous symphysis pubis allow little or no movement. Synovial joints are complex and allow more movement. They have: a cavity, ends of adjacent bone covered in avascular hyaline cartilage and a lining of synovial membrane surrounded by a tough fibrous capsule. The synovial lined bursa reduces friction around the joint. There are six types of synovial joint each allowing different planes of movement.

Patients present acutely to the acute physician with painful joints, loss of mobility or falls either as part of a local/systemic inflammatory process or due to osteoarthritis (or combination of both). Trauma, sepsis and fractures can complicate this further. Good history taking can distinguish degenerative from inflammatory joint disease, optimizing management.

Scenario 37.1

A 75-year-old inpatient receiving treatment for Hodgkin's lymphoma develops an extremely painful swollen right knee. On examination he is clearly in considerable pain. There is marked erythema and swelling of the joint with severe restriction of movement. He is pyrexic at 39°C. This elderly man receiving immunosuppression has a hot swollen joint likely due to a septic arthritis. The white blood cell count and CRP were both markedly elevated. Blood cultures were taken. Joint aspiration confirmed Gram-positive cocci and he was commenced on parenteral antibiotics.

The hot swollen joint

This is one of the most urgent musculoskeletal scenarios. If left untreated, a septic joint is rapidly destroyed.

Factors helping to distinguish a septic joint from an inflammatory or degenerative joint include:

- recent onset of pain
- quality of the pain (severe, unrelenting, often preventing sleep)
- marked warmth
- restriction of movement
- reluctance to weight bear.

Inflammatory markers are usually elevated. Prompt joint aspiration is essential *before* treatment with antibiotics and the synovial fluid should be examined as quickly as possible.

Differential diagnosis for a hot swollen joint

- *Septic arthritis* is commonly mono-articular but poly-articular in 22% of cases and has an 11% mortality. It occurs at the extremes of age, the young and the elderly, otherwise other risk factors are necessary. Up to 80% of cases are due to staphylococcal (60%) or streptococcal (20%) infections but Gram-negative infections are found in the elderly and neonates. Infection with *Neisseria gonorrhoeae* should be considered in the sexually active, mycobacterial infection in those from endemic areas, atypical mycobacterial infection in HIV infection and very rarely fungal infections in the immunocompromised.
- *Crystal arthritis*: gout or calcium pyrophosphate arthropathy (pseudogout). Gout is very rare in premenopausal women but will be found in young men and pseudogout is found in older patients often coexisting with osteoarthritis.
- *Haemarthrosis*: post-traumatic, bleeding disorder, pigmented villonodular synovitis, sickle cell.

Acute Medicine, ed. Stephen Haydock, Duncan Whitehead and Zoë Fritz. Published by Cambridge University Press. © Cambridge University Press 2015.

- Cellulitis.
- Bursitis (e.g. olecranon bursitis, pre-patellar bursitis).
- Post-traumatic effusion/underlying fracture.

Risk factors for joint sepsis

- Pre-existing rheumatoid arthritis (RA) or osteoarthritis
- Prosthetic joints
- Intravenous drug abuse
- Alcoholism
- Diabetes
- Previous intra-articular corticosteroid injection
- Cutaneous ulcers
- Immunosuppression

Clinical features for joint sepsis

- Increased pain, swelling, warmth and restriction, of recent onset (<2 weeks)
- Large joints (knee, hip, wrist, ankle and shoulder)
- Rigors, sweats, confusion, +/– fever
- Septic pustules and tenosynovitis are characteristic of gonococcal infection which can cause both a septic monoarthritis and a polyarthralgia
- Sternoclavicular joint involvement is particularly seen in IV drug abusers

Immediate investigations

Blood tests

- FBC (a high white count is not always found)
- CRP: can be very elevated in sepsis and crystal arthritis (in inflammatory arthritis the CRP is usually only moderately elevated: <100 mg/mL)
- Urea, electrolytes and creatinine
- Liver function tests
- Blood cultures
- Calcium (if calcium pyrophosphate arthritis suspected)
- Urate (can be normal during acute gout)

Radiology

- Chest film
- Plain views of joint:
  - A baseline but likely normal or soft tissue swelling only

Table 37.1 Procedure for arthrocentesis of the knee (medial approach)

Consent	Complications are rare with occasional bruising and minor bleeds into joint Risk of introducing infection is very low (0.01%)
Equipment	21-gauge needles 10–20 mL syringes, gloves, sterile pot Antiseptic (i.e. alcohol wipes) Ethyl chloride (EC) spray (optional) 1% lidocaine (LA) *single* dose ampoules Depo-Medrone 40 mg/mL *single* dose ampoules
Procedure	Check patella freely mobile (quadriceps relaxed) Aseptic 'no-touch' technique Clean the area Infiltrate with LA first or use EC and single needle approach Pull back on plunger frequently until synovial fluid aspirated Aspirate almost to dryness Do not touch open needle hub or injection site during syringe changeover If injecting: mix 40–80 mg Depo-Medrone with 2 mL LA Do not inject against resistance

- Osteomyelitis – bone oedema and periosteal reaction
- Pseudogout – may reveal chondrocalcinosis in the knee or triangular cartilage of the wrist
- Gouty erosions take many years to appear

Microbiology

- Throat/cervical/rectal swabs and pustular fluid culture: Only 50% of joint cultures are positive in gonococcal arthritis (consult genitourinary clinic).

Synovial fluid examination (see Table 37.1 and Figure 37.1):

- Anticoagulation is *not* a contraindication to joint aspiration.
- *Do not attempt joint aspiration of a prosthetic joint.* Refer to orthopaedics urgently.
- *Do not aspirate through overlying soft tissue infection.*
- The hip requires aspiration under ultrasound guidance.
- Sternoclavicular joints may require surgical exploration.

269

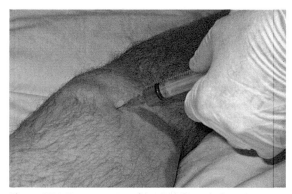

Figure 37.1 Demonstration of the medial approach.

- Pus means sepsis and/or crystal arthritis.
- Send fluid for Gram stain, microscopy, culture, sensitivity and polarizing microscopy. (Direct inoculation of synovial fluid into blood culture bottles is not necessary.)

Additional investigations

- Early morning urine/sputum culture if *Mycobacterium tuberculosis* is suspected.
- Synovial polymerase chain reaction (PCR) if sepsis is suspected and culture is negative.

Management

Septic arthritis

- Intravenous antibiotics to treat likely pathogen according to local microbiological guidelines: 2 weeks IV plus 4 weeks oral, adapted once sensitivities are known.
- Contact orthopaedic department for surgical lavage (it remains unclear whether this is superior to regular closed drainage).
- Splinting/bed rest/DVT prophylaxis.
- Analgesia (NSAID provided no contraindications/codeine/paracetamol).
- Monitor progress with CRP.
- Physiotherapy for passive stretches and later rehabilitation.

Crystal arthritis

Acute calcium pyrophosphate arthropathy

- Responds rapidly (within 24–48 hours) to an NSAID (naproxen plus proton pump inhibitor or cox-II inhibitor).

- If elderly, renal impairment, heart failure or anticoagulated then intra-articular corticosteroids or low dose prednisolone (15–20 mg prednisolone for 3–5 days).
- Check ferritin (haemochromatosis), and thyroid function.

Acute gout

- *Full dose NSAID* (ibuprofen is insufficient) *plus proton pump inhibitor.*
- *Or colchicine* 500 µg qds then tds then bd reducing course.
- Reduce the dose by 50% if eGFR <60 mL/min or avoid if <30 mL/min.
- *Or corticosteroid*: intra-articular, intramuscular (80–120 mg depot triamcinolone) or oral prednisolone (0.5 mg/kg for 7–10 days).
- *Reduce risk factors*: cut alcohol intake, particularly beer, switch diuretic to ACE inhibitor if possible (losartan is mildly uricosuric), reduce fructose intake, check fasting lipids.
- *Refer if frequent attacks or tophi* for urate lowering therapy.

Haemarthrosis

- May need arthroscopic lavage. Consult orthopaedics.

Scenario 37.2

A 35-year-old male IT worker presents to Accident and Emergency with a 2-week history of a swollen right knee. He now cannot weight bear. He feels unwell but is not acutely ill. His general practitioner suggested ibuprofen 400 mg qds. He has no other significant illnesses, lives alone and drinks beer at the weekends. He reported no rash or prodromal illness. On examination the right knee is warm, swollen, painful and restricted but the left ankle is additionally found to be warm and swollen and he has a temperature of 37.5°C.

This man has an asymmetric oligo-arthropathy. The white cell count was normal but CRP markedly elevated. The serum urate was not elevated. Plain radiology showed soft tissue swelling at the knee and ankle and chest film showed no evidence of hilar lymphadenopathy. Aspiration of his knee and ankle were negative for Gram stain and culture but positive for intracellular urate crystals. He improved after naproxen and a PPI and subsequent intra-articular corticosteroid injections. He was advised to reduce his beer intake. He was referred to rheumatology for his polyarticular gout.

Inflammatory arthritis

History

Features suggestive of any inflammatory arthritis

- Onset sudden or gradual over several weeks
- Joints painful, warm and swollen
- Early morning stiffness
- Inactivity stiffness
- Improvement with exercise and movement
- Inability to close fist in the mornings (stiff hands)
- Significant improvement with NSAIDs and or corticosteroids
- Systemic symptoms: fever, lethargy and weight loss

Joints affected may give a clue to diagnosis

- An asymmetric oligoarthropathy suggests a seronegative spondylo-arthropathy (SSPA):
  - psoriatic arthritis
  - reactive arthritis
  - arthritis related to inflammatory bowel disease
  - ankylosing spondylitis.
- Early hip involvement or lower back stiffness with enthesitis (plantar fasciitis, tendo-achillitis, chest wall pain) also suggests an SSPA.
- Dactylitis (sausage toe) suggests psoriatic or reactive arthritis and is never seen in RA.
- Psoriatic arthritis is very common and can present as:
  - an asymmetric oligo-arthropathy
  - a mono-arthritis
  - DIP joint involvement with adjacent nail dystrophy
  - a symmetrical polyarthritis identical to rheumatoid arthritis but without rheumatoid factor
  - sacroiliitis with spinal involvement similar to ankylosing spondylitis
  - you do not need to have psoriasis to have psoriatic arthritis, a family history of psoriasis or nail pits is sufficient.
- Symmetrical polyarthropathy (hands and wrists) with early metatarsophalangeal joint involvement (walking on pebbles) suggests RA.
- Sparing of the distal interphalangeal (DIP) joints suggests RA.

Other associated features relating to inflammatory joint diseases

- A reactive arthritis typically occurs within 2 weeks of a diarrhoeal or genitourinary infection. Refer to a genitourinary clinic if in doubt.
- Any inflammatory bowel symptoms.
- Family history: psoriasis, gout, spinal disease, osteoporosis and RA.
- Excess alcohol (particularly beer), diuretic use, hypertension, diabetes, obesity and CKD. All are risk factors for gout.
- Eye inflammation: iritis is associated with SSPAs, particularly ankylosing spondylitis; acute conjunctivitis with reactive arthritis; episcleritis and scleritis with RA and more rarely systemic vasculitis.
- Raynaud's syndrome, hair loss, photosensitive rashes, mouth or genital ulcers, serositis, headaches, fatigue, muscle weakness and sicca symptoms (dry eyes and mouth) suggest a connective tissue disease. These are linked to a non-deforming non-erosive arthropathy.

Rare associated findings

- Request serology (*Borrelia burgdorferi*) if a history of tick bite (60% do not recall a bite) or spreading rash (erythema chronicum migrans) and an intermittent large joint monoarthritis in Lyme prevalent areas.
- Erythema nodosum (nodules on shins and forearms) is associated with the arthritis of inflammatory bowel disease and acute sarcoid arthropathy (Lofgren's syndrome). The latter causes brawny swelling of the ankles and bilateral hilar lymphadenopathy on chest film. It has an excellent prognosis but may require low dose corticosteroids.
- If there is marked weight loss, haemoptysis or dysphagia, a polyarthritis can be paraneoplastic or part of a pulmonary osteodystrophy.
- Transient self-limiting joint effusions can occur following meningococcal sepsis, rubella, parvovirus, hepatitis B and C infection.
- Endocarditis can present rarely with arthralgia and joint swelling.

271

- Palindromic rheumatism (migratory joint inflammation lasting 24 hours to several days) and periodic fever syndromes are causes of intermittent joint swelling. Refer to rheumatology.
- Migratory polyarthritis approximately 2 weeks after group A streptococcal pharyngitis presenting with fever, rash and a cardiac murmur could be rheumatic fever. Post-streptococcal reactive arthritis may be migratory and self-limiting. Consider cardiac surveillance and antibiotic prophylaxis.
- Keratoderma blennorrhagicum (palmar plantar scaly rash), circinate balinitis (rash on the glans penis): rare and linked to reactive arthritis.

Examination

Follow: *Look, Feel, Move, Function.*

A guide to recap a regional examination of the musculoskeletal system (REMS) can be found at www.arthritisresearch.org.uk, with helpful videos. The GALS screening tool is less suitable for ill, perhaps confused, bed-bound patients. Starting at the soles of the feet and working upwards a systematic and thorough examination can be achieved. If the patient can stand, assess gait and mobility. *Note*: a positive MTP and metacarpophalangeal (MCP) joint squeeze indicates an inflammatory arthritis; if the patient reports knee pain always examine the hip.

Investigations

- Basic blood tests as described previously; in addition basic immunological testing may be indicated.

Interpretation of basic immunological tests in joint swelling

Rheumatoid factors: any antibody which binds IgG (Fc region) is called a rheumatoid factor (RF). Mildly raised levels without a clinical picture of joint swelling are irrelevant. *This is not a specific test for rheumatoid arthritis* as these antibodies are found in normal people and those with other diseases such as SLE and primary Sjögren's syndrome. RF positivity with typical joint inflammation is associated with disease severity and extra-articular manifestations such as nodules, lung and cardiac involvement.

Anti-cyclic citrullinated peptide antibodies (anti-CCP): a newly available and more specific test for rheumatoid arthritis which is rarely positive in other rheumatic diseases and normal people.

Anti-nuclear antibody test (ANA): a screening test looking for anti-nuclear antibodies in the test subjects' serum by indirect immunofluorescence. Dilutions greater than 1/80 are considered positive (i.e. 1/160 and above). Like RF this test is not specific for SLE and must be used in combination with suggestive clinical symptoms. A positive test in the absence of symptoms or signs is irrelevant. Positive ANAs are found commonly in:

- normal older women
- 98% of SLE patients
- primary Sjögren's syndrome
- scleroderma
- autoimmune liver disease
- other connective tissue diseases.

Those with active SLE may have a raised ESR, thrombocytopenia, lymphopenia and *depressed complement levels* (complement consumption) and sometimes have raised antibodies to double-stranded DNA. These parameters normalize when the disease is in remission (apart from lymphopenia).

Radiology in inflammatory joint disease

- Early in disease radiographs will be normal or show soft tissue swelling and may be periarticular osteopenia.
- Joint space loss and erosions take several years to develop, appearing first in the feet in RA, with subsequent bone destruction, subluxation and deformity.

Scenario 37.3

A 75-year-old woman presents to the MAU unable to walk with worsening knee pain. She usually walks the short distance to the local shop using a stick. On examination her left knee was swollen, slightly warm, very painful to move with a valgus deformity and she cannot weight bear. She has swelling of all her fingers. Temperature is 36.6°C. X-rays of the left knee show loss of joint space medially and calcification of the articular cartilage, hands show loss of joint space at PIP and DIP joints. Left knee aspirate showed crystals of calcium pyrophosphate suggesting acute pseudogout complicating osteoarthritis. The painful knee rapidly responded to an intra-articular injection of corticosteroid. The CRP quickly normalized. Her pain and her mobility improved with physiotherapy.

Osteoarthritis

Typical features in the history

- Age >50 years.
- Family history: nodal osteoarthritis is familial.
- Gradual rather than sudden onset.
- Pain is worse with activity and relieved by rest.
- A good discriminatory question: When is your worst time of day? 'It's painful all the time', 'in the evening after activity'.
- Stiffness is usually less than 30 minutes.
- Involvement of the hip restricts activities such as putting on socks.
- Knee pain is worse going up and particularly down stairs.
- Simple analgesia is more effective than NSAIDs. Corticosteroids are not beneficial.

  Commonly involved joints include:
- knees
- hips
- first MTP joint
- PIP and DIP joints (Bouchard's and Heberden's nodes)
- base of the thumb (carpo-metacarpal joint)
- second and third MCP joints
- lumbar and cervical spine.

  Less commonly involved joints include:
- ankle, mid-tarsal, sternoclavicular and shoulder joints.

Investigations

- CRP is usually normal.
- Radiology may show loss of cartilage, subchondral sclerosis, osteophyte formation and subarticular cyst formation.

Scenario 37.4

A 60-year-old woman with a 20-year history of RF-positive RA presents to the MAU unwell with a disease flare. She had a knee replaced one month ago. Her RA had been well controlled with weekly oral methotrexate (15 mg) and etanercept injections SC (an anti-TNF inhibitor). The latter has just been restarted after surgery. However, she now has fever, chills with painful stiff shoulders, wrists, fingers and a productive cough. She has lost her appetite.

Many of her joints feel warm and swollen and there were a few basal crackles heard in the left lung.

This woman has a postoperative flare of RA complicated by infection. Her methotrexate and anti-TNF therapy were temporarily discontinued. Her chest infection was treated by antibiotics and she was referred to the rheumatology team who injected the worst affected joints.

Important acute considerations/ complications of drugs used in RA

RA patients with active disease, taking corticosteroids and anti-TNF inhibitors, have an increased incidence of infections. *Biologics* (anti-TNF, IL-6 inhibitors) but not disease-modifying drugs (DMARDs) are discontinued during routine surgery. *Biologic therapy should always be stopped during any significant infection.*

Rarely *methotrexate* causes an acute pneumonitis presenting with high fever (>38°C), cough, breathlessness, hypoxia, and bi-basal lung crackles. There are bilateral lung infiltrates on chest film and maybe an eosinophilia. This responds to drug withdrawal, high dose corticosteroids and intensive respiratory support. It can be difficult to distinguish from infection in the absence of eosinophilia.

Methotrexate-induced bone marrow toxicity (often precipitated by acute renal impairment or intercurrent illness) requires drug withdrawal and folinic acid rescue.

Leflunomide, a DMARD with a long half-life, can cause toxicity (rash, diarrhoea, mucositis, bone marrow suppression). It requires accelerated drug removal with activated charcoal or cholestyramine. Refer to rheumatology for advice.

Further reading

Bardin T (2003) Gonococcal arthritis. *Best Pract Res Clin Rheumatol* 17(2):201–208.

Coakley G, Mathews C, Field M, Jones A, et al (2006) BSR & BHPR, BOA, RCGP and BSAC guidelines for management of the hot swollen joint in adults. *Rheumatology* 45:1039–1041.

Chapter

38

Unilateral limb pain and swelling

Stephen Haydock

Introduction

The patient with a painful, swollen leg is a common presentation. Most are referred for investigation and management of suspected deep vein thrombosis or cellulitis. Although these conditions are increasingly being managed through ambulatory pathways within primary care, many such patients continue to be referred to the hospital acute medical take.

Causes of an acutely painful swollen leg

We most commonly see:

- deep vein thrombosis
- cellulitis
- ruptured Baker's cyst
- superficial thrombophlebitis.

In addition, local bone and joint problems may be referred:

- joint effusion or haemarthrosis
- acute arthritis
- undiagnosed fracture.

Local damage to the muscles of the calf are sometimes seen:

- haematoma
- gastrocnemius muscle tear

... and finally most physicians can recall at least one occasion when they have been asked to exclude a DVT in a patient with:

- acute arterial ischaemia.

History

Enquire regarding:

- Speed of onset
- Whether really unilateral or bilateral and worse in one leg:
  - bilateral is more suggestive of an underlying systemic problem, e.g. cardiac failure, hypoalbuminaemia
- Swollen or painful joints
- Previous history of:
  - renal or cardiac disease
  - cellulitis
  - recent surgery/immobilization
  - thromboembolic disease
- Family history of thromboembolic disease
- Risk factors for thromboembolic disease (see later)
- Risk factors for cellulitis (see later)

Examination

Take note of:

- Localized or generalized swellings
- Localized tenderness
- Discoloration/erythema
- Pitting oedema
- Associated systemic features

Scenario 38.1

A 65-year-old man is referred by his general practitioner because of a painful swelling of his right calf. His GP informs you that this was present on waking and is sufficiently painful to be limiting mobility. Examination shows the right calf to be 3 cm larger than the left and pitting oedema is present. He is concerned that the patient has a deep vein thrombosis and wishes this to be excluded. He has otherwise been fit and well and is on no regular medication.

Acute Medicine, ed. Stephen Haydock, Duncan Whitehead and Zoë Fritz. Published by Cambridge University Press. © Cambridge University Press 2015.

Factor	Points
Active cancer (treatment within last six months or palliative)	1
Calf swelling ≥3 cm compared to asymptomatic calf (measured 10 cm below tibial tuberosity)	1
Collateral superficial veins (non-varicose)	1
Pitting oedema (confined to symptomatic leg)	1
Swelling of entire leg	1
Localized tenderness along distribution of deep venous system	1
Paralysis, paresis, or recent cast immobilization of lower extremities	1
Recently bedridden ≥3 days, or major surgery requiring regional or general anaesthetic in the previous 12 weeks	1
Previously documented deep vein thrombosis	1
Alternative diagnosis at least as likely as DVT	−2

Figure 38.1 Modified Wells criteria for diagnosis of deep vein thrombosis [2]. Interpretation: for dichotomized evaluation (likely vs. unlikely): score of 2 or higher: DVT is 'likely'
score of less than 2: DVT is 'unlikely' [2].
In patients in whom both legs are symptomatic, the more symptomatic leg is used.

Investigation and management of deep vein thrombosis of the leg

Deep vein thrombosis of the lower limb has an incidence of approximately 1 in 1000 per annum of the population in the UK. The basic pathophysiology of thrombus formation is frequently referred to as Virchow's triad and comprises:

- hypercoagulability of blood
- damage to the endothelium of the vessel wall
- stasis of blood.

  Risk factors therefore include:

- prolonged immobilization
- recent surgery
- pregnancy
- combined oral contraceptive pill
- obesity
- smoking
- inherited disorders of coagulation
- cardiac failure
- nephrotic syndrome.

Clinical assessment

(*See above for general approach to the patient with swollen/painful leg.*)

Current guidelines such as the NICE Clinical Guideline [1] for determining the likelihood of deep vein thrombosis require:

1. Clinical assessment score using the Wells two-level clinical scoring system (likely and unlikely) (Figure 38.1).
2. Quantification of circulating D-dimers.

If DVT is unlikely on Wells scoring and the D-dimer test is negative, then a DVT is excluded. For all other situations, patients are referred for diagnostic imaging by Doppler ultrasound scanning. If this test is not available within 4 hours, then an initial dose of low molecular weight heparin (e.g. Clexane 1.5 mg/kg) should be given.

Homans' sign: pain in the calf on dorsiflexion of the foot with the knee fully extended is obsolete as it lacks both sensitivity and specificity and may precipitate a pulmonary embolism.

The D-dimer test

The measurement of circulating D-dimers is a highly sensitive but relatively non-specific test for the presence of thromboembolic disease. A deep vein thrombosis results from activation of the clotting cascade with the generation of thrombin, which polymerizes soluble circulating fibrinogen (consisting of three subunits

D-E-D) into the insoluble fibrin chains. These chains are then cross-linked by factor XIII. The end product of plasmin degradation of the cross-linked fibrin is a trimer consisting of two D subunits and one E subunit cross-linked together (the 'D-dimer'). These are detected using a monoclonal antibody. D-dimers are not normally found in plasma in the absence of activation of the clotting system. Elevated levels are therefore found in thromboembolic disease and disseminated intravascular coagulation.

The D-dimer test is only useful as a diagnostic tool when the possibility of thromboembolic disease is being actively considered. Acting on the basis of random D-dimer tests performed without a clinical indication is clearly inappropriate. False positive elevations occur in many circumstances including:

- recent surgery
- trauma
- infection
- pregnancy
- liver disease.

Radiological imaging

The venous drainage of the lower limb is by the superficial and deep venous systems. The principal superficial veins are the great (or long) and small (or short) saphenous veins. They arise at the level of the ankle and enter the deep system at the groin and popliteal fossa, respectively.

The principal deep veins are the femoral and popliteal veins. The popliteal vein arises behind the knee from the junction of the anterior and posterior tibial veins of the calf and receives the peroneal vein, subsequently forming the femoral vein as it exits the adductor canal. The femoral vein receives the profunda femoris and great saphenous vein before forming the external iliac vein at the inguinal ligament. The presence of clot in any of these veins constitutes a deep vein thrombosis.

Confusion can arise by the use of the term 'superficial femoral' vein in imaging reports by radiologists when referring to the distal part of the femoral vein and this has led to patients not receiving anticoagulation due to the mistaken belief that the clot is not within the deep venous system.

Duplex ('two part') ultrasound imaging is now the preferred imaging modality for the diagnosis of proximal (above the knee) deep vein thrombosis.

1. *B-mode* (brightness-modulated) ultrasound uses the reflections of high energy sound waves from internal tissues to identify the venous system. Pressure is applied to the skin in an attempt to collapse the underlying vein. Presence of clot prevents complete compression.
2. *Doppler shift* of the frequency of the ultrasound waves identifies abnormal blood flow.

Lack of compressibility and absent blood flow confirms the diagnosis of a deep vein thrombosis with both 95% specificity and sensitivity for above the knee and is both non-invasive and cost effective. Distal (below knee) clot is much harder to reliably detect with this technique. Sensitivity and specificity is only about 65% and scanning is very time-consuming due to the increased number and variability of the calf veins.

Contrast X-ray venography was traditionally the gold standard imaging technique. Contrast medium is injected into a vein on the dorsum of the foot and a filling defect in a deep vein identified. It is increasingly rare for radiology departments to offer this investigation with the advent of ultrasound imaging, as the study requires the administration of iodinated contrast media and radiation exposure. It can be useful in assessment of patients with recurrent DVTs where the venous anatomy may be complex.

Other techniques include MR venography or CT venography. The former is preferred as this avoids the use of iodinated contrast media and radiation exposure. They are occasionally employed when ultrasound is equivocal and venography is not readily available. Advantages include a better estimation of the overall clot burden, especially when clot extends into the pelvis and better information on extravascular anatomy and identification of a potential alternative diagnosis.

Management

The management will depend on the outcome of the duplex ultrasound scanning study.

1. Above knee DVT

Such patients do not generally require admission and are managed according to an ambulatory pathway.

- Check for anaemia, thrombocytopenia, abnormal clotting and assess renal function.
- Treat as soon as possible with a low molecular weight heparin (e.g. Clexane 1.5 mg/kg).
- Commence warfarin within 24 hours of diagnosis and counsel regarding potential risks of treatment.

- Continue low molecular weight heparin for 5 days or until the international normalized ratio (INR) is 2 or above for 24 hours.
- Continue warfarin for period of 3 months (relative risks and benefits of continuing treatment beyond this time will be discussed with the patient).
- Patients with severe renal impairment (eGFR <30 mL/min) or increased bleeding risk may require unfractionated heparin with monitoring of the APTT.
- Patients with active cancer are treated with a low molecular weight heparin alone for a period of 6 months. (The risks and benefits of continuing anticoagulation after this time should also then be discussed with the patient.)
- Offer all patients a below knee graduated compression stocking exerting pressure at the ankle >23 mmHg a week after diagnosis or when swelling has reduced sufficiently. Advise patient to wear the stocking (on the affected leg – I have seen them wear it on the normal leg!) for at least 2 years. They need replacing 2–3 times each year.

2. Below knee DVT

These are less commonly identified as the sonographer may only scan above the knee and, even if they do examine the calf veins, the sensitivity is low and operator dependent. The management remains unclear as studies in this area are not of good quality.

- *Against anticoagulation*: risk of pulmonary embolism is considerably lower than for above knee DVT and there are known risks from anticoagulation to consider.
- *For anticoagulation*: still a significant risk of pulmonary embolism and treatment may also reduce the persistent swelling and discomfort of the post-phlebitic syndrome.
- Some advocate a repeat scan after 7 days to determine if clot has propagated above the knee with subsequent anticoagulation if this has occurred.

3. Negative scan

- Repeat scan after 7 days if D-dimer is positive as might have calf venous clot that was not detected on the initial scan. If after 1 week no clot can be detected above the knee, then even if clot was present but not detected by the initial scan, its

failure to propagate means that the individual risk for embolization is low.
- There is no requirement for anticoagulation during the period between scans.

Newer anticoagulant agents

Until recently the coumarin (e.g. warfarin) and non-coumarin (e.g. phenindione) vitamin K 'antagonists' have been the only oral treatment option. These drugs act by inhibiting vitamin K epoxide reductase, the enzyme responsible for recycling vitamin K epoxide back to the reduced active form of vitamin K.

The newer agents are:

- thrombin (factor IIa) inhibitors, e.g. dabigatran
- factor Xa inhibitors, e.g. rivaroxaban, apixaban.

Rivaroxaban is currently the only new agent both licensed for the treatment of deep vein thrombosis and recommended by NICE as an option for the treatment of deep vein thrombosis. Other agents are likely to follow in the near future.

The newer agents have *advantages*:

- They do not require monitoring by INR as for vitamin K antagonists whose dose is highly variable and dependent on the vitamin K content of the diet, alcohol intake and co-administered drugs.
- They have rapid onset and therefore co-administration of low molecular weight heparin is not required after the initial diagnosis.

They also have *disadvantages*:

- Lack of information on long-term dosing.
- Lack of immediate reversibility when the patient is admitted with a bleeding complication. Most acute Trusts have, however, developed protocols that involve administration of blood products such as prothrombin complex concentrate to address this. Fortunately the half-life of these newer agents is short and there is also very active research under way to develop specific agents to rapidly reverse their action.
- less able to identify poor compliance.

It is likely that the lack of requirement for INR testing and consequent benefits to patient and cost savings will mean that these newer agents will become established as the first-line drugs of choice for the treatment of deep vein thrombosis.

Duration of therapy

There remains considerable uncertainty regarding the optimum period of anticoagulation.

- Consensus that those patients with a clearly identifiable and reversible cause (e.g. surgical immobilization) require 3 months anticoagulation.
- The 10-year recurrence rate after stopping anticoagulation is 52% for an idiopathic DVT and 22% for a provoked DVT.
- 2–3% per year risk of a significant haemorrhagic event from anticoagulation and this increases with increasing age.
- Factors thought to be associated with a high risk of DVT recurrence are:
  - active malignancy (10% per annum on stopping therapy)
  - known thrombophilia
  - idiopathic clot
  - proximal clot
  - older age, male sex, elevated BMI
  - elevated D-dimer 4 weeks after stopping treatment
  - persistent clot on USS scanning.

  A reasonable approach is:
- Long-term treatment with low molecular weight heparin for all patients with active malignancy.
- For others a clinical decision based upon the thorough discussion with and evaluation of risk for the individual patient (including known heritable thrombophilia).
- Treatment beyond 3 months should therefore be considered for patients with:
  - unprovoked proximal DVT
  - high risk of VTE recurrence
  - no additional major bleeding risk.

Screening for malignancy

For

- Approximately 10% of patients presenting with an unprovoked DVT will have an underlying malignancy.

Against

- Cost
- Demand on clinical/diagnostic services
- Lack of robust evidence that detection impacts on survival.

Current NICE recommendations suggest that patients with an *unprovoked* DVT undergo:

- physical examination
- plain chest radiograph
- blood tests (FBC, U&E, calcium)
- urinalysis.
  In addition:
- CT scanning of abdomen and pelvis (and mammography for women) *should be considered* for all patients over 40 years of age with no evidence of malignancy on initial screening above.

Thrombophilia screening

Expert opinion does not support 'indiscriminate' thrombophilia testing after a first DVT.

- Patients with a provoked DVT do not need testing.
- Unprovoked DVT with a first degree relative with a previous DVT or PE should be considered for testing only if it is planned to stop anticoagulation, to inform the risk/benefit analysis for extending treatment.

Superficial thrombophlebitis

Thrombosis with inflammation of superficial veins presents as a hard, painful swelling with overlying erythema. There is no consensus on best treatment.

- Both NSAIDs and low molecular weight heparin (prophylactic and therapeutic doses) reduce extension and recurrence of superficial thrombophlebitis.
- Topical non-steroidal gels improve symptoms.
- Fondaparinux is associated with a significant reduction in symptomatic venous thromboembolism, extension and recurrence of superficial thrombophlebitis, with comparable rates of major bleeding relative to placebo.
- Compression stockings are beneficial.
- Lesions close to the saphenofemoral junction, associated with pain or varicose veins, may require surgical excision.

Thrombolysis

There is some evidence that the incidence of severe postphlebitic syndrome associated with extensive proximal clot might be reduced by catheter-directed thrombolysis. This treatment should be considered for:

- symptomatic iliofemoral DVT with symptoms less than 14 days duration
- good functional status

- life expectancy greater than one year
- low risk of bleeding.

Post-phlebitic/thrombotic syndrome

This term refers to chronic leg swelling with pain, induration and venous ectasia.

- Onset is usually within 2 years of a DVT.
- Risk of intractable leg ulceration and consequent impairment of mobility.
- True prevalence is uncertain (figures between 17% and 50% are quoted).
- More likely with proximal and recurrent disease.
- It may be associated with obesity and female sex.

The use of compression stockings is helpful in preventing development of the syndrome. The use of thrombolytic therapy for proximal DVTs may be an option.

Ruptured Baker's cyst

A Baker's cyst (after William Morrant Baker, 1839–1896, surgeon to St Bartholomew's Hospital, London) is a common cystic swelling behind the knee that arises as an enlargement of the gastrocnemius-semimembranosus bursa. It usually remains in contact with the bursa via a narrow neck.

- Commonly a history of joint trauma or joint disease.
- Usually asymptomatic but can cause knee discomfort and a popliteal swelling.
- Corticosteroid injection can be helpful.
- May mimic a deep vein thrombosis by enlarging into the calf, compressing venous return or by rupturing. The rupture of large cysts can be associated with haemorrhage and risk of compartment syndrome.
- Can be identified on ultrasound scanning for deep vein thrombosis.
- Treatment of a ruptured cyst is by analgesia, bed rest and elevation of the limb.

Scenario 38.2

A 50-year-old man attends his general practitioner for review. The previous day he was treated for a cellulitis of the calf associated with a local puncture wound. He is taking penicillin V 500 mg qds and flucloxacillin 500 mg qds. The leg remains painful and the previously marked area of erythema has extended 1–2 cm beyond the skin marking. He is systemically well. His general practitioner requests admission for IV antibiotics to treat his worsening cellulitis.

Cellulitis of the lower limb

Cellulitis is a non-contagious spreading bacterial infection of the dermis and subcutaneous tissues. Traditionally:

- Cellulitis of the skin was a deep infection with a diffuse edge to the visible erythema.
- Erysipelas was a superficial infection of the dermis and upper subcutaneous tissues with a characteristic well-defined, raised edge.

However, this distinction is no longer thought to be useful. For the purpose of this account the term cellulitis refers to both superficial and deep infection.

Cellulitis, mostly affecting the lower limb, is a common problem in the UK:

- 70 000 emergency department attendances per annum
- 2–3% of all hospital admissions
- 360 000 bed days per annum.

Despite the scale of the problem, very few adequately powered studies have addressed the principal issues of the relative benefits of specific antibiotic regimens (including which drug to give, for how long and by what route).

History and examination

(*See above for general approach to the patient with swollen/painful leg.*)

Cellulitis is characterized by the following features:

- Acute onset of pain, swelling, erythema and tenderness.
- Almost always unilateral.
- Evidence of systemic upset with malaise and fever.
- The edge of the erythema can be well demarcated or more diffuse.
- May be blister and bullae formation and haemorrhage into bullae.
- May be lymphangitis and painful groin lymphadenopathy.

Table 38.1 The Eron classification of the severity of cellulitis. Adapted from Eron et al. [4]. Class I and II may be suitable for outpatient management. Class III and IV require inpatient management

Class I	Have no signs of systemic toxicity, no uncontrolled co-morbidities
Class II	Systemically well or ill but with a co-morbidity which may complicate resolution of infection
Class III	Systemic upset such as confusion, tachycardia, tachypnoea, hypotension, unstable co-morbidities or vascular compromise to limb
Class IV	Sepsis syndrome or severe life-threatening infection

A number of co-morbid medical conditions have been suggested to predispose for an initial episode and recurrence.

- Skin breakage including minor trauma, insect bites and tinea pedis
- Obesity
- Diabetes mellitus
- Lymphoedema
- Venous insufficiency
- Immunosuppression
- Intravenous drug abuse
- Previous cellulitis.

It is usual to draw round the area of erythema with an indelible marker pen with date and time so that spread of the skin involvement can be noted.

Classification of severity

The Clinical Resource Efficiency Support Team (CREST) guidelines [3] refer to the Eron classification [4] (Table 38.1) for the severity of cellulitis and this is the most widely quoted system and has been used to triage patients to inpatient or outpatient management.

Laboratory investigation

- ESR or CRP and white cell count are usually abnormal and useful if the diagnosis is in doubt and in monitoring response to therapy.
- Most studies of cellulitis management report relatively poor microbiological identification and this does not appear detrimental to treatment. Swabs can be taken from appropriate sites. Blood cultures are not indicated in uncomplicated cases.

Antimicrobial therapy

The management requires treatment with oral or systemic antimicrobial therapy together with conservative measures.

The limited clinical data on the management of cellulitis was considered in a Cochrane review of 2010 [5]. Amongst their conclusions were:

- It was not possible to define the best treatment for cellulitis.
- Most studies address patients admitted to hospital and do not look at those patients managed exclusively in primary care.
- Interviews with patients identify that the time to the resolution of unpleasant symptoms is the important patient outcome, yet few studies address this as an endpoint.
- Most regimens involve the administration of a penicillin as first-line agent. A macrolide or clindamycin is an alternative for the penicillin allergic patient.
- Little evidence supports any particular duration of treatment and opinion suggests that residual symptoms may persist due to inflammation, rather than active infection. One small study supported this and suggests that 5 days treatment is as effective as 10 days.
- When oral antibiotics were compared with intravenous for moderate to severe cellulitis, the oral route appeared to be *more* effective than intravenous but these results were inconclusive in view of the small number of studies.
- Without firm evidence of the benefit of parenteral antibiotics, the need for outpatient parenteral therapy has not yet been established for this condition.

The Cochrane review demonstrated that the treatment of cellulitis lacks any sound evidence base. It does, however, suggest that received wisdom in this area may be incorrect and that the common practice of admission to hospital for the benefits of parenteral administration of antibiotics and long treatment durations *are not supported* by the limited available evidence.

All Trusts will have local antimicrobial guidelines based upon knowledge of local antimicrobial resistance and these should be consulted:

- Not systemically unwell and do not require hospitalization, it is usual to treat with a high oral dose of flucloxacillin as monotherapy.
- Penicillin allergic patients can be treated with either oral clarithromycin, clindamycin or doxycycline according to local resistance profiles.
- Systemically unwell or have co-morbidities that necessitate admission, then 24–48 hours of maximum parenteral therapy with flucloxacillin followed by a rapid switch to oral therapy is appropriate.

Adjunctive therapy

- Rest and elevate affected limb. Some clinicians believe that a considerable part of the benefit of hospitalization and parenteral antibiotic use is due to this imposed rest and elevation.
- Adequate analgesia.
- Prophylaxis with low molecular weight heparin considered for those with co-morbidities and markedly reduced mobility.

Apparent slow resolution may not necessarily be indicative of inadequate response to antibiotics. The infection produces considerable tissue damage and inflammation that takes time to resolve.

- In one study, the addition of high dose oral steroids reduced the length of hospital inpatient stay by one bed day without significant side effects. More evidence is required before this could be adopted as a standard strategy.
- Another small study considered the speed of resolution of cellulitis in patients treated with a combination of parenteral and oral antibiotics for 10 days, half of whom were supplemented with a non-steroidal anti-inflammatory drug. The NSAID-supplemented group had markedly more rapid rates of improvement and resolution than the control group. The routine use of NSAIDs as adjunctive therapy in cellulitis has not become routine. It has been proposed (with some evidence) that NSAID therapy in treatment of cellulitis may be associated with increased risk of developing a severe life-threatening necrotizing fasciitis.

Long-term complications

- Most people have no long-term problems after successful treatment.

- 10% of hospitalized patients may suffer from persistent leg swelling and venous ulceration.
- Recurrent cellulitis; evidence suggests the risk is about:
  - 10% at 1 year
  - 30% at 3 years.

Antibiotics for the Treatment of Cellulitis at Home – PATCH I and PATCH II studies suggest a probable benefit from low dose prophylactic penicillin V therapy for those patients with recurrent (PATCH I) and a first episode (PATCH II) of cellulitis.

Lipodermatosclerosis

This condition can be mistaken for cellulitis and is sometimes referred to as 'cellulitis refractory to treatment'. It is characterized by

- Unilateral or bilateral severe pain localised to the lower third (especially medially) of the leg.
- Accompanying erythema with a burning sensation and localised tenderness.
- Absence of pyrexia with no systemic evidence of cellulitis and normal CRP and white cell count.
- Patients are commonly obese with a history of varicose eczema.

The aetiology is poorly understood but is thought to relate to venous hypertension (raised pressure in the leg veins), venous incompetence (leaky valves) and obesity. The acute inflammatory stage of lipodermatosclerosis can occur before there are obvious signs of venous disease. It may progress over months/years to extensive fibrosis or sclerosis (scarring) in the skin and subcutaneous tissue.

Necrotizing fasciitis

Necrotizing fasciitis is a rare bacterial infection of the soft tissue and fascia that usually follows a break in the skin. It can affect previously healthy patients but is more common in intravenous drug users. It is caused by various organisms including the group A streptococcus which is associated with a particularly severe form of necrotizing fasciitis. It may be due to infection with gas-forming organisms. There are an estimated 500 cases of necrotizing fasciitis per year in the UK, with around 70–100 caused by group A streptococci.

It can be distinguished from cellulitis by:

- pain with marked local tenderness and swelling that appears disproportionate to the injury
- rapid progression of skin changes

- erythema
- large dark blotches, that will turn into blisters and fill up with fluid
- a mottled, flaky appearance at the trauma site, as underlying tissue undergoes necrosis +/– crepitus if due to gas-forming organisms

- marked systemic upset with diarrhoea, vomiting and signs of severe sepsis.

But:

- The presenting signs of necrotizing fasciitis can be non-specific and may resemble cellulitis.
- Always consider the diagnosis and if you suspect the diagnosis get a senior to review immediately – this is a major emergency and there is no time to lose!

The Laboratory Risk Indicator for Necrotizing Fasciitis (LRINEC) score [6] can be calculated to risk stratify patients presenting with cellulitis to help identify those patients with necrotizing fasciitis using CRP, WBC, haemoglobin, sodium, creatinine and glucose. A score greater than 6 has a positive predictive value of 92.0% and negative predictive value of 96%. An online calculator is available at www.mdcalc.com/lrinec-score-for-necrotizing-soft-tissue-infection/.

References

1. Venous thromboembolic diseases: the management of venous thromboembolic diseases and the role of thrombophilia testing, Clinical Guideline 144. Published by the National Institute for Health and Care Excellence. Available as a download at www.nice.org.uk/nicemedia/live/13767/59711/59711.pdf.

2. Wells PS, Anderson DR, Rodger M, Forgie M, Kearon C, Dreyer JD, Kovacs G, Mitchell M, Lewandowski B, Kovacs MJ (2003) Evaluation of D-dimer in the diagnosis of deep vein thrombosis. *N Engl J Med* 349: 1227–1235.

3. CREST guidelines. Available at www.crestni.org.uk/publications/cellulitis.html.

4. Eron LJ (2000) Infections of skin and soft tissues: outcome of a classification scheme. *Clin Infect Dis* 31: 287.

5. Kilburn SA et al., for the Cochrane Collaboration (2010) Interventions for cellulitis and erysipelas (Review). Published by John Wiley and Sons. Available as a download at http://onlinelibrary.wiley.com/doi/10.1002/14651858.CD004299.pub2/pdf.

6. Wong CH, Khin LW, Heng KS, Tan KC and Low CO (2004) The LRINEC (Laboratory Risk Indicator for Necrotizing Fasciitis) score: a tool for distinguishing necrotizing fasciitis from other soft tissue infections. *Crit Care Med* 32(7): 1535–1541.

Further reading

Keller EC, et al. (2012) Distinguishing cellulitis from its mimics. *Cleve Clin J Med* 79(8): 542–552. Available as a download at www.ccjm.org/content/79/8/547.long.

Puvanendran R, et al. (2009) Necrotizing fasciitis. *Can Fam Physician* 55(10): 981–987. Available as a download at www.cfp.ca/content/55/10/981.long.

Chapter 39

Loin pain

Duncan Whitehead and Stephen Haydock

Introduction

Loin pain is a common presentation to both primary and secondary care with a wide differential diagnosis. Patients are usually referred to the medical team when the diagnosis is suspected to be acute pyelonephritis. The differential diagnosis of flank or loin pain is best thought of based on where the pain originates:

- *Kidneys and ureters*
  - urinary tract infection
  - pyelonephritis
  - renal calculus
  - clot colic
  - papillary necrosis
  - renal infarction
  - renal vein thrombosis
  - renal abscess
  - renal tumours
  - loin pain haematuria syndrome
  - pelviureteric junction obstruction
  - polycystic kidney disease
  - Page kidney (subcapsular perinephric bleed, compressing the renal parenchyma)
- *Abdominal wall*
  - muscular pain
  - rib pain
  - radiculopathy
  - herpes zoster
- *Chest pathology causing pleural irritation*
  - pneumonia
  - pulmonary embolism
- *Other upper abdominal pathology*

- abdominal aortic aneurysm (dissection or rupture)
- retroperitoneal haemorrhage
- retroperitoneal fibrosis
- cholecystitis
- diverticulitis
- *Gynaecological problems*
  - ectopic pregnancy
  - endometriosis
  - pelvic inflammatory disease
  - rupture/torsion of an ovarian cyst.

This list is far from exhaustive, but includes *the common and serious causes*.

Flank pain due to urinary tract pathology is generally due to an acute stretching of the renal pelvis or capsule or distension of the ureter; these tissues have significant sensory innervation compared to the renal parenchyma. The more rapid the distension, the more severe the resulting pain.

Sudden ureteric distension caused by passage of a calculus makes this one of the most severe acute pains one can experience, often leaving the patient writhing in extreme discomfort; contrasting with the patient who has a longstanding severely dilated hydronephrotic kidney when the slow progressive distension is commonly painless.

> **Scenario 39.1**
>
> *A 30-year-old woman is referred by the emergency department with right-sided abdominal pain. She has been unwell for 24 hours with fever, rigors, nausea and vomiting. On examination she is pyrexial at 39°C and has pain and tenderness in the right flank, particularly on bimanual palpation. Bloods show a leucocytosis and significantly elevated CRP.*

Acute Medicine, ed. Stephen Haydock, Duncan Whitehead and Zoë Fritz. Published by Cambridge University Press. © Cambridge University Press 2015.

History

A full history is required as for any patient presenting with an acute pain syndrome. Regarding loin pain you should obtain and document the following information:

- Speed of onset, quality, duration, location and radiation of the pain including relieving and aggravating factors.
- Associated features of infection such as fever and rigors.
- Presence of dysuria, polyuria or suprapubic pain.
- History of visible haematuria.
- History of the following risk factors for lower urinary tract infections to ascend and involve the renal parenchyma (which complicate management/response to treatment):
  - previous pyelonephritis
  - renal calculi
  - vesicoureteral reflux
  - congenital anomalies of the urinary tract
  - known single kidney
  - altered bladder function
  - diabetes mellitus.
- Any bleeding disorder or anticoagulation increases the risk of spontaneous bleeding into the kidney or retroperitoneum.
- Pre-existing prothrombotic condition increasing the risk of renal infarction or renal vein thrombosis.
- Excessive fluid intake within a short duration, possibly precipitating uretero-pelvic junction obstruction?
- Family history including of renal calculi and ADPCKD.
- Drug history noting in particular:
  - analgesics (paracetamol, NSAIDs and aspirin) – might suggest papillary necrosis
  - bromocriptine, beta-blockers, methysergide and methyldopa (all associated with retroperitoneal fibrosis)
  - anticoagulant drugs (as above).

Examination

In a patient with loin pain perform a complete examination; during the abdominal component:

- Consider the possibility of pain due to an abdominal aortic aneurysm, especially if the patient is over 50 years old or has vascular risk factors; AAAs are easily missed.
- Renal pain may cause localized tenderness in the costovertebral angle, lateral to the sacrospinalis muscle, below the twelfth rib. Percuss this area with the fist.
- Enlarged kidneys are palpated by bimanual ballotment; a palpable and/or tender kidney is abnormal, although the right kidney may be felt in thin individuals.

Investigation

In all patients with loin pain include:

- urinalysis
- urine culture
- full blood count
- urea and electrolytes
- liver function tests
- CRP.

Patients with loin pain have a significant risk of associated AKI so alongside baseline creatinine in unwell patients commence a fluid balance chart on admission; oliguria often occurs before a creatinine rise.

If the history suggests renal colic include:

- calcium
- urate.

If the history includes infective features or pyrexia is present include:

- blood cultures.

In all female patients of childbearing age include:

- beta-HCG.

Radiological imaging

KUB plain radiograph may identify calcium-containing stones (85% of stones) but uric acid, cysteine and indinavir-induced stones are radiolucent. It is a useful adjunct to more complex imaging modalities and can be used to track the passage of a calculus. False positives may result from calcification in close proximity to the ureters. False negatives arise with radiolucent stones and small stones obscured by gas, faeces or bone.

Ultrasonography is a readily available, inexpensive modality without radiation or contrast exposure; it is therefore the imaging modality of choice in pregnancy. It is useful in patients with loin pain as it can identify abdominal aortic aneurysms and free intra-abdominal fluid. Pyelonephritis can be identified but mild changes may be missed, and disease severity and perinephric extension may be underestimated. A renal tumour or abscess can be identified as can hydronephrosis and ureteric dilatation. It has limitations in detection of small stones in the distal ureter.

Intravenous urography (IVU) was the traditional investigation for loin pain. It can identify: factors predisposing to developing ascending infection of the kidney (congenital abnormalities of the urinary tract); factors that can delay response to treatment (urinary tract obstruction); and abscess formation (renal or perinephric). Ureteric calculi are detected directly in 40–60% cases, and can be inferred from tract dilatation to detect 80–90% of all calculi. It does not identify renal inflammation and carries the risk of contrast administration. An IVU examination results in 1.5 mSv radiation exposure.

CTKUB is the most sensitive and useful imaging modality in patients with loin pain. It is an unenhanced scan, so carries no intravenous contrast risk. It is more sensitive than ultrasound in diagnosing inflammatory changes in the kidney and provides useful anatomical and diagnostic information on other abdominal structures. It is more specific (97%) and sensitive (100%) than IVU in detecting of ureteric stones. It takes minutes to perform compared to several hours for an IVU. Conventional CTKUB results in 4.7 mSv radiation exposure. Ultra low dose CT reduces the radiation exposure to less than an IVU but is significantly worse in detection of small ureteric stones (<3 mm). Contrast-enhanced CT has similar sensitivity and specificity to conventional CTKUB with the same radiation exposure as IVU and the risks of contrast exposure.

Magnetic resonance imaging techniques may be used when further imaging is required during pregnancy.

Iodinated contrast risk

- *Contrast-induced nephropathy* is defined as a creatinine rise of 44 µmol/L from baseline within 72 hours of administering IV contrast [1], incidence ≈1–2%. Risk factors include:
  - volume of contrast
  - intra-arterial administration
  - AKI risk factors (see Chapter 6).
- *Allergic reactions* are rare with modern non-ionic iodinated contrast agents [2], incidence of severe reaction ≈0.04%. Risk factors include:
  - previous contrast reaction

- clear history of multiple allergies or a very severe allergy (*shellfish or topical iodine allergy confers no greater risk than other allergies*)
  - asthma (six-fold increase in risk of adverse reaction)
- *Metformin*: there is a theoretical increased risk of lactic acidosis (but lack of evidence base); however, the Royal College of Radiology [2] advises:
  - no requirement to stop metformin if creatinine in the normal range and eGFR >60 mL/min
  - in those with a raised creatinine or eGFR <60 mL/min consider (risk vs. benefit of) stopping it for 48 hours.

Differentiating loin pain

In patients presenting with acute loin pain:

- *In the absence of fever* the likely diagnosis is *renal colic.*
- *In the presence of fever, pyelonephritis* is the probable diagnosis.
- Ureteric obstruction due to stone or other cause predisposes to ascending infection so both conditions may coexist.

Renal colic

- Acute onset of severe flank pain; surprisingly it is most commonly constant in nature.
- Pain may radiate to groin and testes in males and labia in females.
- Patients are restless, *unable to obtain a comfortable position.*
- Half of patients have associated nausea and vomiting.
- Urinary frequency and dysuria can occur if a stone lodges distally.
- Lifetime risk of renal calculi is 10–15% in developed countries
- Male preponderance, prevalence ♂4:1♀.

Pathophysiology of renal stone disease [3]

- The most important risk factor is a concentrated urine; this can result from many causes of note:
  - dehydration
  - hypercalcaemia (caused by hyperparathyroidism or sarcoidosis, for example)

- hyperglycaemia
- gout
- high salt (Western) diet
- high protein diet
- hot climate.
- Most stones are of mixed composition although predominantly calcium oxalate.
- Every solutes' solubility is affected by many variables; of note regarding the urine are:
  - pH
  - concentration of other species (the common ion effect).
- If a solute becomes supersaturated, salts are precipitated out which can form a nidus for stone formation.
- Advise to reduce future risk:
  - high fluid intake (2.5–3 litres per day)
  - neutral pH beverages (*Cola pH* ≈ 2.5)
  - low salt diet (<5 g per day).
- High risk or recurrent stone formers require formal specialist assessment by either urologist or nephrologist depending on local arrangements.

Pyelonephritis

- Pain is less severe than for renal colic and often a dull ache.
- Flank and costovertebral angle *tenderness* is characteristically more severe than with renal colic.
- Fever and rigors are common.
- Nausea and vomiting are common.
- Patients tend to lie motionless, contrasting with the restless behaviour of those with renal colic.
- Suprapubic pain with urgency, dysuria and urinary frequency are commonly seen but can occur in renal colic.

Pathophysiology of pyelonephritis

- Infection within the renal pelvis and parenchyma, usually resulting from ascending infection from the lower urinary tract, therefore much more common in women.
- 80% of infections are due to *E. coli*; other pathogens include *Proteus*, *Klebsiella*, *Staphylococcus* and *Pseudomonas*.

- Inadequate or inappropriate treatment can result in an acute renal abscess that may rupture into the perinephric space forming a perirenal abscess.

Management

Any patient in pain should be offered and administered appropriate analgesia as soon as possible; the doctor who leaves their patient suffering while asking about the home situation has become confused about the key priorities!

- Severe pain may require steady titration of intravenous morphine to comfort for rapid adequate pain control, while slower acting oral preparations take effect.
- Ensure adequate analgesia with paracetamol and opioids according to response.
- See Chapter 6 for safe prescribing of analgesia in those who have AKI or CKD.

Pyelonephritis

- Systemically unwell patients require resuscitation with early administration of intravenous fluids and parenteral antibiotics (severe pyelonephritis).
- European Association of Urology (EAU) [4] recommends IV co-amoxiclav +/– gentamicin *or* cephalosporin *or* carbapenem (consult local antimicrobial guidelines) for severe or complicated pyelonephritis.
- Uncomplicated, non-severe pyelonephritis can be treated with *7–10 days of ciprofloxacin or co-amoxiclav* as recommended by the EAU (consult local antimicrobial guidelines).
- Patients requiring parenteral antimicrobials can be switched to oral therapy within 72 hours when pyrexia settles, according to culture sensitivities, to complete 10–14 days.
- Uncomplicated pyelonephritis typically shows improvement within 48–72 hours of commencing an appropriate antibiotic.
- The ease, availability, low cost and absence of radiation exposure has led to the generally accepted practice of early ultrasound imaging for *all patients* with suspected pyelonephritis.
- The clinical presentation of renal colic associated with a significant pyrexia (>38°C) is an indication for *urgent CTKUB*.
- Early CTKUB imaging should be considered for pyelonephritis when complications are more likely:

- very unwell
- history of flank pain suggestive of renal colic in the days prior to admission
- known renal tract abnormality (e.g. single kidney)
- male
- diabetes mellitus.
- If the patient fails to respond to appropriate antimicrobial therapy (confirmed by culture sensitivities) within 72 hours, a CTKUB should be performed to:
  - definitively exclude obstruction
  - rule out pyonephrosis or perinephric abscess
  - exclude emphysematous pyelonephritis.
- Young female patients who are not systemically unwell can generally be managed on an outpatient basis.

Pyelonephritis with ureteric obstruction

- Maintain a high degree of suspicion: effective treatment requires early identification, with *ultrasound within 6 hours* of assessment (NICE Clinical Guideline 169, on AKI) or CTKUB if available.
- Parenteral antibiotics as for complicated pyelonephritis.
- Obstruction prevents adequate antibiotic penetration and is very unlikely to resolve with antibiotics alone.
- Increased risk of renal and perinephric abscess formation.
- Urgent urological referral for specialist management, commonly with percutaneous nephrostomy.
- Without prompt drainage alongside appropriate antibiotic treatment *patients can rapidly develop septic shock and die* from what is often treatable sepsis.

Renal colic

- Appropriate analgesia is important; evidence suggests that non-steroidal anti-inflammatory drugs are highly effective. Diclofenac suppositories or IM/IV provide good analgesia (once AKI and CKD has been excluded). Oral analgesia according to the WHO analgesic ladder can be added.

- CTKUB is the investigation of choice and should be performed as soon as possible; if not immediately available (out of hours) it can wait until the next day. Patients over 50 years old should have urgent ultrasound imaging if CTKUB is delayed, to exclude aortic aneurysm and other significant pathology.
- Patients may be discharged home if all the following apply:
  - ureteric calculus confirmed on CTKUB
  - minimal evidence of obstruction
  - stone is near bladder
  - normal renal function
  - no evidence of infection
  - pain is adequately controlled.
- Advise to return urgently if symptoms deteriorate.
- They should be followed up by urology.
- Admission is indicated for patients who are systemically unwell with sepsis or if pregnant, elderly or suffering from co-morbidities that may complicate management (e.g. diabetes, immunosuppression).
- Alpha-1-blockers such as tamsulosin increase the probability of stone passage.
- Most stones that will be passed naturally do so by 4 weeks.

Other causes of acute loin pain

Acute papillary necrosis

- Results from acute ischaemic necrosis of the renal papilla.
- Mimics renal colic/pyelonephritis with loin pain, pyrexia, haematuria +/− slough in urine.
- Several aetiologies:
  - pyelonephritis
  - obstruction
  - sickle cell disease
  - tuberculosis
  - chronic liver disease
  - abuse of analgesics or alcohol
  - renal transplant rejection
  - diabetes mellitus
  - systemic vasculitis.
- May result in ureteric obstruction and secondary infection.

- Characteristic appearance of renal pelvis filling defect on IVU or CTKUB.
- Requires treatment of underlying condition and bypassing of obstruction.

Pelviureteric junction obstruction

- Produces similar pain to renal colic.
- Usually following the ingestion of large fluid volumes *(an evening in the pub!)* causing a marked diuresis and subsequent acute dilatation of the renal pelvis and colicky pain.
- Diagnosis is confirmed by diuretic-enhanced nuclear medicine imaging or diuretic-enhanced IVU.
- May require surgical relief of obstruction.

Polycystic kidney disease

- Flank, abdomen or back pain is commonly due to:
  - haemorrhage into a cyst
  - gross cystic enlargement
  - infection of cyst
  - associated stone formation.

Loin pain requires a methodical assessment to clarify the diagnosis, which may be benign muscular pain or a life-threatening condition requiring urgent management to ensure a successful outcome for your patient.

Urgent involvement of surgical colleagues may be required depending on initial findings and investigation results.

References

1. Royal College of Radiology website: Prevention of contrast induced acute kidney injury (CI-AKI) in adult patients. www.rcr.ac.uk/docs/radiology/pdf/2013_RA_BCIS_RCR.pdf.

2. Royal College of Radiology website: Standards for IV contrast agent administration to adult patients, second edition. www.rcr.ac.uk/docs/radiology/pdf/BFCR(10)4_Stand_contrast.pdf.

3. European Association of Urology online guidelines: Guidelines on Urolithiasis. www.uroweb.org/gls/pockets/english/22%20Urolithiasis_LR.pdf.

4. European Association of Urology online guidelines: Guidelines on Urological Infections. www.uroweb.org/gls/pdf/18_Urological%20infections_LR.pdf.

Chapter

40

Lymphadenopathy

Deepak Mannari

Introduction

Lymphadenopathy is a frequent presentation to both primary and secondary care. The ability to correctly assess, examine, arrange appropriate investigations and obtain a suitable differential diagnosis is vitally important. Patients are often anxious, particularly regarding the diagnosis of 'cancer', and a confident assessment with appropriate reassurance or prompt referral and empathy are key to a good consultation. In addition, the ability not to misdiagnose or miss a communicable disease plays an important role in public health surveillance.

Anatomy and physiology of the lymphatic system

A basic understanding of the anatomy and physiology of the lymphatic system is helpful although detailed anatomy is unnecessary.

The functions of the lymphatic system include:

- reabsorbing interstitial fluid
- transporting fatty acids
- transporting white cells to lymphoid organs.

It performs these functions through a highly organized, extensive open system running in conjunction with the vasculature and eventually drains into the thoracic ducts and subsequently into the subclavian veins.

Lymphocytes develop and mature in the primary lymphoid organs.

- B-lymphocytes complete the whole process in the bone marrow.
- T-cells undergo further maturation in the thymus.

The highly organized processes involved in adaptive immunity take place in the secondary lymphoid structures:

- lymph nodes
- organized lymphoid follicles found in tonsils, spleen, intestines, etc.

Superficial lymph nodes are accessible to physical examination whilst deeper intrathoracic and intra-abdominal nodes require further investigations.

- The cervical lymph nodes drain the scalp, skin, oral cavity, larynx and neck.
- Supraclavicular lymph nodes drain the gastrointestinal tract, genitourinary tract and the lungs.
- Axillary nodes drain the upper extremities, breast and thorax.
- Epitrochlear lymph nodes drain the ulna, forearm and hand.
- Inguinal lymph nodes drain the lower abdomen, external genitalia (skin), anal canal, lower third of the vagina and lower extremities.

> **Scenario 40.1**
>
> *You are contacted by the GP of a 35-year-old man. He has been unwell for several weeks with a low-grade fever, malaise and weight loss. Examination has revealed supraclavicular lymphadenopathy. His GP wants advice on further investigation and management. The patient is extremely anxious and concerned that this could be cancer.*

Clinical approach

As in all assessments, a clear logical framework using the history, examination and investigations to guide the process offers a great deal of success.

The initial history volunteered by the patient may give significant clues and is often sufficient to yield a diagnosis.

Is the lymphadenopathy *generalized* or *localized*?

Acute Medicine, ed. Stephen Haydock, Duncan Whitehead and Zoë Fritz. Published by Cambridge University Press. © Cambridge University Press 2015.

Localized lymph nodes

Examine the lymph node, to define its size, mobility and consistency, followed by the regional area.

- If a diagnosis can be made on the history and examination then further testing is often not required. Treatment can be initiated and follow-up arranged.
- If on initial assessment there is no overt pathology and the lymphadenopathy is very small (<10 mm) then reassurance is often all that is required. An appropriate follow-up at 1 month is recommended for most cases.
- Further investigations are likely to be required for persistent, unexplained lymph nodes larger than 10 mm, where significant pathology or malignancy is not excluded.

Generalized lymphadenopathy

Usually requires further investigation.

Causes of generalized lymphadenopathy

Some of the common causes are listed below but this is not exhaustive. A sensible approach paying attention to common causes at specific regions is less daunting and may yield more results. In general practice infections are by far the commonest cause of lymphadenopathy; it is also worthwhile noting that malignant causes are less frequent than infective causes, even at referral centres.

Infective

- Bacterial:
  - tuberculosis (TB)
  - lymphogranuloma venereum (LGV (*Chlamydia*))
  - cat scratch fever (*Bartonella*)
  - typhoid fever
- Viral:
  - HIV/AIDS
  - infectious mononucleosis (Epstein–Barr virus (EBV))
  - Rubella
- Fungal
- Protozoal
- Toxoplasmosis

Neoplastic

- Metastatic malignancy
- Haematological malignancy

Others

- Sarcoidosis
- Amyloidosis
- Drugs
- Immune – lupus, hypothyroidism
- For cervical lymphadenopathy consider local oral infections, TB, head and neck and thyroid cancers and lymphoma. Other causes of masses in the neck such as cysts, salivary glands and thyroid goitres should also be considered.
- Supraclavicular lymph nodes should raise the suspicion of malignancies including lymphomas, bronchogenic and breast carcinomas and abdominal neoplasms (Virchow's node/ Troisier's sign)
- For axillary lymphadenopathy consider local infections including cat scratch disease or streptococcal/staphylococcal skin infection or metastatic breast carcinoma.
- Inguinal lymphadenopathy although often a normal finding is associated with STDs, and venereal disease including LGV should be considered. Other causes include cellulitis and squamous cell carcinoma (metastatic from the penile or vulvar regions).
- Splenomegaly may be associated with lymphadenopathy especially with lymphomas, but may also be seen with EBV, TB, HIV and collagen vascular disease.

History

Often the patient will volunteer diagnostic information. Some aspects to look for in the patient's history are highlighted below but very few are specific and a broad approach is required.

1. Age. Although certain types of malignancies and lymphomas can be more common in younger patients, overall this is uncommon and a young patient is much more likely to present with infection rather than malignancy.

2. Duration. An acute lymphadenitis is of brief duration and usually due to infection/inflammation. In contrast chronic lymphadenopathy can be indicative of chronic infection such as TB, underlying malignancy or collagen vascular disease.

3. Pain. This can be a feature of acute or chronic lymphadenitis but is very rarely a feature of carcinoma or lymphoma. In Hodgkin's lymphoma the onset of pain in the lymph node with the ingestion of alcohol is an infrequent symptom but virtually pathognomonic when it does occur.

4. Associated symptoms. B symptoms: at least one of a triad of symptoms which may be presenting features in lymphoma and are important as part of disease staging.

- Fever greater than 38°C which is often a periodic fever; if associated with Hodgkin's lymphoma it is referred to as a Pel–Ebstein fever.
- Unexplained weight loss of greater than 10% of body weight over 6 months.
- Drenching night sweats.

However, these symptoms can also be found in patients with infections and metastatic malignancy.

Symptoms of infection: especially with regard to localized lymphadenopathy including:

- pharyngitis
- conjunctivitis
- skin ulceration
- localized tenderness
- genital sores or discharge.

Symptoms of metastatic malignancy: constitutional symptoms of malignancy such as:

- weight loss
- localized symptoms according to site of malignancy such as dysphagia, hoarse voice, haemoptysis, etc.

Symptoms of collagen vascular disease: arthralgias, rash and myalgias.

5. Epidemiological clues. Travel history, exposure to pets, occupational exposures or high risk behaviours may suggest specific disorders and need to be specifically queried.

6. Medication history. Drug hypersensitivity (e.g. phenytoin), although often overlooked, can cause lymphadenopathy.

7. Family history. This is particularly helpful regarding malignancies especially breast cancer. In addition, anxiety regarding a family history of cancer may well be the underlying reason for the presentation with patients looking for reassurance.

Examination

The 'lymph node system' is rarely tested or taught at undergraduate level but a good technique not only prevents missing pathology but greatly speeds up the process and gives confidence to be able to reassure the patient that no significant pathology is present.

Examination should include the following:

- Checking oropharynx, cervical chains, axillary, epitrochlear and inguinal lymph nodes.
- Hepatosplenomegaly.
- Breast examination should always be considered and performed in an appropriate and sensitive manner with a chaperone.

Important physical examination findings include:

- lymph node size
- consistency
- mobility
- distribution.

Once again while generalizations are useful in forming a differential diagnosis; there are no specific criteria.

1. Size. Generally lymph nodes are deemed to be clinically insignificant if less than 10 mm and often reassurance is sufficient. In slim individuals, normal small nodes may be easily appreciable, particularly in the cervical regions. In contrast, lymph nodes greater than 20 mm suggest pathology. However, normal inguinal lymph nodes may be as large as 20 mm.

2. Consistency. In general hard nodes are seen more commonly with malignancies; tender nodes often suggest an inflammatory disorder; rubbery or firm nodes are associated with lymphomas. Once again, whilst helpful, these generalizations should not be used to distinguish between malignant and benign aetiologies.

3. Mobility. Fixed or matted nodes suggest metastatic carcinoma, whereas mobile nodes may occur in infections, collagen vascular disease and lymphoma.

4. Distribution. As discussed previously, differentiation between systemic and localized lymphadenopathy is very useful.

- In most cases, generalized lymphadenopathy is a sign of systemic disease.
- Enlarged supraclavicular nodes raise a strong suspicion for malignancy. Specifically, Virchow's node (pathological enlargement of left supraclavicular lymph node) is associated with the presence of an abdominal or thoracic neoplasm.
- Epitrochlear lymphadenopathy is a rare finding in healthy people.
- By contrast, inguinal lymph nodes may occasionally be enlarged in healthy individuals. In addition, biopsy of inguinal lymph nodes offers the lowest diagnostic yield.

- The finding of lymphadenopathy with hepatosplenomegaly is highly suspicious for lymphoma.

Investigations

If the history and physical examination suggest a diagnosis, further testing may not be necessary or appropriate; focused testing may confirm the diagnosis promptly. Where the diagnosis is not apparent the initial tests to perform should include:

- full blood count (FBC) with differential and blood film
- EBV serology and Monospot test.
  If this is not diagnostic consider the following tests:
- inflammatory markers (ESR/CRP)
- liver function tests
- blood cultures
- throat swab for culture
- chest X-ray
- TB testing (sputum, early morning urine)
- serum ACE, which may be elevated in active sarcoidosis
- anti-nuclear antibody (ANA)
- syphilis serology (VDRL)
- hepatitis serology (hepatitis B surface antigen)
- HIV serology.

It is important to ensure that appropriate informed consent has been obtained prior to the latter three tests.

Further assessments are listed below and include:

- ultrasound (US) scan
- computed tomography (CT) scan of chest, abdomen and pelvis
- mammography
- bone marrow biopsy
- fine needle aspiration (FNA)
- core biopsy
- excision biopsy.

Consultation with senior colleagues or referral to specialist services should be performed prior to requesting these latter tests. Often many of these cases will be discussed at an appropriate multidisciplinary team (MDT) meeting. The MDT can provide an expert opinion on the most timely and appropriate further investigations as well as providing initial treatment plans.

- A US scan is particularly useful in investigation of focal lymphadenopathy, providing a quick, cheap and non-invasive assessment. As well as confirming that lumps are lymph nodes and measuring their sizes, US is able to detect the presence of focal nodal necrosis, an excellent indicator of likely pathology.
- A CT scan is more useful in the presence of generalized lymphadenopathy and particularly if a diagnosis of lymphoma is suspected.

If a CT scan is not rapidly available, US scan with a diagnostic biopsy may enable a more timely diagnosis.

Fine needle aspiration

There are many advantages of performing FNA:

- Minimally invasive.
- Quick.
- Cheap.
- Can be performed in outpatients.
- Low risk of complications, although rarely vascular and nerve injuries can occur.
- Samples can be sent for full microbiological analysis including ZN stain and for flow cytometry.
- Can confirm that a mass is a lymph node and differentiate between neoplastic and non-neoplastic, lymphoid and metastatic disease and specific and non-specific infection.

However, there are drawbacks with the use of FNA:

- Quality of the sample can vary and is operator dependent. As it is a small sample it may be unsuitable for heterogeneous masses where a diagnosis may be missed due to sampling error.
- FNAs should be performed on supraclavicular or cervical lymph nodes and not axillary or inguinal where the yield is low.
- FNAs do not provide information on lymph node architecture, essential for accurate lymphoma diagnosis. As this is likely to result in diagnostic and treatment delays for lymphoma patients, FNAs should not be performed in cases with a strong suspicion of lymphoma; rather a core or preferably an excision biopsy should be performed in the first instance.

High-grade lymphomas are potentially highly curable if diagnosed and treated in a timely manner. Great efforts should be made to obtain an adequate tissue biopsy as early as possible. Again, due to the excellent prospects with therapy for many subtypes, lymphoma should be considered even in atypical cases. For example, where there has been a high clinical suspicion of TB causing lymphadenopathy but cultures are non-confirmatory, a biopsy of the nodes should be sought.

Whilst a diagnosis of adenocarcinoma or differentiated squamous cell carcinoma can be made on an FNA sample, it is imperative to obtain a tissue sample for the diagnosis and grading of Hodgkin's and non-Hodgkin's lymphoma. Excision node biopsies are preferred to Trucut samples as the architecture of the intact node is easily assessed and there is no sampling error. However, a core biopsy under radiological guidance may be the most practical option when nodes are not easily accessible, for example in patients with retroperitoneal lymphadenopathy.

Biopsies should be obtained from the largest or most abnormal lymph node site, preferably avoiding inguinal nodes due to lower diagnostic yield. It is vitally important that empirical corticosteroid therapy is avoided prior to biopsy as it may confound the results due to a lympholytic effect. For patients in whom suspicion for an underlying malignancy is high, an unrevealing lymph node biopsy or one with atypical lymphoid hyperplasia should be considered non-diagnostic rather than negative for malignancy, and further work-up including re-biopsy pursued.

Referral guidelines

NICE guidelines have been produced to guide appropriate referral for suspected malignancy [1]. Referral may be considered if at least one of the following lymph node features is present:

- non-tender nodes of firm or hard consistency
- greater than 20 mm in size
- progressively enlarging lymph nodes
- features of ill health such as weight loss
- presence of axillary nodes (in the absence of local infections)
- presence of supraclavicular nodes
- persistent lymphadenopathy for more than 6 weeks.

Guidelines on communicable diseases

Notification of infectious diseases in England and Wales has been a statutory requirement for nearly 100 years [2], providing key surveillance data as well as prompt early intervention to prevent and control the spread of disease. Although not without its drawbacks, comprehensive data is available for many diseases. The most important of these that cause lymphadenopathy is tuberculosis although other diseases that may present with lymphadenopathy include rubella, mumps, measles and typhoid.

Mycobacterial infections

The commonest form of extrapulmonary tuberculosis is tubercular cervical lymphadenitis [3] (scrofula). This commonly presents as unilateral painless matted cervical adenopathy most commonly in the posterior triangle. Ziehl–Neelsen (ZN) staining with material obtained from FNA is a simple and cost-effective investigation. An early diagnosis is readily obtained, allowing initiation of treatment prior to a final diagnosis by biopsy and culture or molecular testing by PCR.

HIV

Lymphadenopathy in a patient with HIV causes unique diagnostic difficulties [4]. It is common in most stages of the disease from early seroconversion adenopathy to end-stage disease. Benign causes need to be differentiated from serious pathology.

Persistent generalized lymphadenopathy (PGL) is a reactive follicular hyperplasia from chronic HIV infection and is very common. However, as HIV is a risk factor for infections and malignancy, lymphadenopathy cannot be presumed to be due to PGL. In non-TB endemic regions, malignancy appears to be more common than infections.

When assessing these patients, the approach outlined in this chapter still applies and the same investigative clues need to be teased out with similar causes borne in mind. CD4 count and viral load should be performed in addition to the general screen outlined. Observation or a trial of antibiotics may be appropriate in some cases. FNA and biopsies should be obtained for more sinister symptoms after discussion with senior colleagues. Often the key assessment is in defining the most likely lymph node to yield a diagnosis. Generally the largest, most abnormal node, most recently changed and ideally not from the inguinal or axillary regions should be targeted.

Emergencies

Lymphadenopathy may cause significant complications from compression of adjacent structures and organs. In this context two medical emergencies need to be highlighted:

- Mediastinal lymphadenopathy can cause superior vena cava (SVC) obstruction.

- Masses in close relation to the spinal cord can lead to spinal cord compression (SCC).

Patients with lymphoma may present with impending SVC obstruction or neurological symptoms suggestive of SCC. The disease is very likely to be treatable and even curable, but therapy may need to be commenced within 24 hours to preserve life and neurological function. *Every effort should be made to obtain tissue* for diagnosis and accurate subtyping of the lymphoma, as this greatly affects the choice of best therapy. Once a tissue biopsy has been obtained, likely from several Trucut biopsies, steroid therapy can be started. This often rapidly eases compression of structures and definitive treatment can then await the histological diagnosis.

References

1. NICE Guidelines. Referral Guidelines for Suspected Cancers (CG27), June 2005.

2. McCormick A (1993) The notification of infectious diseases in England and Wales. *CDR Rev* 3(2): R19–24.

3. Bayazit YA, Bayazit N, Namiduru M. (2004) Mycobacterial cervical lymphadenitis. *ORL J Otorhinolaryngol Relat Spec* 66(5):275–280.

4. Jacobs W (2010) The problem of HIV-related lymphadenopathy. *CME* 28(8) 364–366.

Medical complications during acute illness and following surgical procedures

Zoë Fritz

Introduction

It comes as no surprise that surgical patients are just as likely as everyone else to get 'medical' problems and a medical registrar will spend a considerable part of his or her on-call shift dealing with them. As well as their usual baseline predisposition to illness, surgical patients have additional risks associated with:

- the surgical procedure
- immobility
- pain
- medications.

These can also result in atypical presentations of common medical problems.

There has been a move towards *proactive* regular medical reviews of surgical patients in addition to the current *reactive* medical review when something goes wrong. Many hospitals now have orthogeriatricians, and the possibility of acute medicine taking on the role of a 'hospitalist' looking after such patients has been suggested.

Particular factors in the surgical patient predisposing to medical illness

Blood loss

A lower haemoglobin means poorer tissue oxygenation causing increased risk of ischaemic events, in particular acute coronary syndrome and stroke.

How to minimize the risk:

- There is evidence from retrospective studies that patients with known ischaemic heart disease should have their haemoglobins kept above 100 g/L with transfusions.

- However, this has been questioned by other studies [1,2] and the general advice is to *treat according to physiological need rather than a targeted number*.

Pain

Pain causes changes in blood pressure, tachycardia and an elevated respiratory rate. The danger is that doctors seeing these abnormal physiological markers attribute them to pain alone, rather than looking for other causes. Patients compensating for pain (particularly intra-abdominal pain) may breathe more shallowly and thus be predisposed to hospital-acquired pneumonias.

How to minimize the risk:

- Ensure adequate pain relief by regular review.
- Emphasize to patients that we are not just being 'kind' wanting them to be pain free but it will lead to a faster recovery and fewer complications.
- Ask the physiotherapist to give deep breathing exercises to any patient whose breathing you think might be compromised by pain.

Medication

Opiates can cause respiratory depression, drowsiness and constipation. It is important to remember that some regular prescriptions may have been omitted preoperatively and there may be physiological withdrawal. Of note: remember to double regular steroids since anyone who is on long-term steroids will have a diminished 'stress reaction', and will therefore need pharmacological help. Alcohol withdrawal should always be considered in anyone with postoperative confusion. Consider how parkinsonian medications are being administered in the postoperative period.

How to minimize the risk:

Acute Medicine, ed. Stephen Haydock, Duncan Whitehead and Zoë Fritz. Published by Cambridge University Press.
© Cambridge University Press 2015.

- Tell patients common side effects of drugs, so that they are reported early.
- Prescribe laxatives alongside opiates.
- Monitor respiratory rate closely for anyone on opiates.
- Ensure that a co-lateral drug history is taken *with specific questions about steroids and Parkinson's medication*.

Infection

Both superficial and deep infections can occur. Intra-abdominal collections can present with swinging pyrexias. Remember that postoperative pyrexia is common due to the release of cytokines (interleukin-6 is thought to be particularly important), and so a fever and raised inflammatory markers immediately after surgery do not necessarily indicate a new infection.

How to minimize the risk:

- Surgeons strive to minimize infective complications with sterile technique and perioperative use of prophylactic antibiotics, both included in the World Health Organization's 'Surgical Checklist' [3]. Check temperatures and inflammatory markers regularly, and be particularly alert to a change in trend.

Hypoalbuminaemia

Surgery is planned trauma, and the body responds accordingly with an acute phase response; CRP rises and albumin falls (possibly further diminished by capillary leak). Hypoalbuminaemia can lead to oedema and delays in mobility, and puts patients at heightened risk of infection.

How to minimize the risk:

- Albumin decreases are compounded in abdominal surgery, when absorption is decreased.
- Early referral to a dietitian is helpful.
- Studies show *parenteral albumin is ineffective*.

Hypothermia

Perioperative hypothermia is associated with worse surgical outcomes and is particularly common in those with combined regional and general anaesthesia.

How to minimize the risk: NICE Clinical Guideline 65 [4] suggests:

- simple measures (e.g. extra blankets)
- active external warming if temperature is below 36°C perioperatively (see Chapter 32).

Immobility

Patients are completely immobile during surgery. They also have reduced mobility in their recuperative phase, which puts them at higher risk for PE and DVT (an estimated 25 000 people die from preventable hospital-acquired venous thromboembolism per annum in the UK).

How to minimize the risk:

- All patients should be assessed for pharmacological or other prophylaxis, and indeed this has become a 'CQUIN' (Commissioning for Quality and Innovation), with hospitals needing to risk assess over 95% of their patients to receive their CQUIN payment. As a result, most hospitals have strict proformas for assessing the risks and benefits of starting one of
  - fondaparinux
  - low molecular weight heparin
  - unfractionated heparin for patients with renal failure.

Surgical thromboprophylaxis

Comprehensive guidance has been given in NICE Clinical Guideline 92 [5]. Thromboprophylaxis is recommended:

- If total anaesthetic + surgical time >90 minutes
- If surgery involves pelvis or lower limb and total anaesthetic + surgical time >60 minutes
- If acute surgical admission with inflammatory or intra-abdominal condition
- If expected to have significant reduction in mobility
- If any other VTE risk factor present:
  - active cancer or cancer treatment
  - age >60 years
  - critical care admission
  - dehydration
  - known thrombophilia
  - obesity (BMI >30 kg/m²)
  - one or more significant medical co-morbidities
  - personal history or first-degree relative with a history of VTE
  - use of HRT
  - use of oestrogen-containing contraceptive therapy
  - varicose veins (with phlebitis).

The risks of thromboembolism need to be balanced against the risks of bleeding. Patients who are at a higher bleeding risk (again from NICE guidance) are those with:

- active bleeding
- acquired bleeding disorders (such as acute liver failure)
- concurrent use of anticoagulants known to increase the risk of bleeding (such as warfarin with INR >2)
- lumbar puncture/epidural/spinal anaesthesia within the previous 4 hours or expected within the next 12 hours
- acute stroke
- thrombocytopenia (platelets $<75 \times 10^9/L$)
- uncontrolled hypertension ($\geq 230/120$ mmHg)
- untreated inherited bleeding disorders (such as haemophilia or von Willebrand's disease).

Treatment should be continued as long as the patient is immobile. Patients discharged home with pharmacological VTE prophylaxis should also be given written information about the signs and symptoms of DVT and PE and side effects of the drugs they are being given. NICE has published algorithms (www.nice.org.uk/nicemedia/live/12695/47197/47197.pdf) for initiation of pharmacological VTE and the duration required depending on surgical procedure and patient characteristics. In addition to prescribing pharmacological VTE prophylaxis, there are several other measures which are important to be aware of including:

- Keeping patients well hydrated at all times.
- Encouraging early mobilization.
- Stopping oestrogen-containing oral contraception or HRT one month before elective surgery.
- Stopping (or considering stopping) antiplatelet therapy one week before surgery. This decision needs to be balanced against risks and may require discussion with cardiology.

Assessing the sick surgical patient

As with any patient, follow ABC then history, examination, and review of documentation. However, there are certain elements to pay particular attention to, and these will be emphasized.

Initial assessment

Assess ABC and level of consciousness. If you are concerned about any of these, call for help: the outreach team if you think you will need an extra pair of hands stabilizing the patient (see peri-arrest section in Chapter 14) or the hospital arrest team if necessary.

If the patient is conscious and stable

Introduce yourself and explain that you have been asked to come and assess the patient's medical problems; you are going to look at their observation charts and notes, and then come back and ask them some detailed questions and examine them.

Ask them what their main problem is: their perspective may be different from what you have been told in the referral!

Look at the observation charts. Pay particular attention to:

- *Temperature*: remember 'postoperative' pyrexia is common. Look for a temperature which has fallen and is rising again, or a swinging pyrexia, suggesting an abdominal collection. A postoperative pyrexia may also be associated with a postoperative haematoma.
- *Respiratory rate*: opiates can cause respiratory depression, and a raised respiratory rate is an early indicator of hypovolaemia.
- *Urine output*: patients should be passing at least 0.5 mL/kg per hour; less than this may suggest either hypovolaemia or hypoperfusion (e.g. from sepsis).

Look at the notes. Check their:

- *Surgery*, and the date.
- *Anaesthetic chart* and any significant events, e.g. blood loss, hypoxia.
- *Past medical history*: in particular checking for cardio- and cerebrovascular disease, and previous gastric ulcers.
- *Past drug history*: check for steroid use.
- *Drug chart*: ensure prescribed antibiotics have been given (and not omitted due to lack of cannula). Check VTE prophylaxis has been considered, prescribed where appropriate, and given. Check for opiates, both prescription and use. Assess analgesia prescription and use.

Take a history: on systems review remember to ask questions particularly pertinent to their operation, e.g. *Since the operation have you…*

- Opened your bowels? Passed wind? Have you been eating? (considering ileus and mechanical obstruction)

- Have you had a catheter? Have you passed urine since it was taken out? Do you have any pain on passing urine? (considering urinary tract infections and bladder obstruction)
- Are you feeling breathless? Have you had a cough? Have you coughed up any blood? Have you had any chest pains? Have you been feeling dizzy? Have you had any palpitations? (considering MI, pneumonia, PE, arrhythmias).

Perform a full examination. In particular:

- Assess for fluid status: Are they under-filled?
- Ensure that they have good air entry in both lungs, and there are no signs of pneumonia or pneumothorax.
- Assess their abdomen.
- Look at the surgical site.
- Assess any drains, lines and catheters.
- Ensure not in retention.

Undertake appropriate investigations. Further general investigations should be carried out:

- *Basic blood tests*: U&Es, CRP, FBC and LFTs. It may be appropriate to also send blood cultures, troponin, group and save, magnesium and bone profile.
- *Arterial blood gas analysis* is an exceptionally helpful test in the sick patient; you will get a rapid haemoglobin, electrolytes and, importantly, lactate: high lactate can indicate hypoperfusion (either through impaired blood supply, e.g. in an infarct, hypovolaemia, or peripheral vasodilatation), and is a sensitive but non-specific marker of a patient being physiologically unwell.
- *A CXR*: if concerns about the breathing.
- *A 12-lead ECG*: looking for ischaemia and new AF.
- *Specific additional investigations*: where particular diagnoses are likely or need excluding, e.g. chest pain, fever, breathlessness, reduced consciousness, GI haemorrhage (see appropriate chapter).

Scenario 41.1

You are asked to see a 76-year-old woman who has become short of breath 3 days after a Hartmann's procedure. She had an uncomplicated procedure, with usual levels of blood loss, and her urinary catheter was removed 24 hours postoperatively. She has had some abdominal discomfort since surgery.

Initial assessment

On assessing ABC, you note a mildly elevated respiratory rate of 18, and a blood pressure on the low side of 110/70 and tachycardia of 120 beats per minute. She is conscious.

On direct questioning: her main symptoms are dizziness and breathlessness.

On review of her observation chart: she has been tachycardic (rate approx. 100) since day one after the operation.

On review of her drug card:

- She had her aspirin stopped one week before coming into hospital.
- She has been on VTE prophylaxis, which has been appropriately given.

On review of her medical record:

- She had an MI 3 years ago.
- Her tachycardia has been noted and has been ascribed to abdominal pain.
- Her last ECG was preoperatively and showed normal sinus rhythm.
- Her preoperative haemoglobin was 109 g/L; postoperatively it was 91 g/L.

On full history:

- Her 'abdominal pain' she describes as a 'pressure' and indicates to her sternum/epigastric area.
- She has had palpitations before, but has never seen a doctor; they have always lasted only a few minutes.
- The rest of the history confirms what you have gleaned from the notes.

On examination:

- She is clammy.
- Her pulse is 105.
- Heart sounds are normal.
- Breath sounds are vesicular.
- JVP is not raised.
- Her calves are soft, non-tender.

Problem list:

- Chest/abdominal pain
- Tachycardia
- Palpitations
- Dizziness
- Haemoglobin of 9.1.

Differential diagnosis:

- AF

- MI
- Anaemia
- Postoperative pain and dehydration.

  Investigations and interventions needed:
- Adequate analgesia (ensure pain free)
- Fluid balance chart (recatheterize if necessary)
- 12-lead ECG
- Blood tests: FBC, U&E, CRP, troponin, TFTs, clotting, cross match 2 units of blood.

Discussion

- If the ECG shows atrial fibrillation, the precipitant factors need to be treated. It may be caused by a combination of pain and dehydration, but MI, PE and infection need to be considered; a troponin, FBC and CRP should be sent.
- Although haemoglobin only dropped by 1.8 grams, this patient has known ischaemic heart disease and sternal pressure; whatever the cause of her AF, she should be transfused at least one unit. Her rate should be controlled; the normal choice would be a beta-blocker (bisoprolol 2.5 mg od) unless there are contraindications.
- You should call the surgical specialist registrar to discuss what you have found so far, and what you suggest in terms of management. If the patient has had an MI, a decision will need to be made as to whether to start her on fondaparinux or equivalent.

It is good practice to speak to the team in charge of any patient about any changes you have made in medication or management.

Scenario 41.2

An 82-year-old man has had hip surgery following a fractured neck of femur. He was previously fit and well, and living independently. He has not yet been able to mobilize (6 days postoperatively). You are asked to come and see him because of a tachycardia of 120 and a blood pressure of 90 systolic.

Initial assessment

ABC: the patient is maintaining his airway, and is drowsy but rousable. He is not orientated in time or place. He is tachycardic and hypotensive. He is not catheterized.

This patient is at risk of rapid deterioration; he will need several investigations and interventions done quickly. Communication and getting help are key.

Find the nurse in charge. Tell him or her that:

- The patient is unstable, and that you will need help: Ask if a nurse is free to assist you.
- To contact 'Outreach' and suggest a 'back-up' if they will be unable to attend within 10 minutes, e.g. the ICU core trainee (CT), another medical CT, the surgical CT or the medical specialist registrar.
- To inform the relatives that the patient has deteriorated, and give them the opportunity to come into hospital.

On review of his observation chart:

- He is pyrexial at 38.5°C.
- He was pyrexial for 2 days postoperatively, but following this his temperature has run between 37 and 37.6 until last night.
- His blood pressure was running at 130 systolic, and dropped to 105 yesterday.

Sepsis is high on this man's differential diagnosis: giving antibiotics and fluids quickly is important (see Chapter 55). The following should be performed quickly, either by you or whoever can help:

- Two cannulae should be inserted, taking bloods for FBC, CRP, U&E, blood cultures, LFTs.
- Start 500 mL normal saline.
- Give a stat dose of broad spectrum antibiotics (e.g. piperacillin 4.5 g), given that this is a hospital-acquired infection.
- Take a blood gas.

On review of his drug card:

- He is on antihypertensives (ramipril and diltiazem) which have been given.
- He has been on VTE prophylaxis, which has been appropriately given.
- He has opiates prescribed as required; he has had oromorph three times today.

Cross the antihypertensives off his drug chart. Consider prescribing naloxone to reverse the effect of the opiates, in case they are contributing to his drowsiness.

On review of his medical record:

- He is hypertensive, but has no other significant problems.
- His last ECG showed normal sinus rhythm.
- His preoperative haemoglobin was 13; postoperatively it was 12.
- His creatinine has been rising since admission, from 150 to 210.

On examination he is:

- Pyrexial at 38.5°C.
- Tachycardic, at 120.
- Heart sounds are normal.
- Breath sounds are vesicular.
- JVP is not raised.
- Abdomen is soft, non-tender.
- His calves are soft, non-tender.
- There is no rash.
- The surgical site looks clean.
- All other joints are pain free, and not swollen.
- He has no lines or catheter in situ.
- On rolling, you see a sacral sore with pus.

Problem list:

- Pyrexia
- Hypotension
- Pressure sore
- Worsening renal failure
- Possible opioid toxicity
- Recent hip operation

Differential diagnosis

- *Sepsis*: possible sources include pressure sore, and hip.
- *Pre-renal failure*: secondary to hypovolaemia (contributed to by diuretics and ACE inhibitor).

Investigations and interventions needed

- *ABG*: lactate >2.2 suggests severe sepsis and should be referred to ICU.
- *CXR*: although there were clinically no localizing signs, he could have developed a hospital-acquired pneumonia.
- *ECG*: ensure that he has no arrhythmia or ischaemic changes.
- *Laboratory blood tests* were sent when cannulae were placed previously.
- *Catheter* for careful fluid balance.

He needs to be discussed with the surgical team looking after him both to inform them of what you have found/planned, and to see what other imaging they might want (e.g. ultrasound of hip looking for a collection).

This patient will probably best be managed in an HDU environment; he will need a catheter and hourly observations, as well as repeat gases to ensure that he is responding to therapy.

Make a plan with the surgical team/ICU team as to who will next review him, and make sure the nursing staff have instructions on when to bleep (e.g. if BP goes below 90 again); see 'deteriorating patient' section of Chapter 14.

References

1. Wu WC, Rathore SS, Wang Y, Radford MJ, Krumholz HM (2001) Blood transfusion in elderly patients with acute myocardial infarction. *N Engl J Med* 345(17):1230–1236.

2. Rao SV, Jollis JG, Harrington RA, Granger CB, Newby LK, Armstrong PW, Moliterno DJ, Lindblad L, Pieper K, Topol EJ, Stamler JS, Califf RM (2004) Relationship of blood transfusion and clinical outcomes in patients with acute coronary syndromes. *JAMA* 292(13): 1555–1562.

3. Haynes AB, Weiser TG, Berry WR, Lipsitz SR, et al. for the Safe Surgery Saves Lives Study Group (2009) A surgical safety checklist to reduce morbidity and mortality in a global population. *N Engl J Med* 360: 491–499.

4. NICE Clinical Guideline 65: Management of inadvertent perioperative hypothermia in adults. http://guidance.nice.org.uk/CG65.

5. NICE Clinical Guideline 92: Venous Thromboembolism – reducing the risk. www.nice.org.uk/guidance/index.jsp?action=byID&o=12695.

Chapter 42

Medical problems in pregnancy

Nic Wenninke

Introduction

Medical emergencies during pregnancy pose particular challenges to the physician. Remember that any woman of childbearing age could be pregnant and that either over- or under-investigations and treatment will have an impact on the mother and fetus. Medical emergencies in pregnant women can be due to:

- an exacerbation of an established medical problem condition
- a condition which is unique to pregnancy
- a new condition unrelated to, or that has an increased frequency during, pregnancy.

The Eighth Report on Confidential Enquiries into Maternal Deaths in the United Kingdom (2011) identified that 'medical causes' remain the leading cause of death during pregnancy in the UK [1]. Although potential fetal risks must be carefully considered, it is essential that potentially life-saving investigations and treatments are not inappropriately denied to the mother.

General considerations in pregnancy

- Inform the mother of the potential risks and benefits when undertaking investigations and treatments, accepting the lack of definitive information on safety of many drugs in pregnancy.
- Remember that the risks of specific investigations and treatments will vary with gestational age.
- Use a multidisciplinary approach with involvement of obstetric and neonatal teams as appropriate.
- Recognize that women are becoming pregnant at a later stage of life and thus the number of chronic conditions (e.g. diabetes, hypertension and kidney disease) may be more common and their sequelae may be more prominent.

  - Ideally, a preconception discussion should be undertaken including a medication review ensuring good disease control with minimal teratogenic exposure to the fetus. This should lead to improved medication compliance as well as targeted modifications of remediable risk factors.
  - Subsequent regular multidisciplinary antenatal reviews with close fetal monitoring should occur.

- Large physiological changes occur in pregnancy including an increase in circulatory volume, cardiac output and glomerular filtration rate of ~50%. This leads to haemodilution (physiological anaemia of pregnancy) and reduced plasma protein binding of drugs.
- Great care must be taken when interpreting haematological and biochemical results and they should be interpreted only in the context of modified reference ranges for the appropriate stage of pregnancy.
- Cardiopulmonary resuscitation follows the Resuscitation Council (UK) guidelines with the addition of a wedge to maintain the patient in the left lateral position at ~30° to relieve compression on the inferior vena cava by the fetus and improve venous return. Haemorrhage is a major cause of cardiovascular collapse in this group of patients; thus alongside the common medical causes always consider:

  - placental/uterine abruption
  - placenta praevia
  - ruptured ectopic pregnancy requiring early obstetrician and neonatology involvement

Acute Medicine, ed. Stephen Haydock, Duncan Whitehead and Zoë Fritz. Published by Cambridge University Press. © Cambridge University Press 2015.

- in cases where the fetus is >24 weeks, emergency delivery should be considered if resuscitation is unsuccessful within 5 minutes to relieve caval compression and improve the outcome for the fetus and mother.

Scenario 42.1

A 27-year-old woman who is 32/40 weeks pregnant is referred to the acute medical unit with sudden onset of sharp pleuritic chest pain. On examination she is alert and orientated with a mild tachycardia of 90 bpm in sinus rhythm, BP 120/72, respiratory rate of 30/min and saturation on air of 94%. She has a mild dry cough, a temperature of 37.5°C and mild decreased air entry at the left base.

Infection versus infarction

This is a common presentation to the AMU and the most likely diagnoses are a pulmonary embolism (PE) or lower respiratory tract infection. However, it is important to be aware that other differential diagnoses should be considered which are more common in pregnancy compared to the non-pregnant population and include:

- *Myocardial infarction*: treat as for non-pregnant patients.
- *Aortic dissection* is more common in pregnancy with significant co-morbidity. Early CXR, echocardiography and CT aortography is essential in patients with a good history. Treatment is strict BP control (systolic BP <130 mmHg) and cardiothoracic surgical input. Patients with risk factors for aortic dissection (e.g. hypertension, connective tissue disorders) who are planning on pregnancy should be considered for prophylactic propranolol preconception.
- *Peripartum cardiomyopathy*: occurs in the last 12 weeks of pregnancy up to 3 months postpartum with dyspnoea, palpitations and peripheral or systemic emboli. Emphasis is on delivery of the baby, conventional cardiac failure therapy, thromboprophylaxis and immunosuppression. Mortality is 30% with 35% of patients making a complete recovery with the cardiac function returning to normal.
- *Amniotic fluid embolism* presents in labour or just shortly after classically with sudden cardiovascular collapse, cyanosis and DIC. The emphasis is on supportive care but despite this mortality is 70%.

History

- The history should focus on the differentiation between PE or infection and the exclusion of other causes of chest pain. PE should be high on the differential list as the *risk increases six-fold in pregnancy*.
- Emphasis is placed on risk factors for PE including a positive personal or family history.
- A detailed obstetric history is essential to ascertain whether there have been previous miscarriages suggestive of systemic lupus erythematosus.
- Significant events during the current pregnancy should be explored including the development of the fetus.
- Any concerns warrant early involvement of the obstetric team.

Examination

- A focused ABCDE approach is essential to assess the severity of the medical condition, initiating treatment at the relevant stage if indicated.
- The aim is to confirm or refute the clinical suspicion.
- None of the classical features of PE have a strong predictive value and the Wells score for PE is not validated in pregnancy.

Investigation

The aim is for focused investigations with optimal safety for the mother and fetus (Figure 42.1). In this instance the following blood tests are required:

- Full blood count
- Electrolytes including urea and creatinine
- Liver function tests
- Clotting
- A D-dimer *is not indicated* in this instance as pregnancy is a high risk factor for PE. If there is a clinical suspicion of PE, further investigations via imaging are required.
- ECG and arterial blood gas will aim to reinforce the diagnosis and exclude other causes of this patient's symptoms.
- CXR is helpful for excluding other diagnoses and the radiation exposure is negligible.

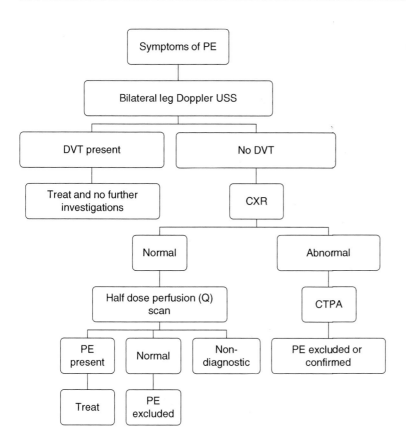

Figure 42.1 Algorithm for the investigation of pulmonary embolism in pregnancy.

- The Royal College of Obstetricians (2010) [2] recommend:
    - if patient has leg symptoms request for ultrasound and if deep vein thrombosis present for treatment
    - if normal CXR for half dose Q scan
    - if equivocal for CTPA.

Scenario 42.1 continued

This woman had a normal CXR, was started on Clexane, and a half dose Q scan was ordered.

Clexane is safe in pregnancy.
- It does not cross the placenta or breast milk.
- Due to the altered pharmacokinetics during pregnancy a slightly higher dose of 1 mg/kg bd is indicated.

This woman now needs further imaging with radiation exposure and it is important to formally obtain her consent for the risks.

- CXR and V/Q scan equilibrates to 1% and 50% of the background radiation exposure during pregnancy, respectively.
- This is 50 times less than the theoretical risk of malformations and radiation-induced malignancies from retrospective analysis studies.
- The mother should also be consented for the increased risk of radiation-induced malignancy to breast and lung tissue, which is substantially higher for CTPA than V/Q.

However, it is important to stress that exclusion/confirmation of PE is essential as undiagnosed PEs have a significant morbidity and mortality for the fetus and mother.

A half dose Q scan was undertaken confirming a PE.

She was continued on Clexane until at least 6 weeks postnatally and for a total of 3 months. At the end of this period a risk assessment needs to be undertaken to ascertain other risk factors for PE which would necessitate a prolonged period of anticoagulation. Routine thrombophilia screens are not indicated unless there is a strong clinical suspicion or family history. Due to the risk of teratogenicity during the first trimester and subsequent risk of haemorrhage at delivery, warfarin is contraindicated and newer anticoagulants such as rivaroxaban are not licensed in pregnancy. For patients with coexisting DVT, grade 2 stockings are also indicated for 2 years to reduce post-thrombotic syndrome.

Other important medical conditions presenting in pregnancy

1. Cerebral venous sinus thrombosis (see also Chapter 30)

This is an uncommon presentation in the general population but the incidence increases 100-fold during the second and third trimesters of pregnancy as well as postpartum up to 1 per 10 000. The typical presentation is:

- severe headache (may mimic subarachnoid haemorrhage)
- photophobia
- symptoms suggestive of raised intracranial pressure
- focal neurological deficit in up to two-thirds of patients though not normally in a specific arterial territory.

Risk factors include:

- pregnancy-induced hypertension
- recent sinus infections
- recent delivery by caesarean section.

Examination should focus on:

- signs suggestive of raised intracranial pressure, especially a change in mental state, seizures or coma
- papilloedema
- neurological signs such as diplopia, sixth cranial nerve palsy or paresis
- pyrexia and leucocytosis, and thus meningitis or encephalitis also needs to be considered.

Emphasis is on early imaging, with MRI venography being the ideal modality. Availability may be an issue and CT venography and lumbar puncture can be useful in exclusion of other causes such as subarachnoid haemorrhage, encephalitis/meningitis, idiopathic intracranial hypertension and space-occupying lesions.

Treatment focuses on supportive measures:

- Rehydration.
- Monitoring of visual acuity/fields and, if there is any impairment, LP is warranted to reduce intracranial pressures.
- Anticoagulation using enoxaparin 1 mg/kg bd during pregnancy and then converting to warfarin postpartum for 3 months is required, and a thorough history to ascertain whether other risk factors for thrombosis are present is essential as this would indicate a prolonged period of anticoagulation.

Despite these measures there is still a 10% mortality and 40% restrictive living amongst survivors.

2. Epilepsy/gestational epilepsy

Epilepsy in pregnancy may be more frequent due to the:

- reduction in seizure threshold
- sudden cessation of medication on discovering conception due to maternal concerns of teratogenicity.

Traditional antiepileptics such as carbamazepine carry a 5% risk of teratogenicity though recent evidence shows no significant increase with newer antiepileptics such as levetiracetam. However, this must be seen in the context of a background rate of teratogenicity in the general population of 2% and 3–4% for patients with untreated epilepsy.

This should be balanced against the risks to the mother and fetus of uncontrolled epilepsy, which carries significant morbidity and mortality.

Preconception counselling is essential for the mother to make an informed decision with an explanation that organogenesis of the three main organs affected by anticonvulsants develops by 13 weeks of gestation. Regular joint neurology and obstetrician review in clinic with ultrasound is essential for this group of patients.

An acute presentation of epilepsy during pregnancy should be treated as per protocols for non-pregnant patients with early involvement from neurology and obstetrics for ongoing treatment and follow-up.

3. Pre-eclampsia/eclampsia

This is a multi-organ disorder which is specific to pregnancy and occurs after 20 weeks gestation and up to

2 weeks postpartum with hypertension >140/90 mmHg and proteinuria >300 mg/24 hours.

Risk factors include:

- age >40 years
- obesity
- personal/family history of pre-eclampsia
- chronic medical conditions such as diabetes, hypertension, chronic renal failure and connective tissue disorders
- primiparity, multiparity or a long inter-pregnancy interval.

In the early stages the patient may be asymptomatic but as the disorder progresses into the severe category the patient may experience:

- headaches
- visual disturbances
- epigastric pain with nausea/vomiting
- facial/peripheral oedema.

It is important to note that the British Eclampsia Survey revealed that at the time of the last antenatal visit:

- 57% had hypertensive proteinuria
- 32% had *either* hypertension or proteinuria
- 11% had neither.

In practice pre-eclampsia cannot be excluded by a normal blood pressure and no proteinuria!

Warning signs suggestive of the development of severe pre-eclampsia and subsequent eclampsia are:

- headaches, visual disturbances and abdominal pain
- worsening hypertension >160/90 and proteinuria >5 g/24 hours
- worsening oedema, oliguria
- hyperreflexia
- acute kidney injury
- HELLP syndrome.

The development of severe pre-eclampsia is grave: for the mother there are risks of intracranial haemorrhage; for the fetus there are risks of stillbirth, placental abruption and intrauterine growth retardation. This is a medical and obstetric emergency with the emphasis on urgent delivery of the fetus and blood pressure control with intravenous labetalol or hydralazine aiming for a blood pressure <140/90.

The aim is to prevent eclampsia, which still occurs in 1 in 200 pregnancies with 2% mortality. In these circumstances a multidisciplinary approach including obstetricians and intensive care focuses on emergency delivery of the baby and supportive measures for the mother including intravenous magnesium sulphate for 24–48 hours if there is evidence of seizure activity.

Pre-eclampsia/eclampsia has a risk of recurrence of 25% in subsequent pregnancies in addition to an increased risk of:

- hypertension
- ischaemic heart disease
- strokes
- venous thromboembolism.

Thus follow-up and assessment of risk factors is essential postpartum and re-emphasizes the need for a thorough obstetric history.

4. Hyperemesis gravidarum

This is a serious condition (0.5% of all pregnancies) which results in significant weight loss (5–20%) and ketosis with nutritional and electrolyte depletion. A thorough history and examination is essential to exclude other causes such as space-occupying lesions and gastrointestinal causes. Treatment focuses on rehydration and careful electrolyte replacement with early thiamine (Pabrinex) to reduce the risk of Wernicke's encephalopathy, and antiemetics such as cyclizine, metoclopramide, prochlorperazine and parenteral hydrocortisone. Early nutritional support via nasogastric or parental route with intravenous insulin to reduce ketosis is essential to reduce the risk of intrauterine growth retardation.

5. Acute fatty liver disease of pregnancy

This is rare (1 per 10 000) but grave and occurs in the last trimester with vague symptoms of right upper quadrant pain, nausea and malaise for a few weeks and then progresses to fulminant liver failure. Diagnosis is via the Swansea criteria [3] and emphasis is on supportive therapy especially for hypoglycaemia. Treatment is emergency delivery of the fetus and involvement of intensive care and hepatology. In practical terms, if an acute physician is managing a pregnant woman with vague abdominal pain, urgent liver function tests and obstetrician input are essential.

6. HELLP syndrome (haemolysis, elevated liver enzymes and low platelets)

This is a serious complication of pre-eclampsia and presents with epigastric pain, nausea and vomiting. The deterioration is less rapid and the severity of liver failure is milder but the main mortality is from intra-hepatic or intracerebral haemorrhage, liver capsule rupture or placental abruption, complications of pre-eclampsia and disseminated intravascular coagulopathy (DIC). The severity of the syndrome depends on the platelet count as per the Mississippi classification [4]. Management is on emergency delivery of the baby and control of hypertension via intravenous labetalol or hydralazine with supportive measures and early suspicion of life-threatening complications.

7. Obstetric cholestasis

Obstetric cholestasis presents with debilitating pruritus, especially of the feet and hands. There is no progression to liver failure but it is essential to exclude more serious conditions. Emphasis is on emollients and antihistamines with induced labour after 37 weeks to reduce fetal mortality. There is some evidence for the use of ursodeoxycholic acid for symptom control.

Summary

Due to excellent antenatal and postnatal care, pregnancy in the UK is very safe with a mortality of 6 per 100 000 pregnancies. The vast majority of pregnancies are uneventful and most symptoms are non-sinister in nature. However, we need to be aware of specific conditions that are unique or more common in pregnancy which can have an impact on the mother and fetus. Investigations should not be avoided due to anxiety of fetal exposure and it is essential for the mother to be adequately informed so as to improve treatment adherence. For this group of patients there should be a low threshold for early admission and involvement of obstetricians.

References

1. Centre for Maternal and Child Enquiries (CMACE). Saving Mothers' Lives: reviewing maternal deaths to make motherhood safer: 2006–08. The Eighth Report on Confidential Enquiries into Maternal Deaths in the United Kingdom. *BJOG* 2011; 118(Suppl. 1): 1–203.

2. Royal College of Obstetricians and Gynaecologists. The Acute Management of Thrombosis and Embolism during Pregnancy and Puerperium. 2010.

3. Ch'ng CL, Morgan M, Kingham JG. Acute fatty liver of pregnancy in South Wales, UK. *Gastroenterology* 2002; **123**:(1 Suppl 1): 53.

4. Martin JN, Rose CH, Briery CM. The spectrum of severe preeclampsia: comparative analysis by HELLP (hemolysis, elevated liver enzyme levels, and low platelet count) syndrome classification. *Am J Obstet Gynecol* 180 (6 Pt 1): 1373–1384.

Memory loss (progressive)

Matthew R. Hayman

Introduction

The commonest cause of progressive memory loss presenting on the acute medical 'take' is *dementia*. It is often associated with delirium but importantly *persists after the delirious episode resolves and does not impair consciousness*.

- Approximately 8–10% of people over the age of 65 in the developed world have dementia.
- The prevalence rises from approximately 2% of those aged 65 to more than 35% of those aged over 85, a doubling in prevalence for every 5-year increase in age.
- In 2008 there were an estimated 700 000 people with a diagnosis of dementia in the UK; this number is predicted to increase to 1.4 million by 2038.

Dementia needs to be differentiated from the process of natural, cognitive ageing.

- Cognition is the ability to think, understand and reason. Cognitive functions include memory, orientation, language (verbal fluency, receptive and expressive communication), praxis (doing things), recognition, visuospatial ability, abstract thought, executive function (decision making, planning, judgement) and insight.
- Age-related changes to the nervous system include neuronal death and demyelination such that by the age of 85 around 20% of brain weight and volume are lost – commonly seen as global cerebral atrophy on brain CT scans.
- Factors that differentiate 'normal' age-related memory loss from dementia include the ability to maintain function in normal life through aids

(lists, calendars, etc.) or adaptations and a very long time scale of decline (years to decades).

Dementia is not *solely progressive memory loss* but is defined as a:

> *serious loss of global cognitive ability (usually memory plus at least one other domain) in a previously unimpaired person (i.e. it is acquired), beyond what might be expected from normal ageing that is not better explained by another diagnosis and that persists for more than 6 months.*

It may be static, the result of a unique global brain injury, or progressive, resulting in long-term decline due to damage or disease in the body. Although dementia is far more common with increasing age, it can occur before the age of 65, in which case it is termed 'early onset dementia'.

Scenario 43.1

An 85-year-old man is admitted to the medical assessment unit after being found wandering in the street by a neighbour. He appeared much more 'confused' than usual. His general practitioner visited and felt that an infection was worsening his normal level of confusion due to his dementia and requested admission. Since arrival he has been continuously wandering around the assessment unit, is uncooperative and insisting on going home.

History

Taking a history from a patient with progressive memory loss can be challenging and it is critical to gain a collateral or supporting history from a carer/relative. The key areas to cover include:

- The rate of onset and progression
- The specific cognitive problems:

Acute Medicine, ed. Stephen Haydock, Duncan Whitehead and Zoë Fritz. Published by Cambridge University Press. © Cambridge University Press 2015.

Table 43.1 Drugs on the anticholinergic burden (ACB) scale (a total score of ≥3 is significant)

ACB score 1 (mild)	ACB score 2 (moderate)	ACB score 3 (severe)
Atenolol	Amantadine	Amitriptyline
Beclometasone dipropionate	Carbamazepine	Chlorpheniramine
Codeine	Oxcarbazepine	Clomipramine
Colchicine	Pethidine hydrochloride	Darifenacin
Diazepam	Pimozide	Doxepin
Digoxin		Hydroxyzine
Dipyridamole		Imipramine
Fentanyl		Oxybutinin
Furosemide		Paroxetine
Loperamide		Procyclidine
Nifedipine		Tolterodine
Prednisolone		Trifluoperazine
Warfarin		Trimipramine

- forgetfulness
- repetition
- accusations
- Any behavioural changes:
  - personality
  - sleep patterns
  - food preferences
  - sexuality
  - delusions and hallucinations
  - continence
- Comprehensive social and functional history:
  - who else is at home
  - what kind of accommodation
  - ability to perform personal and domestic activities of daily living
  - do they drive
  - what support and care arrangements are in place
  - does the patient smoke or drink

The past medical history provides clues to *alternative diagnoses* (a history of depression) or *subtypes of dementia* (vascular disease or risk factors) and a thorough medication history including a check on compliance may reveal a *reversible element to memory problems* (anticholinergic drugs in particular [1], see Table 43.1).

Formal cognitive assessment

- In the acute setting the 10-item Abbreviated Mental Test Score (AMTS) is a widely used screening tool.
- More recently this has been revised to a four-item subset (age, date of birth, place and year) which appears to have *similar sensitivity* (aprox. 80%) and *specificity* (approx. 90%) to the AMTS.
- More detailed testing is generally better suited to an outpatient setting where the likelihood of intercurrent delirium is low:
  - Folstein Mini-Mental State Examination (MMSE, 10–15 minutes)
  - the clock drawing test
  - Addenbrooke's Cognitive Examination (ACE-R, 20+ min)
  - formal neuropsychological testing (1–2 hours).

Examination

Although there are no specific diagnostic signs on clinical examination in early-moderate dementia, examination should focus on signs suggestive of:

- vascular disease (cardio-, cerebro- and peripheral vascular disease)
- neuropathy

- parkinsonism
- thyroid disease
- malignancy
- dehydration
- (alcoholic) liver disease.

In advanced dementia of any type, the following may be present:

- primitive reflexes (glabellar tap, grasp, palmar-mental and pout/snout)
- global hyperreflexia
- upgoing (extensor) plantars.

Investigations

While the diagnosis of dementia is still currently a clinical one there are some relatively simple investigations that will exclude potentially reversible causes of dementia or dementia mimics and may assist with diagnosis.

- *Blood tests*: FBC, ESR, B$_{12}$, folate, U&E, LFTs, Ca^{2+}, TSH, CRP, glucose (HIV and syphilis serology if atypical features in the presentation)
- *ECG*: suggesting evidence of vascular disease
- *CXR*: possible malignancy
- *Neuroimaging*: generally to exclude alternative diagnoses (subdural haematoma, normal pressure hydrocephalus, etc.) for which CT may be sufficient. (MRI may help establish the subtype of dementia and SPECT is used in some specialist centres.)
- *Lumbar puncture*: generally considered only for atypical presentation or research purposes.
- *EEG*: sometimes used if seizure activity is suspected or for unusual presentations (when fronto-temporal dementia or Creutzfeldt–Jakob disease is suspected).

Differential diagnosis

Having excluded normal ageing the two most important differential diagnoses of dementia in the elderly are *delirium* (see Chapter 16) and *depression*. The key distinguishing features are:

- *Onset and course of the condition*:
  - dementia is insidious and progressive
  - delirium is acute and fluctuating
  - depression is rapid and stable.
- *Impaired consciousness*:
  - present in delirium

- absent in depression and dementia.
- *Presence of biological symptoms*:
  - presence of early morning wakening, poor appetite, psychomotor retardation and diurnal variation of mood in depression
  - absent in dementia and delirium.

BUT: Dementia and delirium can coexist and it is not uncommon for patients with early dementia to suffer significant depression.

Common subtypes of dementia

Alzheimer's disease (AD)

- The commonest type and accounting for approximately 55% of dementia in the population.
- Characterized by early short-term memory loss and *slow but relentless* progression.
- Familial forms exist, showing an autosomal dominant pattern of inheritance. These cases tend to present at a younger age (<65) and are a tiny proportion of total cases (<1%).
- Classic pathological changes include beta-amyloid plaques (neuritic plaques) and neurofibrillary tangles (tau protein hyperphosphorylation).
- The parietal and temporal lobes are most frequently involved.

Vascular dementia (VaD)

- Prevalence of 5–15% but very commonly a mixed pathology with AD features at post-mortem.
- Presents with *stepwise and irregular progression* often in the form of 'crises' (sudden worsening of confusion, falls, immobility or incontinence) leading to hospital admission; often associated with intercurrent delirium and explains the much greater prevalence of VaD patients seen in an acute hospital than its population prevalence would predict.
- VaD encompasses a wide range of presentations:
  - sudden onset cognitive impairment associated with classic stroke features (hemiparesis, etc.)
  - multi-infarct dementia mimicking AD-type cognitive decline
  - small vessel ischaemia (leukoaraiosis) resulting in 'subcortical' dementia with clinical features of Parkinson's disease or normal pressure hydrocephalus (gait

abnormalities, executive and information-processing problems).

Mixed aetiology

- There is significant overlap between the dementia disorders and their presentations. Many neurodegenerative diseases have common pathological findings.
- The most common variant is mixed AD-VaD. Estimates of prevalence vary depending on diagnostic criteria and are in the range 20–40%. A mixed aetiology is suggested by a pattern of stepwise deterioration in combination with a progressive decline.

Dementia with Lewy bodies (DLB)

- Accounts for approximately 5% of patients with dementia.
- A syndrome of cognitive impairment, parkinsonism, fluctuation in alertness or cognition, delusions and hallucinations and increased sensitivity to neuroleptic drugs.
- Is characterized neuropathologically by spherical, eosinophilic, intracytoplasmic inclusion bodies most commonly in the basal ganglia and limbic system.
- The term Parkinson's disease dementia (PDD) is used when motor symptoms precede cognitive impairment by more than 12 months.

Fronto-temporal dementia (FTD)

- Accounts for 2–5% of patients with dementia.
- Up to 40% of patients may have an affected first-degree relative (autosomal dominant pattern of inheritance).
- Patients are often relatively younger with mean age of onset 56–61 years and present with problems involving initiative and planning, disinhibition and poor language (economy or stereotypy – patterns of repetition).
- Relatives may describe a change in personality, but simple cognitive assessment (e.g. MMSE) may be normal.
- Neuropathological findings in the commonest variant (Pick's disease) are of Pick bodies, argentophilic intracellular inclusions.

Cortical versus subcortical

A very broad division of dementia subtypes into 'cortical' and 'subcortical' is sometimes used. There is considerable overlap between these broad categories but the division may help an initial assessment:

Cortical (AD, FTD, CJD). Deficits in specific cortical domains (memory, aphasia, apraxia, visuospatial impairment, dyscalculia and agnosia) with otherwise 'spared' cognition.

Subcortical (VaD, movement disorders (Parkinson's disease, progressive supranuclear palsy, multisystem atrophy), normal pressure hydrocephalus, AIDS dementia complex). Deficits in the circuits of the basal ganglia and thalamus affecting information retrieval and storage leading to reduced speed of thought (bradyphrenia) and frontal-executive features (perseveration, sequencing and reduced fluency but *not* aphasia).

Reversible presentations

Hypothyroidism: profound hypothyroidism is often associated with memory impairment, psychomotor retardation and visuospatial impairments. Treatment may only partially reverse these severe symptoms.

Vitamin B$_{12}$/folate deficiency: present (but undiagnosed) in up to 2% of adults over 60 years of age. Cerebral involvement in the associated neuronal lesions can rarely cause progressive personality change and/or memory loss. Replacement therapy may not reverse such advanced neurological complications.

Alcohol-related dementia (Wernicke–Korsakoff syndrome, Marchiafava–Bignami disease): whilst mild-moderate alcohol intake may be protective against dementia, alcohol abuse appears to confer an increased risk. Treatment is thiamine replacement and abstinence which may improve, or at least stabilize, cognition.

Syphilis: frequently part of a dementia 'work-up', neurosyphilis is now an extremely rare presentation of cognitive impairment in the elderly. It is most commonly seen in association with HIV infection with a median age of onset of 39. Clinical features are reduced attention, memory and executive abilities. There may be associated (classically grandiose) delusions, hallucinations and confabulation. With adequate (and sensitive) antibiotic treatment 50% will improve.

Uncommon dementia subtypes

Creutzfeldt–Jakob disease (CJD)

- A prion protein disease causing spongiform degeneration and astrogliosis.
- Most commonly sporadic in nature but familial and infective (including new variant (nvCJD) related to the ingestion of infected animal products).
- Incidence is rare (1 per million per year).
- Key features are rapidly progressive subcortical dementia, myoclonus, ataxia, pyramidal or extrapyramidal signs.
- Diagnosis is on the basis of clinical findings, EEG (periodic sharp wave complexes) and the presence of 14-3-3 protein in the CSF.
- There is no effective treatment.

Neurodegenerative dementia

- Seen in progressive conditions such as multiple sclerosis, motor neurone disease, corticobasilar degeneration, Huntington's disease and in HIV-related dementia.

Treatment (pharmacological and non-pharmacological)

Dementia is currently an incurable condition. While there are modest benefits to be gained from some treatments (see below), the emphasis of care efforts today is directed at maintaining and prolonging independent living and the quality of that life.

A standard geriatric approach to a chronic progressive condition recognizes phases of a disease:

early: emphasis on diagnosis, information, support and advance planning

middle: as disability and/or dependency increases

late: severe disability requiring intensive support and care or institutionalization

end of life/terminal care.

Treatments for cognitive function

Treatments aimed at stabilizing and/or improving cognitive function are most appropriate relatively soon after a confirmed diagnosis.

Non-pharmacological treatments include simple measures such as encouraging the maintenance of daily routines and using written 'to-do' lists. Interventions such as 'brain gym' or a course of occupational therapy sessions have been shown to improve cognitive function and carer well-being.

Cholinesterase inhibitors (donepezil, rivastigmine, galantamine)

- The most commonly prescribed drug treatment for mild-moderate dementias.
- Whilst initial studies showed some positive results, increasing evidence suggests that the effects of these drugs are relatively mild (roughly a 1 point improvement in MMSE versus placebo over a 3-year period).
- All of the cholinesterase inhibitors have side effects (cardiac, GI and urinary symptoms) consistent with their enhanced cholinergic effects and these can be significant enough to discontinue treatment.

Memantine

- Is a glutamate antagonist that acts at the NMDA receptor and may reduce excitatory neurotoxicity in dementia.
- Trials have suggested a modest benefit in moderate to severe dementia and patients sometimes receive dual treatment with a cholinesterase inhibitor.

Prescribing and monitoring of both cholinesterase inhibitors and memantine should be performed via a formal *memory service* with joint care between specialist and GP. Importantly for the hospital doctor there is no evidence of harm from temporary cessation of medication during acute illness (*note*: cholinesterase inhibitors can be applied as transdermal patches which may need to be removed promptly if significant side effects occur).

Treatment of behavioural and psychological symptoms of dementia (BPSD)

- BPSD is the preferred term to describe symptoms such as agitation, fidgeting, wandering, verbal and physical aggression, some of which frequently occur in patients with advanced dementia.
- Whilst often challenging to relatives and caregivers a significant number of such behaviours

will resolve spontaneously and a 'watch and wait' policy for some weeks is appropriate.

- Given the verbal fluency problems that patients with dementia suffer, such challenging behaviours may represent an unusual response to a physical problem such as pain, hunger, cold, etc. and identifying and remedying such ailments is an important intervention.
- Pharmacological treatments should always be seen as a last resort in the management of BPSD.
- Antipsychotics are often poorly tolerated (particularly in DLB and PDD) and increase the risk of falls and infection (due to oversedation).
- Very similar risks apply to the use of benzodiazepines.
- In simple terms the lowest dose of the shortest acting drug should be used *only* when a patient's behaviour is such that they or their carers are at risk of physical injury/harm.
- Repeat dosing should be held off for as long as possible and certainly not before adequate time for a previous dose to reach its target with the least invasive route (oral) always preferable:
  - minimum 10 minutes for IV route
  - minimum 20–30 minutes for IM
  - minimum 30–40 minutes for SC
  - up to 1 hour for oral.

How to communicate with someone with dementia

- Even in patients with severe cognitive impairment implicit memory may be relatively well maintained. Implicit memory is responsible for motor activities such as walking, but also in recognizing emotions and threats.
- Friendliness (facial expression and eye contact), courteousness (voice characteristics – volume and tone; 'safe' physical gestures such as a handshake or hand on the shoulder/elbow) and non-confrontation can be disarming in a tense situation.
- *Speak gently and slowly*, wait for recognition and/or a response before ploughing on.
- *Do not get frustrated*. Remember that the patient with dementia may have visual, perceptual and hearing difficulties.
- *Avoid challenging, arguing or reasoning* with dementia patients.

- *Be patient*, it takes time to build up trust when your title ('Doctor') no longer commands respect.
- *Go with the flow of their conversation*. It can be impossible to gain an answer to a specific question so a classical medical history may be impossible (use carers/relatives for this).
- *Non-verbal cues* can help identify a patient's mental state and how they are feeling.
- *A medical examination can be a very invasive process* so explain and use visual cues or gestures (holding the stethoscope up, exaggeratedly breathing in and out, etc.).
- *Use relatives to help keep the atmosphere calm* and give yourself and the patient pauses in the consultation. A relative or carer may understand a patient's movements or phrases and help you interpret.

Dementia patients in the acute hospital

- Approximately 25% of patients in acute hospitals have dementia.
- The vast majority of such patients are admitted appropriately for an acute deterioration that cannot be managed in the community (intercurrent illness, acute worsening of the condition, e.g. the step-wise deterioration of VaD, or complications/side effects of medications).
- On average patients with a pre-existing diagnosis of dementia are more physiologically unwell for a given acute illness than would be expected for an age-matched control without dementia due to reduced homeostatic/physiological reserve.
- Therefore, an acute admission for a patient with dementia is a *medical emergency*. The vital first step in such a patient's care is accurate diagnosis and prompt treatment. This can be achieved through a medical admissions unit but much of the standard organization of acute medical admissions works against ideal care for a dementia patient. Noise and the loss of a normal routine, multiple bed/ward moves, a lack of continuity of care and limited time from caregivers all conspire to exacerbate the symptoms of dementia and the acute illness.
- Patients often become much more dependent than their baseline and this loss of function associated with being unwell can cause worsening of BPSD. Knee-jerk treatment with antipsychotics

to manage these symptoms can exacerbate this situation.

Reference

1. Campbell N, Boustani M, Limbil T, Ott C, et al. The cognitive impact of anticholinergics: a clinical review. *Clinical Interventions in Aging* 2009; 4(1): 225–233.

Further reading

Burns A, Iliffe S. Dementia (Clinical Review). *Br Med J* 2009; 338: b75.

Living well with dementia: A National Dementia Strategy. Department of Health, 2009. Available to download at www.gov.uk/government/uploads/system/uploads/attachment_data/file/168220/dh_094051.pdf.

Ritchie K, Lovestone S. The dementias. *Lancet* 2002; 360: 1759–1766.

Supporting people with dementia and their carers in health and social care. Issued: November 2006, last modified: October 2012. NICE CG42. Available to download at www.nice.org.uk/nicemedia/live/10998/30318/30318.pdf.

Micturition difficulties

Duncan Whitehead

Introduction

Common causes of micturition difficulties and urinary tract obstruction are best divided by anatomical site.

Urethral

- Stricture:
  - tumour
  - instrumentation/trauma
  - radiotherapy
  - infection
- External urethral compression:
  - constipation
  - benign prostatic hypertrophy/carcinoma
  - vaginal, vulva or rectal tumours

Bladder

- Calculi
- Tumour obstructing ureteric or urethral orifices
- Clot retention
- Neuropathic bladder
- Drug side effects (anticholinergics, antihistamines, antispasmodics and anaesthetics)

Ureteric

- External compression, e.g. retroperitoneal fibrosis
- Ureteric tumours
- Benign strictures
- Pelviureteric junction obstruction
- Stones

Renal

- Stones obstructing the renal pelvis
- Papillary necrosis

Psychological

- Lack of privacy
- Fear of pain on micturition
- Enforced bed rest postoperatively or trauma

Scenario 44.1

The nurses contact you regarding an 80-year-old man, admitted earlier that day with confusion. They are concerned that he has not passed urine since admission some 12 hours earlier. He is becoming increasingly agitated and distressed. There was a telephone discussion with the FY1 doctor earlier that evening who suggested a fluid challenge of 250 mL of intravenous Hartmann's. On assessment you find he is hypertensive, tachycardic, acutely confused and distressed. He has a palpable distended bladder which a bladder scan reveals contains 900 mL of urine.

Clinical assessment

In every patient with oliguria, urinary tract obstruction should be considered as a cause. The following assessment will aid in distinguishing the causes:

History

- Lower urinary tract symptoms:
  - poor stream
  - hesitance
  - post-micturition dribble
  - nocturia
  - frequency
  - urgency
  - incontinence
- Suprapubic pain
- Duration from last micturition
- Thirst

Acute Medicine, ed. Stephen Haydock, Duncan Whitehead and Zoë Fritz. Published by Cambridge University Press. © Cambridge University Press 2015.

Examination

- Palpable bladder
- Loin tenderness
- Ballot kidneys
- Fluid status
- Cardiac output (BP, heart rate, peripheral perfusion)

Treat reversible causes that become apparent.

Investigation

- Bladder scan
- USS KUB:
  - hydronephrosis is seen in high pressure urinary tract obstruction; in rare cases the renal pelvis may be restricted and unable to expand (retroperitoneal fibrosis)
- Urinary flow studies:
  - rate of flow demonstrates bladder function and outflow resistance
  - good for assessing chronic retention

Management

- Urethral catheterization if:
  - proven or continuing concern of bladder outflow obstruction
  - monitoring of hourly urine output in the unwell patient
- Suprapubic catheterization:
  - if urethral catheterization is impossible
  - experienced operator should always be present

If an obstructive cause for oliguria is excluded refer to 'Prescribing fluids in AKI, oliguria and polyuria' in Chapter 6.

Investigation and management of prostate cancer

Digital rectal examination

- Palpate prostate for masses and normal central sulcus.
- Suspicious digital rectal examination with a PSA <4 ng/mL has a positive predictive value for prostate cancer of up to 30% [1].

Prostate specific antigen (PSA)

- Is *not a screening test*, but an adjunct to diagnosing prostate cancer.

- False positives occur with prostatitis, BPH and prostatic trauma.
- Clear value in staging and monitoring prostatic cancer progression.

Clinical suspicion of prostate cancer is an indication for referral to urology for further evaluation:

- transrectal prostatic biopsy under ultrasound guidance
- radioisotope bone scan
- pelvic MRI or CT.

Management of prostate cancer should be by urology or oncology. Treatment depends on stage of tumour and metastatic spread. NICE management guidance varies from watchful waiting to radical therapies such as prostatectomy or radiotherapy with adjuvant hormone agonist. These radical treatments are decided in a multidisciplinary team (MDT) setting.

Prescribing for prostatic symptoms

Alpha-blockers

- α_{1A} receptor blockade causes smooth muscle relaxation in the prostate and bladder neck, reducing resistance to urinary flow within days.

Anti-androgenic medications

- 5α-reductase inhibitors (finasteride); blocks conversion of testosterone to dihydrotestosterone.
- Dihydrotestosterone promotes prostatic growth; reducing production causes gradual reduction in prostatic size, increasing urethral diameter.
- Can be used in combination with an α-receptor blocker.

Anticholinergics/spasmodics

- Bladder stabilizers reduce symptomatic urinary frequency and urgency.
- Use only when obstructive features have been excluded; they can precipitate urinary retention.

Initial treatment of bladder outflow obstruction

- Urethral catheterization (bladder volume >400 mL/hydronephrosis on USS)
  - Monitor urine output for polyuria post catheterization.

Diagnose and treat reversible factors:

- UTI
- constipation
- stop drugs affecting bladder emptying
- commence alpha-blocker when BPH is suspected.

Trial without catheter if any reversible factors have been treated within a few days; if there is no clear reversible cause or very large residual bladder volume leave with catheter in situ and refer for urological assessment.

Urological referral

Certain situations with an obstructed urinary system should prompt urgent urology referral:

- Obstruction at a level above the urethra:
  - hydronephrosis from urethral obstruction will resolve with catheterization
  - decompression of the upper tracts requires nephrostomy or ureteric stent insertion; the cause also requires investigation and management.
- Infected obstructed urinary system:
  - is a *life-threatening situation requiring urgent drainage*; see Chapter 39 on loin pain.
- Renal tract calculi should be referred non-urgently if neither infected nor obstructive.

Urethral catheterization

This should be performed aseptically (Figure 44.1).

Complications of urethral catheterization

Infection

- Bacteraemia and rapid onset of septic shock can occur in the context of a pre-existing urinary tract infection – 'septic shower'.
- Symptomatic UTI rate is high; ≈30% of all hospital-acquired infections are catheter related – early catheter removal is recommended.
- Asymptomatic bacteriuria is nearly universal in long-term (>28 days) catheterized patients.

Prophylactic antibiotics (gentamicin) are often advised pre-catheterization in specific settings such as a recent joint prosthesis; however, the evidence base is limited.

Paraphimosis

- Occurs when foreskin is not reduced post catheterization.
- Blood outflow from the foreskin is reduced by pressure of the catheter reducing venous drainage; foreskin becomes oedematous and difficult to reduce.

Creation of false passage

- Catheter tip pressure on the prostate gland can cause indentation; with continued increased pressure it results in a false passage, more likely with a narrower catheter (higher pressure exerted with same force).

Urethral strictures and perforation

- Trauma to the urethra can result in perforation or more commonly scarring and stricturing.

Bleeding

- Bladder wall irritation.
- Traction on catheter causing trauma.

Oliguria and shock

When assessing a patient with oliguria, consider the following points:

- Oliguria is abnormal and requires prompt assessment: unless in the setting of ESRF.
- Reduced urine output <0.5 mL/kg per hour urine output for ≥6 hours is *AKI*.
- Reduced urine output is commonly due to renal hypoperfusion and often the first sign of *shock* – inadequate tissue perfusion.
- *Shock is a medical emergency* and appropriate early treatment saves lives.
- Loop diuretics are the *treatment for fluid overload NOT oliguria.*
- Obstructive causes need exclusion and early treatment prevents CKD.
- AKI and oliguria are often part of the dying process and appropriate level of intervention should be carefully considered early in the care episode.

If you cannot rapidly restore normal urine output liaise with your senior colleagues: if the cause is obstructive urology should be involved, otherwise consider nephrology or intensive care referral.

Figure 44.1 Procedure for urethral catheterization.

1. Explain the procedure including the risks and benefits

2. Ensure patient is comfortable in a supine position at optimal bed height

3. Arrange equipment on a sterile trolley

4. Expose external genitalia

5. Put on sterile gloves

6. Open inner plastic catheter pack onto the sterile field; *best done before you have lubricant gel on your gloves*

7. Hold the penis in your left hand (now non-sterile hand)

8. Retract the foreskin and clean glans

9. Introduce 5–10 mL of lignocaine gel into urethral meatus and ***allow 5 minutes*** to take effect

10. Insert catheter tip covered in anaesthetic gel into urethral meatus

11. Advance catheter with gentle pressure holding the penis with traction at 90° to the bed

12. If significant resistance is met, several manoeuvres can assist in passing the catheter:

    - ask the patient to cough as you proceed

    - apply peritoneal pressure to guide the catheter tip

    - a larger diameter catheter

    - excessive force ***must be avoided***

If unsuccessful ask for help rather than causing trauma to the urethra or prostate

13. When inserted to the diversion point inject 10 mL of sterile normal saline into the inflation port and release the penis from your left hand

    - if pain is experienced stop and aspirate the balloon

    - ensure the catheter tip is in the bladder

14. Attach the urinary collection bag to the catheter drainage port

15. Slowly draw back the catheter until you feel resistance of the balloon at the bladder neck

16. Replace the foreskin in normal position

17. Keep the catheter bag below the level of the pelvis to avoid retrograde urinary flow, clamp the catheter before lifting higher

Reference

1. Carvalhal GF, Smith DS, Mager DE, Ramos C, Catalona WJ. Digital rectal examination for detecting prostate cancer at prostate specific antigen levels of 4 ng./ml. or less. *Journal of Urology* 1999; 161(3):835–839.

Further reading

Hooton TM et al. Diagnosis, Prevention, and Treatment of Catheter-Associated Urinary Tract Infection in Adults: 2009 International Clinical Practice Guidelines from the Infectious Diseases Society of America. *Clin Infect Dis* 2010; 50(5): 625–663. Available to download at http://cid.oxfordjournals.org/content/50/5/625.full.

Neck pain

Catherine Laversuch

Introduction

Pain localized to the neck results from disorders within the cervical spine itself or is a manifestation of a more generalized condition. Having determined if the problem is localized to the cervical spine it is important to detect involvement of the central cervical cord, peripheral nerve roots or both. The investigation and management of neck pain in the context of suspected meningitis is discussed in Chapter 23.

Anatomy

C1 and C2 (atlas and axis)

- The atlas is a ring structure with no body but two lateral masses.
- The atlanto-occipital joint allows the head to nod and the head pivots left and right around the odontoid peg (or dens) protruding from the axis (C2) into the central foramen of the atlas.
- These vertebrae are held in place by tough ligaments, particularly the transverse ligament posterior to the dens (which articulates with the anterior arch of the atlas).
- Trauma and inflammation (e.g. from RA) can disrupt this arrangement leading to instability. Erosion of the lateral masses over many years allows upward migration of the odontoid peg and pressure on the brainstem. Whiplash injury can also strain the ligaments, particularly the alar ligaments between the dens and medial occipital condyles.

The lower cervical spine (C3–7)

- The intervertebral discs connect the bodies of the vertebrae and additional posterior facet joints articulate at an angle of 45 degrees. These latter joints allow a gliding movement.
- The vertebral bodies are held together by the anterior and posterior longitudinal ligaments and the supraspinous and interspinous ligaments connect the spinous processes.
- The elastin-rich ligamentum flavum joins the laminae of adjacent vertebrae and the adjacent facet joint capsules, lying posterior to the spinal canal. Thickening of this ligament with age contributes towards spinal stenosis.
- Unlike the rest of the vertebral column, the transverse processes of the cervical vertebrae have a foramen allowing the vertebral arteries to reach the brain (Figure 45.1).

Pathophysiology

- Degenerative disc disease or prolapse can lead to loss of joint space.
- Osteophytes narrow the exit foramina for nerves to the arms and more rarely compromise the cervical cord. This is usually a slowly progressive process, called *cervical spondylosis* or more specifically:
  - *cervical radiculopathy* if the exiting nerve roots are compressed
  - *cervical myelopathy* if the cord itself is compromised.

Acute Medicine, ed. Stephen Haydock, Duncan Whitehead and Zoë Fritz. Published by Cambridge University Press. © Cambridge University Press 2015.

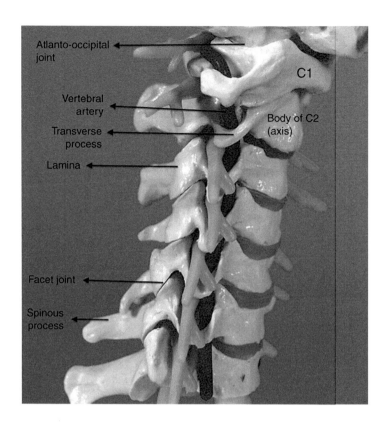

Figure 45.1 Anatomy of the cervical spine.

- The transverse foramen may be disrupted, compromising the vertebral arteries and leading to symptoms from *vertebro-basilar insufficiency* on head movement.
- Posterior rami from C2, C3 and C4 supply the back of the neck and head. This area may be painful as a result of nerve root impingement.
- Bony damage from malignant infiltration, infection and trauma (fracture) can cause rapid involvement of adjacent neurological structures.
- Involvement of blood vessels can accelerate the process, the anterior spinal artery in the central sulcus supplying the anterior two-thirds of the cord and the paired posterior spinal arteries supplying the posterior third.
- Fracture can disrupt the anterior, middle or posterior segments; if two of these are disrupted or C1 and C2 are involved, the fracture is more likely to be unstable.

Scenario 45.1

A 66-year-old woman presents to the MAU. She has a 6-month history of intermittent numbness and tingling in the hands. More recently she has found walking more difficult and now is struggling to walk several hundred yards and her legs feel heavy, like lead. She has a long history of a painful neck and low back pain. The pain is giving her a headache and radiates down to both shoulders and into both arms at times. She sleeps reasonably well provided she can get into a comfortable position. She has no problems elsewhere, is systemically well but is constipated. She has been taking regular paracetamol with added codeine for pain relief. General examination is unremarkable but her neck is restricted and painful. There is no marked muscle wasting, muscle power is good. Tone and reflexes in the legs appear increased. Her left supinator jerk is inverted. Sensory loss in the arms and fingers is patchy and not reproducible.

Important features in the history

- Neck pain due to *cervical spondylosis* is felt in the neck and across the shoulders; additionally, pain and dysaesthesia may be felt up into the back of the head. It is worse on movement and there may be a grinding sensation.

- Numbness and paraesthesia will be felt in the arms and fingers if there is cervical root entrapment or irritation.
- Simple or *non-specific neck pain* produces pain and tenderness in the neck muscles, muscle spasm and pain on particular head movements. It is probably postural in origin.
- Stiffness and abnormal leg movements may suggest *cervical myelopathy*.
- Weakness and wasting of the forearm or muscles in the hand (clumsiness) suggests significant *cervical radiculopathy*.
- Dysphagia may rarely result from extrinsic pressure on the oesophagus by large osteophytes.
- Pain from the shoulder joint is also felt mainly in the upper arm. Movement of the shoulders will be restricted and related to the pain.

Red flags for neck pain

(Suggesting that urgent imaging or senior review is needed, usually plain film and MRI.)

- Pain that is of recent onset (weeks to one or two months), severe, continuous and preventing sleep may indicate tumour or infection.
- Severe neck pain with a history of cancer, particularly those metastasizing to bone (bronchus, breast, kidney, prostate and thyroid).
- Neck pain with other systemic features (unintentional significant weight loss).
- Significant muscle wasting of forearm and hand muscles.
- *Lhermitte's phenomenon*: electric shock like sensations down the spine on neck movement, maybe into the arms and legs, are indicative of pressure on the cervical cord or intrinsic problems within the cervical cord (*demyelination, vitamin B$_{12}$ deficiency*). This warrants further investigation and imaging (usually MRI).
- Neck pain (as with any other spinal pain) in the setting of *staphylococcal septicaemia* should prompt a search for discitis/paravertebral abscess.
- Osteoporotic collapse of the cervical vertebrae is rare without trauma. Therefore a collapsed cervical vertebra should prompt a search for *myeloma or tumour*.
- *A history of significant trauma* and resultant neck pain should prompt a search for a fracture. The majority of cervical fractures occur in young adults, most commonly involving C6 and C7 and

then C1 and C2. Orthopaedic review should be sought urgently.
- *Internal carotid artery dissection* is a difficult diagnosis to make and can present with ipsilateral neck pain. It also occurs after blunt trauma or deceleration injury which can be minor. If spontaneous, it is associated with disorders of connective tissue (Ehlers–Danlos type IV, Marfan's) and hypertension. It is a predominant cause of ischaemic stroke in young patients. Additional features can include headache and a partial Horner's syndrome.

Yellow flags (psychosocial) for the development of chronic neck pain

These should be corrected where possible and may require referral to a pain clinic.

- Associated depression, low mood
- Fear and avoidance response to pain and exercise
- Abnormal belief that pain and exercise can be harmful
- Unrealistic expectations
- Poor job satisfaction
- Over-attentive family or poor social support
- Ongoing litigation

Other systemic diseases presenting with neck pain

- The neck can be stiff and restricted as part of an inflammatory arthropathy (*RA, psoriatic, juvenile inflammatory arthritis*). Ankylosing spondylitis usually begins with low back pain and stiffness before the age of 40 but often involves the cervical spine.
- The neck is often painful and stiff in *polymyalgia rheumatica*. However, the range of movement is usually full and the stiffness improves as the day goes on and with movement. There is limb girdle stiffness and often difficulty turning in bed. This is in contrast to *cervical spondylosis* where pain is produced by movement at any time.
- Widespread soft tissue tenderness and pain from *fibromyalgia* is found across the neck and shoulders but also further down the spine in the paravertebral muscles. It is worse with and after exercise and has a strong association with poor non-restorative sleep and fatigue.

- *Temporal arteritis* can rarely present with occipital and neck pain in those over 55 years. There may be features such as temporal tenderness, jaw claudication and visual loss with raised inflammatory markers.

Rare but important causes of acute neck pain

- *The crowned dens syndrome (or acute pseudogout of the neck).* Severe neck pain, restriction and fever in the elderly. This is associated with calcification around the dens best visualized by CT (visible calcium pyrophosphate or hydroxy-apatite deposition). There is usually a very high CRP. The shoulder can be involved and there may be evidence of chondrocalcinosis elsewhere. This responds to an NSAID or a short course of steroids. It can mimic meningitis, sepsis and rarely temporal arteritis, which need to be considered.
- *A retropharyngeal abscess* may cause pain and severely restrict movements of the neck. More common in children, it is becoming increasingly common in adults.
- *Syringomyelia* can present with pain in the neck and shoulders (shawl-like distribution). Loss of pain and temperature sensation (disruption of decussating spinothalamic fibres) in upper limbs and torso with preservation of joint position, vibration and light touch is known as dissociated sensory loss. Additional lower motor neurone involvement with reduced upper limb reflexes and long tract symptoms and signs can occur.

Torticollis

- Some of the above can present as torticollis, including retropharyngeal and soft tissue abscess, acute cervical disc prolapse, but also vertebral fracture/dislocation, spinal haematoma and epiglottitis (an ill, drooling patient with stridor).
- Imaging (plain film and MRI/CT) will be required to exclude these causes.
- Urgent ENT assessment will be necessary to protect the airway *before* imaging if suspected epiglottitis.
- Drug-induced acute dystonia can be treated with biperiden 5 mg IM.
- Idiopathic intermittent torticollis should be referred to a neurologist.

Acute whiplash injury

- Caused by acute sudden hyperextension, hyperflexion or rotation of the neck most commonly during a car accident.
- This can cause painful self-limiting soft tissue injury to the neck and the majority of cases resolve by 3 months.
- Obtain plain radiology of the neck (and possibly further imaging) particularly if:
  - midline point tenderness (possible fracture/dislocation)
  - restriction of lateral rotation to <45 degrees
  - abnormal neurology or other red flags
  - significant trauma (fall >1 metre)
  - age >65 years.
- Management includes:
  - analgesia (NSAID and/or paracetamol with additional codeine phosphate)
  - early mobilization and resumption of normal activities improves outcome
  - advise against the use of soft collars.
- *Late whiplash syndrome* occurs when symptoms persist after 6 months (often characterized by neck pain, dizziness (vertebro-basilar insufficiency), headache, paraesthesia in upper limbs, and psychological disturbances).
- Whiplash injury with a summary of the evidence for the above can be found in a Clinical Knowledge Summary (CKS) from NICE [1].

Important examination findings

- Palpate for abnormal swellings, including temporal tenderness in the elderly and check the range of movement, noting any pain and limitation.
- Examine the gait.
- Assess the nervous system, particularly for increased tone in the legs, brisk reflexes and upgoing plantar response and lower motor neurone signs in the arms. Generally motor signs are more helpful than sensory signs in cervical disease but remember dissociated sensory loss suggesting syringomyelia.
- Remember cerebral causes of increased tone in the legs and poor gait:
  - Normal pressure hydrocephalus
  - Parasagittal tumours.

Inverted supinator reflex explained

- Pathognomonic for cervical myelopathy at C5/6, the narrowest part of the cervical canal, and is usually due to cervical spondylosis.
- The supinator jerk, brachioradialis (C5 and C6), produces flexion of the fingers (C8) instead of the expected elbow flexion and wrist extension, the biceps jerk (C5 and 6) is diminished and the triceps jerk (C7) brisk or exaggerated.
- Osteophyte and/or cervical disc disease will produce narrowing of the exit foramen at C5 and C6 and thus lower motor neurone deficits.
- Additional pressure on the cord causes upper motor neurone signs below this level. Recruitment of hyperactive lower reflex arcs produces the finger flexion and elbow extension. Additionally tone is likely to be increased in the legs and lower limb reflexes may be brisk, perhaps with clonus. One or both plantars may be upgoing.

Investigations

Blood tests

- FBC, CRP, LFT, urea and electrolytes if systemic disease is suspected.
- Myeloma screen if there is unexplained vertebral collapse.
- Additionally blood cultures/throat swab/Paul–Bunnell test if infection is suspected.

Imaging

- *Plain cervical film*. Not indicated in simple neck pain; may show:
  - loss of normal lordosis (muscle spasm)
  - loss of disc height and osteophytes in cervical spondylosis
  - loss of pedicles on AP view if tumour
  - disruption of both vertebral endplates in infection
  - Soft tissue mass in infection
  - fracture/dislocation after trauma.
- *MRI* is indicated if there is any suggestion of:
  - myelopathy

  - significant radiculopathy
  - tumour
  - infection.
- *CT scan* may demonstrate calcification 'crowning' the dens if acute pseudogout suspected.

Nerve conduction studies

- These may be necessary to exclude other causes of weakness and wasting in the hands (e.g. double crush syndrome).

Management

Uncomplicated cervical spondylosis and most cases of radiculopathy:

- Reassurance, simple analgesia, weight loss and low dose amitryptiline (or gabapentin) for dysaesthesia.
- Referral to physiotherapy for neck exercises and local treatments.
- Suggest a neck pillow for nocturnal use. Cervical collars should be avoided in the daytime and can lead to wasting of the neck muscles.

  Refer on to a spinal team:

- Anyone with significant radiculopathy (weakness or wasting) or myelopathy.

  Refer urgently to spinal team:

- Anyone with cervical fracture, tumour or infection (discitis/abscess).

Scenario 45.1 continued

This woman had cervical myelopathy secondary to cervical spondylosis. CRP was normal. Cervical film demonstrated loss of cervical lordosis, osteophytes and multiple areas of reduced disc height. MRI scan confirmed significant pressure on the cervical cord from osteophytes and calcified thickened ligamentum flavum. Amitryptiline was prescribed to reduce paraesthesia in her hands before surgery to relieve her cervical cord compression.

Reference

1. NICE. Clinical Knowledge Summary. Neck pain – whiplash injury. http://cks.nice.org.uk/neck-pain-whiplash-injury.

Chapter

46

Palliative and end of life care

Marianne Tinkler

Introduction

Despite the great medical advances of the last century, cures for many diseases remain elusive. Chronic progressive illnesses such as dementia and chronic organ failure continue to cause significant disability and suffering. Palliative care had its origins in the provision of excellent end of life care to patients with malignant disease but has since expanded to encompass the whole chronic disease spectrum. Almost 500 000 people died in 2011 in the UK. The minority are sudden and unexpected. Most (90%) are preceded by a gradual physical and mental decline due to:

- cancer (25%)
- frailty and dementia (35%)
- chronic organ failure (30%).

In 2010, 53% of all deaths in the UK occurred in hospital, with a significant proportion on the medical wards, despite the fact that surveys consistently show that it is the least preferred place of death for patients. Failure to recognize and manage the dying process can result in significant suffering, with inadequate symptom control, poor quality of life, inappropriate admissions and invasive treatments. A study in patients with metastatic non-small-cell lung cancer showed that early palliative care led to significant improvements in quality of life and mood. As compared with patients receiving standard care, patients receiving early palliative care had less aggressive care at the end of life but longer survival [1]. Early recognition expertise in palliative care should therefore be a key component of the clinical practice of all physicians.

In the following scenario the acute presentation is of GI haemorrhage but the approach is appropriate to all patients presenting with a chronic incurable disease.

> **Scenario 46.1**
>
> *An 80-year-old woman is referred to the medical assessment unit by the emergency department with 'melaena'. She has a history of dementia and is in a nursing home. She is haemodynamically stable and ED have sent bloods, although had difficulty taking them as she was distressed and hitting out. They were unable to get any history from the patient.*

Clinical assessment

- Obtain a history from the patient as you would for any patient presenting with acute GI haemorrhage.
- In a patient such as this, also assess the functional status as the baseline performance status is strongly associated with survival time in patients with advanced illness (Table 46.1).
- If it is not possible to obtain a history directly from the patient, *a collateral history* from relatives or carers is vital, including the existence of advance decisions to refuse treatment (ADRT), 'preferred priorities of care' documents, or a lasting power of attorney (LPA) for health and welfare.

> **Scenario 46.1 continued**
>
> *Collateral history from the nursing home reveals she has been less well over the last 2 weeks, sleeping more and eating less. She is dependent on assistance with all care and has been bedbound for the previous 6 months. She is unable to communicate. She is incontinent of both urine and faeces. Her carers noticed dark offensive stools when they were changing her and called out-of-hours GP who advised calling 999. Her next of kin is a niece in France. Current medications are aspirin 75 mg od, simvastatin 40 mg od, ramipril 5 mg od.*

Acute Medicine, ed. Stephen Haydock, Duncan Whitehead and Zoë Fritz. Published by Cambridge University Press. © Cambridge University Press 2015.

Table 46.1 WHO performance status

0	Asymptomatic (fully active, able to carry on all activities without restriction)
1	Symptomatic but completely ambulatory (restricted in physically strenuous activity but ambulatory and able to carry out work of a light or sedentary nature, e.g. light housework, office work)
2	Symptomatic, <50% in bed/chair during the day (ambulatory and capable of all self-care but unable to carry out any work activities; up and about more than 50% of waking hours)
3	Symptomatic, >50% in bed, but not bedbound (capable of only limited self-care, confined to bed or chair 50% or more of waking hours)
4	Bedbound (completely disabled; cannot carry on any self-care; totally confined to bed or chair)
5	Death

> *Examination reveals a frail woman sleeping but rousable. She is not hypotensive or tachycardic with normal respiratory rate. Examination is normal but difficult as she becomes distressed when woken up. Bloods reveal a haemoglobin of 90, urea elevated at 16 and creatinine 150 (usual for patient).*

Management

Before simply embarking on the familiar risk stratification and management of the suspected upper GI haemorrhage:

STOP and *THINK.*

Consider: 'Is this appropriate for the patient under my care?'

Aggressive investigation may not be appropriate in this patient as she has severe dementia, poor functional status and has been deteriorating over the previous 6 months. A holistic approach is needed as it appears that this patient is reaching the *terminal phase of life.*

The Department of Health End of Life Care Strategy (2008) [2] identifies that:

> *for many people suffering from a chronic illness a point is reached where it is clear that the person will die from their condition.*

Recognition of terminal phase

It can be extremely difficult to identify patients who may be nearing the end of their lives, but identification is the first and most important step in planning for the end of life period. For many people who die each year, death is associated with preventable physical and psychosocial suffering.

> *Earlier recognition of people nearing the end of their lives leads to earlier planning and better care (GSF prognostic indicator guidance; see Further reading)*

Prognostication in non-malignant diseases is inherently more difficult than in malignant diseases, which tend to have a more predictable decline (Figure 46.1).

The last few years of chronic organ failure are characterized by multiple life-threatening exacerbations. Often the final illness in patients with chronic illness comes as a surprise to relatives, who although aware of their disease were not expecting their death. This can significantly impact on their psychological well-being and grief process. Identification of patients reaching end of life can facilitate open communication between families, allowing a 'time to say goodbye' and affirmation of relationships.

The Gold Standards Framework prognostic indicator guidance can help identify patients who may be in the final 6–12 months of their life.

1. *The surprise question* 'would you be surprised if this patient were to die in the next 6–12 months?'
2. *Clinical indicators of advanced disease* (Figure 46.2).

> **Scenario 46.1 continued**
>
> *The scenario patient meets both the surprise question and has dementia-specific indicators of end of life.*

Advance Care Planning whilst patients retain capacity is vital and enables patients and relatives to discuss their wishes and preferences of care at the end stages in life [3]. *Discussion around:*

- fears and concerns
- symptoms
- admission to hospital
- resuscitation
- preferred place of care (at time of death).

  The goal of care can be formulated:
- preservation of life at all costs

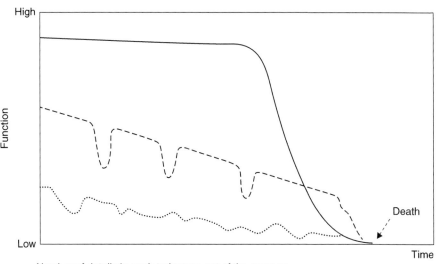

Number of details in each trajectory, out of the average
20 deaths each year per UK general practice list of 2000
patients

——— Cancer (n=5)   – – – · Organ failure (n=6)

·········· Physical and cognitive frailty (n=7)
Other (n=2)

Figure 46.1 Disease trajectory for organ failure, frailty and dementia and incurable cancer. Reproduced from *British Medical Journal*, Murray S and Sheikh A 'Care for All at the End of Life', BMJ 336(7650):958–95, copyright 2008 with permission from BMJ Publishing Group. Patients with malignant disease usually show progression over a few years with a predictable terminal decline over several months. Patients with organ failure (e.g. significant cardiac failure/COPD) are characterized by acute deteriorations associated with increasing dependence over 2–5 years. Patients with physical and cognitive frailty (e.g. dementia) show a prolonged and gradual decline until death.

General indicators:

- Co-morbidity
- Weight loss >10% in 6 months
- General physical decline
- Poor or declining performance status
- Dependence in most ADLs

Dementia*

All of:

- Unable to walk without assistance
- Urinary & faecal incontinence
- No consistently meaningful conversation
- Unable to dress without assistance

And one of:

- 10% weight loss
- Urinary tract infection
- Aspiration pneumonia
- Severe pressure ulcers
- Reduced oral intake
- Recurrent fevers

Figure 46.2 The Gold Standards Framework: *'General indicators'* and *'Dementia specific indicators'* to identify patients in the last 6–12 months of life. Reproduced with permission from Prognostic Indicator Guidance (PIG) 4th Edition Oct 2011 © The Gold Standards Framework Centre In End of Life Care CIC, Thomas K et al.

*See www.goldstandardsframework.org for other chronic conditions.

- preservation of function and quality of life
- comfort care only.

Such important discussions need a sensitive approach and are best undertaken by a familiar clinician, outside a time of crisis, whilst appreciating that some patients may not want to discuss such issues. They cannot be undertaken in a single discussion as patients need time to think over things. We have an important role as hospital clinicians to start or continue this process.

> **Scenario 46.1 continued**
>
> *Unfortunately in this case no identification or advance care planning discussions had occurred.*

All clinical decisions must be made around an ethical framework that guarantees the patient's best interests. Beauchamp and Childress' 'four principles' described below are a commonly used framework.

1. Respect for autonomy

Decide if the patient has mental capacity (as defined by the 2005 Mental Capacity Act) to make a reasoned informed choice regarding treatment (see Chapter 59).

If the patient lacks capacity is there:

An advance decision to refuse treatment: legally binding signed, dated and witnessed documents made by patients when they have capacity (note in the USA these are called Advanced Directives; in the UK, where patients have the right to refuse but not demand treatments they are called 'advance decisions to refuse treatment').

A lasting power of attorney: ensure 'health and welfare' attorney rather than 'property and finance', who can make decisions in the '*best interests*' of the patient.

If not then the medical team must make decisions in the patient's best interests with the involvement of relatives. If there are no next of kin then an *Independent Mental Capacity Advocate (IMCA)* should be involved.

In order to make 'best interest' decisions the following must be considered:

- All relevant circumstances.
- If the patient is likely to regain capacity could decision wait until then?
- Involve patient as fully as possible.
- Withdrawal of life-sustaining treatments must not be motivated by a desire to bring about the person's death.

2. Beneficence

Any treatment plan should benefit the patient. Benefits must be weighed against risks.

3. Non-maleficence

Avoiding harm to patient by treatment. 'Primum non nocere' – *first do no harm*. The risks of treatment must be weighed against the possible benefits.

4. Justice

Patients in similar positions should be treated in a similar manner and not discriminated against.

> **Scenario 46.1 continued**
>
> *Applying these criteria to the patient scenario and after discussion with relatives and GP:*
>
> - *Invasive gastroscopy would not be appropriate. The patient cannot consent and would require heavy sedation with increased risk.*
> - *She should be transferred back to her care home as hospital admission was felt to cause her more distress.*
> - *Aspirin and simvastatin were discontinued as secondary prevention was inappropriate.*
> - *Discharged with a 'just in case' box (see below) and a GP follow-up visit.*
> - *Nursing home staff updated and supported.*
>
> *Unfortunately this patient and family were denied the opportunity to be involved in advance care planning earlier whilst capacity was retained.*

'Just in case' boxes

These are sealed containers containing a range of medications that might be required in emergency and not otherwise immediately available in the primary care setting. They are prescribed by the patient's GP/hospital doctor according to the likely needs of the patient. The medication can be accessed by GPs or appropriately trained nursing staff in the patient's home if required. A 'typical' box would contain:

- diamorphine for analgesia
- cyclizine for nausea and vomiting
- midazolam for agitation
- hyoscine for respiratory secretions.

Ensure that patients on oral opioids are discharged with adequate amounts via subcutaneous form to allow conversion from oral and provide adequate equivalent

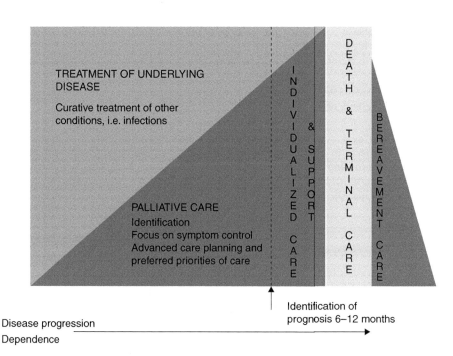

TREATMENT OF UNDERLYING DISEASE

Curative treatment of other conditions, i.e. infections

PALLIATIVE CARE
Identification
Focus on symptom control
Advanced care planning and preferred priorities of care

INDIVIDUALIZED CARE

& SUPPORT

DEATH & TERMINAL CARE

BEREAVEMENT CARE

Identification of prognosis 6–12 months

Disease progression
Dependence

Figure 46.3 Shifting emphasis for treatment and care in terminal illness.

analgesia. The availability of the 'just in case' medication is designed to enable urgent symptom control in the home and prevent an otherwise distressing hospital admission.

Concluding remarks

As clinicians we are all exposed to death and the end of life period and therefore must have generalist experience to identify patients and provide this care. The expert input of specialist palliative care teams when specialist difficulties arise is always available to support us.

The Liverpool Care Pathway (LCP) was designed with the intention of supporting hospital clinicians to provide the excellent levels of palliative care that were available in hospices. In an attempt to ensure that patients who were dying (in the few last hours to days of life) were recognized as requiring a different kind of care, a 'pathway' was created which included prompts to stop unnecessary treatments, and to ensure that palliative ones were given. Significant media attention to instances where the LCP had been poorly applied (e.g. cases where food and water had been withheld, even when the patient wanted them) led to an independent report led by Julia Neuberger. Drawing on evidence [4], she concluded that there were sufficient such instances that the pathway should be phased out. Part of the problem with the LCP being poorly used may have been that

it segregated patients into those who were being treated and those who were being palliated; patients on the LCP stopped having their medical notes used and instead had only the LCP booklet. It is important to emphasize that patients who require palliative treatment still require full medical and nursing attention; we should seek to provide excellent symptom control alongside active disease management with increasing emphasis on palliation as the disease progresses (Figure 46.3).

At the end of life we are not denying treatment but focusing on those that will bring benefit without undertaking futile treatments. It is not appropriate to prolong life at all costs with no regard to its quality or to the potential burdens of treatment for the patient. Many patients wait for us as healthcare professionals to initiate discussions around the possible long-term course of the disease. If we don't broach this important subject they are denied involvement in discussions of their end of life wishes. We should adopt a strategy of:

Planning for the worst, but hoping for the best.

References

1. Temel JS, Greer JA, Muzikansky A, Gallagher ER, Admane S, Jackson VA, Dahlin CM, Blinderman CD, Jacobsen J, Pirl WF, Billings JA, Lynch TJ. Early palliative care for patients with metastatic non-small-cell lung cancer. *N Engl J Med* (2010) 19:363(8):733–742.

2. Department of Health. End of Life. Available to download at www.gov.uk/government/uploads/system/uploads/attachment_data/file/136431/End_of_life_strategy.pdf.

3. GMC. Treatment and Care Towards the End of Life: Good Decision Making. www.gmc-uk.org/End_of_life.pdf_32486688.pdf.

4. Parry R, Seymour J, Whittaker B, Bird L, Cox K. Evidence briefing pathways for the dying phase in end of life care. March 2013. www.gov.uk/government/uploads/system/uploads/attachment_data/file/212451/review_academic_literature_on_end_of_life.pdf.

Further reading

Murray S, Sheikh A (2008) *Care for all at the end of life. BMJ* 336(7650): 958–959.

The GSF Prognostic Indicator Guidance, 4th edn. 2011. Available to download at www.goldstandardsframework.org.uk/cd-content/uploads/files/General%20Files/Prognostic%20Indicator%20Guidance%20October%202011.pdf.

Addendum
Prescribing in palliative care

Stephen Haydock

Most hospitals have access to excellent palliative care services who will advise and support the management of patients at the end of life and suggest appropriate regimens for symptom control.

Opioid analgesia

Opioids: synthetic or semi-synthetic narcotics with opiate-like activity that are not derived from the opium poppy, e.g.:

*   diamorphine
*   buprenorphine
*   oxycodone
*   fentanyl *and many others.*

Opiates: naturally occurring narcotics that are derived from the opium poppy (*Papaver somniferum*):

*   morphine
*   papaverine
*   codeine
*   papaveretum (omnopon) is a mixture of the above three compounds.

The term *opioid* is now incorrectly used to describe all medicinal opioids and opiates and will also be used here (*to prove that the author is not a complete pedant!*).

Oral opioid therapy

Initiate treatment for patients with advanced or progressive disease with *twice daily modified release morphine preparations with immediate release morphine for breakthrough pain.* Titrate dose, balancing symptom control and side effects. If no associated hepatic and/or renal dysfunction then initially:

Opioid naive patients

*   10–15 mg *modified release* morphine sulphate bd; e.g. Zomorph, MST Continus, Morphgesic SR and Filnarine SR *plus*
*   Up to 5 mg *immediate release* morphine prn (1/10th to 1/6th of regular 24 hour dose), e.g. Oramorph, Sevredol.

Patients already taking weak opioids

*   20–30 mg *modified release* morphine sulphate bd *plus*
*   Up to 10 mg *immediate release* morphine prn.

    Up-titrate the morphine dose according to analgesia and side effects:

*   Aim for less than two breakthrough doses per day.
*   Increase regular medication by no more than one-third to one-half in any 24-hour period.

Transdermal opioids

Transdermal opioid patches are an alternative if the oral route is not appropriate *and analgesia requirements are stable.* The conversion factor is as follows:

*   12 µg fentanyl patch equates to about 45 mg oral morphine daily.
*   20 µg transdermal buprenorphine patch equates to about 30 mg morphine daily.

Parenteral opioids

Subcutaneous administration is appropriate for those patients where the oral route is inappropriate and analgesia requirements are not stable (see below).

Side effects of opioids

The following side effects are common.

Constipation: give regular laxatives when starting treatment with opioids. Use a combination of

Table 46.A1 Oral management of other common symptoms of advanced malignant disease

Symptom	Treatment
Breathlessness	• Regular morphine initially 5 mg 4-hourly • Diazepam 5–10 mg daily in divided doses if associated anxiety • Dexamethasone 4–8 mg daily if bronchospasm or obstruction
Hiccups	• Metoclopramide 10 mg 6–8 hourly
Muscle spasm	• Diazepam 5–10 mg daily • Baclofen 5–10 mg three times daily
Nausea and vomiting*	• Metoclopramide 10 mg three times daily • Haloperidol 1.5 mg once or twice daily • Cyclizine up to 50 mg three times daily • Levomepromazine 6 mg once daily increasing to 24 mg twice daily
Restlessness and confusion	• Haloperidol 2 mg and repeated at 2-hourly intervals as required • Levomepromazine 6 mg and repeated at 2-hourly intervals as required
Raised intracranial pressure	• Dexamethasone 8 mg bd (before 6 pm due to insomnia) for 4–5 days • Reduce to 4–6 mg daily

*Not directly related to chemotherapy. (For chemotherapy related nausea and vomiting see Chapter 65.)

a faecal softening agent and a drug that stimulates peristalsis, e.g.:

- co-danthramer
- lactulose plus senna.

Nausea: common in initial stages but usually self-limiting. Treatment with an antiemetic for first 5 days may be required, e.g.:

- metoclopramide.

Sedation: common in early stages and usually improves. If persistent and pain controlled then reduce opioid dose. If pain not controlled then *consider change of opioid with advice from palliative care*.

Other common symptoms

Other common symptoms are shown in Table 46.A1.

Continuous subcutaneous infusions in palliative care

Indications

- The patient is no longer able to take oral medication due to nausea, vomiting, dysphagia, weakness or reduced conscious level (and analgesic requirements are not stable such that the transdermal route can be used).

- Inoperable bowel obstruction.
- In accordance with patient's wishes.
- When other access not suitable, e.g. reduced venous access secondary to chemotherapy; reduced intramuscular access due to loss of muscle bulk.

Advantages of subcutaneous route

- Easier to manage in the home setting in comparison to intravenous. Small calibre butterfly needles can be left in situ for several days.
- Reduced risk of haematoma formation and nerve damage in comparison to intramuscular.
- Slower absorption than IM route allowing smoother 24-hour cover.

Commonly used medications

Subcutaneous infusion using a syringe driver and butterfly needle is set up to administer medication for a 24-hour infusion period. It can be used to control a range of symptoms when the patient cannot take corresponding oral formulation.

Pain:

- Morphine and diamorphine are commonly used.
- Diamorphine has the advantage of greater water solubility over morphine and is preferred as this

avoids need for subsequent conversion from morphine to diamorphine if high opioid doses are then required.

- The *parenteral morphine* dose (IM, SC and IV) is about *half the oral dose of morphine*.
- The *parenteral diamorphine* dose is about *one-third of the oral dose of morphine*.

Confusion and restlessness

- Dopaminergic D2 antagonists (haloperidol and levomepromazine preferred). Metoclopramide can be used but more commonly causes skin reaction.
- Haloperidol 5–15 mg over 24-hour period.
- Levomepromazine (Nozinan) 12.5–50 mg over 24 hours but causes sedation and occasionally a reaction at the infusion site.
- Midazolam if very restless can be used in addition to the above initially at 10–20 mg over 24 hours and up-titrated to a maximum of 60 mg/24 hours.

Nausea and vomiting

- Dopamine D2 receptor antagonists blocking dopamine action in chemoreceptor trigger zone of vomiting centre.
- Haloperidol 2.5–10 mg over 24-hour period.
- Levomepromazine (Nozinan) 5–25 mg over 24 hours but causes sedation.

Excess respiratory secretions

- Anticholinergics (muscarinic) are preferred agents and are also useful for bowel colic.
- Hyoscine hydrobromide 1.2–2 mg over 24-hour period but is sedating.
- Hyoscine butylbromide 20–120 mg over 24-hour period and is less sedating.

Convulsions

- Midazolam at initial dose of 20–40 mg over 24 hours and is useful for prevention of seizures

in patients with cerebral primary or secondary tumours and/or those previously requiring oral antiepileptics.

Some comments on preparing and monitoring the infusion

- Drugs can be dissolved in either water or saline. The latter is less likely to cause pain at the injection site (may be due to hypotonicity of water-based infusions). Drugs are more likely to precipitate out of solution in saline and hence diamorphine concentrations 40 mg/mL should only be made up in water for injection.
- Several different drugs can be mixed in one syringe. Diamorphine is compatible with:
  - haloperidol
  - dexamethasone
  - hyoscine butylbromide or hydrobromide
  - levomepromazine
  - midazolam
  - metoclopramide.
- Pain and inflammation at the injection site merits change of infusion site. Swelling alone does not require a site change.
- Infusions require frequent monitoring for rate, drug precipitation or discoloration.

Further reading

British National Formulary. Prescribing in Palliative Care section.

Opioids in palliative care: safe and effective prescribing of strong opioids for pain in palliative care of adults. (2012) NICE Clinical Guideline 140. Available to download at www.nice.org.uk/nicemedia/live/13745/59285/59285.pdf.

Palpitations

Darshan H. Brahmbhatt and Peter J. Pugh

Introduction

Palpitations are described as *the abnormal sensation and increased awareness of one's own heart beating*. They can occur with a normal cardiac rhythm, or can signal an arrhythmia. Palpitations are a common acute presentation and occur in a range of clinical scenarios from isolated atrial ectopics to life-threatening arrhythmias such as ventricular tachycardia. Palpitations, even when benign, often result in considerable distress and anxiety for the patient.

In the acute setting, the *clinical status of the patient* with particular attention to their *haemodynamic stability* and the *initial ECG findings* are used to risk stratify and guide the urgency of investigation and management:

High risk: those with current haemodynamic compromise require urgent treatment with senior support and specialist advice where needed.

Intermediate risk: patients are at significant risk of deterioration; initiate treatment and arrange admission for cardiac monitoring.

Low risk: patients are haemodynamically stable with minimal risk of deterioration; they are safe to discharge home with review in the outpatient or ambulatory care setting with appropriate planned investigations.

Scenario 47.1

A 72-year-old man is referred due to 'rapid atrial fibrillation'. He has had previous episodes that have lasted a few hours, but this one has persisted for over 12 hours. He had a myocardial infarction 3 years earlier, and admits to being 'fond of a drink'. His regular medications are aspirin 75 mg and simvastatin 40 mg daily. He feels unwell, breathless and light-headed on exertion. Examination reveals an irregularly irregular pulse at a rate of 155 beats per minute. His supine blood pressure is 105/60. ECG confirms atrial fibrillation with fast ventricular response.

Referrals due to atrial fibrillation with fast ventricular rate are very common. Management requires decisions regarding urgency of treatment, and regarding rhythm or rate control, anticoagulation and appropriate lifestyle advice. Further investigation and appropriate follow-up should be planned following discharge.

Clinical assessment

History

Palpitations can mean something different to patient and physician, therefore find out the exact nature of the patient's symptoms.

- Enquire regarding speed and regularity. Ask the patient to tap out the rhythm. Occasional 'thumps' suggest ectopic beats.
- How frequently do the palpitations occur and how long do they last for?
- How are they impacting on the patient's life?
- When do they occur and does anything precipitate them or terminate them, e.g. coughing or breath holding?
  - Exercise-induced palpitations and presyncope need to be investigated thoroughly to exclude underlying structural heart disease, such as hypertrophic cardiomyopathy or arrhythmogenic right ventricular dysplasia.
- Is there a history of syncope?
- Consider and exclude '*arrhythmia-mimics*' such as vertigo, angina, pleurisy, dyspnoea and postural hypotension.
- Ask about onset and offset of symptoms.
  - Abrupt onset and offset suggest AVRT or AVNRT.
  - If in atrial fibrillation, the time from onset will determine how it will be managed.

Acute Medicine, ed. Stephen Haydock, Duncan Whitehead and Zoë Fritz. Published by Cambridge University Press. © Cambridge University Press 2015.

- The frequency of recurrences or paroxysms will help to gauge symptom burden.
- Enquire regarding associated symptoms of chest pain, breathlessness and hypotension.
  - Associated symptoms may help determine if palpitations are causing compromise: *angina, hypotension, symptoms of heart failure and fluctuating conscious level* should all trigger consideration for immediate treatment by direct current cardioversion.

Take a detailed drug history; enquire regarding contributory ingestion of known precipitants of palpitations and arrhythmias:

- Caffeine (increases heart rate and increases ectopics)
- Alcohol (increases risk of atrial fibrillation)
- Illicit substances (especially ecstasy, cocaine and amphetamines)
- Over-the-counter or prescribed medications (especially beta-agonists, theophyllines, calcium channel blockers and drugs prolonging QT interval).

Take a detailed past medical history; particularly consider:

- Anxiety and depression (often associated with palpitations)
- Cardiac disease (acquired or congenital) as arrhythmias are more common in structurally abnormal hearts
- Other conditions which may affect treatment; for example: asthmatics may not tolerate beta-blockers, those with risk factors for stroke are likely to need anticoagulation in atrial fibrillation
- Endocrine syndromes: phaeochromocytoma, thyrotoxicosis, hypothyroidism and carcinoid syndrome, should be given consideration initially with a focused history.

A careful family history must be taken:

- Enquire regarding close relatives with early onset cardiac disease, atrial fibrillation or implantable devices.
- Ask specifically regarding instances of sudden cardiac death, or unexplained deaths of close relatives under 40 years of age.
- If close relatives have a diagnosis of epilepsy this may be relevant as it can be a misdiagnosis for cardiac arrhythmias which cause syncope.

Examination

Examination should focus on:

- Signs of cardiac compromise
- Ensuring there are no obvious precipitating causes for palpitations. In particular a thorough cardiovascular examination should elicit signs of heart failure or valvular disease. Be alert to evidence of current infection.
- Thyroid status
- Anaemia.

Investigations

12-lead ECG

During symptoms this is the investigation of choice; if the arrhythmia has terminated the ECG may still have important features:

- Cardiac conduction abnormalities
- Signs of previous myocardial infarction
- Left ventricular hypertrophy
- Signs of pre-excitation (short PR interval and delta waves)
- QT prolongation.

Blood tests

- Urea and electrolytes
- Mg^{2+}
- Ca^{2+}
- FBC
- TFTs
- CRP

Electrolyte imbalances can frequently drive arrhythmias, as can anaemia, infection or volume depletion. Serum potassium, magnesium and calcium should be checked and corrected, alongside a full blood count with transfusion if necessary.

Cardiac monitoring

Recorded rhythm strips from cardiac monitoring can be helpful in identifying the underlying rhythm disturbance with symptoms. The most common in-hospital methods of monitoring are:

- bedside monitor
- telemetry, which allows patients to be ambulatory whilst having their rhythm monitored.

Both options can be helpful in making a diagnosis, especially if the symptoms are debilitating and may be causing compromise. They can also guide treatment titration, preventing iatrogenic bradycardia. Ambulatory inpatient monitoring can help confirm that patients do not develop arrhythmias during normal daily activities.

Ambulatory ECG monitoring

Ambulatory monitoring can detect changes in heart rhythm and rate while the patient performs their usual activities. For patients who do not have any concerning features of compromise, outpatient Holter monitoring can be very useful. A small monitor records a 24-hour ECG to be analysed later.

Ambulatory ECG reports will report maximum and minimum heart rates and the mean heart rate. This can be valuable for reviewing rate control therapy in atrial fibrillation. If *symptomatic pauses >3 seconds occur the patient should be considered for a pacemaker*, especially if they have periods of poor rate control at other times, allowing a 'block and pace' approach.

Many people have ectopic beats, and a frequency chart of aberrant complexes is often reported, but investigation is only warranted when they account for >5% of total heart beats. Runs of aberrant ventricular origin complexes, salvos of non-sustained ventricular tachycardia, should be investigated for underlying structural heart disease and treated with beta-blockers to reduce the risk of developing a sustained ventricular arrhythmia.

Exercise ECG

This is an underused test that can act as a diagnostic tool and afford patient reassurance. It commonly takes the form of treadmill testing, but exercise bikes which monitor heart rhythm and rate are available.

If investigating frequent ectopic beats, the burden of abnormal heart beats should reduce with exercise; *an increase in ectopic burden would warrant further investigation and referral*. For investigating patients whose symptoms occur with exercise, physician supervision of the test is important in case a ventricular arrhythmia is triggered.

Echocardiography

Echo is a useful tool to look for underlying structural heart disease; *it is rarely required as an inpatient*, and can be organized before follow-up review as an outpatient. Reports can be comprehensive, often with too much detail for the non-specialist. The most important aspects to review are the chamber descriptions:

- *Left ventricle*: assessment of systolic function is important as it will guide therapy, negatively inotropic medications generally being avoided in heart failure. Regional variations in wall motion suggest an ischaemic cause of the impairment in function. Dilatation suggests a higher propensity of ventricular arrhythmias, as does an increased wall thickness and hypertrophy, especially in hypertrophic cardiomyopathy.
- *Left atrium*: dilatation is a good predictor that atrial fibrillation will be longstanding and difficult to return to sinus rhythm.
- *Right ventricle*: Dilatation can be a sign of pulmonary disease causing pulmonary hypertension with strain on the right ventricle. *The sensitivity and specificity for predicting acute pulmonary embolism is low*. Right ventricular regional wall motion abnormalities may suggest arrhythmogenic right ventricular dysplasia, a diagnosis not to miss in a young patient with palpitations, as it can progress to be fatal.

Slowing AV nodal conduction

For patients in suspected supraventricular tachycardia (SVT), diagnosis can be unclear with higher ventricular rates, the QRS complexes on the ECG being too close to determine atrial activity. In this situation, using vagal stimulation to slow AV nodal conduction can be helpful for diagnosis and may cardiovert the patient; failing this a pharmacological approach can be employed.

Vagal manoeuvres

- *Valsalva manoeuvre*: raising intrathoracic pressure by exhaling against a closed glottis; 'popping your ear drums' as though on a plane landing or asking them to blow hard into a 20 mL plastic syringe also gives the desired effect.
- *Carotid sinus massage*: first check the patient has *no history of carotid artery disease or CVE or TIA*. Next *ensure the contralateral artery is not obstructed*, by palpating the carotid pulsation. The area for massage is just lateral to the thyroid cartilage; deep circulating pressure on this area should result in a reflex cholinergic inhibition of the AV node, slowing conduction down to enable deciphering of atrial activity.

Pharmacological approach

- *Adenosine* is the commonest drug used at 6 mg and 12 mg doses, although this should not be attempted without medical support and only when the patient is *attached to a defibrillator capable of transcutaneous pacing*. Pre-warn the patient they may feel their heart rhythm change and some have the feeling of '*impending doom*'. Then a rapid intravenous bolus of adenosine is delivered through a large cannula, followed by a 20 mL saline flush. During this procedure a continuous printed ECG recording should be made.
- Adenosine has a short half-life, but will transiently inhibit the AV node to allow atrial fibrillation or flutter to become more obvious, or terminate AVRT and AVNRT, helping make the diagnosis. Rarely the sino-atrial node may take some time to recover, and the ensuing asystole may require external pacing to bridge that gap.
- *Verapamil* is used in those with asthma, allergies or other contraindication to adenosine. Unlike adenosine, verapamil 5 mg is given by *slow intravenous injection over several minutes*.

Indications for admission

- Any patient who has suffered haemodynamic compromise should be admitted to hospital to a ward with static ECG monitoring, possibly with early involvement of the cardiology team.
- *This is especially true for ventricular arrhythmias*; these patients are at high risk of recurrence and treatment of underlying causes may require specialist intervention.
- Any patients with red flag symptoms (exertional syncope and palpitations) should not be discharged without cardiology assessment and review plan.
- Most patients with first presentations of atrial arrhythmia *without compromise or ventricular ectopy* can be managed as outpatients after careful explanation and commencement of medications to settle their symptoms, as needed.

Indications for cardiology review

It is perhaps easier to define those patients that do not need to be seen by a cardiologist, since all ventricular arrhythmias and patients requiring admission due to a primary disturbance of cardiac rhythm should be seen by the cardiology team. Many hospitals now have a dedicated cardiac rhythm management team, with specialist nurses who manage arrhythmia services. Those patients who do not require cardiology referral include:

- When palpitations are secondary to another medical problem causing an arrhythmia, such as sepsis or hyperthyroidism leading to atrial fibrillation, treating the underlying cause will often resolve the arrhythmia. These patients only require cardiology review if the initial management of the rhythm disturbance is unsuccessful.
- Young patients (under 65 years old) with AF or where management is difficult should be considered for referral on to cardiology for outpatient review following discharge, likewise patients with pre-excited ECGs (*delta waves present on ECG*) and those with other troublesome supraventricular tachycardias. It is often helpful to organize echocardiography and Holter monitoring for these patients to review how successfully current treatment is controlling their arrhythmia.

Classification and management of common arrhythmias

All patients should be counselled, regardless of their arrhythmia, on preventing recurrence by adherence to their maintenance medications. They should also be given advice to reduce stimulants, such as caffeine, alcohol and illicit medications, which may trigger palpitations and arrhythmias.

Supraventricular arrhythmias

1. Ectopic beats

These are the commonest form of palpitation; patients may describe a 'skip' or 'jump' within their body, and feel that their heart rhythm is irregular. A series of intermittent ectopic beats can cause a great deal of distress due to the 'thumping' sensation created by the variable volume of blood ejected by the left ventricle, which results from the varying time period for diastolic filling. Isolated ectopic beats are not in themselves dangerous, but frequent ectopics might suggest the need for longer monitoring to look for the total burden of ectopic beats.

A common problem can be that the perception of an 'abnormal' heart beat by the patient increases their vigilance for further ectopic beats which, when they occur, cause increased anxiety levels. Ambulatory ECG monitoring can be a very useful diagnostic tool here to correlate symptoms with ectopic beats, especially if they do not occur very frequently. Atrial bigeminy, where a sinus beat is followed by a premature atrial ectopic beat before another sinus beat and the same again, is benign and does not require any treatment more than ensuring haemodynamic stability and normal electrolyte levels.

2. Atrial fibrillation and flutter

Overall this affects 1.5–2% of the general population.

Atrial fibrillation (AF) is a disorder where the intrinsic heart beat generation of the sino-atrial node is overwhelmed by disorganized electrical activity, often from the atrial tissue around the pulmonary veins. The resulting atrial activity is uncoordinated, and the rate at which the impulses are conducted through the AV node determines the ventricular response, and so apical heart rate.

Atrial flutter is a similar arrhythmia of the atrium that involves a self-perpetuating circuit of electrical activity that causes rapid depolarization of the atria, with the ventricular response being governed by the conductance through the AV node. Flutter tends to degenerate into atrial fibrillation, so is managed as one would manage atrial fibrillation.

The classification of atrial fibrillation is determined by its time course. Regardless of the time of onset, *the first presentation* is nominated as first diagnosed AF. This is independent of the severity and duration of symptoms.

- *Paroxysmal* denotes intermittent AF often with short episodes of arrhythmia with symptoms, which may terminate spontaneously or with medication.
- *Persistent* indicates AF ongoing for more than 7 days; either rate or rhythm control may be appropriate strategies, dependent on the clinical situation.
- *Permanent AF* is when it is accepted, by both the patient and treating physician, that return to sinus rhythm is unlikely and the focus of treatment is on rate control rather than rhythm control.

AF can be secondary to other medical conditions/ specific triggers: pneumonia and other infections, lung tumours, thyrotoxicosis, hypertension, valvular heart disease, ischaemic heart disease, caffeine and alcohol. Looking for these causes is an important part of the clinical work-up for AF, but often no specific cause is found.

Management

The natural history of the condition is of one that recurs after a variable period of time, with subsequent episodes becoming more frequent and lasting for longer periods of time; paroxysmal progresses to persistent, and eventually permanent AF. For younger patients initial treatment should be aimed at trying to return the patient to sinus rhythm (*rhythm control*) to minimize symptom burden from AF and medications. Where this is not possible, the aim should be to prevent an accelerated ventricular rate that causes symptoms and possible compromise by sufficiently blocking AV nodal conduction with medications (*rate control*). If a fast ventricular rate is left untreated then a rate-related cardiomyopathy can develop. There is no demonstrated survival benefit for rhythm over rate control.

Determine time of onset

- If <48 hours, or if well anticoagulated (INR >2 for 4 weeks), consider rhythm control with medical or DC cardioversion. Patients who are not anticoagulated should be commenced on therapeutic dose low molecular weight heparin and considered for formal anticoagulation.
- If >48 hours since onset, but rhythm control is preferred option, commence LMWH and consider referral to cardiology for transoesophageal echocardiogram to exclude intracardiac thrombus, before cardioversion.
- For those without clear onset of symptoms, aim to achieve rate control using a beta-blocker (bisoprolol 2.5 mg od) or rate-controlling calcium channel antagonist (verapamil 40 mg tds or diltiazem MR 90 mg od) if beta-blockers are contraindicated. Aim for a ventricular rate <110 beats/minute. This can be done either as an inpatient or through an ambulatory care clinic with further review and titration of medication done by the GP. Digoxin can be used in addition if required or first line in sedentary patients or when hypotension is a concern; it offers poor rate control during exertion.
- For those in whom sinus rhythm is restored, beta-blockers are recommended, unless there was a clear reversible precipitant (pneumonia). If there is a recurrence of AF on a beta-blocker,

Table 47.1 CHA$_2$DS$_2$VASc score for thromboembolic stroke risk in AF

Risk factor	Score
Congestive heart failure	1
Hypertension	1
Age ≥75 years	2
Diabetes	1
Stroke, transient ischaemic attack, or thromboembolism	2
Myocardial infarction, aortic plaque or peripheral arterial disease	1
Age 65–74 years	1
Female sex	1
Maximum CHA2DS2-VASc Index score	**9**

Table 47.2 Observed annual stroke risk from calculated CHA$_2$DS$_2$-VASc Index score

CHA$_2$DS$_2$-VASc score	Annual stroke risk (%)	Guideline
0	0	No treatment recommended
1	1.3	No treatment or oral anticoagulation (anticoagulation preferred option)
2	2.2	Oral anticoagulation recommended
3	3.2	
4	4.0	
5	6.7	
6	9.8	
7–9	9.6–15.2	

pharmacological options to prevent further episodes include sotalol and flecainide in those with structurally normal hearts or amiodarone if there is structural heart disease or impaired left ventricular systolic function.

Anticoagulation and newer anticoagulants

Atrial fibrillation/flutter carries a significant risk of systemic thromboembolism. 12 500 strokes each year in the UK are due to atrial fibrillation. Previously aspirin was advised as an antithrombotic in this group of patients, but it is no longer included in the European guidelines as thromboprophylaxis in atrial fibrillation, as it only gives a relative risk reduction of 20–30%.

Another paradigm shift in AF management is that risk stratification should be used to decide who will not need to be anticoagulated, *with routine thromboprophylaxis being the standard of care* [1]. The current recommended risk assessment tool is the CHA$_2$DS$_2$-VASc Index (Table 47.1), which identifies those who have low risk of having stroke, dependent on the score:

- 0: no thromboprophylaxis advised.
- 1: preference for oral anticoagulation but no thromboprophylaxis is an option.
- 2 or higher: commence anticoagulation with warfarin (target INR 2–3) or equivalent anticoagulant. (See Table 47.2.)

Anticoagulation always has a risk. The risk of severe bleeding can be estimated using the HAS-BLED [2] scoring system (see Tables 47.3 and 47.4).

Novel oral anticoagulants [3] with the aim of having more predictable pharmacokinetics and pharmacodynamics than warfarin are increasingly used. Dabigatran, rivaroxaban and apixaban all have UK licences for non-valvular atrial fibrillation with an additional risk factor (heart failure, hypertension, age>75, diabetes or previous stroke/TIA). The different medications are summarized in Table 47.5. It is important to remember that, unlike warfarin, none of these medications currently have a specific antidote.

3. Atrioventricular re-entrant and atrioventricular nodal re-entrant tachycardias

Although atrioventricular re-entrant tachycardia (AVRT) and atrioventricular nodal re-entrant tachycardia (AVNRT) are less common than AF, they affect a disproportionately larger number of young patients, and are more common in women than men. The presence of an accessory pathway either between the atria and ventricles (AVRT) or within the AV node (AVNRT) allows re-entry of depolarization to perpetuate a cycle of depolarization.

AVNRT is the commonest cause of a regular SVT, resulting in a regular tachycardia with narrow QRS complexes, sometimes with retrograde atrial depolarization, confirmed by *P-waves after the QRS complex.*

Wolff–Parkinson–White syndrome is characterized by an accessory pathway that allows pre-excitation and can lead to AVRT; this accessory pathway can often be seen on an ECG as a slurred upstroke of the QRS complex (delta wave) and a shortened PR interval. AV

Table 47.3 HAS-BLED risk factors for bleeding

Risk factor	Score
Hypertension history (systolic blood pressure >160 mmHg)	1
Abnormal renal (dialysis, transplant, creatinine >200 μmol/L)	1
or liver function (cirrhosis, bilirubin >2× normal, AST/ALT/AP >3× normal)	1
Stroke history (previous stroke)	1
Bleeding previously or predisposition to bleeding (major bleeds)	1
Labile INR (unstable/high INRs)	1
Elderly (>65 years old)	1
Drugs predisposing to bleeding (antiplatelet agents, NSAIDs)	1
or Alcohol usage history? (≥8 alcoholic drinks per week)	1
Maximum HAS-BLED score	9

Table 47.4 Bleeding rates according to HAS-BLED score (note that the numbers of patients in some groups were low, and the number of bleeds was also low, so this is a guide and not a precise bleed risk)

HAS-BLED score	Bleeds/100 patients
0	1.13
1	1.02
2	1.88
3	3.74
4	8.70
5	12.50

nodal blockade should be avoided in these patients. Flecainide can be a useful agent.

The fast heart rate can cause symptoms itself, and often patients describe the retrograde atrial activation against a closed tricuspid valve causing '*neck pulsations*'. Patients can also report dizziness and light-headedness, related to the reduced cardiac output.

Management

These rhythms rarely cause compromise, and treatment aims to break the cycle of activation through blocking of either the AV node or the accessory pathway; (refer to the earlier section 'Slowing AV nodal conduction'). If vagal manoeuvres fail to cardiovert the patient, use intravenous adenosine up to a maximum dose of 18 mg, or IV verapamil 5 mg. These measures should interrupt true AVRT and AVNRT; if they do not, an alternative diagnosis, such as atrial flutter or sinus tachycardia, is likely. Often, the reentrant tachycardia may recur, and in these cases, long-acting medications that block the AV node should be used, such as beta-blockers or calcium channel blockers.

Ventricular arrhythmias

The AV node offers protection to the ventricles by limiting conduction of supraventricular arrhythmias, preventing an excessive ventricular rate, thus allowing adequate ventricular filling time during diastole. When the arrhythmia is ventricular in origin, this protection is removed and accelerated rates are more likely to result

Table 47.5 Novel oral anticoagulants

Drug	Mechanism	Doses	Bleeding	Contraindications	Notes
Dabigatran	Pro-drug dabigatran etexilate metabolized to active compound, dabigatran, a direct thrombin inhibitor	150 mg bd (superior to warfarin) 110 mg bd (non-inferior to warfarin)	Higher GI bleeding risk at 150 mg dose, lower bleeding risk at 110 mg dose, lower intracranial bleeding at both doses	Creatinine clearance <30 mL/min	Dose 150 mg if <75 years old; 110 mg if >75 years old or other risk factors that increase bleeding
Rivaroxaban	Direct factor Xa inhibitor	20 mg od (non inferior to warfarin)	Similar bleeding risk to warfarin, although lower intracranial bleeding risk	Creatinine clearance <15 mL/min	Reduce dose to 15 mg if Cr Cl 15–49 mL/min
Apixaban	Direct factor Xa inhibitor	5 mg bd (non-inferior to warfarin)	Reduced major bleeding	Creatinine clearance <15 mL/min	Reduce dose to 2.5 mg if Cr Cl 15–29 mL/min or if two of age >80 years, weight ≤60 kg, or creatinine >133 μmol/L

Table 47.6 The Vaughan-Williams classification of anti-arrhythmic agents. Digoxin and adenosine were never included in the original classification

Class	Mechanism	Comments
1	Sodium channel blockers	Further divided into subgroups 1a, 1b and 1c based on their effect on the action potential duration (e.g. flecainide and propafenone)
2	Beta-blockers	Act to slow conduction, by blocking sympathetic activity throughout all cardiac tissue, in particular the sino-atrial and atrioventricular nodes (e.g. bisoprolol and metoprolol)
3	Potassium channel blockers	Delay repolarization, effectively increasing the action potential duration and therefore prolonging the effective refractory period (e.g. amiodarone)
4	Calcium channel blockers (non-dihydropyridines)	Block L-type voltage-gated calcium channels, reducing the activity of the sino-atrial and atrioventricular nodes, with negative inotropic effects (e.g. diltiazem and verapamil)

in reduced ventricular filling and cardiac output and so potentially in cardiovascular compromise and collapse.

The commonest forms of ventricular arrhythmia are isolated ectopic beats, monomorphic and polymorphic ventricular tachycardia. Ventricular fibrillation more frequently presents as collapse and cardiac arrest (see Chapter 14).

1. Ventricular ectopy

Assess and treat in a similar way to atrial ectopy. Only when the ectopic burden is significantly raised (at least 5% of total beats) can it lead to deleterious long-term effects such as left ventricular dysfunction and potentially indicates underlying cardiac disease. At levels less than 5%, they can be treated purely for symptom relief. Ventricular bigeminy or trigeminy can be treated conservatively if there is no haemodynamic compromise, correcting electrolyte imbalances and any underlying hormonal imbalances.

2. Ventricular tachycardia

Ventricular tachycardia is usually caused by an area of abnormal or scarred tissue that conducts electrical impulses more slowly than healthy myocardial tissue and can set up a delay in conduction to facilitate a circuit of activation. This can lead to very fast ventricular rates, which are likely to cause syncope and cardiac arrest.

Paroxysmal non-sustained ventricular tachycardia can be a warning sign for prolonged VT and should be further investigated by looking for underlying ischaemia and structural heart disease. Treatment should focus on reducing the ectopic activity that may be setting off the arrhythmia, and to reduce the excitability of the scar tissue.

Management

In patients who had features of compromise according to the Advanced Life Support guidelines, emergency *synchronized DC cardioversion* should be undertaken. If after three attempts, cardioversion has not been successful, the patient should be loaded with 300 mg IV amiodarone over 10–20 minutes before further attempts at cardioversion.

In the patient with no signs of compromise, amiodarone should be commenced at 300 mg IV over one hour, before continuing 900 mg IV over 23 hours. There should be a low threshold for cardioversion after the first hour of therapy, as the longer the patient remains in an accelerated ventricular rhythm, the more likely they are to deteriorate haemodynamically.

After return to sinus rhythm, the patient should be commenced on regular oral amiodarone (200 mg tds for 7 days, then 200 mg bd for 7 days and then continue on 200 mg od as a maintenance dose) and concomitant beta-blocker therapy. These patients should be considered for a secondary prevention implantable cardioverter defibrillator.

Polymorphic ventricular tachycardia

'*Torsades de pointes*' can result from frequent ventricular ectopy and the 'R on T' phenomenon, whereby the R wave of an ectopic depolarization occurs on the T wave of a preceding sinus conducted depolarization, setting up a ventricular re-entrant circuit of depolarization and causing the arrhythmia.

Management

Unstable polymorphic ventricular tachycardia is treated with unsynchronized DC cardioversion.

Both monomorphic and polymorphic VT can be caused by pre-existing conditions and looking for these should be part of the investigation. *Other than isolated ventricular ectopy, all ventricular arrhythmias warrant inpatient specialist cardiac review and treatment.*

Common anti-arrhythmic agents

The **Vaughan-Williams Classification** (see Table 47.6) categorized anti-arrhythmic drugs by method of action:

Beta-blockers: useful first-line anti-arrhythmic as the newer preparations such as bisoprolol and metoprolol are highly beta-1 selective and without many of the side effects of beta-2 receptor blockade. Even so, they can lead to bronchospasm and should be avoided in patients with asthma.

- Slow AV conduction to reduce the ventricular response in AF.
- Suppress ectopic beats which may initiate re-entrant tachycardias.
- Dampen down the sympathetic, adrenergic drive to the heart, further reducing the risk of ventricular dysrhythmias.
- They should be used with caution in those with significant airways disease as they can lead to bronchospasm, particularly in those with brittle, or poorly controlled asthma.

Calcium channel blockers: frequently used as second-line drugs in rate control strategies. They do not cause bronchospasm and are often used where beta-blockers are contraindicated. Due to their negative inotropic effects, they should be avoided in patients with left ventricular impairment or a history of heart failure.

Amiodarone is perhaps the most widely used intravenous anti-arrhythmic in the acute presentation of tachyarrhythmias. It can settle most arrhythmias by stabilizing the action potential and lengthening the refractory period. It can cause chemical injury to smaller veins and tissue necrosis if it extravasates; therefore after the initial loading dose, longer infusions should be *administered through a long-line or central venous catheter*.

The initial treatment dose for stable tachyarrhythmias is 300 mg over 1 hour, followed by 900 mg over 23 hours. It can cardiovert atrial fibrillation, so should always be used with anticoagulation. It should not be used when *polymorphic VT* is the culprit, nor should it be considered when there is a prolonged QT interval as it may precipitate 'R on T' phenomenon and worsen ventricular tachycardia.

Flecainide and propafenone: should probably be discussed with cardiology teams before commencement. It may be advisable to exclude significant coronary artery disease and undertake echocardiography before commencing these medications.

Flecainide can be administered as an intravenous injection (usually 2 mg/kg over 10 minutes, up to a maximum of 150 mg) and is a good choice for achieving rhythm control in those with *structurally normal hearts and no history of ischaemic heart disease*. It must be co-prescribed with an AV node blocker if atrial flutter is present, as it may slow down the flutter rate within the atrium to 200/min which could be conducted to the ventricles 1:1 and lead to worse symptoms. Oral flecainide (100–200 mg twice daily) can work to restore sinus rhythm; it also works as a 'pill-in-the-pocket' remedy for patients with paroxysmal AF.

Propafenone (also 2 mg/kg over 10–20 minutes IV) also achieves rapid cardioversion of recent onset AF. Similarly to flecainide, it can be pro-arrhythmic in patients with underlying ischaemia or structural abnormalities.

Digoxin: similar to beta-blockers and calcium channel blockers, it is an AV node inhibitor. It slows down conduction to the ventricle to achieve rate control in atrial fibrillation. It does not have as significant a blood pressure lowering effect as the other two classes of drugs do, and it is a weak positive inotrope, allowing its use in heart failure. It can be used intravenously or orally, and is often used in elderly and more sedentary patients where there is concern that beta-blocker may cause symptomatic hypotension.

References

1. Lip GY, Nieuwlaat R, Pisters R, Lane DA, Crijns HJ. Refining clinical risk stratification for predicting stroke and thromboembolism in atrial fibrillation using a novel risk factor-based approach: the Euro Heart Survey on atrial fibrillation. *Chest* 2010; 137(2): 263–272.

2. Pisters R, Lane DA, Nieuwlaat R, de Vos CB, Crijns HJ, Lip GY. A novel user-friendly score (HAS-BLED) to assess 1-year risk of major bleeding in patients with atrial fibrillation: the Euro Heart Survey. *Chest* 2010; 138(5): 1093–1100.

3. EHRA. Practical Guide on the use of new oral anticoagulants in patients with non-valvular atrial fibrillation: executive summary. *Eur Heart J* 2013; doi: 10.1093/eurheartj/eht13.

Further reading

Advanced Life Support (6th edn) (2011) Resuscitation Council (UK).

Atrial Fibrillation (Management of) 2010 and Focused Update (2012). *European Heart Journal* 2012; 33: 2719–2747.

NICE: CG36 Atrial fibrillation: full guideline. http://guidance.nice.org.uk/CG36/Guidance/pdf/English.

Supraventricular Arrhythmias (ACC/AHA/ESC Guidelines for the Management of Patients with) ESC Clinical Practice Guidelines. *European Heart Journal* 2003; 24: 1857–1897.

Ventricular Arrhythmias and the Prevention of Sudden Cardiac Death (ACC/AHA/ESC 2006 Guidelines for Management of Patients With). *Europace* 2006; 8: 746–837.

Chapter

48

Physical symptoms in absence of organic disease

Marguerite Paffard

Introduction

The document outlining the government's strategy for mental health, *No Health without Mental Health* [1], suggests that patients with medically unexplained symptoms (MUS) may consult their GP at least 50% more frequently than the general population and may have up to 33% more secondary care consultations, resulting in a cost to the NHS in England of £3 billion per year.

> **Scenario 48.1**
>
> *You are asked to review a 60-year-old man on the MAU who has been admitted with chest pain and collapse. He attends regularly and his last discharge was 2 weeks previously after a prolonged admission under the cardiologists. During that admission he had intermittent pain without ECG changes or troponin elevation and was reluctant to be discharged. He had a non-ST-elevation MI about 10 years previously. There is a past history of IBS. Recent extensive investigations have included coronary angiography, CTPA, ECHO and oesophageal manometry. He is on numerous medications including a complex analgesic regime. He is refusing to leave hospital as he is afraid he 'will drop dead', although the nurses insist that 'there is never anything wrong with him'.*

Definition of MUS

MUS arise in any bodily organ or system, making classification problematic and leading to the current confusing terminology of the ICD-10, DSM-IV and DSM-5 classificatory systems. In addition many patients with MUS also have coexisting significant symptoms of anxiety and depression.

A modern definition of MUS should recognize that the symptoms experienced by the patient are:

- distressing and/or result in significant disruption of functioning
- *either* cannot be medically explained

  or
- where there is established physical illness (e.g. cardiac disease, asthma or epilepsy), the nature or severity of the symptoms cannot be accounted for by the underlying condition.

Creed et al. [2] have suggested the adoption of the alternative term '*bodily distress syndrome*', the advantages being:

- It encompasses the myriad of different conditions thereby avoiding specialty-specific terms and allowing clinicians to communicate between specialties more easily.
- It emphasizes the presence of physical symptoms without the negative connotation of no explanation, making it more acceptable to the patient.
- There is no aetiological inference including a psychological one which is unacceptable to some patients.

Functional somatic syndromes (FSS) with characteristic features are frequently encountered on the general medical take including:

- IBS, functional dyspepsia
- premenstrual syndrome, chronic pelvic pain
- fibromyalgia, repetitive strain injury, chronic lower back pain
- atypical chest pain
- atypical facial pain
- tension headache, non-epileptic seizures
- whiplash disorder

Acute Medicine, ed. Stephen Haydock, Duncan Whitehead and Zoë Fritz. Published by Cambridge University Press. © Cambridge University Press 2015.

- chronic fatigue
- hyperventilation
- irritable bladder.

There is a significant overlap in symptoms between the various FSS and only a few individuals present within a single syndrome, suggesting that the separation of these conditions into individual syndromes simply reflects specialization within health services.

Factitious disorder describes patients who present with psychological or physical symptoms which have been fabricated. There appears to be no motive other than the desire to adopt the sick role.

Malingering applies when there is some secondary gain such as obtaining benefits or avoiding prison.

In both these latter conditions it can be difficult to prove either the fabrication or the ulterior motive. Individuals are unwilling to accept psychological help and if challenged are likely to re-present elsewhere.

Pathophysiology

- Experiencing the emotion of stressful life events as both a bodily sensation and a psychological phenomenon is normal and is reflected in the simultaneous activation of the somatic and emotional processing areas of the brain.
- These bodily sensations only become symptoms when interpreted either by the patient or the doctor as an illness.
- Which physical symptoms develop in response to stressful life events, and their persistence, depends on complex interactions between the physiology and psychology of the individual.
- The symptoms may have been present for some while but presentation is triggered by a particularly stressful life event, with the patient taking into account the existing:
  - symptom severity
  - symptom chronicity
  - perceived threat to self that the symptom poses.

Prognosis

Spontaneous remission can be expected in approximately 70% of people. Although there are some patients who stick rigidly to a somatic explanation, especially at the more chronic and disabled end of the spectrum, the majority of sufferers are in fact willing to accept a multifactorial cause for their symptoms.

Where symptoms persist, there is often a history of:

- childhood physical or sexual abuse
- underlying psychiatric disorder
- ongoing severe psychosocial stressors.

In addition, certain cognitions and behaviours appear to predispose to the development of troublesome MUS.

Body scanning describes a tendency to check parts of the body for signs of malfunction. This attention to somatic perceptions tends to amplify normal sensations and bodily feedback leading to misinterpretation (*catastrophizing*) that in turn increases the tendency to self-monitor, leading to constant rumination about physical complaints and illness. However, although health anxiety is a frequent occurrence in patients, it is not a prerequisite as reassurance that no serious illness is present can be accepted but somatic symptoms can still persist.

A *negative self-view* incorporating ideas of being weak, unable to tolerate stress or any physical demands upon them results in avoidance of physical activity or stress-inducing situations. Lack of physical activity leads to muscle and cardiovascular deconditioning which in turn enhances the perception and the reality of bodily frailty.

'*Safety behaviours*' are common, whereby people, places, TV programmes, etc. are avoided if it is anticipated that they will provoke symptoms. The memory of symptoms and increased expectation of renewal can in itself trigger symptom recurrence.

Interpersonal problems are a prominent feature for some patients, often manifest as dissatisfaction with the care being given and frequent change of care provider. Disturbed attachments to caregivers in childhood due to some form of physical or emotional maltreatment result in troubled relationships in adulthood whereby trust is difficult to establish and attempts by others to help are experienced as inadequate.

General principles of the approach to MUS

(i) *The reattribution model for somatoform disorders* was described in 1989 by Goldberg et al. [3].

Stage 1 – feeling understood:

- Take full history of the symptoms.
- Explore emotional cues.
- Explore social and family factors.

- Explore the patient's health beliefs.
- Brief focused physical examination if indicated.

  Stage 2 – broadening the agenda:
- Feed back the results of the examination.
- Acknowledge the reality of the symptom.
- Reframe the complaints: link physical, psychological and life events.

  Stage 3 – making the link:
  Use simple explanations:
- Explain how anxiety causes physical symptoms.
- Explain how depression lowers the pain threshold.
- Give practical example of how pain results from tensed muscles.
- Link to life events (how pain is worse on days with stress).
- Here and now (how the pain is at the moment and enquiry about feelings).
- Project or identify (ask if anyone else in the family or amongst friends has suffered from similar symptoms).

(ii) Patient-centred care is a guiding principle of modern psychiatry. It is defined by the Institute of Medicine as providing 'care that is respectful of and responsive to individual patient preferences, needs and values, and ensuring that patient values guide all clinical decisions' [4].

(iii) The biopsychosocial model recognizes the contribution of physical, psychological and social components of the presentation. A doctor offering only a biomedical model is less likely to be given clues to psychological stressors and underlying issues will be missed and the ultimate outcome and patient satisfaction will both be adversely affected.

Assessment

In secondary care, symptoms are likely to have become more persistent and a more detailed assessment is required than would be appropriate in primary care.

- A collateral history from a relative may be useful.
- A review of previous notes will indicate any illness in the past, which investigations have been carried out and whether there have been any identified episodes of MUS.

The assessment should be carried out in a way that facilitates acceptance of and working within a psychological framework by:

- Using a biopsychosocial approach that recognizes the complexity of the pathogenesis:

- be vigilant for emotional cues given by the patient related to areas of psychological stress
- Adopting a supportive, non-judgemental approach
- Eliciting concerns and gaining an understanding of the patient's views of their symptoms.

  In order to:
- Establish whether an individual is suffering from MUS either with or without an accompanying physical or psychiatric disorder
- Determine the severity of the condition. People presenting for the first time with mild symptoms may be far more open to a psychological explanation than those who have chronic, disabling symptoms.

Key information to be obtained

- History of the current problem
- Previous investigations or treatments
- The patient's opinion about the nature and causation of the symptoms and any concerns about their significance; the views of other family members may be important and more influential than the doctor's
- The degree of impairment or disability, including ruminations and catastrophic thinking and the general level of functioning
- Family history of physical or mental illness, especially during their childhood
- Childhood experiences including disrupted relationships and any abuse
- Current family/work situation and any stressful life events or long-term stressors
- Symptoms of anxiety, panic, depression or other mental health problem:
    - the *Hospital Anxiety and Depression Scale (HADS)* or the PHQ-9 for depression and PHQ-7 for anxiety may help identify those patients suffering from anxiety or depressive disorder in addition to MUS

- Drug or alcohol use
- Avoidant or safety behaviours
- Abnormal illness behaviours:
    - repeatedly returning to symptoms throughout the interview in an attempt to convey their severity might indicate abnormal illness behaviour

- hostility towards previous doctors and blame for making the symptoms worse
- expression of discomfort either greater or less than might be expected from the symptom (especially when the patient knows they are observed)
- repeated checking of body part

- Any compensation or legal case related to the symptoms
- Expectations of the consultation and motivation for change
- Degree of denial of the psychological aspect of the problem:
  - patients with the most intractable symptoms are often convinced of the physical nature of their symptoms despite extensive negative investigations; they are unlikely to accept referral for psychological intervention.

Taking a full history in this way gives the patient a sense of having been listened to and understood, an important first step in patient-centred care.

Cultural differences

MUS occur in all cultures with explanatory models varying between cultures. Asking about illness beliefs is a vital part of the assessment. Challenges posed by different cultural backgrounds include:

- appropriate form of address of the patient
- the family structure and who makes decisions
- perception of the doctor as the person who makes the decisions with no expectation of negotiation around diagnosis or treatment
- perception of illness as a matter of fate and not accessible to intervention
- different attitudes to complementary medicines but where appropriate, advantage can be taken of these in the management plan, e.g. attending yoga classes for relaxation and increased physical exercise
- taboos on talking about certain topics particularly if the doctor's gender is an issue.

Management

A comprehensible explanation and logical management plan are essential. In addition, it is vital to acknowledge the reality of the symptoms and the suffering they cause. Telling a patient there is 'nothing wrong with them', in the expectation that this will be reassuring when this is so obviously in conflict with their experience, immediately alienates them and reduces the credibility of any treatment plan suggested.

- Explanations of the problem must include the physical, psychological and behavioural factors involved.
- Recognize and acknowledge the disability and suffering experienced by the patient. Labels based simply on pathology and the absence of organic disease are often unhelpful, leaving the patient with the feeling that the doctor has not understood and believes there is nothing wrong. Giving examples of normal bodily reactions to stress may help the patient understand and accept the explanation.
- Avoid investigations unless clear clinical indication. Manage expectation by explaining likely negative result given the overall picture.
- Relevant educational material and self-help sites are helpful for some people, as is keeping a diary (helps establish the link between physical symptoms and emotional/behavioural triggers).
- A healthy lifestyle should be promoted with particular attention to diet and exercise. The latter may be deliberately avoided because of health anxieties related to exertion.
- Stress reduction through relaxation or meditation may be advocated.
- Where significant depression or anxiety have been identified, antidepressants in full dosage may be helpful; sufferers of IBS and fibromyalgia may also benefit from antidepressants in low doses. Physical symptoms should be reassessed after successful treatment of depression.

Psychotherapy may be helpful where symptoms are persistent.

- Attitudes to referral will range from complete acceptance to total opposition, the former being more likely if psychological factors have been given sufficient weight during the assessment.
- Cognitive behaviour therapy (CBT) has been found to be of benefit in MUS. Funding for CBT for MUS has been provided via the 'Improving Access to Psychological Therapy' programme.
- Graded exercise therapy, effective in chronic fatigue, often accompanies CBT, the latter being necessary in tackling catastrophic interpretations of the physical consequences of increased activity.

Case management can be employed for more complex/chronic cases where multiple body systems are involved.

- Aim to reduce disability and healthcare utilization rather than cure.
- Referral to a psychiatrist may be helpful, particularly if there is a liaison service based at the hospital.
- An overall view of the problem can be gained and communication between various departments involved with the patient facilitated.
- Ideally, with repeat admissions an identified physician will take overall charge of care to establish a good working relationship and to avoid unnecessary investigations.
- The GP may be in the best position to case manage by offering regular appointments to avoid new symptoms and avoiding unnecessary onward referral.

Through a positive doctor–patient relationship, the patient can be encouraged to re-evaluate the nature of their condition, to develop new coping strategies and thereby reduce disability and healthcare usage.

References

1. No Health without Mental Health: A Cross-Government Mental Health Strategy for People of All Ages. (2013) Available to download at www.gov.uk/government/uploads/system/uploads/attachment_data/file/216870/No-Health-Without-Mental-Health-Implementation-Framework-Report-accessible-version.pdf.

2. Creed F, Henningsen P, Fink P. *Medically Unexplained Symptoms, Somatisation and Bodily Distress. Developing Better Clinical Services.* Cambridge University Press; 2011.

3. Goldberg D, Gask L, O'Dowd T. The treatment of somatization: teaching techniques of reattribution. *J Psychosom Res* 1989; 33(6): 689–695.

4. Institute of Medicine of the National Academies. *Crossing the Quality Chasm: A New Health System for the 21st Century.* Released 1 March 2001.

Further reading

Hatcher S, Arroll B. Assessment and management of medically unexplained symptoms. *BMJ* 2008; 336(7653): 1124–1128.

Poisoning

Stephen Haydock

Introduction

The UK has one of the highest rates of deliberate self-harm in Europe. Accidental or deliberate poisoning is responsible for over 150 000 hospital attendances per annum in England and Wales. In a 24-hour period the medical team working in an average sized district general hospital will admit 1–2 patients with drug overdose. Older patients have greater access to prescribed medications and overdoses of anxiolytics and antidepressants are common. Teenagers more frequently overdose on over-the-counter analgesics, in particular paracetamol, which is currently responsible for almost half of all poisoning admissions in the UK. Deliberate drug overdose is often accompanied by excess alcohol consumption. Deaths from poisoning in England and Wales *had* been consistently falling but recent data have shown an upward trend. The number of drug poisoning related deaths was just under 3000 in 2008. Most patients who die from drug overdose do so before reaching hospital, inpatient deaths being uncommon and most frequently involve paracetamol, tricyclic antidepressants and benzodiazepines.

Scenario 49.1

A 25-year-old woman is referred to the medical assessment unit by the emergency department following 'another overdose'. They give a history of several previous attendances at the emergency department with self-mutilation and self-poisoning with both prescribed and over-the-counter medications. The paramedics were called to her flat after she texted her mother to tell her that she had taken another overdose but did not specify the medications taken. At the time of referral she is tachycardic, hypotensive and has a reduced level of consciousness.

This is a common referral to the on-call medical team. The patient has a previous history of self-poisoning with a range of drugs. The history of prescribed drugs suggests coexisting physical or more likely, in view of her age, coexisting mental health issues. The specific agents ingested are not known. There is evidence of central nervous system and cardiovascular dysfunction.

Although the scenario appears straightforward we should always remember that situations can be more complex than they at first appear. All experienced physicians can recall cases where the '*obvious diagnosis*' at presentation was partly or entirely misleading. It is always important to keep an open mind in order to avoid missing important clues that could lead to alternative or additional diagnoses that might otherwise be overlooked. The depressed conscious level is likely due to alcohol and CNS depressant medication BUT has the patient fallen and sustained a head injury due to confusion resulting from drug/alcohol intoxication…?

The management of self-poisoning requires a systematic approach to both the clinical assessment and management. Most patients can in fact be safely discharged after a period of observation combined with simple medical management, good nursing care and an appropriate psychiatric assessment. *A small number can become very unwell indeed!*

History

What is the key information?

- Identities and doses of the substances taken.
- Time since ingestion.
- Was alcohol also taken?

Acute Medicine, ed. Stephen Haydock, Duncan Whitehead and Zoë Fritz. Published by Cambridge University Press.
© Cambridge University Press 2015.

Figure 49.1 Common toxidromes.

Cholinergic drugs produce diaphoresis, diarrhoea, urination, small pupils, bradycardia, bronchosecretion, emesis, excess lacrimation, hypersalivation
examples
Anticholinesterases such as organophosphate insecticides, carbamate insecticides, Alzheimer's drugs such as galantamine and donepezil

which are the opposite of

Anticholinergic drugs producing hyperthermia, urine retention, large pupils with blurred vision, constipation, tachycardia, dry skin, delirium and hallucinations
examples
Antipsychotics, tricyclic antidepressants, antispasmodics, antihistamines, many plant toxins

which are sort of similar to

Sympathomimetic drugs producing diaphoresis, large pupils and blurred vision, hypertension, tachycardia, hyperthermia and seizures
examples
Salbutamol, amphetamine, methamphetamine, cocaine, ephedrine, pseudoephedrine, phenylpropanolamine

Opiate drugs produce pinpoint pupils, hypoventilation, coma, hypotension, bradycardia, pulmonary oedema (look for injection marks)
examples
morphine, diamorphine, buprenorphine, codeine, papaveretum, methadone

- Has the subject vomited since ingestion?
- Whether the overdose was staggered.
- Whether there is a history of psychiatric illness, drug or alcohol abuse.
- Whether there is a history of previous or ongoing physical illness.
- Are there children who need to be cared for and who might be identified as 'at risk'?
- Is there ongoing suicidal ideation and need for supervision? Occasionally patients are admitted 'under section' and it is important to understand what section is in place, its duration and what the implications are with regard to treatment (see Chapter 59).

How do we obtain this information?

- By direct questioning of the patient if conscious, always keeping in mind the fact that information so obtained may not be entirely reliable. This is particularly the case if the patient is suicidal, suffering from serious psychiatric illness or following use of recreational drugs.
- Discharge letters or case notes indicate recent prescription drugs.
- Empty drug containers in pocket or at the scene.

- Paramedics who attended the scene should be questioned and will often have recovered medication containers from the scene.
- Family or friends of the patient (within limits of confidentiality).
- The patient's general practitioner or pharmacy.

Examination

- The principal focus of the clinical examination should be in identifying life-threatening complications (always remember ABCDE) such that these can be rapidly corrected.
- A full clinical examination seeks to identify any clinical features that are not consistent with the presentation and alert us to consider other diagnoses contributing to the clinical state.
- The examination can provide clues to the nature of the drug(s) ingested. Many substances used in accidental or self-poisoning produce recognizable clinical manifestations. These are frequently referred to as 'toxidromes'. However, considerable overlap exists between toxidromes and overdoses with several drugs from different drug classes are common. Both factors limit the usefulness of recognizing toxidromes in everyday clinical

practice. The more important are shown in Figure 49.1.

Under certain circumstances, the response to a specific antidote may provide a diagnosis. Such an approach is frequently used but it is important to appreciate the potential risks.

- Dilatation of constricted pupils and increased respiratory rate after intravenous naloxone in patients with opiate poisoning

  BUT

  Naloxone has a relatively short half-life compared with several opiates, in particular methadone. This is compounded if there is also acute or chronic kidney injury. Bolus injections of naloxone can produce a marked improvement in conscious level and respiratory rate. Such patients can be deemed safe for transfer to a medical bed where they may be a low priority for medical and nursing supervision and quietly lapse back into profound coma and hypoventilation. Patients having ingested long half-life opiates frequently require a continuous infusion of naloxone until the drug has been cleared from their system.

- Arousal from unconsciousness in response to intravenous flumazenil in benzodiazepine poisoning

  BUT

  Although NICE guidance indicates that this approach can reduce the need for ITU admission in benzodiazepine overdose it is an unlicensed indication. NICE highlights that this should NOT be undertaken if the patient is benzodiazepine dependent, after co-ingestion of pro-convulsants, including tricyclic antidepressants, or with a history of epilepsy. It is hard to imagine that any or all of these can be safely excluded for the unconscious patient admitted in the early hours of the morning in a busy emergency department!

Investigations

All patients should have the following baseline investigations:

- electrocardiogram
- serum electrolytes including urea, creatinine and bicarbonate
- full blood count
- liver function tests
- blood glucose

- lactate
- creatine kinase
- clotting
- plasma paracetamol/salicylate levels.

In addition

If patient is a female of childbearing age:

- pregnancy test.

If conscious level is impaired or there is suspicion of hypoxaemia, hyperpnoea or significant acidosis:

- arterial blood gas analysis.

If associated aspiration or other indication is suspected:

- chest radiograph.

If there is still concern or confusion regarding the ingested drug:

- urine rapid qualitative toxicological screening may help to identify cocaine, amphetamine, methamphetamine, cannabis, methadone, benzodiazepines, barbiturates, phencyclidine and opiates
- but studies show that this rarely alters management.

Other specific agents can be measured if indicated to aid diagnosis, quantify risk or as a preliminary to employing specific treatments, commonly:

- iron
- lithium
- digoxin.

Other specific investigations may be indicated depending on the clinical situation. Patients with a reduced conscious level that cannot be explained by the presumed drugs ingested may require cranial CT imaging or diagnostic lumbar puncture to exclude other intracranial pathology.

What is the significance of the high anion gap?

In the presence of a significant acidosis calculating the anion gap can sometimes be diagnostically useful and is still frequently performed in the emergency department. Therefore (at very least in order to maintain your credibility), the derivation and interpretation of this value needs to be understood!

It is given by: plasma *sodium* – (plasma *chloride* + *bicarbonate*).

An anion gap greater than 12 mmol/L *in the context of overdose* suggests poisoning with:

- methanol
- propylene glycol, paraldehyde
- iron, isoniazid
- ethylene glycol, ethanol (due to high lactate)
- salicylates.

Management

Inpatient mortality and morbidity from self-poisoning result from:

1. Respiratory depression, cardiac arrhythmias, convulsions in the acute phase of toxicity; e.g. ventricular arrhythmias due to tricyclic antidepressants.
2. Organ damage due to poor resuscitation; e.g. hypoxic brain injury, hypotensive acute kidney injury.
3. Specific drug toxicity; e.g. paracetamol-induced hepatotoxicity.
4. Subsequent potentially fatal overdose as the significance of this presentation and psychiatric co-morbidity was not fully appreciated and appropriate action taken.

Hence our management of the patient should focus on:

- ensuring adequate tissue oxygenation by managing *airway, breathing, circulation*
- prediction and management of life-threatening complications by close monitoring for cardiac arrhythmias, convulsions and respiratory depression
- preventing further drug absorption, enhancing excretion and administration of specific antidotes
- adequate psychiatric assessment and support.

In the UK, the most up-to-date advice on the management of specific poisoning is available at any time of day.

- *TOXBASE*, the primary clinical toxicology database of the UK National Poisons Information Service, is available on the internet to registered users at: www.toxbase.org. It should *always* be consulted and a hard copy of downloaded information should be inserted into the medical notes.
- In the UK, regional medicines information centres of the National Poisons Information Service

(based in Birmingham, Cardiff, Edinburgh and Newcastle) provide specialist 24-hour telephone advice and information (0870 600 6266).

Resuscitation

Most patients recover from acute poisonings provided they are adequately oxygenated and hydrated and blood pressure is maintained.

Maintenance of an adequate oxygenation

- The airway must be cleared and secured if necessary by using airway adjuncts, e.g. oropharyngeal or nasopharyngeal airways.
- Administer oxygen therapy as needed.
- Mechanical ventilation is sometimes required but rarely needed for greater than 24 hours.

Maintenance of an adequate circulation

- *Shock* in acute poisoning is usually due to vasodilatation and is best managed by head-down tilt combined with IV fluid replacement.
- If such measures are unsuccessful then further management may require admission to the high dependency or the intensive therapy unit to provide for:
  - vasopressor support
  - conventional inotropic agents
  - high dose insulin infusion (0.5–2 units/kg per hour) with euglycaemic clamping (sometimes used for poisoning with agents that are resistant to conventional inotropic agents, e.g. calcium channel blockers).

Cardiac arrhythmias can accompany poisoning with:

- tricyclic antidepressants
- theophylline
- beta-blockers.

Correct acidosis, hypoxia and electrolyte disturbance before using anti-arrhythmic drugs.

Many patients admitted with overdoses are otherwise young and healthy. Cardiac arrest in the context of overdose often involves a drug-induced cardiac arrhythmia or myocardial depression in a heart free from significant coronary artery disease or ventricular dysfunction. Survival with excellent outcomes has been reported after several hours of cardiopulmonary resuscitation. *It is inappropriate to abandon resuscitation* in such patients if cardiac output is not rapidly re-established.

Convulsions frequently accompany poisoning with tricyclic antidepressants, theophylline and cocaine.

- They require treatment if they are persistent or protracted.
- Intravenous benzodiazepine (diazepam or lorazepam) is the first choice.

  Hypothermia:

- CNS depressants may impair temperature regulation.
- A low-reading rectal thermometer can monitor core temperature.
- Heat-retaining 'space blankets', warmed IV fluids and active external warming can be employed.

  Immobility:

- May lead to pressure lesions of peripheral nerves and skin damage.
- Requires prophylaxis with low molecular weight heparin.

  Rhabdomyolysis:

- May result from prolonged immobilization on floor or from agents that cause muscle spasm or convulsions (phencyclidine, theophylline).
- May be aggravated by hyperthermia due to muscle contraction, e.g. with ecstasy.
- Is treated in the conventional way by volume replacement with/without urine alkalinization.

Methods to reduce exposure to the drug and its toxic effects

Several techniques can help reduce the exposure of the patient to the toxic effects of the ingested drug. In implementing these procedures we should always remember that the most efficient eliminating mechanisms are *the patient's own physiology*, which will, given time, inactivate and eliminate all the poison. Our focus should always be on *ensuring adequate resuscitation* so that this can happen. Specific methods employed for individual drugs are implemented according to the nature and severity of poisoning as recommended by *TOXBASE*.

(a) Prevention of further absorption of the poison

From the environment

When a poison has been inhaled or absorbed through the skin, the patient should be taken from the toxic environment, the contaminated clothing removed and the skin cleansed.

From the alimentary tract ('gut decontamination')

Gastric lavage and *induced emesis* are no longer employed. Clinical studies have shown no benefit and identified potential harmful effects. Antiemetics are in fact commonly given to reduce vomiting, hence improving patient well-being and reducing risk of aspiration. This is probably appropriate but the effects have not been studied.

Oral adsorbents: activated charcoal consists of a very fine black powder which has an enormous surface area in relation to weight ($1000 \ m^2/g$). This binds to, and thus inactivates, a wide variety of compounds in the gut. Important *exceptions* include:

- iron
- lithium
- cyanide
- alcohols (ethanol and methanol).

An initial adult dose of 50 g is usual, repeated if necessary. If the patient is vomiting, the charcoal should be given through a nasogastric tube. In volunteers, administration within 1 h prevents up to 40–50% of absorption. There are no clinical trial data in patients. It is advised for substances that bind to activated charcoal (most ingested drugs but excluding the above list) within one hour of poisoning, or sometimes longer as recommended by TOXBASE.

Activated charcoal, although unpalatable, appears to be relatively safe but in drowsy patients there is a risk of lung aspiration. It should not be used if there is concern regarding protection of the airway. Constipation or rarely mechanical bowel obstruction is described with large repeated doses.

Whole-bowel irrigation should not be employed routinely. Activated charcoal in frequent (50 g) doses is generally preferred. Irrigation with large volumes of a polyethylene glycol–electrolyte solution, e.g. Klean-Prep, by mouth causes minimal fluid and electrolyte disturbance. Magnesium sulphate may also be used. Volunteer studies shown marked reductions in the bioavailability of ingested drugs but there is no evidence from controlled clinical trials in patients. It may be used for the removal of sustained-release or enteric-coated formulations from patients who present more than 2 h after ingestion and for the removal of ingested packets of illicit drugs. It is contraindicated in patients with:

- bowel obstruction
- perforation or ileus
- haemodynamic instability

- compromised unprotected airways
- the elderly or debilitated.

It may reduce effectiveness of activated charcoal.

(b) Acceleration of elimination of the poison

Such methods depend on removing drug from the circulation and successful use requires that the poison:

- has a high plasma concentration relative to the rest of the body (i.e. a small volume of distribution)
- binds only weakly to plasma proteins
- has effects that relate to its plasma concentration.

Repeated doses of activated charcoal by mouth not only prevent absorption into the body (see above), but also adsorb drug that diffuses from the blood into the gut lumen when the concentration there is lower. As binding is irreversible, the concentration gradient is maintained and drug is continuously removed ('intestinal dialysis'). Charcoal may also adsorb drugs that secrete into the bile by interrupting an enterohepatic cycle.

In adults, activated charcoal 50 g is given every 4 hours. Vomiting should be treated with an antiemetic drug because it reduces the efficacy of charcoal treatment. Where there is intolerance, the dose may be halved and the frequency doubled. It is useful in managing poisoning with:

- carbamazepine
- phenytoin
- salicylate
- tricyclic antidepressants
- warfarin
- theophylline
- verapamil.

Altering the pH of the glomerular filtrate can increase ionization of a weak electrolyte, thus lowering lipid solubility and causing retention in renal tubular fluid and therefore enhanced excretion. Maintenance of a good urine flow (e.g. 100 mL/h) facilitates this. Forcing diuresis with furosemide and large volumes of intravenous fluid is ineffective, dangerous and obsolete.

Urinary alkalinization involves maintaining a urine pH of 7.5–8.5 by an intravenous infusion of sodium bicarbonate. Preparations of sodium bicarbonate vary between 1.2% and 8.4% and the concentration used will depend on the patient's fluid needs. It may be useful for poisoning with:

- salicylates
- phenobarbital
- phenoxy herbicides.

Urinary acidification is rarely used. The objective is to maintain a urine pH of 5.5–6.5 by giving an intravenous infusion of arginine hydrochloride followed by repeat doses of oral ammonium chloride. It is sometimes indicated for severe, acute poisoning with:

- amphetamine
- dexfenfluramine
- phencyclidine.

Haemodialysis requires a temporary extracorporeal circulation. A semipermeable membrane separates blood from dialysis fluid; the poison passes passively from the blood, where it is present in high concentration to enter the dialysis fluid, which is flowing and the concentration gradient is therefore constantly replaced. It may be used in poisoning with:

- salicylate
- isopropanol (aftershave lotions and window-cleaning solutions)
- lithium
- methanol
- ethylene glycol
- ethanol.

Haemofiltration brings blood via an extracorporeal circulation into contact with a highly permeable membrane. Water is lost by ultrafiltration (the rate being dependent on the hydrostatic pressure gradient across membrane) and solutes by convection.

Haemofiltration is readily available but is a less efficient method of drug elimination (one-half to one-third depending on the specific drug that has been ingested) than haemodialysis. Both are invasive, demand skill and experience on the part of the operator and are costly in terms of staffing. Their use is confined to cases of severe, prolonged or progressive clinical intoxication, when high plasma concentration indicates a dangerous degree of poisoning, and their effect constitutes a significant addition to natural methods of elimination.

(c) Specific antidotes

TOXBASE recommends a range of drug-specific antidotes and associated treatment regimens for commonly ingested drugs. The principal mechanisms are summarized below.

Direct removal of ingested drug from plasma

- Chelating agents are charged organic molecules that can bind to oppositely charged drug molecules and enhance their excretion in urine;

example: intravenous desferrioxamine is used to treat acute iron poisoning.

- Antibodies bind specifically to the drug to form inactive complexes that are removed by the kidneys;
  example: digoxin-specific antibody fragments (Digibind) in the treatment of digoxin toxicity.

Blockage of formation/inactivation of a toxic metabolite of the ingested drug

- Antidote prevents generation of toxic species within the body from an inactive ingested poison;
  example: use of ethanol to block the conversion of methanol to the toxic metabolite methanoate (formate).

- Antidote chemically inactivates a toxic metabolite of the ingested drug;
  example: use of N-acetylcysteine as a sulfhydryl group donor in paracetamol poisoning. This augments the depleted glutathione that inactivates the extremely cytotoxic free radical compound NAPQI (N-acetyl-p-benzoquinonimine).
  This is generated by liver metabolism of excess paracetamol using the mixed function oxidase system.

Opposing action of ingested drug

- Antidote competes for the receptor that is blocked by the ingested poison;
  example: use of the beta-agonist isoprenaline in the management of beta-blocker overdose.

- Antidote opposes the action of the ingested drug by a mechanism other than directly stimulating the blocked receptor;
  example: use of glucagon in beta-blocker overdose. cAMP acts as the second messenger of both the beta-adrenoceptor and the glucagon receptor. Stimulation of the glucagon receptor raises cAMP levels resulting in an indirect positive inotropic and chronotropic effect.

- Antidote competes for the receptor that is occupied and stimulated by the ingested drug, hence reducing binding of the ingested drug and blocking its effects;
  example: use of naloxone to reverse effects of opiate poisoning; use of flumazenil to reverse effects of benzodiazepines.

- Affinity of drug for receptor may be pH dependent and occurs in competition with natural ligand;
  example: the use of bolus injections of sodium bicarbonate to raise plasma pH and reduce pH dependent binding and blockade of tricyclic antidepressants to the sodium channel.
  The sodium load may also help by raising concentration of the natural ligand sodium.

Psychosocial assessment

Patients who have attempted deliberate self-harm will need assessment by the liaison psychiatry service. The mental state assessment and the statutory framework regarding such assessments is described in detail in Chapter 59.

Further reading

American Society of Toxicology. Position statements of the American Society of Toxicology. Available as downloads from www.clintox.org/positionstatements.cfm.

Haydock SF (2012) Poisoning, overdoses and antidotes. Chapter 20. In: Bennet, Brown and Sharma, eds. *Clinical Pharmacology*, 11th edn. Elsevier.

NICE (2004) The short-term physical and psychological management and secondary prevention of self-harm in primary and secondary care. National Institute for Health and Care Excellence Clinical Guideline 16. Available as a download from www.nice.org.uk/nicemedia/pdf/CG016NICEguideline.pdf.

Polydipsia and polyuria
Water and sodium homeostasis; hypo- and hypernatraemia

John Kalk

Scenario 50.1

A 78-year-old woman is admitted to the MAU after a fall at home. She lives alone but is usually independent, with only the support of her family who live close by. The history suggests that she tripped over a rug in her living room and was subsequently unable to get up as she was wedged between her coffee table and sofa. She was on the floor for several hours. She has a history of hypertension, a previous NSTEMI some 2 years previously and mild depression. Her medication includes amitryptiline 50 mg nocte, bendroflumethiazide 2.5 mg od, aspirin 75 mg od and bisoprolol 5 mg od. Investigations are essentially unremarkable except for a plasma sodium of 120 mmol/L. The sodium was normal at the time of her previous NSTEMI.

Introduction

Disturbances of fluid and sodium homeostasis are common in acutely ill patients and may be either a consequence or a cause of the acute illness:

- Severe diarrhoea and/or vomiting are frequent causes of dehydration and acute hospital admission.
- Any illness may reduce fluid intake in the frail elderly who may then become dehydrated. In addition, the sensation of thirst may be blunted in the elderly and dehydration may be further amplified by the continuation of diuretic therapy in the face of reduced fluid intake. Acute kidney injury can be exaggerated by commonly prescribed agents such as non-steroidal anti-inflammatory drugs and ACE inhibitors.
- Hyponatraemia is the commonest electrolyte disturbance in hospitalized patients, is associated

with increased mortality, and requires careful management.
- Hypernatraemia occurs less frequently, but it too can be life-threatening.

Physiology of fluid balance

(See also Figure 50.1.)

- Water makes up 50% of body weight in adult females and 60% in males:
  - intracellular fluid (ICF; cytosol) is 27–33%
  - extracellular fluid (ECF):
  - 18–22% is interstitial fluid
  - 4.5% is plasma (together with the interstitial fluid = the ECF)
- The remaining fraction is made up of body solids.
- For normal functioning the body must maintain normal volume and composition of both the ECF and ICF compartments.
- The major ions in the ECF are sodium, chloride and bicarbonate, and in the ICF are potassium, magnesium and phosphate plus large amounts of negatively charged proteins. The osmotic concentrations of the ECF and ICF are the same in normal circumstances.
- The homeostatic mechanisms that maintain fluid homeostasis respond *only to changes in ECF*.
- Normally, fluid and electrolyte homeostasis is maintained by a balance between water intake determined by thirst, and water from food and metabolism, insensible fluid loss (sweating, respiration, faeces, and obligatory urine production), and the ability of the kidneys to concentrate or dilute urine. Disturbance at any level may disturb the balance.

Acute Medicine, ed. Stephen Haydock, Duncan Whitehead and Zoë Fritz. Published by Cambridge University Press.
© Cambridge University Press 2015.

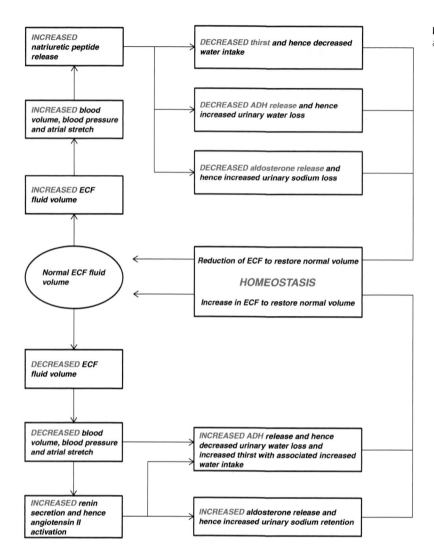

Figure 50.1 Regulation of salt and water balance.

Fluid and electrolyte homeostasis is regulated by:

- *antidiuretic hormone* (ADH, also known as vasopressin)
- *renin-angiotensin-aldosterone* system (RAAS)
- *natriuretic peptides* (atrial natriuretic factor (NF), and brain NF produced by ventricular myocardium).

Antidiuretic hormone

- Regulates renal free water clearance and thirst.
- Is synthesized by neurones in the hypothalamus and is secreted via their axons from the posterior pituitary into the systemic circulation.

- ADH secretion is controlled by impulses from osmoreceptors in the hypothalamus, and via baroreceptors located in the carotid sinus, aortic arch and pulmonary veins. The normal range for plasma osmolality is 275–295 mOsm/kg.
- A *rise* in plasma osmolality (e.g. by dehydration) stimulates the release of ADH, which increases the permeability of the distal nephron and collecting ducts to water (via the aquaporin system), increasing water reabsorption and leading to more concentrated urine, and to increased thirst.
- Conversely, a *fall* in plasma osmolality will reduce ADH secretion, resulting in reduced permeability

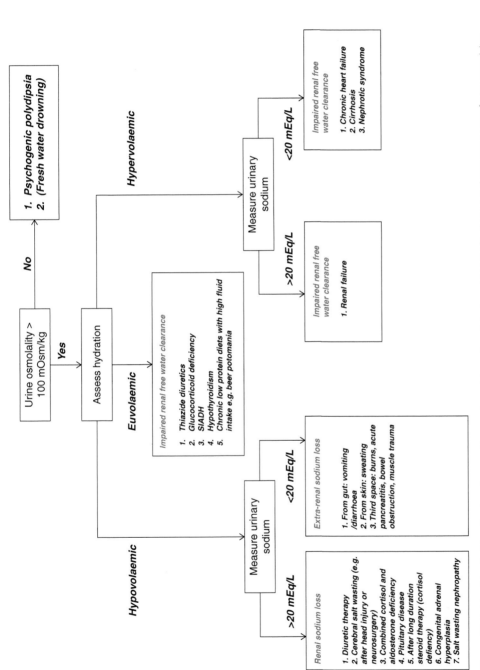

Figure 50.2 Algorithm for identification of cause of hyponatraemia based on clinical assessment of hydration and measurements of urine osmolality and urinary sodium concentration.

to water in the distal nephron and collecting ducts and therefore reduced water reabsorption, leading to the production of dilute urine; thirst will also be reduced.

- Failure of hypotonic plasma to appropriately inhibit ADH secretion results in the *syndrome of inappropriate ADH* secretion (SIADH), the most frequent cause of hyponatraemia, which may also contribute to diluted serum sodium levels in subjects with hypovolaemia (e.g. cirrhosis).

Renin-angiotensin-aldosterone system

- Is stimulated by a reduction in effective renal plasma flow and in response to sympathetic stimulation (e.g. fall in blood pressure), a low osmotic concentration in the glomerular filtrate, and changes in sodium and potassium concentrations in the distal nephron.
- The resulting increase in *aldosterone* secretion promotes renal tubular sodium resorption, and with it water (thereby increasing plasma volume), and potassium loss.
- Activation of the RAAS also stimulates ADH secretion.

Natriuretic peptides

- Secreted by the atrial and ventricular myocardium in response to excessive stretch (e.g. from an increase in blood volume).
- Both peptides cause a sodium and water diuresis, and inhibit ADH and aldosterone secretion.

Hyponatraemia

- Hyponatraemia is the commonest disorder of electrolytes in clinical practice and is found in 15–30% of acutely or chronically hospitalized patients.
- Although most cases are mild and asymptomatic, it is associated with substantial mortality.
  - Severe '*acute*' (known duration <24–48 h) hyponatraemia can cause significant mortality and morbidity from cerebral oedema.
  - In '*chronic*' hyponatraemia (≥48 h), over-rapid correction can cause neurological damage and death.
- In many patients hyponatraemia is an unexpected diagnosis found during routine testing, and is

usually then classified as 'chronic' as the precise duration is unknown.

Causes of hyponatraemia

(See also Figure 50.2.)

A. Sodium depletion (hypovolaemia)

Renal sodium loss

- Diuretic therapy
- Cerebral salt wasting (e.g. after head injury or neurosurgery)
- Steroid deficiency (cortisol and aldosterone) – primary adrenal disease (combined cortisol and aldosterone deficiency); pituitary disease or after long duration steroid therapy (cortisol deficiency)
- Congenital adrenal hyperplasia
- Salt wasting nephropathy

Extra-renal sodium loss with water retention

- From the GI tract – vomiting, diarrhoea
- Sweat losses – endurance exercise
- Third space loss – bowel obstruction, acute pancreatitis, burns, muscle trauma

B. Dilutional hyponatraemia (euvolaemia)

With impaired renal free water clearance

- SIADH – tumours, CNS disorders, drug induced, pulmonary diseases, AIDS, hypothyroidism
- Glucocorticoid deficiency
- Chronic low protein diets with high fluid intake (e.g. beer potomania)

C. Dilutional hyponatraemia (hypervolaemia)

With impaired renal free water clearance

- Chronic heart failure
- Cirrhosis
- Nephrotic syndrome
- Renal failure

With excessive water intake

- Primary polydipsia
- Freshwater drowning

Pseudohyponatraemia can occur in the presence of very high concentrations of lipoproteins (severe hyper-triglyceridaemia) or proteins (e.g. untreated myeloma).

History

- Obtain careful medication history – diuretics, steroid therapy, agents known to cause SIADH.
- Symptoms depend on the cause and severity of the hyponatraemia:
  - mild degrees of hyponatraemia (<135, ≥130 mmol/L) are often asymptomatic
  - most patients will have some symptoms at serum sodium levels <125 mmol/L, whatever the cause.
- Symptoms include weakness and fatigue, poor concentration and memory, confusion, delirium, nausea and vomiting, muscle cramps, gait disturbances (high risk of falls); seizures can occur with extreme hyponatraemia.

Signs

- Look for evidence of hypovolaemia and hypervolaemia (see above list of causes). If the patient is euvolaemic the likely diagnosis is SIADH in the presence of normal renal function.

Investigations

- Plasma glucose, serum electrolytes, and creatinine and urea concentrations, and serum osmolality, with urine sent for sodium level and osmolality *at the same time*.
- In subjects with SIADH, serum *osmolality* will be subnormal (<275 mOsm/kg) and urine osmolality relatively high, above the minimum expected for the hypo-osmolar serum (>100 mOsm/kg).
- Urine sodium concentrations are usually relatively high. A useful cut-point for urine sodium is 20 mmol/L: in the presence of hyponatraemia a urinary sodium concentration at or above 20 mmol/L suggests the inability to increase free water clearance, and is suggestive of the diagnosis of SIADH.
- Urine sodium concentrations below 20 mmol/L, especially if very low (<10 mmol/L) favour body sodium depletion. Some patients with SIADH may have urine sodium below 20 mmol/L if they are also sodium depleted or have become hypovolaemic, e.g. from fluid and sodium restriction.
- Hyponatraemia with urinary sodium >20 mmol/L also occurs in patients taking diuretics (thiazides

account for ≥80% of these patients, frequently elderly women, who often have hypokalaemia as well), hypoadrenal states (may also have high normal potassium concentrations or hyperkalaemia), during osmotic diuresis (e.g. hyperglycaemia).
- To diagnose/exclude hypoadrenalism, measure serum cortisol concentrations: in a stressed patient levels should be high normal or supranormal for the time of day; if in doubt do a short Synacthen test.
- Hypothyroidism is often considered as a cause of hyponatraemia and serum TSH should be measured. However, the validity of this association has been challenged.

NB. The diagnosis of SIADH is made by the above investigations *and by the exclusion of other causes of hyponatraemia*. If SIADH is diagnosed, seek the cause (see list above), and treat it.

Treatment of hyponatraemia

Basic principles

- The brain is vulnerable to rapid changes in serum sodium concentrations irrespective of the cause of the hyponatraemia, especially in malnourished individuals, e.g. patients with alcoholism, cirrhosis.
- For patients with significant hyponatraemia-related neurological symptoms (e.g. stupor, coma, fits, often with very severe hyponatraemia, e.g. serum Na <105 mmol/L), the use of *intravenous hypertonic saline (3%)* is indicated (*only with senior input and is best done in the ICU*).

1. Acute hyponatraemia (e.g. postoperative; uncommon)

- The osmotic pressures within the cells of the brain tend to equilibrate with the osmotic pressure of the ECF and plasma. If the ECF becomes acutely hypotonic, in <24–48 hours, water enters the brain leading to acute cerebral oedema, which can cause death by brainstem herniation.
- Such patients present with the rapid onset of neurological symptoms and signs (from headache, nausea and vomiting, to stupor, coma, convulsions). *This is a medical emergency and requires treatment with intravenous hypertonic (3%) saline.*

- Thus in patients with significant *symptoms induced by rapid onset hyponatraemia, especially those with seizures or coma, a bolus infusion of 100 mL of 3% NaCl should be administered immediately, followed by one or two further infusions at 10-minute intervals if there is no initial clinical improvement.* This regimen will raise serum sodium by a maximum of 5–6 mmol/L, and is usually sufficient to reduce cerebral oedema and improve symptoms rapidly (e.g. convulsions stop); further hypertonic saline may not be immediately necessary.

2. Chronic hyponatraemia (common)

- In practice the rate of development of hyponatraemia is not known: therefore most patients should be regarded as having *chronic* hyponatraemia.
- During more prolonged hyponatraemia (≥48 hours) sodium and organic solutes leave the brain and its osmolar pressure equilibrates with that of the ECF, so brain swelling is minimized, and symptoms are usually less acute.
- Symptoms include weakness, confusion, delirium, nausea, vomiting, muscle cramps, gait disturbances (high risk of falls); seizures can occur with extreme hyponatraemia.
- However, because the brain regains sodium rapidly, but organic osmolytes slowly, rapid correction of the hyponatraemia in this context can lead to an *osmotic demyelination syndrome* (probably a breakdown of the blood–brain barrier, damage to oligodendrocytes, leading to delayed pontine and extra-pontine demyelinosis, which typically develops 1–7 days after the rapid correction of chronic hyponatraemia).
- This syndrome is defined clinically – patients present with slowly evolving symptoms which include movement disorders, behavioural disturbances, quadriparesis, pseudobulbar palsy, seizures and death. MRI in the acute phase may or may not show pathology; some recovery can occur, but the syndrome is often permanent. Patients with malnutrition, alcoholism, or liver cirrhosis appear to be especially susceptible to this complication.
- *In conscious subjects* the major therapeutic approach should be continued *fluid restriction* (600–1300 mL water per 24 hours) (see below).
- Irrespective of the cause, the rate of correction of severe hyponatraemia (serum Na <120 mmol/L)

should be slow. In patients with severe *chronic* hyponatraemia and significant symptoms (especially neurological symptoms), start with IV infusion of 3% NaCl at 15–30 mL/hour; check serum electrolytes 2-hourly initially. Discontinue the infusion once serum Na has increased by 4–6 mmol/L. The hypertonic saline can induce a diuresis in some patients; therefore all patients should be catheterized and urine output monitored hourly. *If a diuresis is induced, stop the hypertonic saline infusion.*

- Aim to raise serum sodium concentrations *by no more than 6–8 mmol/L per 24 hours, 12–14 mmol/L in 48 hours, and 14–18 mmol/L in 72 hours.* Serum Na concentrations should be frequently monitored to prevent too rapid correction. If hypokalaemia is also present, conventional correction with intravenous infusion of KCl will help correct the hyponatraemia.
- *The 3% sodium infusion rate should be stopped if the increase in serum Na is greater than 0.5 mmol/L per hour.* (It can then be resumed at a slower infusion rate if still indicated.)
- *A guide to a safe infusion rate*: 35 mL/hour of 3% sodium infusion for a 70 kg man will increase serum Na by about 0.5 mmol/L per hour.
- *This acute IV treatment should also be interrupted if any of three end-points is reached*:
  - the patient's symptoms improve considerably
  - serum sodium levels become 'safe' (≥120 mmol/L)
  - total correction of 16 mmol/L has been achieved over 72 hours.

Correction of SIADH without major neurological symptoms

- For all patients with chronic SIADH without major neurological symptoms *fluid restriction* is the treatment of choice – restrict total fluid intake (includes water in food) to between 600 and 1300 mL in 24 hours.
- The degree of effective fluid restriction will depend on urine output. Therefore *monitor urine output* carefully and *aim for about 500 mL intake less than urine output each day.*
- Do not restrict sodium intake in food. Several days of water restriction may be needed to initiate a rise in serum sodium concentrations – the degree of fluid restriction may have to be adjusted.

- Failure of proven, tight fluid restriction to raise sodium significantly should prompt the reconsideration of the diagnosis of SIADH.

Over-correction of serum sodium concentrations

- Some patients with moderate to severe hyponatraemia (e.g. *serum sodium <115 mmol/L*) can rapidly '*autocorrect*':
  - patients with volume depletion given IV saline
  - steroid replacement in hypoadrenalism
  - discontinuation of thiazide or desmopressin therapy
  - preventing psychogenic polydipsia.
- They are potentially vulnerable to the osmotic demyelination syndrome complication as serum Na levels can rise by as much as 2 mmol/L per hour (i.e. resulting in too rapid correction of the deficit – within 12 hours).
- If the rise in serum sodium exceeds those itemized above, *lower the sodium levels with intravenous 5% dextrose infusions, and consider using desmopressin to induce water retention* so as to slow down the rate of rise of sodium, e.g. 2 µg subcutaneously (can be repeated).

Treatment of hyponatraemia from diuretic therapy

- Commonly elderly women; about 90% associated with thiazides; often serum K is also low.
- Stop diuretics; *slow IV 0.9% saline infusion (e.g. 1 litre in 12/24 hours).* If [Na] is <120 mmol/L, monitor serum Na 2–4-hourly, avoid rapid correction – follow the SIADH guidelines for the safe rate of increase of sodium.

Treatment of hyponatraemia in hypoadrenal states

- If this diagnosis is suspected, measure serum cortisol levels, resuscitate as clinically indicated, and *immediately* administer IV hydrocortisone 100 mg (repeat 6-hourly). *Do not wait for lab cortisol results.* This approach can be life-saving, and is harmless if it proves to have been unnecessary.
- In patients with serum sodium concentrations <120 mmol/L, measure serum Na 4-hourly, and avoid too rapid correction – follow the SIADH guidelines for the safe rate of rise of Na – *it is easy to rapidly overcorrect the hyponatraemia in these circumstances.*

Cerebral salt wasting (CSW)

- Occurs after head injury or neurosurgery. Its aetiology is unclear, but results in renal sodium and chloride loss, leading to hypovolaemia and baroreceptor-mediated ADH release and water retention.
- The differentiation of CSW from CNS-associated SIADH is difficult and depends on noting urinary volume and Na loss and evidence of volume depletion (accurate fluid balance and evidence of volume depletion before and during the development of hyponatraemia).
- Treatment is sodium replacement which will correct the Na deficit (in SIADH IV saline will not correct the hyponatraemia).

Dilutional hyponatraemia

Treat the oedema

- *Heart failure*: loop diuretics, and other conventional medications.
- *CKD with fluid overload*: fluid restriction; consider loop diuretics.
- *Cirrhosis with portal hypertension*: spironolactone as first-line therapy.
- *Hypoalbuminaemia*: spironolactone as first-line therapy.

In all of the above monitor renal function frequently, for the development of hypokalaemia (loop diuretics) or hyperkalaemia (spironolactone), and for deteriorating renal function.

> ### Scenario 50.2
>
> *An 85-year-old man is admitted from a local residential home as he has become increasingly drowsy and confused over the previous week. He has been refusing to eat and drink and is now unable to get out of bed. His GP has treated him for a presumptive urinary tract infection without improvement. On admission he has a reduced GCS and is very dehydrated. Investigations reveal a hypernatraemia with a plasma sodium of 155 mmol/L.*

Hypernatraemia

- Hypernatraemia is defined as serum sodium concentration >145 mmol/L, and is often associated with dehydration.
- It is a consequence of *inadequate water intake*.

- Severe symptoms occur with large, acute increases in serum sodium concentrations above 160 mmol/L.

Causes

- *Reduced water intake*: hypernatraemia most commonly occurs in adults when thirst is impaired, or when an individual no longer has independent access to water, or both. Patients at risk include the infirm elderly, often with fever; those with altered mental status; rarely in the presence of hypothalamic lesions which reduce the sense of thirst.
- *Hypotonic fluid loss*: burns; excessive sweating (e.g. endurance sports).
- *Gastrointestinal loss*: laxative abuse; non-secretory diarrhoea; vomiting; nasogastric drains; GI fistula.
- *Renal loss*: diuretic abuse; osmotic diuresis (e.g. hyperosmolar non-ketoacidotic diabetic states).
- *Hypertonic sodium-containing fluids*: IV hypertonic saline infusion; IV sodium bicarbonate; IV sodium-containing antibiotics; tube feeding.
- *Hyperaldosteronism*: causes minimal hypernatraemia.

Symptoms

- If the patient is conscious: typically thirst with polyuria and polydipsia; lethargy, weakness.

Signs

- Confusion, myoclonic jerks, evidence of dehydration and hypovolaemia.

Investigations

- Usually an unexpected finding on routine testing.
- Check serum calcium, glucose, lithium (if appropriate) concentrations.
- If diabetes insipidus is suspected, check serum and urine osmolarities (in diabetes insipidus the serum osmolality >300 mOsm/kg, with an inappropriately low urine osmolarity).

Management

- Urgently check the laboratory results.
- Assess the severity, and the duration of hypernatraemia. Assume it is a chronic state (duration >24 hours) unless there is good evidence for acute hypernatraemia.
- Seek senior advice if sodium concentration ≥155 mmol/L.
- Correct dehydration by replacing free water; correct hypovolaemia by the administration of electrolytes; treat the cause, if possible.
- Ideally the patient should be encouraged to drink water – satisfactory for mild hypernatraemia in conscious subjects. Nasogastric fluids can be used in patients unable to drink; hypotonic intravenous infusions may be necessary for unconscious patients (see below).
- *Appropriate fluids*: if the patient is hypotensive/hypovolaemic, 0.9% saline to restore circulation. If BP is satisfactory, oral water; 0.45% saline; 5% dextrose.
- *Calculate the approximate water requirements*: water deficit (litres) = TBW × ((serum Na mmol/L ÷ 145) – 1), where TBW is total body water = lean body weight (kg) × Y (Y = 0.6 for men; 0.5 for women and elderly men; 0.45 for elderly women).
- *The rate of correction of hypernatraemia* is important in *chronic* states: the rise in sodium be no more rapid than 0.5 mmol/L per hour (i.e. 10–12 mmol/L in 24 hours).
- *The key to successful treatment* of hypernatraemia lies in frequent assessments of the patient and serum sodium concentrations, and the adjustment of the rate of hypotonic fluid administration.
- *Prevention*. Be alert to the possibility of hypernatraemia in the frail elderly in care and in hospital, and in critically ill patients; careful monitoring of fluid balance; if in doubt, check renal function tests.

Further reading

Martini FH. *Fundamentals of Anatomy and Physiology*, 7th edn. Pergamon, Penguin, Cummings; 2006.

Spasovski G, et al. Clinical Practice guideline on diagnosis and treatment of hyponatraemia. *Eur. J. Endochrinol* 2014; 170: G1–G47.

Sterns RH, Nigwekan SU, Hix JK. The treatment of hyponatraemia. *Seminars in Nephrology* 2009; 29: 282.

Chapter

51

Polydipsia and polyuria
The patient presenting with polydipsia and/or polyuria

Stephen Haydock and John Kalk

Introduction

Polyuria is usually defined as passing ≥3 litres of urine in 24 hours (a 'normal' volume is 1–2 litres per day) and is usually accompanied by passing urine more frequently than usual, including nocturia.

Polydipsia is an abnormally increased intake of fluids and its causes are usually also the causes of polyuria. The exceptions to this rule are *psychogenic polydipsia*, and the imbibing of large volumes of fluids, usually associated with a low protein diet (e.g. *beer potomania*, or the '*tea and toast*' diet sometimes observed in the elderly).

Conditions of polydipsia and polyuria may be associated with significant hypo- and hypernatraemia, the management of which is described in the previous chapter.

Causes of polydipsia/polyuria

Driven by primary increase in water intake

- *Psychogenic polydipsia* (compulsive water drinking), sometimes associated with severe psychotic illness with *severe polydipsia*
- *Alcohol excess – especially large volumes of beer* (beer potomania)
- *Prescription of agents that reduce saliva secretion* and cause a dry mouth (e.g. tricyclic antidepressant agents, an antimuscarinic effect)

Driven by osmotic diuresis

- *Diabetes mellitus*
- *'Post obstruction'* (e.g. of ureters) diuresis

Driven by loss of renal concentrating ability

Inadequate production of antidiuretic hormone

- *Neurogenic diabetes insipidus*
    - congenital (in children, rare)
    - acquired:
        - head trauma
        - tumours and granulomas of the hypothalamus or pituitary
        - complicates brain death in up to 80% of cases

Inadequate response to antidiuretic hormone

- *Nephrogenic diabetes insipidus*
    - congenital (in children, rare)
    - acquired:
        - lithium therapy (in 10–20% of patients)
        - hypercalcaemia (serum calcium concentrations usually >3.0 mmol/L) – hyperparathyroidism; tumour-related (parathyroid-like hormone secretion, bone metastases), myeloma, sarcoidosis
        - chronic potassium depletion – chronic diarrhoea, purgative abuse, diuretic therapy, diuretic abuse, primary hyperaldosteronism
        - chronic kidney diseases (e.g. polycystic kidneys)
        - diuretic phase of recovery from acute kidney injury
        - post obstruction diuresis

Acute Medicine, ed. Stephen Haydock, Duncan Whitehead and Zoë Fritz. Published by Cambridge University Press. © Cambridge University Press 2015.

History

It is important to differentiate urinary frequency, with frequent voiding of a normal daily urine volume, from true polyuria.

Ask about

- When did the symptoms begin, did they begin suddenly or gradually?
- How often do you pass urine during the day?
- How often do you pass urine at night?
- What volumes of urine are passed on voiding?
- What volume of urine is passed in 24 hours?
- What volumes of fluid are drunk during the day?
- What volumes of fluid are drunk at night?
- Family history of diabetes.
- Family history of polyuria.
- Past history of head trauma, malignancy, renal disease, psychiatric illness.
- Current and past medications, e.g. lithium, tetracyclines, diuretics, anticholinergics.

Note

- A low night-time fluid intake, relative to the daytime intake, may be a pointer to psychogenic polydipsia.
- New onset of nocturia in absence of other causes is suggestive of diabetes insipidus.
- Sudden onset is suggestive of cranial diabetes insipidus.
- The effects of lithium can be long lasting after the drug has been discontinued.

Examination

Perform a complete physical examination but in particular *carefully assess fluid volume status*:

Dehydration: hypotension, postural hypotension, tachycardia, reduced skin turgor

Fluid overload: raised JVP, oedema, bi-basal crackles, gallop rhythm, ascites.

Investigations

Uncontrolled diabetes mellitus and *severe hypercalcaemia* are the commonest causes of polyuria (and polydipsia) in patients presenting on the acute medical take. *Obtain*:

- full blood count
- blood glucose and HbA_{1c}
- urea and electrolytes
- plasma calcium and phosphate
- plasma lithium (if relevant)
- urinary glucose and ketones
- serum and concomitant urine osmolalities; *ideally the first urine specimen in the morning.*

Other investigations will be dictated by the above findings. (Refer to information relating to specific conditions at end of this chapter.)

In the absence of glycosuria, a *low* early morning urine osmolarity with a *high* serum osmolality (and high serum Na) favours the diagnosis of diabetes insipidus.

Low serum and *low* urine osmolalities favour psychogenic polydipsia.

If the patient can tolerate it, reduction or deprivation of fluids overnight can be a helpful screening test (e.g. from midnight to 9 am):

- A significant increase in urine osmolality, well into the normal range (e.g. about 500 mOsm/kg), with normal serum osmolality and sodium levels favours the diagnosis of psychogenic polydipsia (or mild diabetes insipidus which should not cause significant symptoms).
- However, the differentiation of these two conditions may be difficult, and formal testing with a water deprivation test can be useful. It is usually carried out by the endocrinology team.

Notes on some important causes of polydipsia and polyuria

Psychogenic polydipsia

Aetiology

- Found in up to 20% of psychiatric patients.

- Particularly associated with schizophrenia, patients with developmental disorders, and middle-aged women with anxiety disorders.
- Aetiology is not fully understood but the following have been implicated:
  - compulsive behaviour
  - increased dopamine receptor sensitivity due to long-term dopamine-2 antagonist use in schizophrenic patients
  - abnormality in hypothalamic thirst centre
  - attempts to counteract anticholinergic side effects of drugs.

Investigation

- Patients may present with acute or chronic hyponatraemia.
- Morning osmolality specimens show *low* serum and *low* urine osmolalities.
- Water deprivation produces a significant rise in urine osmolality.

Treatment

- Behavioural treatments and water restriction.
- Newer antipsychotic agents such as clozapine with lower D2 receptor occupancy appear beneficial compared to older agents.

Diabetes insipidus

Aetiology

Results from impaired action of the hypophyseal hormone ADH (antidiuretic hormone/arginine vasopressin) either due to impaired secretion (*neurogenic DI*) or renal resistance to its action (*nephrogenic DI*):

Neurogenic diabetes insipidus

- Very rare familial cases
- Autoimmune (idiopathic)
- Head trauma, pituitary surgery, hypoxic or ischaemic brain injury

Nephrogenic diabetes insipidus

Mild degrees of ADH resistance are common especially in the elderly, resulting in mild and largely asymptomatic impairment of renal concentrating ability. Symptomatic nephrogenic DI is most commonly due to:

- hereditary nephrogenic DI in children due to mutations in the ADH receptor

- chronic lithium toxicity due to dysfunction of kidney aquaporin-2 water channels in the collecting ducts
- severe hypercalcaemia due to impairment of sodium chloride reabsorption in the thick ascending limb of the loop of Henle, and the inability of ADH to increase collecting tubule permeability.

Investigation

- Diagnosis is suggested by paired serum/urine early morning osmolality. In the absence of hyperglycaemia, urine osmolality is low and serum osmolality is high.
- Overnight fluid deprivation with careful observation.
- Confirmation is by formal water deprivation test, under the care of endocrinology.

Treatment

Neurogenic diabetes insipidus

- Oral or intranasal desmopressin (DDAVP): A long-acting modified ADH that acts as a potent antidiuretic but does not have any vasopressor activity; it is well tolerated and is first-line therapy in symptomatic patients.
- Alternative therapies in patients with very mild disease include:
  - low sodium, low protein diet +/− thiazide diuretic, NSAIDs
  - carbamazepine – increased secretion of ADH and possible increased renal sensitivity to ADH.

Nephrogenic diabetes insipidus

- Usually treat the underlying cause: correct hypercalcaemia, lithium toxicity (renal effects of lithium can be very prolonged, i.e. months, or permanent).
- Low sodium, low protein diet +/− long-acting thiazide diuretic, NSAIDs.
- Desmopressin may be tried if above unsuccessful.

Hypercalcaemia of malignancy

Aetiology

Common: multiple myeloma, breast cancer.

Less common: non-small cell lung cancer, lymphoma.
Rarely: renal cell cancer, colon, small cell lung cancer.

- Hypercalcaemia of malignancy can occur in the absence of bony metastases; 80% of humoral hypercalcaemia of malignancy is due to secretion of PTH-related peptide (PTHrP).
- Significant polydipsia and polyuria tend to be seen at calcium concentrations of 3 mmol/L and greater.

Management

- Check blood levels for vitamin D and PTH (should be undetectable), and PTHrP if indicated.
- Stop drugs which contain calcium or inhibit calcium excretion.
- Administer IV saline at (0.9%) 300–400 mL per hour until euvolaemic (this may be tailored to individual patient as many elderly patients with malignancy are quite frail and may have co-morbid cardiac and renal disease).
- *For hypercalcaemia >3 mmol/L* and when euvolaemia established administer pamidronate 60–90 mg IV in 500 mL normal saline over 2 hours. It takes 1–2 days for serum calcium to decline maximally in response to a pamidronate infusion, *which should not be repeated within 7 days*.
- *For hypercalcaemia >4 mmol/L* give IV fluids and IV pamidronate 90 mg in 500 mL over 2 hours and consider use of calcitonin 4–8 units per kg, which can be given 6- or 12-hourly over 2 days.

New onset diabetes mellitus

New onset diabetes can present on the medical take with varying degrees of severity and urgency. Always perform a full examination including skin (especially feet), perform fundoscopy, check for peripheral neuropathy and always consider possible associated sepsis. Many can and should be managed without recourse to IV insulin infusions.

Patients may be:

- *Asymptomatic* (found on blood or urine testing)
- *Symptomatic* with the classic triad of polydipsia, polyuria and weight loss with varying degrees of dehydration. Some patients will present with extreme manifestations:
    - ketoacidosis
    - hyperosmolar non-ketotic hyperglycaemia (plasma glucose >30 mmol/L).

Investigations

- Urine for glucose, ketones, protein, infection
- Capillary glucose and ketones
- Plasma glucose, HbA_{1c}, renal and liver function, blood count, CRP, TSH, lipids
- CRP, blood culture, urine culture if sepsis suspected
- If type 1 DM considered and plasma ketones ≥3.0 mg/dL or heavy ketonuria:
    - venous or arterial blood gases
    - islet and GAD65 antibodies.

Treatment

Most Trusts will have clinical guidelines prepared by the diabetes team to aid management and these should be consulted. Management and need for admission is guided by:

- clinical status
- level of hydration
- whether able to eat or drink
- plasma glucose
- degree of ketonuria/ketonaemia.

The well patient: is likely to have type 2 diabetes. They will be able to eat and drink and have absent or minimal symptoms. Plasma glucose will be ≤20 mmol/L with absent or mild/moderate ketonuria and ketonaemia <3.0 mg/dL.

- Initiate 'lifestyle' management (dietitian, diabetes specialist nurses).
- Start metformin (500 mg od/bd initial dose).
- If symptomatic, consider also initiating sulfonylurea therapy for rapid improvement in blood glucose (e.g. gliclazide 80 mg bd).
- Monitor blood glucose pre-meal and bedtime if needs to stay in hospital.
- If requires hydration then use IV 0.9% saline.
- Ask GP for further diabetes education and follow-up.

The unwell patient with probable type 2 DM and high plasma glucose: likely to have significant degree of dehydration and may have nausea and vomiting preventing eating and drinking.

- Rehydrate with 0.9% saline, with potassium as indicated.
- *If vomiting, unable to drink and eat, if 'nil per mouth'*:
    - commence variable rate IV insulin infusion, hourly blood glucose monitoring, until eating and drinking

- monitor renal function and potassium at least twice daily
- manage co-morbidities
- request diabetes team advice.

- *If eating, drinking adequately* and *blood glucose <20 mmol/L*:

  - rehydrate with 0.9% saline if needed
  - start sulfonylurea therapy
  - start metformin therapy.

- *If eating, drinking adequately* and *blood glucose >20 mmol/L*:

  - consider initiating subcutaneous insulin therapy, e.g. isophane or biphasic insulin (0.2–0.3 units/kg in 24 hours, in two equal, divided doses given before breakfast and evening meal)
  - monitor blood glucose pre-meal and bedtime
  - request diabetes team advice
  - consider 'correction doses' of rapid-acting insulin (4–6 units), before meals only, for blood glucose >15 mmol/L
  - manage co-morbidities.

The patient with suspected type 1 diabetes not in ketoacidosis

- Rehydrate if needed with 0.9% saline (with potassium supplementation according to plasma electrolyte measurements).
- Urgent diabetes specialist nurse (DSN) input.
- If DSN not immediately available, then initiate basal insulin therapy with isophane insulin, starting at 0.2–0.3 units/kg body weight/day, in two divided, equal doses.
- Consider 'correction doses' of rapid-acting insulin SC (2–4 units) before meals only, if blood glucose >15mmol/L.

The patient with diabetic ketoacidosis or hyperosmolar non-ketotic hyperglycaemia (glucose >30 mmol/L)

- Follow local/national guidelines.

Further reading

Clines GA. Mechanisms and treatment of hypercalcemia of malignancy. *Curr Opin Endocrinol Diabetes Obes* 2011; 18(6): 339–346.

Dundas B, Harris M, Narasimhan M. Psychogenic polydipsia review: etiology, differential and treatment. *Current Psychiatry Reports* 2007; 9: 236–241.

NICE. Diagnosis and management of type 1 diabetes in children, young people and adults; NICE Clinical Guideline 15 (July 2004). Available to download at www.nice.org.uk/nicemedia/pdf/cg015niceguideline.pdf.

Raz I. Guideline approach to therapy in patients with newly diagnosed type 2 diabetes. *Diabetes Care* 2013; 36(Suppl 2): S139–144.

Shapiro M, Weiss JP. Diabetes insipidus: a review. *J Diabetes Metab* 2012; S8: 001. doi:10.4172/2155-6156.S8-001 Available to download at www.omicsonline.org/2155-6156/2155-6156-S8-001.pdf.

SIGN. Management of diabetes; Scottish Intercollegiate Guidelines Network – Guideline 116 (March 2010). Available to download at www.sign.ac.uk/pdf/sign116.pdf.

Pruritus

Penny Williams

Introduction

Pruritus can be defined as an unpleasant, poorly localized sensation that leads to the desire to scratch. It is a symptom that essentially manifests itself in the skin and/or mucous membranes and can be:

- localized or generalized
- intermittent or persistent (chronic pruritus when present for >6 weeks).

Severe pruritus can lead to considerable psychological distress. This must *not be underestimated* by the physician and should be addressed directly. Pruritus can result in significant behavioural adjustments and a withdrawal from social and work life.

Pruritus as a sensation evolved to give awareness to and trigger a response to remove irritants from the skin and mucous membranes, minimizing local damage. The urge to scratch when experiencing pruritus is very hard to suppress when fully alert; when asleep there is no suppression.

Scenario 52.1

A 72-year-old woman is admitted to the MAU with increasing breathlessness. She is clearly distressed by severe pruritus and has a widespread excoriated nodular rash. The history reveals she is an ex-smoker and has been diagnosed with mild COPD and atopy (mild eczema and hay fever). The dyspnoea is of gradual onset over the last few months. She has also developed severe intractable pruritus interfering with her sleep, leading to a low mood. The pruritus developed before her rash. She was recently started on an ACE inhibitor by her general practitioner for hypertension.

Pruritus is common in medical patients and often overlooked, although a cause of considerable distress to the patient and may herald serious systemic pathology.

In this patient we already have several possible aetiologies to explore:

- Eczema: however, a good history will reveal the patient's eczema has always been mild and associated with minimal symptoms of pruritus.
- ACE inhibitors commonly cause a lichenoid drug rash, although the rash can be non-specific; skin biopsy will confirm or refute this suspicion.
- Consider if the skin rash present is primary or secondary to scratching (e.g. nodular prurigo or lichen simplex chronicus).
- The breathlessness raises the possibility of a unifying systemic medical disorder. Investigation revealed severe iron deficiency anaemia, secondary to coeliac disease. Typically the rash associated with coeliac disease presents with herpetiform lesions over the extensor aspects, but iron deficiency can cause pruritus and secondary nodular prurigo in its own right. A biopsy with immunofluorescence will confirm the suspicion of *dermatitis herpetiformis*.

Pathophysiology

The pathways underlying the sensory perception of pruritus are not fully understood. Highly branched nerve endings in the skin are sensitive to histamine and several other mediators. Slow conducting nerve fibres project from these endings, via intermediate neurones to multiple regions of the contralateral cerebral cortex. Pruritus can result from stimulation or abnormalities anywhere along this pathway:

- pruritioceptive (stimulation of skin receptors)
- neuropathic (due to lesions of afferent conduction pathways)
- neurogenic (due to centrally acting mediators)
- psychogenic.

Acute Medicine, ed. Stephen Haydock, Duncan Whitehead and Zoë Fritz. Published by Cambridge University Press.
© Cambridge University Press 2015.

Aetiology

For the non-dermatologist it is diagnostically useful to think of pruritus in terms of the distribution of pruritus and associated dermatosis (primary skin disease). Be careful of secondary changes from scratching.

Localized pruritus without dermatosis

- Xerosis (in older patients, xerosis or dry skin is the most common cause of pruritus without a florid skin eruption)
- Psychogenic
- Neurological (localized to a dermatome):
  - brachioradialis pruritus (involving upper dorsolateral forearm)
  - notalgia paraesthetica (sensory neuropathic syndrome of the mid-back skin, the classic location of which is the unilateral infrascapular area)
  - post-herpetic neuralgia
- Pediculosis (head lice)

Generalized pruritus without dermatosis

- Xerosis
- Drugs (morphine)
- Pregnancy
- Iron deficiency
- Thyroid disease
- Cholestasis
- Chronic kidney disease
- Multiple sclerosis
- Malignant disease:
  - lymphoma
  - polycythaemia rubra vera
  - leukaemia
  - multiple myeloma
  - carcinoid tumours
- Psychogenic [1]:
  - anxiety and depression can manifest with pruritus: somatization
  - often impulsive/habitual scratching behaviour
  - can accompany or result from pruritus of any cause
  - Never underestimate the power of suggestion on the psyche

Localized pruritus with dermatosis

- Eczema
- Contact dermatitis
- Urticarial reaction (often a pressure-induced urticaria)
- Drugs (fixed drug reaction)
- Skin cancer (melanoma)
- Pediculosis (body and pubic lice)
- Dermatophytosis (fungal infection of the skin)
- Lichen planus
- Psoriasis

Generalized pruritus with widespread dermatosis

Common causes

- Eczema
- Contact dermatitis
- Urticaria and angio-oedema
- Drugs (ACE inhibitors and penicillins are common culprits)
- Scabies
- Chickenpox
- Mycosis fungoides (cutaneous T-cell lymphoma)
- Psoriasis

Rare causes

- Lichen planus
- Dermatitis herpetiformis (coeliac disease)
- Bullous pemphigoid

Skin changes due to scratching

Nodular prurigo describes firm, often hyperpigmented, intensely pruritic skin nodules, most commonly found on the arms and legs. Scratching often removes the top of the lesion to give crusting.

Lichen simplex chronicus describes the characteristic skin changes that result from chronic persistent scratching of the skin, in the presence (usually eczema) or absence of an underlying dermatosis. In the former case it will alter the appearance of the characteristic skin lesion. It is characterized by:

- intensely pruritic plaques
- scaling, excoriations, lichenification (skin thickening and increased skin markings)
- commonly calf, back of neck, elbow and genitalia (scrotum or vulva).

History

There are no definite clinical findings related to specific pruritic diseases; the history should clarify:

- duration, quality and localization of itching
- preceding or associated skin changes
- all current and recent medications (prescribed, OTC and illicit), infusions and blood transfusions
- history of alcohol abuse
- systemic features of illness including weight loss, fever, fatigue and night sweats
- medical and psychiatric history
- recent emotional or psychological stress
- contacts affected? (*scabies or other parasites should be considered*)
- impact on quality of life
- the relationship between pruritus and specific aggravators:
  - pruritus during physical activity is common in patients with *atopic eczema* and *cholinergic pruritus*
  - pruritus provoked by skin cooling after bathing should prompt consideration of *aquagenic pruritus*; it may be associated with or precede *polycythaemia vera* or *myelodysplastic syndrome*, and screening for these diseases should be considered
  - nocturnal generalized pruritus associated with chills, fatigue, tiredness and 'B' symptoms (weight loss, fever and nocturnal sweating) raises the possibility of lymphoma; somatoform pruritus rarely disturbs sleep but most other pruritic diseases cause nocturnal wakening
  - seasonal pruritus frequently presents as 'winter itch', which may also be the manifestation of pruritus in the elderly due to xerosis cutis and asteatotic eczema.

Examination

Document carefully any skin changes present (see Chapter 53) and consider if they reflect an underlying skin disease (with reference to the above list of conditions) or are secondary changes resulting from scratching. Always use correct terminology when describing rashes in the notes and when speaking to colleagues.

Generalized pruritus in the absence of a dermatosis requires a full physical examination to exclude a systemic disorder; specifically give attention to finding any lymphadenopathy.

Investigations

Appropriate investigation is dependent upon the findings from the clinical assessment; generalized pruritus without any associated dermatosis should raise the possibility of systemic disease, prompting further investigation:

- FBC
- ferritin (can be low even if Hb normal)
- CRP
- U&E
- LFT
- calcium (and phosphate in CKD)
- TFT
- glucose
- urinalysis
- anti-mitochondrial antibody (to rule out primary biliary cirrhosis)
- CXR (lymphadenopathy)
- immunoglobulins and plasma electrophoresis
- beta-HCG.

Indications for skin biopsy

- May be useful when there is evidence of an unrecognized primary dermatosis or localized pruritic lesions suspicious of malignancy (diagnosis, treatment and staging – see below).
- Generally not useful when either normal skin appearance or extensive secondary changes due to chronic scratching are present.

Skin cancer staging

Basal cell carcinomas rarely spread and do not require specific staging investigations.

Squamous cell carcinomas are locally invasive and may metastasize and therefore require a thorough clinical examination for lymphadenopathy; bear in mind that those greater than 2 cm in diameter, with a depth greater than 4 mm or poorly differentiated have a significantly greater chance of metastatic spread. High risk sites include lip and ear, non-sun-exposed sites (e.g. perineum, sacrum, sole of foot), areas of radiation or thermal injury, chronic ulcers, chronic inflammation, chronic draining sinuses or Bowen's disease.

Melanomas are pathologically staged according to the 2009 American Joint Committee on Cancer (AJCC)

Table 52.1 Relative potency of topical steroids

Class	Potency (versus hydrocortisone)	Examples
I (mild)	×1	Hydrocortisone
II (moderate)	×2–25	Clobetasone butyrate
III (potent)	×50–100	Betamethasone dipropionate, mometasone furoate
IV (highly potent)	Up to ×600	Clobetasol propionate

staging system and the *Tumour Node Metastases* staging [2]. Greater tumour thickness, the presence of ulceration and higher mitotic rate are all negative prognostic factors.

Physical examination with attention to other pigmented lesions, satellite lesions, in transit metastases, regional lymph node and systemic metastases is required. Low risk melanomas require no other investigations but higher tumour stages require imaging in order to allow full staging.

Treatment

- Patients with unexplained generalized pruritus without dermatosis require follow-up as generalized pruritus may predate a diagnosis of malignancy by several years.
- Management of pruritus involves:
  - treating symptoms
  - treating the underlying cause(s) if known.

Symptomatic relief

Recommendations from the European guidelines on chronic pruritus [3] include the following:

Avoid

- Environmental factors which promote skin dryness including: dry climate, heat, ice packs, excessively frequent washing and bathing
- Skin contact with irritants such as alcohol gel
- Oral intake of hotly spiced food and alcohol, large volumes of hot beverages
- Emotional extremes; excitement, significant stress
- Allergens, especially if atopic (house dust mites and dust).

Application

- Mild non-alkaline soaps, emollients for washing in the shower/bath

- Lukewarm, short duration, baths or showers
- If skin changes are present, dab dry after washing to avoid additional friction damage
- Skin emollient/moisturizing daily, especially after washing
- Advise to wear clothing which is permeable to the air (cotton, silver-based textiles)
- At night, topical treatments to reduce pruritus can be very beneficial; in particular, 1% or 2% menthol in aqueous cream is very cooling and may provide good relief.

Pharmacological

- Sedating antihistamine (hydroxyzine) taken in the evening
- Anticonvulsants/pain modulators (gabapentin, pregabalin) are recommended in neuropathic pruritus and pruritus secondary to chronic kidney disease
- Antidepressants can be helpful when pruritus is not responding to other therapies.

After commencing pharmacological treatments for pruritus, it is essential the response and side effects are reviewed and treatment stopped if it isn't beneficial.

Topical glucocorticoids

- Topical glucocorticosteroids can be effective in pruritus secondary to an inflammatory dermatosis; they are *not advised* in the absence of an inflammatory dermatosis.

All topical steroids have the same potential side effects: skin thinning, easy bruising, skin fragility and increased risk of secondary bacterial or fungal infections. The relative potency varies, and probability of side effects is related to relative potency (Table 52.1).

Indications for specialist referral

- When there is diagnostic doubt.

- Where there is treatment failure (*having excluded scabies*).
- When further investigation is warranted for patients with significant weight loss or any red flags that could suggest a paraneoplastic phenomenon or other potentially serious cause.
- Suspected primary cutaneous malignancy; beware amelanotic melanoma which can be skin coloured or red and so hard to diagnose early.

References

1. Schneider G, Driesch G, Heuft G, Evers S, Luger TA, Ständer S (2006) Psychosomatic cofactors and psychiatric comorbidity in patients with chronic itch. *Clin Exp Dermatol* 31: 762–767.

2. Marsden JR, Newton-Bishop JA, Burrows L, Cook M, Corrie PG, Cox NH, Gore ME, Lorigan P, MacKie R, Nathan P, Peach H, Powell B, Walker C (2010) Revised U.K. guidelines for the management of cutaneous melanoma 2010. *Br J Dermatol* 163: 238–256.

3. Weisshaar E, Szepietowski JC, Darsow U, et al (2012) European guideline on chronic pruritus. *Acta Derm Venereol* 92: 563–581.

Further reading

Weisshaar E, Apfelbacher C, Jager G, Zimmermann E, Bruckner T, Diepgen TL, et al (2006) Pruritus as a leading symptom: clinical characteristics and quality of life in German and Ugandan patients. *Br J Dermatol* 155: 957–964.

Rash

Pawel Bogucki

Introduction

Rash is a very broad term used to describe skin eruptions, but generally excluding cancerous lesions. As a physician on the acute medical take you should be able to:

- take a history and perform appropriate examination of the patient presenting with a rash
- accurately describe the distribution and appearance of a rash using appropriate terminology
- recognize rashes requiring urgent medical intervention, in particular:
  - erythroderma of any aetiology
  - rashes complicated by mucosal involvement
  - rashes associated with systemic disorders.

And be aware that:

- rashes can precede, or develop in conjunction with chronic diseases and if correctly identified may help early diagnosis of the underlying condition
- almost every internal malignancy can induce a paraneoplastic skin rash
- certain rashes, although subtle or asymptomatic (especially at early stages), may represent potentially fatal systemic disease requiring prompt identification and action, e.g. the ANCA positive vasculitic rash
- establishing the aetiology may require skin biopsies and clinico-histopathological correlation.

Scenario 53.1

A 52-year-old man is admitted via the emergency department. He is acutely unwell, hypotensive and tachycardic in association with a widespread erythematous rash with peeling of the epidermis. The rash covers almost all his skin surface. He has a past history of psoriasis and gout, and has recently started allopurinol.

This patient is presenting with *acute erythroderma* either due to his psoriasis or his recent medication change. It is a life-threatening condition requiring prompt recognition and management.

History

In relation to the skin condition itself:

- When and where did the rash first appear?
- How did it first appear and how has it developed or changed since initial appearance?
- Does it hurt or itch (see Chapter 52)?
- What makes it worse?
- Are close contacts affected?
- What treatments have been tried and how effective were they?
- Has this rash occurred previously?
- If previous history, what treatments were tried then and how effective were they?
- What does the patient think caused the rash?
- Has the patient used any different products, e.g. makeup, washing powders?
- Have there been any changes in occupation?
- Have there been any new pets?

Enquire carefully regarding other symptoms, in particular the presence of:

- malaise or systemic upset
- fevers/night sweats
- eye problems
- mouth or genital ulceration
- joint problems

Acute Medicine, ed. Stephen Haydock, Duncan Whitehead and Zoë Fritz. Published by Cambridge University Press.
© Cambridge University Press 2015.

Table 53.1 Common dermatological terms and meanings

Macule	Small smooth areas of changed colour <1.5 cm in diameter
Patches	Large areas of colour change, with a smooth surface
Papules	Small raised palpable lesions <1.5 cm diameter
Nodules	Enlarged papules in three planes (height, width, length)
Cysts	Fluid-filled papules or nodules
Plaque	Palpable flat lesions >0.5 cm diameter
Telangiectasia	Dilated superficial blood vessel
Pustules	Papules containing purulent material
Vesicles	Small <0.5 cm diameter papules containing serous fluid
Bullae	Large >0.5 cm diameter vesicles
Wheals	Irregular, usually erythematous raised oedematous areas of skin
The initial appearance of skin lesions can change over time due to scratching, rubbing and secondary infection resulting in:	
Excoriations	Superficial linear skin erosions
Lichenification	Increased skin thickening and skin markings as a reaction to scratching
Atrophy	Skin thinning often due to topical or oral steroids
Scarring	Deposition of fibrous tissue
Hypo- and hyperpigmentation	Reduced or increased melanin pigmentation compared to the patient's normal skin
Crusting	Scab formation
Erosions	Superficial, focal loss of epidermis; heals without scarring
Ulceration	Loss of epidermis and part of the dermis; heals with scarring
Fissures	Deep skin splits including the dermis

- weight loss.
  Document carefully:
- medical history
- medications present and past including OTC preparations, herbal and alternative remedies
- social history including occupation, hobbies, smoking, illicit drug and alcohol use
- travel history
- known allergies.

Examination

Carry out both detailed skin examination and general examination.

In examining the skin:
- expose and examine all the skin
- note the distribution of the lesions (trunk/periphery, flexor/extensor surfaces, sun exposed areas)
- carefully examine both scalp and nails
- describe the observed lesions:

- type(s) of lesion(s) present (see below)
- shape, size, colour/pigmentation of the lesions
- moist or dry
- arrangement of lesions (solitary, grouped, linear, etc.)
- consistency
- secondary changes often due to scratching or secondary infection (thickening, lichenification)

- check mucous membranes, mouth and genitalia (if indicated) for associated lesions.

Describing skin lesions

You should be able to describe the nature and distribution of the rash using appropriate terminology (Table 53.1).

Investigations

These should be guided by the appearance but may include:

- full blood count
- CRP
- urea and electrolytes
- liver function tests
- urinalysis and culture
- chest X-ray
- autoantibody screen/immunology
- skin swab and cultures
- blood cultures
- viral serology
- skin biopsy.

Skin biopsy

Safe to be performed in outpatient or ambulatory setting using local anaesthetic, the sample is transported to the laboratory in an appropriate fixative (usually 10% formalin).

Indications

- Diagnostic evaluation and excision of suspected skin malignancies
- Diagnostic evaluation of rashes of uncertain aetiology
- Confirmation of treatment response

Methods

- Tangential shave
- Punch
- Incisional
- Excisional

Punch biopsy is performed with a cylindrical instrument (2–8 mm diameter) and allows sampling of epidermis, dermis and subcutaneous fat.

Immunofluorescence

In addition to direct histological examination, immunofluorescence of a fresh skin biopsy can be useful in the diagnosis of:

- *bullous disorders*: both intraepidermal, e.g. pemphigus vulgaris, and subepidermal, e.g. bullous pemphigoid
- *connective tissue disorders*, e.g. SLE
- *vasculitides*, e.g. Henoch–Schönlein purpura.

Acute erythema

Remember that anaphylaxis can also be manifest by widespread erythema.

Erythroderma

- Is a generalized reddening of the skin involving >90% of the body surface, often associated with scaling or exfoliation (skin peeling).
- Usually results from either extension of existing inflammatory skin condition, or is drug induced (30% of cases are idiopathic).
- Erythroderma may lead to extensive loss of fluids, electrolytes and proteins as well as problems with thermoregulation resulting in major systemic upset and eventually death.

Management

- Identifying and avoiding/treating the underlying cause is a priority. All *unnecessary medication must be stopped* until the cause is found.
- Prevention and correction of systemic complications, acute and long-term consequences (cachexia, diffuse alopecia, ectropion and nail dystrophy).
- Treat the inflammation and if present secondary infection. Topical and systemic corticosteroids might decrease the degree of inflammation (particularly in drug-induced and idiopathic erythroderma); this should be prescribed and supervised by physicians trained in treating this skin condition. Frequent application of emollients helps to maintain the homeostasis of fluid balance and thermoregulation (*normal functions of healthy skin*).
- Patients with erythroderma require a multidisciplinary approach: acute physicians, dermatologists, ophthalmologists, dietitians, physiotherapists and occupational therapists.
- Appropriate nursing care, often in the ITU or HDU, is of paramount importance.

Toxic epidermal necrolysis (TEN)

- A very rare acute skin reaction with erythema of skin and mucosal surfaces and exfoliation.
- Almost always drug induced.
- TEN is *characterized by ≥30% body surface area involvement* and results from extensive death of keratinocytes (apoptosis) that leads to detachment of epidermis (the top skin layer).

  Stevens–Johnson syndrome:
- Pathophysiology is very similar to TEN, but results in less extensive disease, commonly <10% of body surface affected.

- More frequently caused by infections such as *Mycoplasma* or HSV than by TEN.

Management

- Immediately stop any possible offending drug(s).
- Complete loss of the epidermis in TEN has an even more profound impact on thermoregulation, fluid balance and protein and electrolyte loss than erythroderma; therefore a more 'aggressive' therapeutic approach is required.
- Patients with TEN should be treated as third degree burns victims, ideally in the regional burns unit or centres with experience in treating this condition.
- Effort should concentrate on supportive care (emollients, analgesia, correction of fluid balance and nutrition) and treatment of any secondary infections.
- Early involvement of ophthalmologists is even more important than in case of erythroderma sufferers.
- Specific therapies aiming to stop the apoptosis of keratinocytes are controversial and include intravenous immunoglobulins and in less severe cases ciclosporin.

Drug reaction with eosinophilia and systemic symptoms (DRESS)

- Is also known as *hypersensitivity syndrome*.
- A severe drug reaction which usually begins with high fever and maculopapular erythema.
- Often involves multiple organs, for example: lymph nodes, liver, kidneys, bone marrow, pericardium, gastrointestinal tract and central nervous system.
- Multiple haematological abnormalities are observed, such as: leucocytosis or leucocytopenia, thrombocytopenia, anaemia, eosinophilia (*interestingly eosinophilia is not essential to diagnose DRESS*).
- Deranged liver function tests in more than 70% of cases.
- Most common drug triggers include: allopurinol, antiepileptic drugs and antibiotics.
- Average time between the introduction of the offending drug and DRESS is 2 weeks.
- Mortality rate ≈10%.

Management

- The responsible medication has to be withdrawn.
- Patients require supportive treatment for identified organ dysfunction.
- Skin treatment is based on topical corticosteroids and emollients.
- More severe cases of DRESS can be treated with systemic corticosteroids, but evidence is limited.

Acute exanthematous generalized pustulosis

- Relatively rare (possibly underdiagnosed) drug-related (especially beta-lactam antibiotics) rash presenting as erythema covered with small pustules.
- It tends to begin on the head, in the flexures such as axillae and groins, and then to spread downwards.
- Sometimes associated with systemic symptoms such as fever and malaise, but on the whole patients are rarely unwell.
- Leucocytosis is common.
- Subcorneal pustules on skin biopsy confirm the diagnosis.

Management

- Withdrawal of the responsible medication.
- Symptomatic treatment with topical corticosteroids and emollients.
- Oral antihistamines.
- Analgesia as required.

Maculopapular drug reaction

- The most common rash produced by a drug reaction.
- In contrast to those described above, it is not associated with any systemic involvement (*when systemic features are present consider the diagnosis of DRESS*).
- Usually develops on the trunk initially, and then spreads to the limbs and head in a symmetrical pattern without any mucosal involvement.

Management

- Firstly the possibility of a type I hypersensitivity reaction should be excluded and culprit medications identified and stopped.

- Symptomatic treatment involves antihistamines, emollients and topical or systemic corticosteroids to relieve pruritus and decrease skin inflammation.

Viral exanthema

- Maculopapular reactive rash following viral infections similar to a maculopapular drug eruption.
- It is usually preceded by fever, malaise and arthralgia.

Management

- Commonly self-limiting and short-lived, no specific treatment is required.
- Treatment for pruritus might help to control the symptoms (see Chapter 52).
- Although benign, it often prompts patients or their parents to seek medical attention due to its distressing appearance.

Vasculitic rash

- Very broad term for rashes resulting from the inflammation of blood vessels; when they bleed under the skin this results in petechiae or purpura, livedo reticularis and, in severe cases, ulcers may also occur.
- Inflammation of small calibre vessels typically causes a petechial rash and is often related to viral or bacterial infection and systemic medication.
- The vasculitic rash should trigger investigation for other organ involvement.

Management

- Petechial rashes of drug or infective origin tend to resolve spontaneously after the triggering drug is removed or infection resolved.
- CXR, urine dipstick (*for blood and protein*), U&E, FBC, CRP, LFTs are a good starting point regarding investigation for systemic involvement; autoantibodies are often required.

- If further organ involvement is suspected refer to the appropriate specialist: nephrologist, respiratory physician or rheumatologist.

Bullous skin disorders

- Usually congenital or autoimmune skin conditions which present with rashes accompanied by bullae, vesicles and erosions that can extend to involve mucosal surfaces.
- They develop:
  - *Either* as a result of the absence of specific structural molecules leading to the easy breakdown of the skin (*congenital*); e.g. *epidermolysis bullosa*, where large blisters and erosions can result from minor skin trauma.
  - *Or* due to autoantibodies targeting antigens present within the skin, usually in the epidermis or epidermo-dermal junction (*acquired*); e.g. pemphigus, bullous pemphigoid, dermatitis herpetiformis.
  - *Bullous pemphigoid* is the most common of the immunobullous disorders and affects the elderly. Itchy plaques develop over days to weeks to form tense fluid-filled or haemorrhagic blisters.
  - *Pemphigus vulgaris* can be fatal. It produces *widespread oral ulceration* followed by bullae that easily rupture to give large denuded areas of skin. It may be precipitated by drugs or neoplasia.
- They are rare and patients presenting to the emergency services should *be promptly reviewed* by a dermatologist.

Further reading

Rothe MJ, Bialy TL, Grant-Kels JM. Erythroderma. *Dermatol Clin* 2000; 18: 405–415.

Rothe MJ, Bernstein ML, Grant-Kels JM. Life-threatening erythroderma: diagnosing and treating the "red man". *Clin Dermatol* 2005; 23: 206–217.

Chapter

54

Rectal bleeding

Stephen Haydock and Gareth Walker

Introduction

Rectal bleeding refers to the passage of bright red blood, blood clots or maroon blood per rectum and is indicative of lower GI bleeding, traditionally defined as blood loss from a site distal to the ligament of Treitz, the anatomical landmark of the junction between the duodenum and jejunum. Such blood loss is referred to as *haematochezia* to distinguish it from the passage of black, tarry stools of altered blood (*melaena*) suggestive of upper GI haemorrhage. Lower GI bleeding accounts for 25% of patients presenting to secondary care with GI bleeding. *The bleeding will stop spontaneously in 80–85% of patients.* The mortality rate for patients admitted to hospital with lower GI bleeding is 3.6% overall. Haematochezia can also be seen in severe upper GI haemorrhage and melaena can be seen in lower GI haemorrhage, due to bleeding from the small bowel or proximal colon.

Aetiology of lower GI bleeding

The passing of small amounts of blood per rectum is a very common symptom, usually manifest as blood on the toilet paper after defecation and probably experienced by over 15% of the population. This is usually due to a number of benign problems of the anorectal region that rarely cause bleeding sufficient to result in haemodynamic compromise, but may be due to a colorectal neoplasm. Significant haematochezia prompting emergency referral to secondary care usually results from colorectal bleeding but 11% are still due to severe upper GI bleeding and up to 9% from haemorrhage from the small bowel. Bleeding from diverticular disease and angiodysplasia are the commonest causes of significant lower GI haemorrhage.

Structural

- Haemorrhoids
- Diverticula
- Anal fissures
- Anal polyps
- Colorectal neoplasm

Vascular

- Angiodysplasia
- Radiation:
  - telangiectasia
  - proctitis
- Ischaemic colitis

Inflammatory

(Frequently associated with diarrhoea and abdominal pain.)

- Inflammatory bowel disease:
  - Crohn's disease
  - ulcerative colitis
- Infectious colitis

Coagulopathy

- Disorders of primary haemostasis
- Disorders of secondary haemostasis

Bleeding into the GI tract is more commonly associated with disorders of primary haemostasis (platelet plug formation at site of injury) – see Chapter 13.

Iatrogenic

- Following endoscopic biopsy/polypectomy

Acute Medicine, ed. Stephen Haydock, Duncan Whitehead and Zoë Fritz. Published by Cambridge University Press. © Cambridge University Press 2015.

Scenario 54.1

You are fast bleeped to review a 65-year-old man in the 'resus' bay of the emergency department. He has collapsed at home and his wife has dialled 999. During the journey to hospital he became progressively tachycardic and on arrival has a heart rate of 130 beats per minute and a blood pressure of 95 systolic. On your arrival he passes a large quantity of maroon blood per rectum. His only previous medical history is of atrial fibrillation, for which he is taking warfarin.

This patient is showing signs of shock with the passage of blood per rectum suggestive of bleeding from the lower GI tract. As for upper GI bleeding, the management aims are:

- provide early resuscitation
- elicit a detailed history and physical examination
- arrange appropriate definitive therapy to obtain haemostasis.

Clinical assessment

The approach to the patient with rectal bleeding will clearly depend on the severity of bleeding. The following account describes the management of those patients whose bleeding is *acute and severe* enough to present as an emergency to secondary care. *Patients with severe rectal bleeding will require urgent assessment and resuscitation as a priority.* There are no predictive scoring stools as for upper GI haemorrhage.

History

- When did the bleeding start, how frequent, mixed with or separate from stool, present in toilet pan, present on toilet paper?
- Is there associated pain, tenesmus, diarrhoea, mucus?
- Is there alteration in bowel habit?
- Is there abdominal pain?
- Is there associated vomiting?
- Enquire regarding previous episodes of bleeding and investigations at that time.
- Enquire regarding general health, e.g. malaise, weight loss?
- Take a detailed past medical history, e.g. diverticular disease, IBD, abdominal/pelvic radiotherapy.
- Take a family history: IBD, colon cancer.

- List current medication with particular reference to agents that might interfere with coagulation: antiplatelet (including aspirin and NSAIDs) and anticoagulant drugs (including newer agents).

Remember the risk factors for colon cancer

- Familial polyposis, e.g. familial adenomatous polyposis
- Increasing age and rare under 40 years of age
- Low socioeconomic group
- Personal history of polyp removal
- Personal history of ulcerative colitis (and Crohn's disease), especially if extensive colonic disease (pancolitis)
- Family history of colon cancer (*risk doubles if affected first degree relative*)
- Abdominal/pelvic radiation

Examination

- Assess haemodynamic status for patients with significant acute haemorrhage.
- Look for weight loss and other evidence of malignancy.
- Look for stigmata of chronic liver disease suggesting a possible upper GI origin.
- Abdominal tenderness is suggestive of an inflammatory source of bleeding such as infectious colitis, inflammatory bowel disease or diverticulitis, although ischaemic colitis can also be painful.
- Perform a rectal examination and identify local anorectal pathology and stool/blood.

Initial investigations

Baseline bloods include:

- FBC:
  - may initially be normal until haemodilution occurs
  - microcytosis suggests chronic blood loss
- Urea and electrolytes:
  - elevated urea:creatinine ratio suggests an upper GI source of bleeding
- Liver function tests
- Coagulation studies
- Venous blood gas:

- elevated lactate may indicate sepsis, with perforated viscus or ischaemic colitis
- Group and save serum/cross match as required.

Management

- Decide if patient requires admission (SIGN guidelines 2008 [1]). Patients suitable for discharge or outpatient management:
  - are under 60 years of age
  - are not haemodynamically compromised
  - have no evidence of gross rectal bleeding
  - have obvious anorectal source of bleeding seen on rectal examination.
- In such patients initial investigation by flexible sigmoidoscopy is appropriate. Depending on the findings they may go on to have definitive treatment (e.g. haemorrhoids) or further outpatient investigation including colonoscopy.

For patients with very severe bleeding resulting in haemodynamic compromise

- Appropriate resuscitation for the patient with haemodynamic compromise according to ABC guidelines:
  - oxygen
  - wide bore IV cannulae.
- Rapid volume replacement with crystalloid (normal saline).
- Packed red blood cell transfusion (pRBC) if >30% circulating volume lost:
  - onset of systolic and diastolic hypotension
  - tachycardia >120 (this physiological response may be attenuated in patients taking beta-blockers)
  - tachypnoea >20 breaths per minute.
- Significant blood loss is also indicated by a haematocrit <18% or a fall >6% and requires transfusion. Consider activating major haemorrhage protocol with hospital transfusion laboratory.
- Reverse any coagulopathy:
  - Send bloods for FBC, PT (INR), APTT, fibrinogen, corrected calcium.
  - Give fibrinogen if INR >1.5 with fibrinogen concentrate or cryoprecipitate if fibrinogen concentrate unavailable. Fresh frozen plasma

(FFP) also contains fibrinogen but needs to be given in large volumes (15 mL/kg), which may preclude its use once a coagulopathy has developed in the context of massive haemorrhage. FFP can be used to prevent a coagulopathy occurring and should be given with platelets to prevent haemodilutional deficiencies in platelets and clotting factors during red cell transfusions and volume expansion with crystalloids. A 1:1:1 ratio of pRBC:platelets:FFP is usually reserved for severe trauma cases.

- Thrombocytopenia with platelet infusion. Aim to keep platelets $>75 \times 10^9$/L. Platelets may also be given to reverse antiplatelet effect of aspirin but are only partly effective in reversal of other antiplatelet agents such as clopidogrel.
- Hypocalcaemia, hypothermia and acidosis also all impair coagulation and should be corrected.
- The SIGN guidelines (2008) identified the following as predictive of uncontrolled bleeding and death. These factors should be taken into consideration when deciding the appropriate care setting [1]:
  - increasing age
  - acute haemodynamic compromise and gross rectal bleeding
  - the presence of two significant co-morbidities
  - taking aspirin and NSAIDs
  - inpatients hospitalized for another condition who bleed after admission (mortality 23%).
- Therefore arrange transfer to the intensive therapy unit and involve gastroenterologist and surgical colleagues for:
  - shocked patients
  - patients with continuous active bleeding
  - patients with serious co-morbidities
  - those requiring multiple transfusion
  - haemorrhage in the context of an acute abdomen.

Consider and exclude upper GI haemorrhage

- Up to 15% of patients with severe haematochezia will have an upper GI origin for the blood loss;

such patients will have severe cardiovascular compromise; blood urea:creatinine ratio will be elevated.

- Passing of a nasogastric tube and subsequent aspiration may identify blood in the stomach but a negative aspirate does not exclude an upper GI source of blood loss. Urine dipsticks are not reliable or valid in identifying haematemesis in vomitus.
- Therefore, if there is significant clinical suspicion of upper GI bleeding then organize an urgent upper GI endoscopy as soon as patient is resuscitated.

Determining the cause of acute rectal bleeding

In the context of *acute severe* lower GI haemorrhage:

1. Once an upper GI source of bleeding has been excluded, perform colonoscopy with bowel preparation unless severe bleeding does not permit visualization or patient cannot be haemodynamically stabilized.
2. Perform mesenteric angiography, which may be preceded by CT angiography or radionucleotide scanning depending on local availability and expertise, in those patients not suitable for urgent colonoscopy (as above) or in whom colonoscopy failed to identify a source of bleeding.

Colonoscopy

This is the investigation of choice once upper GI haemorrhage has been excluded by upper GI endoscopy. There remains controversy regarding optimal timing but most would wait for adequate resuscitation and bowel preparation, generally 12–48 hours after presentation.

Advantages

- Is able to identify the bleeding source (89–97% with adequate bowel preparation).
- Direct visualization means bleeding point can be identified in absence of active bleeding.
- Able to identify arterial and venous bleeding points.
- Enables endoscopic haemostasis. If endoscopic therapy fails to achieve haemostasis the placement of an endoclip close to the culprit vessel will aid interventional radiologists with embolization therapy.

- Endoscopic haemostasis is much more difficult than in upper GI haemorrhage.

Disadvantages

- Requires adequate bowel preparation with polyethylene glycol based solutions (3–6 litres).
- Requires sedation.
- Small risk of bowel perforation.
- Unable to visualize small bowel.

Visceral angiography

Is indicated for patients with massive rectal bleeding when colonoscopy is precluded on grounds of visualization or haemodynamic stability, and in those patients in whom endoscopic examination has failed to identify a cause of bleeding.

Advantages

- Sensitivity of 40–86% and specificity of 100% in context of lower GI bleeding.
- Does not require bowel preparation.
- Allows accurate anatomical localization from bleeding from both small and large bowel.
- Enables catheter haemostasis.

Disadvantages

- Requires active bleeding with blood loss of 1–1.5 mL/minute.
- Serious complications including bowel ischaemia and cardiac arrhythmias and complications related to vascular access.
- Generally not available out of hours.
- Potential reactions to contrast material.
- Anatomical vascular variants are common and may lead to false negative findings.
- Does not allow for prolonged imaging times so not useful for intermittent bleeding.
- Exposure to ionizing radiation.
- Images the arterial phase only and does not identify venous bleeding sources.

CT angiography

Multidetector imaging with rapid data acquisition detects focal areas of contrast extravasation into gut following injection of iodinated contrast media. This is compared with a prior unenhanced scan to identify potential false positives (clips, sutures, pills, coproliths, etc.).

Advantages

- 91–92% sensitivity in patients with active lower GI haemorrhage, 100% specificity.
- Does not require bowel preparation.
- Can be performed rapidly.
- Non-invasive.
- Able to image both arterial and venous phase.

Disadvantages

- Requires administration of iodinated contrast media.
- Considerable radiation exposure.
- Diagnosis only and does not allow for haemostasis.

Nuclear scintigraphy

Tc-99m RBC scintigraphy has limited application in the acute setting but can be useful when endoscopy is not readily available or in patients in whom endoscopy is difficult or impossible. It is particularly useful in the investigation of obscure GI bleeding from distal small bowel. It may be performed prior to the more invasive angiography, as it is more sensitive, and if negative, angiography is unlikely to be helpful.

Advantages

- Is non-invasive and most sensitive technique for detecting GI blood loss.
- Detects both arterial and venous bleeding at low rates with little patient preparation.
- Allows prolonged imaging times and therefore useful for intermittent bleeding.

Disadvantages

- Must be actively bleeding (but allows prolonged imaging).
- Imprecise anatomical localization of bleeding.
- High false localization rates.
- Time-consuming.
- Limited availability out of hours.

Haemostasis

It is important to recall that 80–85% of lower GI bleeds will resolve spontaneously. Acute investigation and intervention is required only for those with severe life-threatening haemorrhage.

The selection of colonoscopy and visceral angiography as the initial investigations of lower GI bleeding is due to the abilities of these diagnostic modalities to also enable therapeutic control of the bleeding.

Colonoscopy: is effective means of controlling bleeding from a number of causes including angiodysplasia, diverticula, neoplasms and polyps by means of sclerotherapy, coagulation, clipping and adrenaline injection.

Transcatheter embolization: microcatheters and newer embolization methods give success rates approaching 90% without the major ischaemic complications of older techniques. Better for treatment of diverticular bleeding than from angiodysplasia. Older technique of vasopressin injection associated with systemic complications and high rebleed rate is now rarely used.

Surgery: will not be necessary for the majority of patients. Surgical intervention is indicated for:

- bleeding related to neoplasia
- identified bleeding source not responding to conservative therapy
- unidentified bleeding source associated with fulminant haemorrhage or recurrent bleeding. Aim is to identify bleeding source at surgery by intraoperative endoscopy and perform a segmental bowel resection (4% mortality and 6% rebleed rate), thus avoiding blind segmental colectomy (up to 50% mortality and up to 75% rebleed rate).

Additional investigations if unable to identify bleeding source

No source of bleeding may be identified in those patients who have blood loss from the small bowel (not visualized on colonoscopy) and if bleeding has stopped at time of angiography or nucleotide scanning. Options include:

- Radionucleotide imaging/angiography if further bleeding occurs.
- Examination of the small bowel:
  - *Push enteroscopy* with a paediatric endoscope or enteroscope, allowing examination of the proximal 60 cm of the duodenum
  - *Capsule endoscopy* is non-invasive and allows visualization of most/all of the small bowel. It is contraindicated in people with cognitive impairment (swallowing of capsule), patients

with oesophageal strictures and partial small bowel obstruction. Capsule may be retained due to severe dysmotility or Crohn's strictures. A soluble patency test capsule can be used to check for strictures prior to use of the proper capsule.

Inflammatory disorders causing lower GI bleeding

Patients often present to the medical take with passage of blood per rectum in association with increased bowel frequency, loose stools, abdominal pain and systemic upset. This may be indicative of:

- infectious colitis
- a new presentation of inflammatory bowel disease
- a flare of ulcerative colitis or Crohn's disease in a patient known to have these conditions.

Inflammatory bowel disease (see also Chapter 19)

Those patients presenting with a presumed flare of their existing inflammatory bowel disease should be discussed early with the gastroenterology team. Most Trusts will have an IBD nurse specialist who will be able to offer advice and act as liaison between the acute medical team and the gastroenterology unit. Visible rectal bleeding is more common in patients with ulcerative colitis but can occur in patients with Crohn's colitis as well [2].

- Patients with IBD will usually liaise directly with the IBD nurse specialist in the event of a disease flare. Many such patients are managed in an outpatient setting with a course of oral prednisolone commencing at 20–40 mg/day and tapered according to response.
- Patients with a flare of IBD are admitted to hospital if:
  - condition not responding to outpatient management with oral steroids
  - uncontrolled pain and/or diarrhoea
  - dehydration
  - if considering surgical intervention.
- Patients who are referred for admission require:
  - stool cultures and *C. difficile* toxin
  - request FBC, ESR/CRP, LFTs, serum albumin, glucose, calcium, magnesium, cholesterol and pregnancy test (if applicable). (Low

magnesium and low cholesterol levels are associated with increased toxicity from ciclosporin if this is required as second-line medical therapy.)
- plain abdominal X-ray to exclude toxic megacolon and obstruction
- early discussion with surgeon if severe colitis or obstruction and inform gastroenterology team of situation.
- Involve the gastroenterology team early if evidence of severe colitis (*Truelove and Witts criteria*):
  - frequent bloody stools (6 or more per day), and at least one of the following:
  - pyrexia of >37.8°C
  - tachycardia of >90/min
  - anaemia with haemoglobin <10.5 g/dL
  - ESR >30 mm/h.
- Other indicators of severe disease include:
  - severe abdominal pain
  - rapid weight loss.
- Treatment of severe colitis is with:
  - IV rehydration
  - IV steroids, e.g. hydrocortisone 400 mg per day (in four 100 mg doses) or methylprednisolone 60 mg per day (also give bone protection with calcium and vitamin D)
  - thromboprophylaxis.
- Second-line medical therapy of severe colitis not responding to steroids is with:
  - ciclosporin or if contraindicated …
  - anti-TNFα monoclonal antibodies – infliximab.
- Emergency colectomy may be required for acute severe colitis:
  - stool frequency >8/day or 3–8 stools/day *and* CRP >45 on day 3 of hydrocortisone treatment predicts need for colectomy in 85% of patients (*Travis criteria*).
- Treatment of mild-moderate colitis is with:
  - 5-aminosalicylic acids (5-ASAs), which are useful anti-inflammatory agents in managing mild to moderate flares of UC as well as for long-term maintenance therapy. Mesalazine (also called mesalamine) is commonly used and lacks the sulfapyridine moiety that causes many of sulfasalazine's side effects. Mesalazine high dose therapy is needed for moderately

extensive active UC (>2 g/day). Using a combination of topical mesalazine (enema and suppository) with oral preparations can be effective in the treatment of mild-moderate pancolitis and is more efficacious than oral or topical treatment alone. If patients do not respond within 10–14 days of mesalazine treatment then they should be considered for oral steroids. There is little convincing evidence for commencing 5-ASAs in the induction of remission of Crohn's disease, and only weak evidence for maintenance therapy and only if steroids were not needed to induce remission in the first place. However, studies suggest that mesalazine has a chemoprotective effect in reducing the risk of colorectal cancer in UC and it may also have a similar effect in colonic Crohn's disease as well. All available preparations are derivatives of the parent compound 5-aminosalicylic acid (olsalazine, mesalazine (Asacol, Pentasa), balsalazide).

Patients with a known or suspected diagnosis of inflammatory bowel disease require urgent referral and evaluation by the gastroenterology team. Severe IBD should be managed by joint care between a gastroenterologist and colorectal surgeons.

Infectious colitis

Infectious colitis and bloody diarrhoea may result from infection with the following bacteria:

- *shigellosis* due to e.g. *Shigella sonnei* and *Shigella flexneri*
- *salmonellosis* due to e.g. *Salmonella enteritidis* and *Salmonella typhimurium*.

Severe infection with *Shigella* and *Salmonella* can be treated with a 5-day course of ciprofloxacin 500 mg bd.

- *Campylobacter* due to e.g. *Campylobacter jejuni* and *Campylobacter coli*.

Campylobacter is now the commonest cause of bacterial food poisoning in the UK. Most cases resolve without antibiotic treatment. If necessary it can be treated with a 5-day course of azithromycin 250 mg od.

Before commencing treatment, discuss with the local microbiology department as antibiotic regimens will vary between Trusts.

References

1. Management of upper and lower GI bleeding (2008) SIGN Clinical Guideline 105. Available to download at www.sign.ac.uk/pdf/sign105.pdf.

2. Mowat C et al. (2011) Guidelines for the management of inflammatory bowel disease in adults. *Gut* 60(5): 571–607.

Further reading

Barnet J, Messman H (2009) Diagnosis and management of lower gastrointestinal bleeding. *Nature Reveiws Gastroenterology and Hepatology* 6: 637–646.

Chapter

55

Sepsis

Andrew Thompson

(See also Chapter 23 'Fever' and Chapter 56 'The shocked patient')

Introduction

The human body is continuously exposed to potentially pathogenic bacteria, and other organisms. It has evolved a complex immune-mediated inflammatory response to recognize and destroy pathogens. Both the failure to recognize and/or remove a pathogen and the 'inappropriate' over-production of the immune-mediated response can be detrimental to the host. Although all of us are at risk of sepsis, particular high risk groups are recognized:

- immunosuppressed due to acquired disease (HIV, haematological malignancy) or its treatment and congenital immunoparesis
- the very young and very old
- postoperative patients
- ventilated patients
- patients with indwelling cannulae and catheters.

The majority of cases of sepsis arise from the respiratory tract, gut and urogenital system. More serious infections account for 1–2% of all hospital admissions, and up to 25% of admissions to intensive care, where septic shock has a mortality of 30–70% and requires immediate treatment.

> **Scenario 55.1**
>
> *A 34-year-old woman is admitted with a one-week history of diarrhoea and vomiting which commenced whilst on holiday in Spain, together with a painful left calf. The calf muscle is tender on palpation, and a deep vein thrombosis is suspected. Further examination is unremarkable, her temperature is 38.2 °C, respiratory rate 18, pulse rate 107 and blood pressure is 90/63 mmHg.*

Is this infection?

Infection can be difficult to identify as the symptoms and signs are non-specific and microbiological proof

usually follows significantly later. The Surviving Sepsis Campaign was launched in 2002 to highlight the high mortality of sepsis and to promote evidence-based, time critical interventions to reduce mortality. The campaign standardized the definitions of sepsis (Figure 55.1) and produced guidelines on diagnosis and management [1].

Systemic inflammatory response syndrome (SIRS) is the body's response to insults such as burns, trauma, pancreatitis and infection.

Sepsis is diagnosed if SIRS is due to infection or presumed infection.

Severe sepsis is defined as sepsis with organ-induced dysfunction or tissue hypoperfusion, and for each organ there are defined abnormalities, e.g. renal impairment evidenced by acute oliguria (urine output <0.5 mL/kg per hour for at least 2 hours, despite adequate fluid) or creatinine increase (≥2 mg/dL or 176.8 mmol/L).

Septic shock is defined as sepsis-induced hypotension, with a systolic blood pressure >90 mmHg or a decrease to >40 mmHg below normal, *that persists despite adequate fluid resuscitation.*

Septic shock, oliguria or a raised lactate are all markers of tissue hypoperfusion.

The scenario is consistent with sepsis, where infection is thought to be driving the systemic response, although the source of infection may not yet be apparent. The principles of sepsis management are:

- prompt diagnosis
- rapid resuscitation and organ support
- early (and appropriate) antibiotic therapy and source control.

History

- The history should focus on symptoms consistent with infection. These may be potentially localizing

---

Acute Medicine, ed. Stephen Haydock, Duncan Whitehead and Zoë Fritz. Published by Cambridge University Press. © Cambridge University Press 2015.

Figure 55.1 The spectrum of sepsis.

SIRS	Sepsis	Severe sepsis	Septic shock
2 of: -Temp >38°C or <35.5°C - Respiratory rate >20 or $PaCO_2$ <32 mmHg - Heart rate >90 - WCC >11 000 or <4000/mm³ or >10% immature forms	SIRS + Confirmed or suspected infection	Sepsis + Signs of end organ damage/ hypoperfusion/ hypotension	Severe sepsis + Persistent hypotension despite adequate fluid resuscitation

symptoms, e.g. headache, neck stiffness and photophobia for meningitis, or non-specific symptoms of infection, e.g. feeling hot or cold, shivering and rigors. The very old and very young may present with less obvious symptoms such as confusion.

- The past medical history and drug history may identify risk factors for immunocompromise, e.g. corticosteroid use, alcoholism, malignancy, and alter the response to sepsis, e.g. beta-blockers preventing tachycardia, or a history of untreated hypertension necessitating a higher blood pressure when resuscitating a patient.
- A detailed recent travel, occupation and recreational history is required as this may be the only clue to specific pathogen exposure.

Examination

- The aim is to identify any source of infection, and assess the severity of infection, looking for signs of organ failure.
- As these patients may be very sick this should be performed via the ABCDE approach, initiating treatment at each stage.

Investigations

All patients should have the following baseline investigations:

- Serum electrolytes including urea, creatinine and bicarbonate.
- Full blood count.
- Liver function tests.
- Blood glucose.

- Clotting.
- Lactate is a marker of tissue hypoperfusion:
  - patients with a lactate >4 mmol/L *due to sepsis* have a mortality of 40% compared with a mortality of <15% when the lactate is <2 mmol/L [2].
- CRP is a marker of infection and/or inflammation:
  - it can be used to monitor response to treatment though not to make the diagnosis [3]
  - other biomarkers are being used to try and either improve the sensitivity of infection recognition or guide its treatment, e.g. procalcitonin; however, no markers can currently distinguish between severe infection and other inflammatory conditions.
- Blood cultures should be taken as soon as possible after onset of pyrexia in patients suspected of having bacteraemia. Two sets if there is an indwelling vascular access device, one taken peripherally and one from the line to establish if line sepsis is the source.
- Any microbiological samples (sputum culture, insert urine wound swabs, etc.) that can be sent, should be sent, to establish a microbiological diagnosis, where possible, and ensure the antimicrobial treatment started is appropriate.
- Imaging appropriate to determine the infection source, therefore CXR and/or US or CT.

Management

- A '*care bundle*' is a group of therapies for a given disease that, when implemented together, may result in better outcomes than if implemented individually. The management of sepsis has been grouped into several such bundles of care. The early identification of sepsis, allowing implementation of these bundles, is key to improving sepsis mortality.

- *'Early goal directed therapy'* was a term first coined by a single centre study (Rivers et al.) which reduced the 28-day mortality for septic shock by 15.9% (31% vs. 47%) by targeting resuscitation to several physiological goals in the initial 6 hours [4]. The interventions used to achieve the targets have been reproduced in other studies and form many of the components of the sepsis bundle.
- The *Surviving Sepsis Campaign Bundle* first part is to be completed within 3 hours of sepsis recognition:
  - measure lactate
  - obtain blood cultures prior to antibiotics
  - administer broad spectrum antibiotics
  - administer 30 mL/kg crystalloid for hypotension or a lactate ≥4 mmol/L.
- The second part is to be completed within 6 hours and requires:
  - central venous access and drugs (vasopressors and inotropes) which are only used in higher-level monitored beds.

Resuscitation

Airway
Breathing – high flow oxygen should be applied for patients with severe sepsis. Consider ventilatory support.
Circulation – IV access, and fluid resuscitation.

- Use crystalloid (Hartmann's or equivalent) if hypotension is suspected, then an initial fluid bolus of 30 mL/kg should be used, i.e. 2 L in a 70 kg patient, and started as soon as possible.
- There is no evidence that colloids are superior to crystalloid and they are considerably more expensive. Starch-based colloids may increase risk of acute kidney injury and mortality.
- Similarly a hyperchloraemic acidosis can accumulate with large amounts of 0.9% saline.
- Fluid boluses (e.g. 500 mL) should be used for as long as there are haemodynamic improvements in blood pressure or pulse pressure (5 litres in the first 6 hours was required in sepsis trials).

Adequate intravenous access is important to facilitate resuscitation. Central venous access may be required in a shocked patient if there is an initial poor response to fluid therapy.

If after one hour of fluid resuscitation the blood pressure does not achieve a mean arterial pressure of 65 mmHg, referral to Intensive Care should be considered for invasive monitoring and vasopressor use.

Antimicrobials

- Antibiotics should be commenced within 1 hour of sepsis recognition. The initial antibiotic regimen should cover a broad range of pathogens. Each hour of delay in effective antimicrobial administration is associated with an average decrease of survival of 7.6% in patients with persistent hypotension [5]. Only in patients with no evidence of severe sepsis should a narrower spectrum of antibiotics be used; guided by the presumed source of infection and local hospital policy.
- Septic shock in hospitalized patients is most commonly due to Gram-positive bacteria (e.g. staphylococci or streptococci) followed by Gram-negative bacteria.
- The majority of fungi are not pathogenic to immunocompetent humans, but immunocompromised individuals are at risk for opportunistic infections with fungi such as *Candida* or *Aspergillus*. Therefore antifungal treatment should be initiated if septic shock due to fungal infection is suspected and likewise antiviral treatment during an influenza epidemic.

Scenario 55.1 continued

The patient is commenced on IV fluids with an improvement in the blood pressure, blood cultures are sent and flucloxacillin started for presumed cellulitis. Blood tests showed hyponatraemia 126 mmol/L, acute kidney injury urea 20.2 mmol/L, creatinine 210 mmol/L, creatine phosphokinase 2735 μg/L, WCC 4.7 × 10⁹ L, CRP 378 mg/L, and a lactate of 3.2 mmol/L. At this stage she clearly has severe sepsis, and broader spectrum antibiotics should be considered. A more detailed examination notes an effusion in her right knee, from which pus is aspirated and identified as a group A Streptococcus. In the next 4 hours she rapidly deteriorates, developing septic shock, and is transferred to Intensive Care.

Ongoing management

- The remaining part of the resuscitation bundle is to apply vasopressors to maintain a mean arterial pressure (MAP) ≥65 mmHg and/or if the initial lactate was ≥4 mmol/L to measure:
  - central venous pressure with a target of 8 mmHg
  - central venous oxygen saturation with a target of 70%.

Also to re-measure and normalize the lactate if it was elevated initially.

- The focus on the central venous oxygen saturation (ScvO$_2$) derives from the Rivers study when targeting ScvO$_2$ ≥70% directed therapy. However, in a trial targeting either a lactate clearance ≥10% or an ScvO$_2$ ≥70% for resuscitation there was no difference in mortality, suggesting that lactate clearance criteria may be an acceptable and more easily monitored alternative to ScvO$_2$ criteria [6].
- Early, aggressive fluid therapy is appropriate in severe sepsis and septic shock; however, patients with sepsis typically develop non-cardiogenic pulmonary oedema (acute respiratory distress syndrome), due to increased capillary permeability, increased hydrostatic pressure and decreased oncotic pressure, and further fluids may be harmful when the circulation is no longer fluid-responsive. Therefore these patients will need frequent reviews.
- Vasopressors (drugs that increase the blood pressure by vasoconstriction) are used when the hypotension does not respond to fluid resuscitation:
  - noradrenaline predominantly increases blood pressure by its α-adrenergic effects causing vasoconstriction rather than its β-adrenergic effects of increased contractility and heart rate
  - adrenaline (a non-selective agonist of α and β adrenoreceptors)
  - vasopressin (acting via V-1 vascular receptors).
- Dobutamine inotropic support is recommended if there is evidence of myocardial dysfunction with a low cardiac output or ongoing signs of hypoperfusion despite an adequate MAP. It increases cardiac contractility (and heart rate) via beta-adrenergic effects.

- If fluid resuscitation and vasopressors are unable to establish haemodynamic stability initially then intravenous hydrocortisone 200 mg/day is added.
- Ventilation is often required to treat hypoxia, or failing respiratory muscle function which has attempted to compensate for an increased metabolic acidosis. A low tidal volume of 6 mL/kg predicted weight and limiting the inspiratory pressure ('a lung protective strategy') has been shown to be beneficial [7].
- Surgical removal of infection is also essential – in this scenario knee washout.

Specific infections

Group A streptococcal infections are caused by *Streptococcus pyogenes*, and commonly present as sore throat or skin and soft tissue infections. However, the incidence of invasive infections – defined as the isolation of streptococcus from a normally sterile site – is low, around 3 per 100 000 cases of bacteraemia in 2007 but this rate is increasing (a 62% increase to over 500 cases from November 2008 to February 2009 led to a letter sent to all doctors by the Department of Health) [8].

Streptococci produce superantigens, which cause non-specific activation of T cells resulting in polyclonal T-cell activation of up to 20% of the body's T cells compared to a normal antigen-induced response of 0.0001–0.001% and massive cytokine release. The mortality is between 15% and 25%, and up to 80% for streptococcal toxic shock syndrome. The large immune response is not specific to any particular antigen and thus is not helpful, but leads to septic shock. Human polyspecific intravenous IgG (IVIg) is recommended for severe invasive streptococcal infections if other approaches have failed because of its ability to neutralize a wide variety of superantigens, but is otherwise not recommended for sepsis management [9].

Some bacteria produce toxins which may require changes to antibiotic regimens. For example, staphylococcal infections can occasionally produce the Panton Valentine leukocidin (PVL) phage-mediated toxin which perforates the basement membranes of various cells including neutrophils. Antibiotics which are ribosomally active and switch off toxin production such as clindamycin are therefore particularly useful, and cell wall active agents may be less effective [10].

References

1. Dellinger RP, Levy MM, Rhodes A, et al. Surviving Sepsis Campaign: international guidelines for management of severe sepsis and septic shock 2012. *CCM* 2013; 41(2):580–637.

2. Trzeciak S, Chansky ME, Dellinger RP, et al. Operationalizing the use of serum lactate measurement for identifying high risk of death in a clinical practice algorithm for suspected severe sepsis. *Acad Emerg Med* 2006; 13(Suppl 1):S150-b-1.

3. Chalmers JD, Singanayagam A, Hill AT. C-reactive protein is an independent predictor of severity in community-acquired pneumonia. *Am J Med* 2008; 121:219–225.

4. Rivers E, Nguyen B, Havstad S, et al. Early goal-directed therapy in the treatment of severe sepsis and septic shock. *N Engl J Med* 2001; 345:1368e77.

5. Kumar A, Roberts D, Wood KE, et al. Duration of hypotension before initiation of effective antimicrobial therapy is the critical determinant of survival in human septic shock. *CCM* 2006; 34(6): 1589–1596.

6. Jones AE, Shapiro NI, Trzeciak S, et al. Emergency Medicine Shock Research Network (EMShockNet) Investigators: Lactate clearance vs central venous oxygen saturation as goals of early sepsis therapy: a randomized clinical trial. *JAMA* 2010; 303: 739–746.

7. Acute Respiratory Distress Syndrome Network. Ventilation with lower tidal volumes as compared with traditional tidal volumes for acute lung injury and the acute respiratory distress syndrome. *N Engl J Med* 2000; 342:1301–1308.

8. Health Protection Report, 2007: vol 1 (46). Department of Health.

9. Department of Health. Clinical guidelines for immunoglobulin use. May 2008.

10. Stevens DL, Yongsheng M, Salmi DB, McIndool E Wallace RJ. Impact of antibiotics on expression of virulence-associated exotoxin genes in methicillin-sensitive and methicillin-resistant *Staphylococcus aureus. J Infect Dis* 2007; 195(2): 202–211.

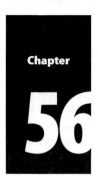

Chapter

56

The shocked patient

Christopher Westall and Kobus Preller

Introduction

Shock describes any pathological state in which *global tissue perfusion is insufficient to support ongoing aerobic cellular respiration*. Shock principally arises from regional mismatch between oxygen demand and delivery resulting in tissue hypoxia, leading to organ dysfunction and death. Shock can occur in the presence of adequate arterial oxygen saturations and adequate arterial blood pressure.

Essential physiology

Shock is managed by maintaining tissue oxygen delivery. This is achieved by optimizing blood oxygen concentration and tissue perfusion.

Oxygen delivery (Box 56.1)

> **Box 56.1 Determinants of rate of oxygen delivery**
>
> $$DO_2 = ([Hb] \times 1.34 \times \%SpO_2) \times CO.$$
>
> DO_2 = oxygen delivery in mL of O_2 per minute.
> [Hb] = blood haemoglobin concentration expressed in g/100 mL.
> 1.34 = Hüfner's constant; theoretical maximal O_2-carrying capacity of the haemoglobin molecule.
> $\%SpO_2$ = arterial oxygen saturation.
> CO = cardiac output expressed in L/min.
> The small role played by oxygen dissolved in plasma is left out for simplification.

Oxygen delivery can be improved by increasing:

- oxygen saturation *but* supra-oxygenation results in only marginal improvement due to the haemoglobin–oxygen dissociation relationship
- haemoglobin concentration *but* increasing concentration increases blood viscosity, eventually impairing blood flow through smaller vessels
- cardiac output (Box 56.2).

Cardiac output

> **Box 56.2 Determinants of cardiac output**
>
> Cardiac output (L/min) = stroke volume
> × heart rate /1000.
>
> Stroke volume = volume of blood ejected by the heart during systole in mL.
> Cardiac output in healthy adults is 4–8 L/min.

Stroke volume is the principal determinant and is dependent upon:

- preload
- myocardial contractility
- afterload

all of which can be therapeutically manipulated.

Preload is the degree of stretch (fibre length) of cardiac muscle immediately prior to the onset of systole.

The Frank–Starling law of the heart states that 'an increase in preload will result in an increase in stroke volume provided afterload and myocardial contractility remain constant'.

This remains true until a point of decompensation whereby increasing preload further results in reduction in stroke volume. Preload cannot be directly measured; clinicians must use surrogate markers such as:

- central venous pressure
- pulmonary artery occlusion pressure
- left ventricular end-diastolic volume.

Acute Medicine, ed. Stephen Haydock, Duncan Whitehead and Zoë Fritz. Published by Cambridge University Press. © Cambridge University Press 2015.

Myocardial contractility (inotropy) describes the 'intrinsic force of myocardial fibres contraction, independent of the influence of preload and afterload', controlled by the sympathetic nervous system. Myocardial contractility is adversely affected by:

- hypoxaemia
- acidaemia
- hypothermia
- hypocalcaemia.

Afterload is defined as the 'tension developed within the left ventricular wall during systole'. This is the resistance that the left ventricle must overcome to eject blood, the systemic vascular resistance. If preload and contractility remain constant, increasing afterload results in reduced stroke volume and increased myocardial oxygen demand, and vice versa.

Pressure and perfusion

Box 56.3 Determinants of mean arterial pressure

Mean arterial pressure $\backsimeq$ cardiac output × SVR.

SVR = systemic vascular resistance in dynes/s/cm^5.

Blood flow = potential difference in blood pressure/vascular resistance.

Perfusion is the flow of blood to tissues determined by blood pressure and vascular resistance. The most important determinant of vascular resistance is the size of the vessel lumen; a decrease in vessel radius results in an increase in resistance to the fourth power.

While flow within the great vessels is pulsatile and systolic, blood flow in arteriolar beds occurs in systole and diastole due to the elastic recoil of the arteriolar wall. Mean arterial pressure (Box 56.3) is a better determinant of flow in these vessels and better represents organ perfusion pressure.

Control of cardiac contractility and systemic vascular resistance

The cardiovascular system is under the control of the sympathetic nervous system, mediated by catecholamines through adrenergic receptors. There are many types of receptor, of which three are key:

- α1: smooth muscle contraction (skin, splanchnic and renal circulation).

- β1: increased chronotropy and inotropy (cardiac tissue).
- β2: smooth muscle relaxation (coronary circulation and airways).

The effect of sympathetic stimulation on an organ system therefore depends upon the type and number of adrenergic receptors found within that tissue.

Adrenaline stimulates both α1 and β2 receptors, causing:

- vasoconstriction within non-essential tissues such as the skin, splanchnic circulation and kidneys where there is a preponderance of α1 receptors
- vasodilation in the coronary circulation and skeletal muscle where there is a preponderance of β2 receptors.

Classification of shock

There is frequently significant overlap between these presentations.

Hypovolaemic

Occurs because of inadequate circulating blood volume. Hypotension is a late sign in previously well individuals.

Pathophysiology

- Reduced circulating volume reduces preload.
- Initially catecholamine release preserves cardiac output by increasing myocardial contractility and heart rate and by causing vasoconstriction.
- Vasoconstriction diverts blood away from non-essential systems to maintain perfusion to the essential systems of the heart, lungs and brain.
- Vasoconstriction of vascular beds in the peripheral and splanchnic circulation results in the return of a significant volume of whole blood to the central circulation.
- Eventually reduced perfusion of non-essential systems results in failure of these organs.
- The heart tolerates prolonged hypovolaemia poorly as vasoconstriction causes increased afterload resulting in persistent tachycardia causing:
    - increased myocardial oxygen demand
    - reduced myocardial perfusion as shortened diastolic times reduce coronary arterial flow.
- Myocardial efficiency is further reduced as organ dysfunction and acidaemia evolve.

- These factors create a pro-arrhythmic state. The development of arrhythmia further compromises the system.

Causes

1. Haemorrhage
   - Overt: e.g. trauma, intraoperative
   - Concealed: e.g. ruptured AAA, splenic rupture, retroperitoneal haemorrhage
2. Plasma loss
   - Overt: e.g. burns, diarrhoea, vomiting, excessive fluid removal during dialysis, excessive environmental loss, iatrogenic including diuretic use
   - Concealed: e.g. 'third space losses' in post-surgical states, pancreatitis

Cardiogenic

Cardiogenic shock is a low cardiac output state due to primary cardiac failure characterized by inadequate stroke volume despite adequate cardiac filling pressures.

Pathophysiology

- Has a poor outcome as there is no effective compensatory strategy.
- The body responds to the low cardiac output as in hypovolaemia.

  But

- Unlike hypovolaemic shock, the myocardium is fundamentally unable to respond to sympathetic stimulation. Decompensation occurs at a much earlier stage.
- Tissue perfusion is extremely poor due to poor cardiac output combined with intense vasoconstriction.

Causes

1. Acute myocardial infarction (AMI)
   - Death of cardiac muscle
   - Structural complication of AMI; e.g. acute valvular regurgitation, ventricular septal rupture, left ventricular free wall rupture
2. Reduced contractility
   - Myocarditis of any cause
   - Cardio-depressant drugs

- Cardiac stunning post-arrest or contusion from blunt trauma
- Stress-induced and acute non-ischaemic cardiomyopathy

3. Mechanical failure
   - Dehiscence of a prosthetic valve
   - Dysrhythmia

Distributive

Distributive shock occurs because of uncontrolled vasodilatation leading to relative hypovolaemia and mismatch between regional blood flow and local metabolic need.

Causes

1. Sepsis (see Chapter 55)
2. Anaphylaxis (see Chapter 9)
3. Acute adrenal insufficiency
4. Neurogenic shock

Obstructive

Obstructive shock occurs because of reduced cardiac output as a consequence of mechanical obstruction to blood flow.

Causes

1. Pulmonary
   - Massive pulmonary embolism
   - Tension pneumothorax
2. Cardiac
   - Tamponade (e.g. traumatic haemopericardium, large volume pericardial effusion from uraemia, streptococcal infection)
   - Acute valvular obstruction (e.g. large vegetation in endocarditis, thrombosis of mechanical valve, atrial myxoma)
   - Type A thoracic dissection affecting the aortic root

Special causes of shock

Acute adrenal insufficiency

- Profound hypotension refractory to initial fluid therapy and/or poorly responsive to vasopressors must always raise the suspicion of adrenal insufficiency.

- It is rare for primary autoimmune hypoadrenalism (Addison's disease) to first present as shock, although an additional acute stressful illness may precipitate overt hypoadrenalism.

Neurogenic shock

- Caused by loss of sympathetic vascular tone due to physical disruption of autonomic outflow by a cervical or high thoracic spinal injury.
- Hypotension with paradoxical bradycardia due to unopposed parasympathetic activity on the heart, exacerbated by any vagal stimulation including airway suctioning.
- Support in the early phase includes early vasopressor use and mitigation of vagal stimulation using anticholinergic drugs.

Scenario 56.1

A 73-year-old man is brought into a resuscitation bay in the ED. He has been found collapsed at home by a neighbour. On arrival he has a GCS of 11/15 and is hypotensive with a blood pressure of 80/40 and tachycardic with a heart rate of 130 beats per minute despite fluid administration en route to hospital. His temperature is 34.5°C and SpO₂ 92% on high flow O₂. His neighbour last saw him 2 days previously and called round as she was becoming concerned as to his whereabouts. She saw a bottle of vodka next to the sofa, which was unusual as he seldom drank alcohol.

Immediate management of the shocked patient

A shock state will only resolve if the underlying cause is treated. Initial management aims to prevent organ dysfunction by:

- optimizing oxygen delivery
- maintaining tissue perfusion.

Assessment and resuscitation should occur in parallel and focus on airway, breathing and circulation. *Resuscitation is goal-directed*; effectiveness is assessed against specific, measurable physiological goals.

Goal-directed therapy: initial resuscitation goals

1. Target SpO_2 ≥94% unless otherwise indicated
2. Mean arterial pressure ≥65mmHg
3. Urine output ≥0.5mL/kg per hour
4. Serum glucose 4–10 mmol/L

5. Serum haemoglobin concentration 70–90 g/L unless otherwise indicated
6. Resuscitative efforts should aim to normalize serum lactate levels to <2 mmol/L

Airway and breathing

- Airway patency must be maintained if unconscious. This may require endotracheal intubation.
- Rapidly institute oxygen saturation monitoring. The patient may be peripherally shut down and oxygen saturation unreliable. If there are concerns regarding the reliability of monitoring, apply high-flow supplemental oxygen and obtain an arterial blood gas urgently.
- Maintain saturations >94% with supplemental oxygen unless there is underlying respiratory disease, which mandates a lower target. If there are unconfirmed suspicions of underlying respiratory disease, aim for saturations >94% until the situation can be clarified.
- Shocked patients may present with coexistent lung injury by many mechanisms including respiratory tract infection or pulmonary contusion. Non-invasive or invasive mechanical ventilation is required where oxygen saturations cannot be maintained despite increasing inspired oxygen concentrations.
- Shocked patients may develop a high work of breathing by trying to maintain oxygenation or compensate metabolic acidaemia. If the patient appears to be tiring or has a rising $PaCO_2$ or lactate level, ventilatory support may be required to prevent decompensation and alleviate significant metabolic burden.

Circulation

- Rapidly institute basic haemodynamic monitoring: BP monitoring (every 5–15 minutes initially) and cardiac monitoring as a minimum. Obtain a 12-lead ECG early.
- Insert two large bore (18G or bigger) cannulae and take blood samples. Insert largest cannula into a proximal peripheral vein (antecubital fossa) and reserve as a 'volume line' for giving fluids. Drugs can be given through the second cannula, which may be smaller.
- Maintain mean arterial pressure ≥65 mmHg.
- Carefully assess and correct volume status.

- Hypotensive patients should receive a crystalloid fluid challenge, unless there is overt haemorrhage where fluid losses should be replaced 'like for like' with blood.
- Vasopressor or inotropic support may be required early in order to stabilize the patient, but every attempt should be made to correct the fluid status beforehand.

Exposure

- A quick global examination may reveal an obvious cause. Special attention should be paid to the abdomen (? intra-abdominal pathology).
- Arrange for a urinary catheter. Note the residual volume and monitor urine output hourly.

Glucose

- Measure capillary glucose as soon as possible.
- Maintain between 4 and 10 mmol/L with a variable rate insulin infusion if necessary [1].
- Hypoglycaemia <4 mmol/L should be treated promptly with intravenous glucose.

Serum lactate concentration

- Rapidly obtain serum lactate from standard blood-gas analysis. Elevated serum lactate levels may indicate a switch to anaerobic respiration due to inadequate oxygen delivery. In the appropriate context this signifies a shock state.
- Elevated lactate levels are associated with poorer outcomes in septic shock. Generally increasing lactate levels are associated with worsening outcome. Using lactate levels as part of goal-directed therapy is associated with improved outcomes.

Clinical assessment of haemodynamic status

- The JVP is commonly used as a non-invasive surrogate for central venous pressure, although assessment can be difficult.
- The volume of a central pulse correlates well with cardiac output.
- Comparing peripheral with central skin colour, temperature and capillary refill time provides a semi-quantitative assessment of vascular tone.

- Blood pressure characteristics can provide markers of vascular tone:
  - high systolic pressure generally indicates good cardiac output but CO may be reduced if high systolic pressure due to high systemic vascular resistance
  - low systolic pressure generally indicates good cardiac output but CO may be increased if low systolic BP due to low systemic vascular resistance
  - narrow pulse pressure with a high diastolic – suggests intense vasoconstriction
  - wide pulse pressure with a low diastolic – suggests widespread vasodilatation.

Initial investigations

Minimum necessary investigations

1. Arterial blood gas
2. Venous blood glucose
3. Serum lactate
4. Haematology: full blood count, clotting profile and group and save; fibrinogen should be added if haemorrhage or concerns regarding coagulopathy.
5. Biochemistry: renal function, liver function tests, electrolytes and CRP
6. ECG
7. Chest radiograph

Recognition of shock is not in itself a diagnosis. Investigations are used to clarify the underlying pathology or else to define the level of organ dysfunction. The classification of shock type will narrow the differential diagnosis, which will determine the plan of investigation.

Ultrasonography

The extended FAST scan (focused assessment with sonography for trauma) includes imaging of the pleural spaces, pericardium, abdomen and pelvis (for free fluid) with or without basic echocardiography and assessment of the abdominal aorta. It is a quick yet sensitive screening tool for major pathology and can be performed in parallel with resuscitation.

If the underlying pathology is unclear, ask an emergency department physician or radiologist to perform a FAST scan as soon as possible.

CT imaging

Has a limited role as it is time-consuming, resource heavy and dangerous to transfer an unstable patient to a CT scanner that is often in a remote location away from resuscitation facilities. There are no absolute indications for CT. In the initial assessment it is only useful when:

- the patient is stabilized
- suspected intra-abdominal pathology which cannot be proven by other imaging techniques and the CT images will change the surgical approach.

If a patient cannot be stabilized for CT and there is a high index of suspicion of pathology requiring surgical intervention, the patient should be transferred for surgery immediately unless this is deemed an inappropriate escalation of care. However, major trauma centres now have procedures in place to allow early rapid access to whole body CT imaging in severely injured patients.

When to involve surgical colleagues

Generally a shocked patient with a 'surgical' pathology can only be stabilized for a period of time inversely proportional to the severity of the insult (consider a ruptured abdominal aortic aneurysm!). Surgical colleagues should be involved immediately when there is:

- major haemorrhage (for source control – including cases of massive upper gastrointestinal bleeding that may not be managed by endoscopic techniques)
- ischaemic tissue (e.g. limb or gut ischaemia)
- intra-abdominal sepsis amenable to surgical source control (e.g. perforated viscus, appendicitis)
- extra-abdominal sepsis requiring surgical source control (e.g. necrotizing fasciitis, debridement of ulcers, septic arthritis)
- acute pancreatitis
- bowel obstruction.

Fluid therapy

Fluid therapy increases cardiac output by delivering more volume to the left ventricle and thereby increasing preload. The goal is to optimize preload without causing decompensation. Simply infusing fluid until the JVP is elevated and the patient is developing signs of pulmonary oedema *is not acceptable*; at this point decompensation has already occurred.

Usually losses should be replaced 'like for like', i.e. if there is major haemorrhage then blood products should be given, otherwise crystalloid is now considered first line.

Crystalloid versus colloid

The perceived benefit of colloid solutions is that they are retained in the intravascular compartment for longer so less volume is needed to achieve the same effect when compared to crystalloid. High molecular weight colloids cannot cross the capillary membrane easily, prolonging the duration of their intravascular colloid-oncotic pressure influence. However, there are persistent concerns regarding the safety profile of colloid solutions:

- increased risk of anaphylactic reactions (gelatins and dextrans)
- impaired haemostasis (gelatins and dextrans)
- emerging evidence that hydroxyethyl starch is associated with an increased risk of acute kidney injury and need for renal replacement therapy.

Meta-analyses comparing colloids with crystalloids for the resuscitation of critically ill patients have found no significant differences in outcomes between the two [2]. Since crystalloids are universally available, standardized, cheap and comparatively safe, crystalloid solutions are generally considered first line.

Human albumin solution

There is no evidence for improved outcome in a general population of patients resuscitated with 4% human albumin solution versus 0.9% sodium chloride [3]. Human albumin solution (HAS) should be considered in shock states associated with:

- large volume paracentesis
- spontaneous bacterial peritonitis
- hepatorenal syndrome
- marked hypoalbuminaemia in cirrhotic patients.

Fluid challenges

A fluid challenge is a therapeutic intervention and dynamic assessment of the volume status of a patient. Its purpose is to assess whether preload is low, intermediate or high and as such determine whether further fluid infusion will improve cardiac output. The principal danger with a fluid challenge is that the response is incorrectly interpreted; this can lead to excessive fluid administration and delay appropriate vasopressor/inotropic therapy. There is no consensus regarding the type or volume of fluid or the infusion rate that should be used. The most widely accepted protocol is conducted thus:

1. Assess the JVP or measure the CVP. Record the heart rate and blood pressure.
2. Infuse 250 mL of crystalloid over a maximum of 10 minutes.
3. Assess the JVP or measure the CVP. Record the heart rate and blood pressure immediately post-challenge and then at intervals of 10 minutes.
4. Urine output does not respond quickly enough and has too many confounding factors to make it a useful marker of response to a fluid challenge, although it may provide useful information regarding fluid balance over the medium term.
5. If cardiac output monitoring is available, direct measurement of cardiac output and other variables can improve interpretation of response.

Interpreting the response to fluid challenges

Interpreting the response to a fluid challenge is a difficult skill requiring attention to the overall clinical picture. There are broadly three responses to a fluid challenge:

- Non-responder (underfilled): there is no rise in JVP/CVP or improvement in blood pressure or reduction in heart rate in response to the challenge. Giving further fluid should convert the patient into a responder.
- Transient responder (requires more filling): there is a rise in the JVP/CVP, improvement in blood pressure and reduction in heart rate immediately after the fluid challenge, but this is not sustained. The duration of response will indicate how far the patient is from 'optimal' filling; briefer responses suggest more marked hypovolaemia. Further challenges are likely to improve cardiac output.
- Persistent responder (filled): there is a persistent rise in JVP/CVP. There may or may not be an improvement in blood pressure or a reduction in heart rate. Further fluid is unlikely to improve cardiac output. If the patient is hypotensive, vasopressor/inotropic therapy is required.

> **Scenario 56.1 continued**
>
> *Initial investigations do not give an obvious cause for his persistent hypotension with moderate elevations of urea, creatinine, WCC and glucose. The ECG is unremarkable. A CXR shows patchy bilateral shadowing. Review of previous medical records indicates that he has been previously well. Discussion with his GP reveals that he had attended rarely but that his wife died recently and that this has hit him very hard. He is known to have hypertension and his current medication is amlodipine 5 mg od, irbesartan 150 mg od and recently temazepam 10 mg nocte. Despite aggressive fluid resuscitation the patient remains drowsy, profoundly hypotensive and anuric. In view of the medication and history of recent bereavement, IV calcium gluconate and flumazenil are administered without benefit. It is felt appropriate to transfer to the critical care unit. It is suspected that his clinical state may be due to an overdose of hypotensive medication that is proving refractory to treatment. The changes on the CXR may be due to cardiogenic or non-cardiogenic pulmonary oedema, but he could also have aspirated his own vomit (overdose and alcohol) and developed septic shock secondary to aspiration pneumonia. It is planned to monitor his airway, and support his breathing while instituting invasive monitoring to guide fluid resuscitation, vasopressor and inotropic support. He will also receive high dose insulin and glucose and the infusion of a lipid solution may be considered. Broad spectrum antibiotics are administered and a septic screen sent to the laboratory.*

Levels of care and referral to critical care

Critical care is not in itself a treatment, it is an integrated system of organ support that stabilizes a patient and attempts to ameliorate further injury while the primary treatment is allowed to take effect. It is a precious resource with limited capacity, and demand constantly outweighs availability. Appropriate allocation of resources ensures the greatest benefit to the greatest number of patients. When referring to critical care ask: *'what exactly do I want critical care to do that cannot be provided elsewhere?'*

The SBAR (Situation, Background, Assessment and Recommendation) communication tool provides a useful framework for referrals; be sure to state what support is required in the 'Situation' report, e.g.

> I am the medical SHO on-call looking after Mr Smith who has septic shock and requires vasopressor support…

- Standard observations and CVP monitoring can be managed in a level 1 environment (ward care with additional support).

- Single organ support (excluding mechanical ventilation) can generally be managed in a level 2 environment (high dependency unit).
- Multi-organ support or mechanical ventilation alone can only be managed in a level 3 environment (intensive care unit).

Advanced haemodynamic monitoring

Monitoring is a continuous process of observation of organ-systems performance with inbuilt triggers for clinical review. Monitoring also allows assessment of response to interventions. Trends are generally more important than single values. Monitoring data should only be interpreted in clinical context; *one of the risks of modern critical care is unnecessary intervention due to misinterpretation of haemodynamic monitoring data.*

Goal-directed therapy that requires advanced support

1. Maintain CVP 8–12 mmHg (contentious).
2. Commence vasopressor/inotropic therapy where MAP remains <65 mmHg despite fluid resuscitation.
3. Maintain $ScvO_2$ >70%.
4. Commence inotropic therapy in patients where MAP is ≥65 mmHg and there is demonstrable evidence of low cardiac output state or signs of persistent tissue hypoperfusion.

Central venous pressure

Central venous access can provide:

- secure route of venous access, for infusion of concentrated solutions and vasoactive drugs
- measurement of $ScvO_2$
- CVP monitoring.

CVP is the intravascular pressure recorded at the junction of the right atrium and superior vena cava. CVP is used as a surrogate measure for left ventricular preload, although it is a poor surrogate as CVP measures intravascular pressure, and pressure and preload do not share a linear correlation.

The value of CVP monitoring is limited by a multitude of factors:

- technical errors (inaccurate calibration and incorrect patient positioning)
- central venous catheter errors (misplacement and occlusion)
- patient factors (valvular heart disease, right ventricular impairment, pulmonary hypertension and pathological changes in ventricular compliance)
- changes with variation in intrathoracic pressure (as seen in positive pressure ventilation).

CVP is increasingly falling out of fashion in critical care medicine. There is no convincing evidence that CVP is a good predictor of preload or fluid responsiveness, either as an absolute value or expressed as change in response to fluid challenge.

Central venous oxygen saturations

Elevated serum lactate signifies global tissue hypoxia, which occurs only once shock is *established.* Central venous oxygen saturations may detect inadequate oxygen delivery before it is clinically apparent and is a more sensitive biomarker than lactate for early shock and a better marker by which to assess resuscitation.

Central venous oxygen saturation ($ScvO_2$) is measured from the superior vena cava using a central venous catheter.

- Normal value is 70–75%.
- Mixed venous oxygen saturation (SvO_2) is measured in the pulmonary artery using a pulmonary artery catheter.
- SvO_2 and $ScvO_2$ give an indication of the balance between oxygen delivery (DO_2) and oxygen consumption (VO_2).
- Under normal conditions arterial oxygen saturations are >94%, the tissues extract around 25% of this and hence the saturation of all venous blood, mixed just before return to the right atrium, is 70–75%.
- If DO_2 is impaired but VO_2 remains constant, the venous oxygen saturation will fall as the oxygen extraction rate of the tissues increases.

Invasive arterial blood pressure monitoring

Invasive arterial blood pressure monitoring (IABP) is no more valid than non-invasive blood pressure monitoring (NIBP), although it does have advantages:

- IABP provides continuous monitoring, essential if using potent vasoactive drugs.
- IABP is more reliable in profound hypotension where automated NIBP monitors are often unable to detect the arterial pulse pressure wave.

- IABP uses an arterial catheter that can be used for arterial gas sampling, phlebotomy and cardiac output monitoring.

Cardiac output monitoring

Cardiac output monitoring is required to guide treatment when the classification of shock is not possible or the patient does not respond to therapy as expected. Several modalities can be used, some more commonly and reliably than others.

Echocardiography is gaining popularity as a means of monitoring, although it is resource-heavy in terms of staff training, equipment and time. Echocardiography can give detailed studies of ventricular end-diastolic volume, ventricular systolic function and volume status in addition to information about valvular pathology and structural defects.

Pulse contour systems analyse the arterial pressure waveform from an arterial line. These systems are relatively non-invasive, provide continuous monitoring of cardiac output and stroke volume and are able to provide analyses for newer markers of fluid responsiveness such as stroke volume variation. However, the data obtained is largely derived from complex algorithms that may substantially magnify error. Their use is limited to mechanically ventilated patients as the algorithms are unable to adjust for the variable relationship between intrathoracic and cardiac transmural pressures seen in spontaneously breathing patients.

Two other methods, the *oesophageal Doppler* and the *pulmonary artery catheter* [4], are available but less commonly used due to the advent of less invasive devices, and full description of their use are beyond the scope of this book.

Vasopressor and inotropic agents

Vasoactive agents are used to optimize oxygen delivery by manipulating cardiac output and systemic vascular resistance (Box 56.4). They should only be infused through a central venous line with adequate monitoring in a high-level care environment.

Vasopressors

Vasopressors increase vascular tone causing vasoconstriction, predominantly of arteriolar beds. There are many classes of vasopressor:

- most commonly α1-adrenergic receptor agonists such as:
  - noradrenaline
  - metaraminol
- arginine vasopressin analogues at the V1 receptor
- agents with both vasopressor activity and inotropic activity, including
  - adrenaline
  - dopamine.

Noradrenaline and dopamine appear equally effective, although dopamine is associated with a greater risk of arrhythmia and has fallen out of fashion [5]. Vasopressin is not recommended as a first-line therapy compared with noradrenaline.

Box 56.4 Overview of haemodynamic support

Hypovolaemic and distributive shock

- Vasopressors are first-line therapy. Noradrenaline is the drug of choice. Titrate to achieve MAP ≥65 mmHg.
- If a patient fails to respond as expected, cardiac output monitoring should be instituted.
- If cardiac output is adequate but SVR remains low, continue to titrate noradrenaline or add steroids and/or vasopressin if septic shock.
- If cardiac output is inadequate, commence inotropes. Dobutamine is first line. If dobutamine causes significant tachycardia or severe hypertension, switch to adrenaline, either in combination with noradrenaline or alone.

Anaphylaxis (see Chapter 9)

- Adrenaline is the drug of choice. It reverses vasodilation (α1 activity) and suppresses release of histamine from degranulated mast cells (β2 activity). It is usually required as a bolus dose only.

Cardiogenic shock

- Inotropic therapy with dobutamine is first line.
- Cardiac output monitoring is required if the patient does not respond as expected.
- A complex regimen of inotropes and vasodilatory drugs may be required.
- Seek advice from specialist centres early.

Noradrenaline

Noradrenaline accounts for approximately 80% of all vasopressor and inotropic drug therapy in the UK and is the drug of choice in vasodilatory states.

- Catecholamine α1-adrenergic receptor agonist with negligible β1 effect and no β2 effect.
- Intense vasoconstrictor predominantly in the skin, splanchnic and renal circulation.
- Increases SVR and increases MAP with little effect on cardiac output.

  BUT

- Reduced splanchnic flow can result in gut ischaemia and reduced skin perfusion can lead to skin necrosis and digital ischaemia, especially if underlying hypovolaemia is not adequately corrected.
- Renal blood flow is reduced but GFR is largely preserved, although the kidneys are vulnerable to superadded hypovolaemia.
- Can decrease insulin secretion resulting in mild hyperglycaemia.

Arginine vasopressin (AVP)

- In septic shock AVP levels are lower than would be expected in stressed states, termed 'relative vasopressin insufficiency'.
- Stimulation of vasopressin receptors, particularly AVPR1a (V1), by exogenous AVP stimulates profound vasoconstriction, but compared with noradrenaline an increase in renal blood flow is observed.
- Synthetic analogues appear to have greater selectivity for the V1 receptor and longer biological half-life.
- Can be given as bolus doses rather than continuous infusions and do not require central venous access.
- Analogues increasingly used with significant liver disease; variceal bleeding, fulminant hepatic failure, spontaneous bacterial peritonitis and hypotension with hepatorenal syndrome.
- May have a role in septic shock as an adjunctive therapy when noradrenaline dose is high (>15 μg/min). Some trial evidence favours better outcome with early use.

Metaraminol

- Metaraminol is a synthetic α1-receptor agonist. It has an action and side effect profile similar to that of noradrenaline.
- It can be given as a bolus into a peripheral vein in 0.5 mg aliquots or by an infusion titrated to response.

Steroids and vasopressors in septic shock

In septic shock cortisol levels are lower than would be expected in similar stressed states, termed 'relative adrenal insufficiency'. There is trial evidence that 50 mg hydrocortisone IV qds results in more rapid reversal of shock, possibly due to endothelial sensitization to vasopressors, though not improved mortality outcomes [6].

Inotropes

Inotropes increase myocardial contractility and chronotropy through β1-adrenoceptor agonism. They can be classified by their secondary actions into:

- Inopressors:
  - adrenaline.
- Inodilators:
  - dobutamine.
  - dopexamine.
- Dopamine shows variable characteristics dependent upon dose.

There are other inotropic agents outside the scope of this book. All β1 agonists increase myocardial oxygen demand and can precipitate myocardial ischaemia and arrhythmia.

Adrenaline is a catecholamine:

- with α1, α2, β1 and β2 activity
- that causes dose-dependent vasoconstriction through α1 stimulation and increased myocardial contractility through β1 stimulation
- that decreases splanchnic and renal blood flow, although GFR is preserved initially.

The metabolic effects of adrenaline are marked.

- Hyperglycaemia is common as a consequence of reduced insulin secretion, increased glucagon release and increased glycogenolysis.
- Adrenaline use results in a rise in serum lactate.

Adrenaline has a wide range of indications:

- Especially depressed myocardial function with severe vasodilation (such as septic shock) where it is as good as noradrenaline and dobutamine in combination [7].
- Adrenaline has a limited role in cardiogenic shock, especially due to acute myocardial ischaemia, as it markedly increases myocardial oxygen demand and may precipitate arrhythmia.

Dobutamine is the drug of choice in cardiogenic shock and as an adjunct to noradrenaline in vasodilatory states where there is depressed myocardial function.

- Synthetic catecholamine-derivative with $\alpha 1$, $\beta 1$ and $\beta 2$ activity.
- Acts mainly via $\beta 1$ agonism to enhance myocardial contractility and causes vasodilation, as affinity for $\beta 2$ receptors is slightly greater than for $\alpha 1$ receptors.
- The combination of increased stroke volume and increased heart rate against decreased SVR results in improved cardiac output, but its use is often limited by the development of significant tachycardia and tachyarrhythmia.
- The concurrent use of a vasopressor may be required to offset vasodilatation and restore mean arterial pressure.
- Dobutamine is contraindicated when there is cardiac outflow obstruction such as severe aortic stenosis, severe mitral stenosis, HOCM or cardiac tamponade.

Dopamine is a naturally occurring catecholamine and precursor to adrenaline and noradrenaline.

- Has dose-dependent activity at D1, D2, $\alpha 1$, $\alpha 2$, $\beta 1$ and $\beta 2$ receptors.
- At doses of 0–5 µg/kg per minute dopaminergic activity predominates resulting in improved renal and splanchnic blood flow.
- At doses of 5–10 µg/kg per minute there is increasing $\beta 1$ activity giving rise to inodilator-type activity.
- At doses above 10 µg/kg per minute there is progressive $\alpha 1$ activity resulting in potent vasoconstriction.

Dopamine use is increasingly less common and is only employed under expert guidance.

Cardiogenic shock: ventricular assistance

When cardiogenic shock has developed secondary to myocardial infarction, emergency revascularization improves outcome [8]. There is no guidance on how to best manage patients who develop cardiogenic shock due to non-ischaemic causes or who are unable to undergo emergency revascularization. Current standard therapy is with careful fluid management and a balanced regime of vasopressors, inotropes and vasodilatory agents, guided by cardiac output monitoring.

Intra-aortic balloon counterpulsation (IABCP) has been used to mechanically support the failing heart in a number of conditions, predominantly following myocardial infarction or structural complication thereof. IABCP does not function as a blood-pump. A polyethylene balloon is placed in the descending aorta via femoral puncture, which rapidly inflates and deflates, triggered by ECG synchronization. This reduces myocardial oxygen demand by reducing afterload; the balloon deflates at the onset of systole creating a vacuum effect in the descending aorta that assists ejection of blood from the left ventricle. IABCP also improves coronary blood flow. The balloon inflates at the onset of diastole; this increases pressure at the aortic root and actively promotes filling of the coronary arteries.

Recent trial data has led to a review of IABCP use; no benefit was found from using IABCP compared to standard medical therapy [9]. The use of IABCP is now largely restricted to expert use in specialist centres. Increasingly new technologies are being evaluated. These include the use of mechanical left ventricular assist devices and veno-arterial extracorporeal membrane oxygenation. The role of these technologies has not yet been fully established and their use is limited to specialist centres.

References

1. Finfer S, Chittock DR, Su SY, Blair D, Foster D, Dhingra V, Bellomo R, Cook D, Dodek P, Henderson WR, Hébert PC, et al. The NICE-SUGAR Study Investigators. Intensive versus conventional glucose control in critically ill patients. *N Engl J Med* 2009; 360: 1283–1297.

2. Perel P, Roberts I, Ker K. Colloids versus crystalloids for fluid resuscitation in critically ill patients. *Cochrane Database of Systematic Reviews* 2013, Issue 2. Art. No.: CD000567.

3. Roberts I, Blackhall K, Alderson P, Bunn F, Schierhout G. Human albumin solution for resuscitation and volume expansion in critically ill patients. *Cochrane Database of Systematic Reviews* 2011, Issue 11. Art. No.: CD001208.

4. Rajaram SS, Desai NK, Kalra A, Gajera M, Cavanaugh SK, Brampton W, Young D, Harvey S, Rowan K. Pulmonary artery catheters for adult patients in intensive care. *Cochrane Database of Systematic Reviews* 2013, Issue 2. Art. No.: CD003408.

5. Havel C, Arrich J, Losert H, Gamper G, Müllner M, Herkner H. Vasopressors for hypotensive shock. *Cochrane Database of Systematic Reviews* 2011, Issue 5. Art. No.: CD003709.

6. Sprung CL, Annane D, Keh D, Moreno R, Singer M, Freivogel K, Weiss YG, Benbenishty J, Kalenka A, Forst H, Laterre PF, et al. The CORTICUS Study Group. Hydrocortisone Therapy for Patients with Septic Shock. *N Engl J Med* 2008; 358: 111–124.

7. Annane D, Vignon P, Renault A, Bollaert PE, Charpentier C, Martin C, Troché G, Ricard JD, Nitenberg G, Papazian L, Azoulay E, et al. The CATS Study Group. Norepinephrine plus dobutamine versus epinephrine alone for management of septic shock: a randomised trial. *Lancet* 2007; 370: 676–684.

8. Hochman JS, Sleeper LA, Webb JG, Sanborn TA, White HD, Talley JD, Buller CE, Jacobs AK, Slater JN, Col J, McKinlay SM, et al. The SHOCK Investigators. Early revascularization in acute myocardial infarction complicated by cardiogenic shock. Should we emergently revascularize occluded coronaries for cardiogenic shock. *N Engl J Med* 1999; 341: 625–634.

9. Thiele H, Zeymer U, Neumann FJ, Ferenc M, Olbrich HG, Hausleiter J, Richardt G, Hennersdorf M, Empen K, Fuernau G, Desch S, et al. The IABP-SHOCK II Trial Investigators. Intraaortic balloon support for myocardial infarction with cardiogenic shock. *N Engl J Med* 2012; 367: 1287–1296.

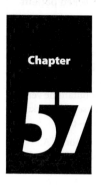

Skin and mouth ulcers

Pawel Bogucki and Tony Coll

Introduction

- Skin ulcers result from destruction of the epidermis and penetration through the basement membrane with loss of at least the upper part of the dermis (Figure 57.1).
- Mucosal ulcers penetrate to the epithelial connective tissue border.

The causes are multiple and identification can prove challenging. History coupled with the ulcer features help to determine the aetiology:

- location
- associated symptoms (pain, pruritus)
- appearance of the wound (border, base, discharge)
- appearance of surrounding and often distant skin and mucosal surfaces
- history of trauma
- past medical history.

Aetiological classification of skin ulcers

Congenital

- Epidermolysis bullosa
- Cutis aplasia

Acquired

- *Traumatic*
  - local trauma and burns
  - pressure ulcers (bed sores)
  - dermatitis artifacta (usually well demarcated and bizarre shape)
- *Infectious*
  - ecthyma
  - chancre
  - Buruli ulcer
  - cutaneous anthrax
  - cutaneous leishmaniasis
- *Neoplastic*
  - melanoma
  - basal cell carcinoma
  - squamous cell carcinoma
- *Vascular*
  - venous
  - arterial
  - vasculitis
- *Associated with systemic disease*
  - neuropathic ulcers (diabetes, alcoholism, spinal cord lesions)
  - calciphylaxis
  - rheumatoid arthritis
  - pyoderma gangrenosum
- *Drug-induced*
  - nicorandil
  - hydroxycarbamide
  - methotrexate
  - interferon

Diabetic foot ulcers

Scenario 57.1

A 65-year-old insulin-requiring type 2 diabetic patient is referred due to an ulcer on the plantar surface of his right foot. He is able to walk on it. On examination the ulcer is deep but painless with surrounding erythema. It has failed to improve with oral antibiotics. The GP thinks that intravenous antibiotics might be appropriate.

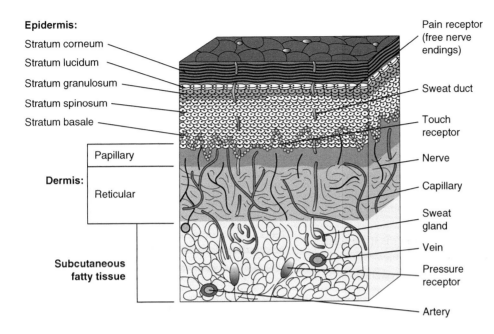

Epidermis:

Stratum corneum

Stratum lucidum

Stratum granulosum

Stratum spinosum

Stratum basale

Dermis:

Papillary

Reticular

Subcutaneous fatty tissue

Pain receptor (free nerve endings)

Sweat duct

Touch receptor

Nerve

Capillary

Sweat gland

Vein

Pressure receptor

Artery

Figure 57.1 Cross-section of human skin.

Over 3 million people in the UK are estimated to have diabetes mellitus. As the prevalence of this multisystem, metabolic disorder increases, so too does the clinical burden of macro- and microvascular complications.

An *acute diabetic foot is a common problem* on the medical take. An evolving foot lesion should be considered an urgent clinical problem which requires thoughtful assessment of all contributing factors.

Patients with diabetic foot disease are typically burdened with a large number of chronic co-morbidities and without care and attention to all systems involved the outcome is often poor. Do not stop thinking once the ulcer has been found but think on as to relevant aetiology – consider always, '*Why that lesion on that foot, and why now?*' Throughout all stages of management *keep as your aim the maintenance of the foot as a weight-bearing unit.*

Pathophysiology

A foot lesion is not an inevitability of diabetes. It typically arises due to several defined pathological processes acting together:

- *Peripheral sensorimotor neuropathy.* Damage to long, unmyelinated fibres results in a loss of protective sensation, meaning even

significant antecedent trauma can go unnoticed. Architectural deformities (e.g. clawed toes and prominent metatarsal heads) driven by the motor component of neuropathy, frequently subject fragile tissue to excessive pressure and stress. Look for callus over prominent areas of tissue – these are a reaction to excessive pressure and friction and require attention.

- *Peripheral vascular disease.* Both large and small vessel disease compromise both the integrity of the foot skin and healing once breached. The typical pain of claudication may be masked by coexisting neuropathy. Medial wall calcification is also common in longstanding diabetes and can make palpation of pulses difficult. A normal foot should have two pulses (dorsal pedis and posterior tibial) – *if you cannot count the pulse, consider that it is absent and that ischaemia is a potential contributor to the problem.*

- *Infection.* Almost all infection arises from direct contiguous spread from organisms on the skin rather than haematogenous spread. Common pathogens in an acute wound include *Staphylococcus aureus* and haemolytic *Streptococcus*, while chronic wounds are often polymicrobial containing both Gram-positive and Gram-negative organisms.

- *The external environment.* All too often lesions are driven by pressure from an external source – ill-fitting shoes, wheelchair footplates and foreign bodies. Look to the environment in which the foot was living when the ulcer started and remove this excess pressure.

Investigation and management

Aim to get the patient under the named care of the multidisciplinary foot team *as soon as possible.* Getting the interventions needed in a timely manner requires coordination and there should be established processes to do this.

However, upon first presentation there is still a need to undertake basic management.

- *Start with the whole patient*: are they systemically unwell?
- Do not be fooled by a lack of pain; neuropathy can mask life-threatening sepsis. *Assess and correct airway, breathing, circulation and hyperglycaemia.* Does this person need intermediate or critical care?
- If the patient is systemically unwell, look specifically for signs of deep-seated infection (e.g. soft tissue collection) and *limb-threatening ischaemia.* If suspected, get *urgent* surgical assistance. *(Now not later!)* A necrotic limb full of pus may be unsalvageable but this should not be allowed to make the patient sicker.
- Once the patient is stable, *consider other aspects of the history.* Worry particularly about the patient who has previously lost tissue to diabetic foot disease – the vascular insufficiency will only have got worse over time. Immunosuppressed patients and patients on renal replacement therapy are at very high risk of a poor outcome.
- *Focus on the index lesion.* Record size, depth, appearance (photos are good – get consent), pulses in foot ('*yes*' or '*no*') and neuropathy ('*Does it hurt?*'). If the foot is insensate, significant injury to bone and/or soft tissue can have occurred without the patient noticing. Always look at the other foot too; it can be a useful control to the index foot but can also reveal other undeclared pathologies.
- Take a *deep tissue swab from the ulcer base*; the microbiology result will help your colleagues later on. Remember both the diagnosis of infection and the decision to start antimicrobials are based on clinical grounds (discharge, erythema,

swelling, odour and discoloration). Cover Gram-positive organisms in acute mild infections but add Gram-negative cover in chronic, deeper infection. Consult your local antibiotic guidelines. Be mindful of resistant organisms (e.g. MRSA) in those previously affected.

- *Always X-ray the affected foot* (weight-bearing views whenever possible). Look for gas in soft tissues, foreign bodies, unsuspected fractures and possible osteomyelitis. A normal plain film on presentation does not exclude osteomyelitis and tells you nothing about the severity of ischaemia.
- *Think about pressure relief now.* Fragile ischaemic feet can develop new ulcers very quickly and hospital beds are hard. Air mattresses and heel troughs offer some protection. Keep swollen infected limbs elevated and make patients with neuropathic plantar wounds 'non-weight bearing'.
- *Keep dressings simple.* Dry necrotic plaques should be left dry, do not try and soak off the eschar. Do not cover wounds with expensive occlusive dressings; these only turn wounds into a soggy playground for Gram-negative organisms. *Iodine-based dressings and gauze are a sensible first choice.* Hold them in place with light circumferential bandaging, *not with adhesive tape to the skin* which is likely to cause more damage when it is removed.

Easily missed foot problems

- *Charcot neuroarthropathy* is a great mimic; consider this in any person with diabetes and neuropathy who has a red, hot swollen foot which 'flares up' with no apparent cause. Left unchecked it can destroy the foot architecture. Be especially worried when a patient walks in on a hugely swollen foot without concern or care; this may not be cellulitis or a DVT and it mandates an X-ray. Alcohol excess and diabetes often combine to give profound neuropathy. Even if the patient goes home, contact the foot team to arrange follow-up as soon as possible.
- '*Collapsed query cause*'. Could there be a problem with this person's feet? All patients with diabetes should have their feet examined on admission. This is especially true in the frail elderly whose sight, mobility and sensation has meant they have long since lost touch with their feet. *Remove those bandages to find the cause of the confusion and fall.*

Preventing problems

Hospitals are full of hazards for the unwary foot, so become 'foot aware' on ward rounds.

- Where are the patient's feet spending the day? Rammed up against the hand wash bottle on the end of the bed, resting on the bare metal of their wheelchair?
- Does the patient have shoes to protect their feet during their stay?
- Antithrombotic compression stockings should be avoided in neuropathic and ischaemic feet.

Other causes of skin ulceration

Managing skin ulcers requires recognition of the aetiology, with leg ulceration of a vascular origin being the commonest. The vascular aetiology of leg ulcers is usually multifactorial with both arterial and venous insufficiency present, often with other factors promoting occurrence of ulcers.

The aim is to establish the leading precipitating problems and balance the therapeutic options, such as compression versus compromise of arterial supply. The commonest and most serious causes include:

Venous ulcers

- Venous ulcers occur on the lower limbs, most commonly over the medial malleolus. The prevalence is as high as 1% in some societies. Risk factors include:
  - old age
  - obesity
  - trauma
  - deep vein thrombosis
  - phlebitis
  - factor V Leiden deficiency.
- A combination of factors leads to delayed venous return and distension of capillaries, resulting in fibrinogen leakage and subsequent fibrin formation which tightens around the capillaries; surrounding tissue is deprived of oxygen and nutrients, resulting ultimately in ulceration.
- Venous ulcers are accompanied by oedema, brown discoloration resulting from haemosiderin deposition and lipodermatosclerosis (tight, leathery skin). Advanced lipodermatosclerosis can result in an 'inverted champagne bottle' appearance of the legs.

- *Frequently large*, they can involve the entire circumference of the leg.
- Patients often describe heaviness of their legs, *but their main concern is pain.*
- Venous insufficiency can also be associated with venous eczema, 'red legs', which is often misdiagnosed as cellulitis.

Management

- Reverse venous hypertension by improving venous drainage with leg elevation and compression hosiery or bandaging after exclusion of arterial insufficiency.
- The compression therapy can be combined with treatment with pentoxifylline in an attempt to improve blood flow.
- Dressing type and frequency of changing depends on the character of the ulcer (heavy exudate, necrotic debris) and associated factors such as a secondary infection. Antimicrobial dressings are preferable; *be aware antiseptics* such as *chlorhexidine can delay healing, inhibiting the re-epithelialization.*
- Topical or oral antibiotics only if a significant infection is identified. There is a high risk of provoking allergic contact dermatitis with topical antibiotics, so they should be used cautiously.
- Healing can be enhanced by surgical, chemical or biological (maggots) debridement of necrotic tissue.
- *Allergic contact dermatitis and venous eczema* respond to short courses of moderate potency topical steroids.

Arterial ulcers

- These almost always develop on the lower limbs as a result of atherosclerotic disease, but can be caused by:
  - cholesterol emboli
  - vasospasm
  - trauma
  - hypothermia.
- Narrowing of the arteries leads to tissue ischaemia, necrosis and ultimately ulceration.
- Patients often report *claudication* pain on walking, relieved by rest.
- Arterial ulcers can be *severely painful* due to ischaemia.

- Tend to develop over bony prominences, often following minor trauma.
- Usually *round, with a sharply demarcated border* and 'dry' wound bed; the skin around the ulcer tends to be hairless and cold to touch.
- Palpation of the peripheral arteries may reveal *diminished or absent pulses*.

Management

- Prompt surgical or radiological intervention to restore adequate blood supply coupled with appropriate wound care may prevent amputation and increases the chance of successful healing of arterial ulcers.
- Wound care should concentrate on keeping the area warm and free of secondary infections.
- Provision of *adequate pain control is crucial*.

Vasculitis

- An inflammation of blood vessels which can occur in the skin, but can affect other organs as well.
- Vasculitis can result from direct injury to the vessel wall, for example caused by infection or induced by antibodies or activated complement.
- Skin findings depend on the size of vessels involved:
  - small vessel vasculitis tends to present as petechiae, macular or palpable purpura which only occasionally develop into ulcerations
  - large vessel vasculitis can present with livedo reticularis, large purpuric often necrotic eruptions and *frequently ulcerations*.
- Systemic symptoms may suggest other organ involvement and should prompt relevant investigations to confirm this.

Investigations

- Urinalysis (proteins and blood).
- Blood tests: FBC, U&E, LFTs, ESR. The full vasculitis screen also includes: anti-nuclear antibodies (ANA), extractable nuclear antibodies, anti-streptococcal antibodies, viral hepatitis screen, anti-neutrophilic cytoplasmic antibodies (ANCA), cryoglobulins, protein electrophoresis.
- Skin biopsy can prove helpful. Incisional biopsy extending from the bed of the wound, through the edge of the ulcer into surrounding, ideally unaffected skin is preferred. Additional biopsy from a non-ulcerated area showing background changes such as livedo reticularis can be considered.

Treatment

- Vasculitis with ulceration requires aggressive treatment with systemic glucocorticoids or immunosuppression.
- Combined with rest, analgesia and, if there are leg ulcers, leg elevation and compression with hosiery or bandaging.

Malignancy

- Melanoma and non-melanoma skin cancers, including basal cell carcinoma and squamous cell carcinoma, can ulcerate or resemble ulceration.
- *All longstanding ulcers* and those refractory to treatment should undergo biopsy to confirm or exclude malignancy.
- In addition, longstanding ulcers can develop malignancy, such as squamous cell carcinoma (Marjolin's ulcer).
- Cutaneous lymphoma; mycosis fungoides can also ulcerate but usually at a later stage.

Management

Surgery if feasible; radiotherapy remains an option for basal and squamous cell carcinomas.

Pyoderma gangrenosum

- A rare ulcerative disorder most commonly associated with inflammatory bowel disease, rheumatoid arthritis and haematological malignancies.
- Fast forming, painful ulcers which tend to have a violaceous undermined edge; the majority develop on the lower limbs and buttocks.

Management

- Analgesia.
- Appropriate dressing (including compression hosiery/bandages).
- Immunosuppression with oral steroids or agents such as ciclosporin. Anti-TNFα monoclonal antibodies are promising alternatives.
- Associated diseases should be sought out and treated.

Calciphylaxis

- Calcification of small vessels leads to tissue necrosis and ulcer formation.
- Although uncommon, it is seen in patients with:
  - chronic kidney disease
  - primary hyperparathyroidism due to hypercalcaemia
  - states of hypercoagulability that may occur in liver failure or diabetes
  - paradoxically in those treated with warfarin.
- *Unbearable pain is the predominant feature.*
- Ulcers develop in areas with a thick layer of subcutaneous tissue such as thighs and flanks.
- Mortality is up to 80% due to secondary sepsis.

Management

- IV sodium thiosulfate or etidronate.
- Antibiotics for secondary infection/sepsis.
- Analgesics.
- Wound care.

Ecthyma

- Deeper form of impetigo, caused by bacteria such as *Pseudomonas*, *Staphylococcus aureus* and *Streptococcus pyogenes*.
- Risk factors include: poor hygiene, high temperature and humidity (hence more common in the tropics) and immunosuppression.

Management

- Improved hygiene.
- Topical antiseptics and antibiotics; several weeks of treatment might be required.

Mouth ulceration

Mouth ulcers occur either due to local pathology or as part of a systemic disorder involving the skin and/or other mucous membranes. Consider:

Aphthous

- Painful, recurrent, round/oval ulcers of the oral cavity. They often have an erythematous halo and white bed.
- 80% are smaller than 5 mm and resolve within 2 weeks (minor ulcers).

- Those larger than 10 mm (major ulcer) might take up to a few months to heal.
- Multiple, herpetiform ulcers may develop due to immune dysfunction.

Management

- Local anaesthetics.
- Superpotent topical corticosteroids applied at the onset (clobetasol propionate), intralesional corticosteroids, topical tacrolimus or systemic therapy with colchicine, dapsone or thalidomide.

Candidiasis 'thrush'

- More than 50% of individuals carry *Candida* (mainly *Candida albicans*) on mucosal surfaces of the oral cavity; candidiasis results from transient or chronic immunodeficiency.
- It presents as erythematous, raw-looking patches on mucosal surfaces often covered by a white coating.
- Angular cheilitis (splits in the corners of mouth) help to establish the diagnosis.
- Ulceration occurs if untreated or in profound immunodeficiency.
- Any suspicion of oral candidiasis should prompt questions and potentially investigations to assess the extent of the gastrointestinal tract involvement and search for the underlying cause.
- Diagnostic difficulty arises as non-fungal oral ulceration can develop secondary, superimposed candidiasis. Skin swabs and scrapings (ideally both) sent for microscopy and culture will aid in the diagnosis.

Management

- Oral candidiasis complicated by ulceration requires systemic oral antifungal: fluconazole, itraconazole or amphotericin in combination with increased oral hygiene.

Herpes simplex virus (HSV) 'cold sores'

- Primary and recurrent HSV infection can present with oral ulcers; in immunocompromised patients these can be extensive.
- Ulcers tend to resolve spontaneously within 5–14 days.
- Atopic patients with active eczema may develop eczema herpeticum.

Management

- Topical antiseptics and soothing preparations are normally all that is needed.
- If there is florid or widespread ulceration in highly symptomatic patients, antiviral medication should be introduced, ideally at the onset.
- Eczema herpeticum requires aggressive treatment with antiviral agents combined with topical or systemic corticosteroids.

Stevens–Johnson syndrome

- Is a rare, most likely delayed hypersensitivity reaction caused by infections such as *Mycoplasma*, HSV and medication.
- Results in extensive erosions and ulcerations of the mucosal surfaces (oral cavity, conjunctiva, genital mucosa) and up to 10% of total body skin surface.
- It overlaps with the life-threatening skin condition called toxic epidermal necrolysis which affects a larger area of skin.
- Identification of the cause is of paramount importance.

Management

- Any potential culprit medication must be stopped immediately.
- Local antiseptics.
- Adequate analgesia.
- Nutrition and hydration often through nasogastric tube or parenterally.
- Systemic therapy with ciclosporin, immunoglobulins and corticosteroids may be used, but benefit is uncertain.
- Patients may benefit from being managed in a centre with experience in this condition or in a high dependency unit/intensive care unit.

Lichen planus

- Very common, inflammatory condition affecting skin and mucosa.
- Presents in the oral cavity as white, linear lesions (Wickham striae) and in severe cases with ulcerations.
- Commonly skin papular, itchy eruptions and nail changes such as pitting can be found.

Management

- Topical corticosteroids (mouth washes) or immunosuppression with systemic corticosteroids or azathioprine.
- Refractory ulcers should be considered for biopsy to exclude malignancy.

Pemphigus and pemphigoid

- Relatively rare blistering, autoimmune disorders affecting skin and mucosal surfaces; they present with blisters, bullae, erosions and ulcerations.
- Diagnosis requires clinico-histopathological correlation.

Management

- Treatment is with immunosuppression.

Any patients with oral ulcerations and blisters affecting the skin should be referred to dermatology.

Behçet's disease

- A rare autoimmune, systemic, small-vessel vasculitis.
- It presents with painful mouth and genital ulcers, eye problems and skin lesions.
- Oral ulcers are usually recurrent and tend to resolve within 1–3 weeks.

Management

- There is *no cure* for this disease.
- Medications that help to control it include:
  - topical anti-inflammatory antibiotics (such as tetracyclines)
  - corticosteroids
  - local anaesthetics
  - systemic corticosteroids
  - immunosuppressants (azathioprine).

Malignancy

- *Oral ulcers that do not heal require investigations to exclude malignancies* such as:
  - squamous cell carcinoma
  - Kaposi's sarcoma
  - leukaemia.

Medication

- Multiple chemotherapeutics may lead to oral ulcerations.
- Rarely requires discontinuation.
- If symptomatic, a topical treatment might be required: mouth washes with antiseptics.

Concluding remarks

Oral ulcers are a common presentation in systemic and gastrointestinal diseases, such as systemic lupus erythematosus and inflammatory bowel disease. Bacterial infections such as *Streptococcus* or *Treponema pallidum* (syphilis) can also induce oral ulceration.

Oral ulcers should not be dismissed as benign aphthous ulcers without proper evaluation and consideration.

Further reading

Brownrigg JR, Apelqvist J, Bakker K, Schaper NC, Hinchliffe RJ. Evidence-based management of PAD & the diabetic foot. *Eur J Vasc Endovasc Surg* 2013; 45(6): 673–681.

Grey JE, Harding KG, Enoch S. Venous and arterial leg ulcers. *BMJ* 2006; 332(7537): 347–350.

National Institute for Health and Care Excellence. Diabetic foot problems: inpatient management of diabetic foot problems. NICE Clinical Guideline 119, March 2011. www.nice.org.uk/cg119.

Powlson AS, Coll AP. The treatment of diabetic foot infections. *J Antimicrob Chemother* 2010; 65 (Suppl 3): iii3–9.

Scottish Intercollegiate Guidelines Network (SIGN). Management of chronic venous leg ulcers. August 2010. www.sign.ac.uk/guidelines/fulltext/120/index.html.

Chapter 58

Speech disturbance

Rob Whiting and Stephen Haydock

Introduction

The production of intelligible speech and language is a highly complex physiological process involving:

Central structures:

- Cerebral cortex
- Basal ganglia and associated nigrostriatal pathway
- Cerebellum
- Brainstem (corticobulbar tracts and cranial nerve nuclei).

Peripheral structures:

- Motor and sensory nerves (vagus, facial, hypoglossal and phrenic)
- Muscles and tissues of the larynx, e.g. vocal cords
- Muscles and structures of the pharynx, palate, tongue and lips
- Muscles of respiration
- Supralaryngeal structures, e.g. mouth and tongue.

Abnormal speech can result from damage to any of these structures, resulting in:

- *Dysphasia*: the disturbance of comprehension (*reception*) and/or production of speech (*expression*) resulting from damage to areas of the cerebral cortex. It is a *disorder of language*.
- *Dysarthria*: the disturbance of speech production resulting in abnormal articulation and slurring of speech due to damage of the motor pathways (brainstem, cerebellum and motor nerves) or muscles of the larynx and supralaryngeal region.
- *Apraxia of speech*: a problem with the programming of the movements of speech (rather than their neuromuscular execution as in dysarthria).

- *Dysphonia*: an alteration in voice production that impairs social and professional communication, resulting from abnormalities of the vocal organs themselves (laryngeal structures and vocal cords). It should be differentiated from 'hoarseness', which describes impaired voice production that does not produce the significant impairment of interaction characterized by dysphonia.

Neuroanatomy of speech and language

An understanding of dysphasia requires some understanding of the anatomical basis of language comprehension and production by the cerebral cortex. Speech is lateralized within the cerebral cortex with the specialized speech/language centres usually residing within the left cerebral hemisphere. There is some variation according to hand dominance, with speech lateralization to the left cerebral hemisphere in:

- 97% of right-handed people
- 81% of left-handed people (those with lateralization to right often have some language ability found in both hemispheres)

Important anatomical areas

Broca's area

Located in the frontal lobe in the region anterior to the motor cortex, it is responsible for speech production in terms of the motor outflow. Impulses are sent to the premotor cortex, resulting in appropriate contractions of the muscles of the larynx, pharynx and mouth. In addition, impulses pass to the primary motor area to ensure that speech is coordinated with respiration (*try breathing in and speaking normally!*).

Acute Medicine, ed. Stephen Haydock, Duncan Whitehead and Zoë Fritz. Published by Cambridge University Press.
© Cambridge University Press 2015.

Patients with lesions localized to this area have defects in speech production, so-called 'expressive dysphasia', 'Broca's dysphasia'. This can vary from complete aphasia to slow, laborious speech with numerous grammatical errors. They are able to comprehend speech, although it appears that there is some grammatical processing that occurs in this region. Patients are therefore prone to make some comprehension errors with more complex grammatical structures, e.g. passive tenses.

Wernicke's area

This area is located in the posterior superior temporal gyrus just posterior to the auditory cortex. It is responsible for speech comprehension. Patients with lesions in this area are able to understand speech but respond to questioning with answers that have grammatical structure but meaningless content with inappropriate words, often referred to as 'word salad'. This is referred to as 'receptive dysphasia', 'Wernicke's dysphasia' or 'fluent dysphasia'. Lesions in this region also produce difficulty accessing the nominal dictionary and so frequently an inability to correctly name objects, using words with similar sounds (e.g. mouse for house) or the names of similar objects (e.g. clock for watch) producing an associated 'nominal dysphasia'.

Arcuate fasciculus

A deep white matter tract that connects Broca's area to Wernicke's area. Damage to the arcuate fasciculus produces a less severe language and speech deficit than those involving Broca's and Wernicke's areas directly. These patients are able to comprehend speech, and with difficulty produce language, but are unable to repeat words or sentences spoken to them.

> #### Scenario 58.1
>
> *Mr HS is a 65-year-old man who has been admitted via his GP with confusion thought to be due to a urinary tract infection. He was started on trimethoprim the previous day but is not improving. On MAU you have the benefit of relatives who explain that Mr HS is usually fit and well (still working as a solicitor) and has been unwell for a few days with headache and general malaise. His family agree that he is a little confused but they also think he is having problems 'finding the right words'. On examination he is pyrexial, with an Abbreviated Mental Test Score of 8/10 with clear evidence of an expressive dysphasia. His bloods are essentially normal.*

Patients with mild dysphasia are not infrequently thought to have confusion that may or may not also be present. Confusion is often attributed to a 'UTI' resulting in correction of a presumed 'acute trimethoprim deficiency'. However, a high functioning 65-year-old would be unlikely to become acutely confused due to a mild urinary infection. The prodrome of headache, mild confusion, pyrexia and onset of expressive dysphasia is highly suggestive of herpes simplex encephalitis. The virus has a particular predilection for the temporal lobes and dysphasia is a common feature of acute CNS infection. Outcome is highly dependent on time from onset of symptoms to first treatment with aciclovir.

Clinical assessment of the patient with speech disturbance

History

This can be taken from the patient but if verbal communication is very limited, written communication may be beneficial, or involve family, friend or carer as available. When encountered on the medical take the onset is likely to be rapid, as gradual onset speech disturbance would generally be referred to outpatient neurology. Elicit:

- speed of onset
- associated headache: onset with or preceding speech disturbance
- associated swallowing difficulties
- associated neurological symptoms
- any previous transient episodes
- systemic features of malignancy: weight loss, fatigue and malaise
- history of vascular risk factors: hypertension, diabetes
- antecedent activities: vertebral artery dissection
- past medical history of migraine, stroke, epilepsy, multiple sclerosis
- medication: anticonvulsants
- social history: smoking and alcohol.

Examination

A full examination is required looking for features of systemic disease and other neurological signs. When assessing speech and language function, there are seven main components that should be tested:

1. Spontaneous (conversational) speech
2. Auditory comprehension
3. Naming
4. Repetition
5. Reading
6. Writing
7. Articulation.

1. Spontaneous speech

- You will have a good idea of this from the history taking.
- There are a number of features to note regarding speech:
  - pronunciation
  - word and sentence formation
  - fluency, cadence, rhythm and prosody (stress and intonation)
  - omission or transposition of syllables
  - repetition
  - circumlocutions (use of unnecessarily wordy and indirect language)
  - paraphasias
  - neologisms (invented words).
- Some patients with non-fluent aphasia may have some preserved 'automatic' speech, usually due to recitation of overlearned items from childhood, or sometimes a specific retained speech fragment; this is often referred to as a verbal automatism. Verbal automatisms occur most frequently in global aphasia; they may be real words, fragments of a word, or a neologism.
- When listening to spontaneous speech, you may detect a paraphasia, a speech defect in which the patient substitutes a wrong word or sound for the intended word. There are two main types.
  Phonemic paraphasia:
  - addition, deletion or substitution of a phoneme (e.g. 'dug' instead of 'jug')
  - more typical of anterior lesions.
  Semantic paraphasia:
  - substitution of the wrong word, but with a similar meaning (e.g. 'cup' instead of 'jug')
  - more typical of posterior, perisylvian lesions.
- When a patient is having difficulty with fluency, it is more difficult to assess spontaneous speech. Normal speech fluency is 100–115 words per minute *(world record >600 words per minute!)*. Speech output may be as low as 10–15 words per minute in non-fluent aphasia. If maximum sentence length is <7 words, *the patient is non-fluent.*

2. Auditory comprehension

- It is important to establish that difficulty with comprehension is not due to impaired hearing.
- Ask the patient to follow commands of increasing complexity:
  - one-step command (e.g. 'close your eyes')
  - two-step commands (e.g. 'touch your right ear then poke out your tongue')
  - three-step commands (e.g. 'stand up, turn around once and then touch your hair').
- Failure to follow commands may not prove comprehension is impaired; patients may not comply if they have a verbal apraxia. Ask simple yes/no questions (e.g. Is England the capital of London? Can cats fly?)

3. Naming

- This requires integration of visual, semantic and phonological aspects of item knowledge.
- Ask the patient to name familiar, common objects (e.g. pen, watch), before progressing to less common items (e.g. nib, winder). Semantic or phonemic paraphasias may be evident.
- If a visual agnosia is present, use auditory/tactile presentation of information for the patient to name (e.g. running a tap, or placing a key in the patient's hand).

4. Repetition

- Ask the patient to repeat well-known phrases, such as:
  - 'No ifs, ands, or buts' (difficult for them to repeat if dysphasic)
  - 'West Register Street' (difficult for them to repeat accurately if dysarthric).

5. Reading

- Ask the patient to read aloud a sentence or paragraph from a newspaper or book.
- Then assess their comprehension of what they have read out.

6. Writing

- Assess spontaneous writing by asking them to write about their family, or where they live.
- Assess dictation; ask the patient to write down a spoken phrase (e.g. 'the quick brown fox jumped over the lazy black dog').
- Assess copying by requesting the patient copies a sentence from newspaper or book.

7. Articulation

Speech alternating motion rates

- From these alternating motion rate tasks one can judge rate, rhythm, precision and range of movements of the lips, jaw and tongue. Normal adults can produce an even rhythm at a rate of about five or six syllables per second.
- Ask the patient to take a deep breath and make these specific sounds as quickly and steadily as possible for 3–5 seconds:
  - labial sounds; say 'puh, puh, puh', which tests orbicularis oris
  - lingual sounds; say 'tuh, tuh, tuh', which tests the anterior tongue
  - Palatal sounds; say 'kuh, kuh, kuh' to test the posterior tongue and palate.

Speech sequential motion rates

- This task assesses the patient's ability to program a sequence of speech movements rapidly and successively. After brief practice at slow rates, normal speakers accomplish this task rapidly and accurately.
- Ask your patient to take a deep breath and make all three sounds 'puh, tuh, kuh' repeatedly over 3–5 seconds.
- Articulation can also be tested by using some of the classic phrases, e.g. *West Register Street*, *British constitution*.

Other sounds

- *Glottal coup*: instruct the patient to cough, or produce a grunt-like 'uh' (the glottal coup); this permits assessment of vocal cord integrity. The cough and coup should be sharp, a gross indication of adequate vocal cord adduction.
- *Vowel prolongation*: ask the patient to take a deep breath and say 'ah' for as long as possible. Many normal adults can do this for 15 seconds or more, but 5 seconds usually suffices. This task allows an evaluation of the respiratory and laryngeal mechanisms and their ability to produce a sustained tone at normal pitch, quality, loudness, duration and steadiness.
- Ask the patient to blow, cough, smack the lips, and click the tongue. This assesses their ability to organize and program some fairly reflexive oromotor movements. If the patient produces odd or inaccurate sounds, or verbalizes the command rather than making the sounds, this might suggest an apraxia.

Commonly recognized dysphasias

(For summary see Table 58.1.)

Expressive (Broca's) aphasia

- Speech is hesitant and lacks fluency.
- There are word-finding difficulties, use of incorrect words and many grammatical errors.
- Comprehension is well preserved.
- Look for other associated neurological signs.

Transcortical motor aphasia

- Similar to Broca's aphasia but repetition is intact.
- Usually due to a lesion in the border zone superior or anterior to Broca's area.

Receptive (Wernicke's) aphasia

- Rapid fluent speech with normal intonation but the speech is meaningless (wrong order and neologisms).
- There may be paraphasias (flow of words interrupted by inappropriate words/sounds/phrases) and neologisms (invented words).
- Repetition is impaired with paraphasia and insertions.
- Comprehension is severely impaired.
- Look for other associated neurological signs.

Transcortical sensory aphasia

- Similar to Wernicke's aphasia, but with intact repetition.
- Often due to a lesion in the border zone posterior and inferior to Wernicke's area.

Table 58.1 Types of aphasia and their characteristic deficits

Type of aphasia	Fluency	Comprehension	Repetition	Naming	Reading	Writing	Lesion localization
Broca's	Poor	Good	Poor	Poor	Poor	Poor	Inferior frontal gyrus
Anomic aphasia	Good	Good	Good	Poor	Good	Varies	
Wernicke's	Good	Poor	Poor	Poor	Poor	Poor	Wernicke's area
Global	Poor	Poor	Poor	Poor	Poor	Poor	Usually large lesion involving Broca's and Wernicke's area
Conduction	Good	Good	Poor	Varies	Good	Good	Arcuate fasciculus
Transcortical motor	Poor	Good	Good	Poor	Varies	Poor	Perisylvian area, superior/anterior to Broca's area
Transcortical sensory	Good	Poor	Good	Poor	Poor	Poor	Parietotemporal region, posterior to Wernicke's area
Transcortical mixed	Poor	Poor	Good	Poor	Poor	Poor	
Apraxia of speech	Poor	Good	Poor	Poor	Poor	Good	

Conduction aphasia

- Spontaneous speech is fluent, and comprehension is preserved.
- There is significant difficulty with repetition.
- May be due to a lesion in the arcuate fasciculus.

Global aphasia

- The close proximity of Broca's and Wernicke's area means that patients rarely have a pure receptive or expressive dysphasia but a mixed problem with either expressive or receptive component most prominent.
- A true global aphasia with severe receptive and expressive problems is associated with large middle cerebral artery infarction (*normally of the left cerebral hemisphere*).
- Look for other associated neurological signs.

Anomic (nominal) aphasia

- Is unusual in isolation and usually part of a more generalized dysphasia.

Common causes of dysphasia

Dysphasia can result from any insult to the cerebral cortex in these areas, but most commonly on the acute medical take is due to:

- stroke
- tumour
- trauma
- infection, e.g. herpes simplex encephalitis
- migraine (transient)
- epilepsy (transient).

Commonly recognized dysarthrias

All types of dysarthria produce altered articulation of consonants and slurring of speech with variable degrees of intelligibility. In a pure dysarthria, the speech content is normal. Patients may have associated respiratory and swallowing problems. Dysarthrias are classified according to the site of the lesion and resulting characteristic manifestations.

Spastic dysarthria (pseudobulbar palsy)

Results from lesions in the pyramidal tract. All of the cranial nerves (except VII and XII) have bilateral inputs from the corticospinal tract, hence bilateral lesions are much more severe than unilateral lesions.

Clinical features:

- Monotonous slurred speech with a harsh, strained quality ('Donald Duck' speech).
- The tongue is small and tense and cannot be protruded.
- The palate does not move.

- May drool saliva while talking.
- There may be swallowing difficulties with nasal regurgitation.
- Patients may have emotional lability.
- There may be exaggerated jaw jerk.
- Look carefully for features of possible causes.
  Causes include:
- cerebrovascular disease (internal capsule, bilateral if severe)
- motor neurone disease (usually mixed bulbar/pseudobulbar palsy)
- multiple sclerosis
- trauma
- syphilis
- high tumours of brainstem.

Flaccid dysarthria (bulbar palsy)

Occurs from damage to the cranial motor nerves which innervate the muscles of speech.

Clinical features:

- Speech is unclear, unmodulated and nasal, with difficulty in articulating consonants.
- Muscles are flaccid, undergo atrophy and fasciculation; these features are most obviously seen in the tongue.
- The palate does not move.
- May drool saliva while talking.
- There may be swallowing difficulties with nasal regurgitation.
- Look carefully for features of other possible causes.
  Causes include:
- motor neurone disease (usually mixed bulbar/pseudobulbar palsy)
- syringobulbia
- Guillain–Barré
- poliomyelitis
- neurosyphilis.

Ataxic dysarthria (cerebellar dysarthria)

Is due to lesion(s) in the cerebellum or/and connections.

Clinical features:

- Speech with excessive and equal stress on all syllables.
- Slurred, scanning staccato speech (sounds as if drunk).
- Respiration and phonation are not well coordinated.

- May be other features of cerebellar disease including:
  - nystagmus
  - past pointing
  - intention tremor
  - dysdidokinesis
  - ataxic gait
  - impaired coordination.
- Look carefully for other features or possible causes.
  Causes include:
- cerebrovascular disease
- tumours (commonly secondary or astrocytomas, haemangioblastomas)
- multiple sclerosis
- toxins (including alcohol and lead)
- hereditary cerebellar degenerative disorders, e.g. Friedreich's ataxia
- Wilson's disease
- *Hypokinetic*: usually seen in patients with PD due to abnormalities in the nigrostriatal pathway. Speech is delayed in onset, slow and of low volume.
- *Hyperkinetic*: due to lesions of the basal ganglia associated with involuntary movement disorders. Consequence is a similar speech quality to spastic dysarthria but of variable severity, and speech may be interrupted by involuntary movements (see also Chapter 35).

Swallowing problems

- Difficulty swallowing is commonly associated with speech disturbance, in particular dysarthria. In particular, approximately *40% of patients will develop difficulties swallowing after a stroke.*
- A number of guidelines recognize the importance of this (ISWP, NICE and SIGN [1–3]) and require that all stroke patients on admission should have a swallow screen by an appropriately trained professional before being given oral food, fluid or medication. If there are concerns a referral to Speech and Language Therapy (SALT) (or other appropriately trained person) should be made ideally within 24 hours but not more than 72 hours.
- Further investigation if required to study the swallow mechanism is by video-fluoroscopy or direct visualization by fibreoptic endoscopic evaluation of swallowing. The latter can be safely performed at the bedside.

- Most hospitals have a multidisciplinary team to assist with patients with significant swallowing difficulties including a gastroenterologist, speech and language therapist, dietitian and nutrition nurse.
- A range of interventions are available from pureed food and thickeners to alternative feeding methods including nasogastric tube and percutaneous endoscopic gastrostomy (see Chapter 67).
- Most patients recover normal swallowing within several weeks of an acute stroke.
- Difficulty swallowing is clearly distressing to both the patient and family and the nature of the problem and associated risks should be carefully explained. A useful leaflet can be downloaded from the Stroke Association at stroke.org.uk.

Speech and language therapy (SALT)

There are currently around 1500 speech and language therapists registered in the UK, most practising within the NHS:

- In addition to the assessment and management of swallowing problems they all provide a range of assessments and interventions for children and adults with a variety of speech problems.
- NICE recommends that SALT referral should be made for all patients following stroke with dysarthria, dysphasia, speech dyspraxia or other communication difficulties despite reasonable cognition.
- SALT are involved in the initial assessment, diagnosis and treatment at all stages of the stroke recovery. They aim to help the patient make best use of their remaining abilities, restore language and compensate for the persisting language deficit by developing new methods of communication. They also work closely with family and carers to help them to communicate with the patient.
- There is as yet no developed evidence base for SALT therapy in patients with speech disorders and NICE have highlighted that such research is needed for interventions for dysphasia following stroke. A Cochrane review in 2012 [4] addressed the evidence for SALT interventions in dysphasia following stroke. It concluded that there was no universally accepted intervention (single or group therapy, skilled or semi-skilled therapist) and that although there was evidence that there might be benefit, there was insufficient evidence to define the best approach.

References

1. Intercollegiate Stroke Working Party (ISWP). National Clinical Guidelines for Stroke, 4th edn. 2012. Royal College of Physicians. Available to download at www.rcplondon.ac.uk/sites/default/files/national-clinical-guidelines-for-stroke-fourth-edition.pdf.

2. SIGN. Clinical Guideline 118. Management of Patients with Stroke: Rehabilitation, Prevention and Management of Complications. 2011. Available to download at www.sign.ac.uk/guidelines/fulltext/118/.

3. NICE. Clinical Guideline 68. Diagnosis and Initial Management of Stroke and Transient Ischaemic Attacks. Available to download at http://guidance.nice.org.uk/CG68/NICEGuidance/pdf/English.

4. Brady MC, Kelly H, Godwin J, Enderby P. Speech and language therapy for aphasia following stroke. *Cochrane Database Syst Rev* 2012; 5: CD000425. Available to download at http://onlinelibrary.wiley.com/doi/10.1002/14651858.CD000425.pub3/pdf/standard.

Further reading

Ashley J, Duggan M, Sutcliffe N. Speech, language and swallowing disorders in the older adult. *Clin Geriatr Med* 22 (2006):291–310.

Campbell WW. *DeJong's The Neurologic Examination*, 7th en. Wolters Kluwer Health; 2012.

Duffy J. Motor speech disorders: clues to neurological diagnosis. In: Adler CH and Ahlskog JE (eds.) *Parkinson's Disease and Movement Disorders: Diagnosis and Treatment Guidelines for the Practicing Physician.* Humana Press; 2000.

Murdoch BE. *Acquired Speech and Language Disorders: A Neuroanatomical and Functional Neurological Approach,* 2nd edn. Wiley-Blackwell; 2009.

Warlow C, et al. *Stroke: Practical Management*, 3rd edn. Blackwell Publishing; 2007.

Chapter

59

Suicidal ideation

Marguerite Paffard

Introduction

Doctors commonly encounter patients expressing suicidal thoughts, and who may have acted upon these thoughts. Self-destructive behaviour can appear in several forms:

- suicide
- attempted suicide
- self-injurious behaviour without suicidal intent.

Completed suicide is relatively rare and can have a profound effect on family and friends. The Office for National Statistics recorded 6045 completed suicides amongst people aged over 15 in 2011, with the highest rate being in middle-aged men [1]. Healthcare professionals may also be deeply affected by a completed suicide, with a sense of guilt and failure. Added to this is scrutiny of the treatment offered through the Serious Untoward Incident review process. Recent case law has found Trusts increasingly liable to protect individuals who present with a '*real and immediate*' risk of suicide [2,3].

Accurate prediction of suicide is notoriously difficult due to the high prevalence of suicidal thinking and many false positive predictions based on risk factors. The downward trend in the rate of completed suicide in the past twenty years contrasts with the rise in the rate of self-harm, particularly amongst young people, with the UK possibly having the highest rate in Europe [4]. Self-harm without suicidal intent can provide a means of escaping from intolerable dysphoric feelings or situations or can be a form of self-punishment. It can act as a means of communicating distress in order to elicit care and attention from families, friends and healthcare professionals.

Scenario 59.1

Miss P is a 23-year-old woman who has been brought to the A&E department by her partner, who smells faintly of alcohol. He reports that he found her at home surrounded by a number of empty medication packets. He had gone out to the shop. She was drowsy and reluctant to come to the hospital.

Considerations

- More history is needed but is she fit to be interviewed given the drowsiness?
- She needs to be assessed physically.

Scenario 59.2

Mr J, a 42-year-old man, was brought into A&E by his parents. He is known to have had alcohol dependence problems in the past to an extent that caused some brain damage leading to cognitive impairment. He lives independently. His parents went to his house as he hadn't answered the phone and they were concerned. They found him lying in bed saying his back hurt. It transpired that he had jumped from his first floor window the previous day in an attempt to kill himself. A spinal X-ray reveals a fracture at C5 and he is admitted to the orthopaedic ward. It is recommended that he has operative stabilization of his fracture but he seems unconcerned about the injury and refuses treatment.

Considerations

- Accessing his medical records to obtain a full past history.
- Full assessment of his mental state including his capacity in relation to treatment.

Acute Medicine, ed. Stephen Haydock, Duncan Whitehead and Zoë Fritz. Published by Cambridge University Press. © Cambridge University Press 2015.

Suicide risk assessment

There is very rarely a single reason why an individual arrives at the point of considering suicide or self-harm; several interacting factors determine the individual process.

Risk factors include:

- increasing age (although increasing suicide rate in young adults over past 40 years)
- male sex
- social isolation
- low social and educational status
- unemployment
- family history of mental disorder
- personal history of or current psychiatric disorder and treatment especially depression
- history of self-harming behaviour (lethality of method is important)
- hopelessness
- drug and alcohol misuse
- poor physical health
- access to lethal methods
- history of abuse
- recent life events
- relationship problems.

These risk factors can be described as:

- *static and stable* (e.g. history of self-harm, gender, family history)
- *dynamic* (e.g. recent life event, hopelessness, recent discharge from hospital)
- *future* (e.g. access to lethal means, support).

In any one individual, personal risk factors may change over time, sometimes quite rapidly, increasing that person's vulnerability from one day to the next. Suicide is a rare event and difficult to predict. However, identifying risk and protective factors (such as supportive family, work) in a systematic way leads to a management plan targeted at those risks which are treatable or modifiable.

The components of a good assessment include:

- obtaining a psychiatric history from the patient
- obtaining collateral information where possible from family, friends, current and previous medical notes, the treating team, police if relevant
- physical examination and appropriate investigations.

Taking a psychiatric history

A psychiatric examination involves taking a detailed history and examining the mental state. Skilfully done,

this forms the basis of a therapeutic relationship in which trust is established and through which negotiations with often reluctant patients can be carried out. A compassionate approach encourages patients to disclose often intimate and painful information which in itself may act as a protective factor.

Before beginning the interview take account of your personal safety. Very few psychiatric patients are violent but simple precautions are sensible (see Chapter 7).

Principal elements of a psychiatric interview

1. *The presenting complaint*: start by asking open-ended questions such as 'can you tell me what the problem is?' Move on to more specific questions to elicit the information you need to know and to keep control of the interview. Ask simple questions and try to pick up on verbal cues (e.g. mentioning stress at work); explore these areas further. It can be helpful to summarize your findings so that the patient can correct any inaccuracies but also to demonstrate that the patient has been heard and understood. This establishes good rapport and deepens the therapeutic relationship.

2. *Precipitants to current crisis*: indicators of risk will be presented throughout the interview. It may be appropriate at this stage of the interview to probe more deeply about the actual suicide attempt/episode of self-harm. However, further on in the interview, after a more complete picture of the person and their life has been obtained, it may be possible to explore difficult topics more sensitively. This may be the first time this person has spoken of these issues and may feel a great sense of relief. They may become more closed to questions in subsequent interviews with professionals – the structure of services being such that people may be asked the same questions many times by different individuals as they move from one team to another. Information gained in the first interview may be invaluable and a truer reflection of how the individual is feeling.

3. *History of mental disorder*: any history of mental disorder is important but in particular of depression, previous suicide attempts or acts of self-harm. Self-injurious acts are strongly linked to emotionally unstable personality disorder but any psychiatric diagnosis elevates the risk.

4. *Drugs and alcohol*: past and present use.

5. *History of violence.*
6. *Brief personal history*: enquire about the quality of care during childhood and of any abuse as a child or adult; employment status; social network; family contacts. Look for protective factors and recent life events, particularly bereavement or other loss event.
7. *Family history of mental disorder.*
8. *Physical health*: particularly chronic painful conditions, disability, incurable.
9. *Mental state examination*:

   - *Appearance and behaviour*. Look for self-neglect, signs of previous self-harm, bizarre behaviour, signs of intoxication.
   - *Speech*: speed, coherence, content.
   - *Mood*: subjective and objective, eye contact, body posture.
   - *Thought*: speed, form, content. Ask about hopelessness. Symptoms of severe depression include guilt and nihilistic delusions. Persecutory or other distressing beliefs occur in psychotic disorders including the transient states experienced by people with personality disorder in acute distress.
   - *Abnormal perceptions*: ask about auditory hallucinations, particularly of a derogatory nature or command. Hallucinatory voices may be telling the patient to kill himself. Assess the degree to which the patient feels he has to obey and the effect on him of trying to resist.

10. *Risk assessment*:

    - Sociodemographic risk factors will have been ascertained. Risk factors associated with this specific attempt should be determined.
    - How serious was the intent?
    - Was there careful preparation or was it impulsive? Both situations carry risk which should be determined by the context, e.g. an impulsive person with access to a lethal method may be as at risk as someone who has made meticulous plans but then informed someone.
    - Relatively harmless attempts do not always mean lack of serious intent *if the patient believed the method would be fatal.*
    - Likelihood of rescue.
    - Access to the means of suicide.

- Sense of relief or regret about outcome of attempt.
- Hopelessness for the future.
- Feelings of guilt, family being better off without them, a burden.
- Recent escalation in self-harming behaviour (many people who complete suicide have a history of self-harm).

Determining the level of risk

The outcome of the assessment should include the main clinical and demographic variables as well as the individual psychological factors increasing or mitigating risk. *Hopelessness and ongoing suicidal intent should have received particular attention.*

In addition to a clinical interview, there are a number of risk assessment scales which can be used. Unfortunately there is no consensus as to the most accurate or effective one [5]. The Beck's Suicide Intent Scale, which is one of the best validated instruments, still only has a low predictive power [6].

Local, non-validated, systems for risk stratification may exist whereby different scores trigger different pathways of management. If using one of these, care needs to be taken to avoid risk assessment becoming a box-ticking exercise with the patient experiencing the interviewer as remote and unempathic, detracting from the quality of the interaction. However, systematizing the risk assessment is helpful in ensuring that all risk and protective factors are considered along with the significance of these factors for the individual.

> **Scenario 59.1 continued**
>
> *Assessment reveals that Miss P is sufficiently alert to be interviewed. She has taken a combination of citalopram and paracetamol. She is well known to psychiatric services but not currently in contact; she has a history of similar behaviour in the past. She and her partner had had an argument earlier in the day. They have a 6-year-old son who was being cared for by his maternal grandmother that day. The partner does most of the talking and is reluctant to allow her to be interviewed alone. Physical examination is unremarkable other than some superficial lacerations to her arm, some scarring from previous cutting and some bruising on her arm, back and neck.*
>
> *Miss P is monosyllabic but has refused any further investigations such as paracetamol levels. Her partner is becoming increasingly agitated and demanding and has been verbally abusive to one of the junior nurses.*

Considerations: Miss P's partner appears to be controlling the interview situation and Miss P may not be able to talk freely with him there. Being able to communicate a non-coerced opinion is one aspect of capacity. Does she have capacity to refuse treatment? The bruising raises the possibility of physical abuse. Although there are no immediate childcare issues, is the 6-year-old at risk of emotional abuse? It would be appropriate to notify the child protection services within the hospital who can further assess the situation.

Scenario 59.2 continued

Mr J's notes reveal that he has a history of alcohol abuse but is currently abstinent. He has regular contact with the mental health services because of recurrent depression and disorganized, sometimes impulsive behaviour. At interview he reports that voices had told him to commit suicide by jumping from the window but he is no longer hearing them. He is vague when asked about current suicidal thinking. Cognitively he has a poor short-term memory, finds it hard to keep to the point and does not seem to grasp the seriousness of his condition. He is agitated and wishing to leave the hospital. He is unwilling to comply with bed rest, the alternative way to manage his spinal fracture. Sedation has been considered but it would involve restraining Mr J; any torsional strain on his spine might dislodge the fracture.

Considerations: Mr J appears to be suffering from a mental disorder and may lack capacity in relation to treatment for his physical condition. He has some high risk indicators for suicide including a history of depression, command hallucinations, poor impulse control, a serious self-harm attempt with failure to inform others and a lack of concern for his well-being.

Management

Once the assessment is completed an evaluation of the information obtained is made. Individual suicide and protective factors should be identified, both long term and acute. Clear documentation of diagnosis, risk and protective factors is essential both as a means of guiding the management plan but also to protect the clinician against subsequent litigation.

Any physical consequences of any self-harming behaviour need to be treated. Doctors are often faced with a situation where a patient has presented to A&E but then refuses treatment. In these cases involvement of the liaison team can be helpful. A longer interview allowing the patient to talk through their issues can result in an agreement to have treatment. If this fails then the patient's capacity should be considered.

In more straightforward presentations the presence or absence of mental illness, the level of risk of repetition and the risk of completed suicide will determine any onward referral. In some cases discharge back to the GP with communication to the GP about the incident will suffice. Signposting to various sources of support may be useful. Links to websites offering support to anyone in distress include:

- Samaritans helpline 08457909090 or www.samaritans.org
- International Association for Suicide Prevention at www.iasp.info/index.php
- Living Life to the Full at www.llttf.com
- The Mood Gym and e-couch at https://moodgym.anu.edu.au/welcome
- Self-help groups at www.patient.co.uk/selfhelp.asp
- The Kevin Hines Story at www.kevinhinesstory.com
- www.connectingwithpeople.org
- www.rcpsych.ac.uk/expertadvice.aspx.

In more serious cases referral to local mental health services may be appropriate. This is usually via the hospital-based liaison service but every hospital will have a referral pathway to the local mental health service.

Legislative framework (Mental Health Act versus Mental Capacity Act)

Mental Capacity Act 2005 Part 1

- The MCA provides a framework for decision making on behalf of people who lack capacity to decide for themselves, where there is an underlying disorder of mind or brain, permanent or temporary.
- The MCA applies to all aspects of life not simply for physical and mental disorder. This Act only applies to those over 16 years of age.
- The MCA is underpinned by *five principles*:
  1. Assumption of capacity
  2. Presumption of incapacity only after all practical steps have been taken to aid decision making
  3. An unwise decision is not necessarily an indication of lack of capacity
  4. Best interests principle

5. Regard to the option which least restricts the individual's rights and freedoms.

- A person will be deemed not to have capacity under the MCA if that person is unable to make the particular decision if, after all appropriate help and support to make the decision has been given to them (principle 2), they cannot do the following things:
  1. Understand the information relevant to that decision, including understanding the likely consequences of making, or not making the decision
  2. Retain that information
  3. Use or weigh that information as part of the process of making the decision
  4. Communicate their decision (whether by talking, using sign language or any other means).

- The capacity of an individual following self-harm may be impaired temporarily due to the presence of drugs or alcohol, their state of distress, confusion, shock, pain or fatigue. Even an apparently calm individual may express a wish to die but you should consider if there is evidence of a deep ambivalence about dying given that they have actually presented to hospital for treatment.

- In depressed individuals, or those who have suffered recent loss, their depressive ideation may cause them to lose touch with the reasons for staying alive, meaning they are unable to weigh information appropriately.

- The more serious the outcome of the decision, the higher the level of capacity needed.

Mental Health Act 1983

- The MHA is used where *further assessment and treatment of a disorder of the mind is required* in the absence of consent, whether due to lack of capacity or valid refusal of treatment.

- Where an individual is considered to have capacity but is thought to be suffering from a mental disorder then assessment under the MHA should be considered. Early involvement of mental health services in these complicated cases is appropriate.

- There are no defined principles underpinning the MHA but the Code of Practice suggests that

decisions made under the Act should promote autonomy and be the least restrictive possible.

- If a person, whom the doctor considers is mentally disordered, is stating a desire to leave hospital, and this would present a risk either to themselves or others, then the doctor can apply *Section 5/2 of the MHA*, which allows the patient to be detained in hospital for 72 hours whilst a Mental Health Act assessment is organized. S5/2 can only be used on *inpatients*. In a similar circumstance in the emergency department a person can only be held in hospital if they lack capacity and it is in their best interests so to do.

- A Mental Health Act assessment, carried out by two doctors, at least one being approved under the MHA as having psychiatric expertise (S12 approved), and an Approved Mental Health Practitioner, usually a social worker, determines whether a patient should be further detained under the MHA or released from the S5/2.

- Any doctor other than F1 grade doctors can detain under S5/2 or be the second doctor in a Mental Health Act assessment.

- *Section 2* of the MHA allows for detention for 28 days for further assessment in hospital and possibly treatment. *Section 3* allows detention for up to 6 months for treatment in hospital.

- The MHA requires specific documentation to be filled in. (There is no equivalent in the MCA unless there is significant deprivation of liberty, for which a set of safeguards has been established.)

- *Part IV (Consent to Treatment)* of the MHA authorizes treatment for mental disorder and for people detained under the MHA (sections 2, 3 for example). The only exception to this is *S5/2, which does not allow treatment* under the MHA. So, for example, if a patient detained on S5/2 were to become so disturbed that sedation was required, assuming they lacked capacity to refuse, *then the sedation could be given under the MCA.*

- Treatment for the *physical consequences of mental disorder, such as the consequences of self-harm, can be given under the MHA.* This is now established in case law [7]. In the case of *B* v. *Croydon Health Authority* (1995), the judge stated:

It would seem strange to me if a hospital could, without the patient's consent, give him treatment directed to alleviating a psychopathic disorder showing itself in suicidal tendencies, but not without such consent be able to treat the consequences of the suicide attempt

- In cases of self-harm by people with a *personality disorder* the decision as to whether they should be placed under the Mental Health Act and given treatment can be a difficult one and a psychiatric opinion should be sought.
- Patients detained under the MHA have an automatic right of appeal and their rights under Part 5 of the Human Rights Act are recognized.
- In some cases a patient might qualify for detention under either Act. In these circumstances, where it is anticipated there will be significant deprivation of liberty or the requirement for repeated restraint, then treatment under the MHA is more appropriate.

Scenario 59.1 continued

Reluctantly Miss P's partner agrees to her to being interviewed alone and then abruptly leaves the department. Careful enquiry reveals that the bruises are the result of physical abuse by her partner. She does not wish to take any action in regard to this. She becomes increasingly distressed and agitated when she learns he has left the hospital and continues to refuse investigation.

After discussion with the liaison team and the duty psychiatrist it is agreed that further investigations and any treatment necessary will be carried out in her best interest under the MCA. Once she is told this, she complies with the management plan. She is deemed to lack capacity on the grounds that:

- Her level of consciousness is slightly impaired.
- She is distressed and therefore unable to consider her actions.
- There may be a degree of coercion involved in her wishing to leave the hospital.

Once medically fit she requires further psychiatric follow-up. She is a vulnerable adult being subjected to physical abuse presenting with signs and symptoms of mental disorder; there is a risk of repetition. The

question of a child at risk also needs to be addressed and this should be flagged up to mental health services and the GP. Further enquiry will determine whether involvement of social services is warranted.

Scenario 59.2 continued

Although Mr J is felt to lack capacity in relation to treatment due to his state of mind, it is felt that a more specialist psychiatric opinion is needed. He appears to need treatment for a mental disorder which may well involve detention in hospital and therefore the MHA is the more appropriate vehicle with which to proceed. A Mental Health Act assessment is requested via local psychiatric services.

References

1. Office for National Statistics (2011) Suicides in the United Kingdom. ONS.

2. *Rabone* v. *Pennine Care NHS Foundation Trust* (2012).

3. *Savage* v. *South Essex Partnership NHS Foundation Trust* (2008) UKHL 74.

4. Royal College of Psychiatrists (2010) Self-Harm, Suicide and Risk: Helping People who Self-Harm (College Report CR158). Royal College of Psychiatrists.

5. Cole-King A, Parker V, Williams H, Platt S (2013) Suicide prevention: are we doing enough? *Advances in Psychiatric Treatment* 19: 284–291.

6. Sarkar J (2013) To be or not to be: legal and ethical considerations in suicide prevention. *Advances in Psychiatric Treatment* 19: 295–301.

7. *B* v. *Croydon Health Authority* (1995) 1 All ER 683.

Further reading

Hines K, Cole-King A, Blaustein M (2013) Hey kid, are you OK? A story of suicide survived. *Advances in Psychiatric Treatment* 19: 292–294.

Royal College of Psychiatrists (2010) Self-Harm, Suicide and Risk: Helping People who Self-Harm (College Report CR158). Royal College of Psychiatrists.

Chapter

60

Swallowing difficulties (dysphagia)

Iftikhar Ahmed and Rudi Matull

Introduction

Dysphagia, commonly referred to in the acute take as 'difficulty in swallowing', is often described as a feeling of food sticking retrosternally or in the neck. It is a common condition reported by as many as 5–8% of the general population aged over 50 years. Other presentations of 'dysphagia' include meal-related regurgitation, a sense of fullness retrosternally, or hiccuping during meals. A significant proportion of patients with stroke are affected by dysphagia, predominantly oropharyngeal, which can be the only presenting feature. It poses an increased risk of aspiration pneumonia, undernutrition and dehydration.

Physiology of swallowing

Oral cavity phase is the voluntary elevation of the tongue against the palate after closing the mouth, which forces the bolus to the pharynx and triggers the swallowing reflex.

Pharyngeal phase is involuntary during which the soft palate is elevated against the posterior pharyngeal wall, sealing the nasopharynx, and the larynx is elevated closing the laryngeal inlet. This prevents aspiration and forces the food to the upper part of the oesophagus, this initiating the:

Oesophageal phase by starting the peristaltic contraction of the cricopharyngeal muscle and opening up the upper oesophageal sphincter (UOS). As the peristalsis progresses further down, the UOS closes and the lower oesophageal sphincter (LOS) opens up, allowing the food bolus to enter into the stomach after which the LOS closes again.

Classification of dysphagia

Oropharyngeal dysphagia is due to disorders of the oropharyngeal musculature:

- peripheral (neuromuscular diseases)
- central (e.g. stroke).

Oesophageal dysphagia is due to disorders of:

- oesophageal motility (e.g. achalasia)
- structural lesions of oesophageal wall or lumen (e.g. stricture, ulcerated tumours).

> **Scenario 60.1**
>
> A 65-year-old man is referred by his GP with a 2-month history of progressive dysphagia for solids and 1 stone(6 kg) weight loss. He is an ex-smoker and previously drank 40–50 units of alcohol per week. He has previously been treated for symptoms of gastro-oesophageal reflux disease. When seen he is only able to swallow liquids.

History

- *Is it true dysphagia or 'globus'?* Globus is a painless sensation of lump or fullness in the throat in the absence of any deglutition impairment, usually present in between meals, often with a feeling of dry mouth and improves with eating [1].
- *Is it oropharyngeal or oesophageal dysphagia?* Symptoms which favour oropharyngeal dysphagia are:
  - presence of cough on swallowing
  - nasal regurgitation
  - frequent throat clearing
  - dysphonia
  - delayed oropharyngeal swallow initiation
  - aspiration is common with excessive coughing or choking when swallowing.
- Neurological diseases (central) are the commonest cause.
- *Is dysphagia acute or chronic?*

Acute Medicine, ed. Stephen Haydock, Duncan Whitehead and Zoë Fritz. Published by Cambridge University Press. © Cambridge University Press 2015.

- Acute dysphagia usually implies mechanical obstruction, more frequently food bolus on the background of some underlying luminal pathology (oesophageal stricture, web, solid lesion) or oesophageal spasm. It can also be a presenting symptom of stroke.
- Chronic dysphagia is often caused by intraluminal pathology such as malignancy or external compression in the case of mediastinal lesions; though a long time line can also be seen with advanced dysmotility, e.g. achalasia.
- *Is dysphagia progressive or intermittent?*
  - Intermittent dysphagia, particularly for solids, is more likely caused by oesophageal web/rings, and in rare cases, eosinophilic oesophagitis (see below). Oesophageal dysmotility, e.g. spasms, can often present with intermittent dysphagia to liquids.
  - Progressive painless dysphagia more likely reflects luminal or extraluminal obstruction, often neoplastic, while progressive dysphagia with pain and regurgitation can be a sign of additional *Candida* infestation or be caused by achalasia.
- *Does the patient have dysphagia for solid only, liquid only or both?*
  - Solids only suggests a structural abnormality.
  - Both solids and liquids suggest a motility abnormality, though advanced, tight strictures will also result in inability to swallow liquids.
- *Is it painful or painless?*
  - Painful dysphagia suggests spasm, severe inflammation or ulcers.
  - Painless dysphagia suggests an intraluminal solid lesion or stricture.
- *Odynophagia* is painful swallowing, even without dysphagia, and suggests:
  - oesophageal spasm
  - severe oesophageal inflammation (e.g. reflux- or *Candida*-related)
  - ulceration
  - oesophageal rupture (Boerhaave's syndrome), a potentially life-threatening condition, when there is acute odynophagia after severe retching or recurrent vomiting.
- *A pharyngeal pouch* ('Zenker's diverticulum') causes:
  - sensation of food sticking in the throat
  - coughing on swallowing
  - regurgitation of undigested food hours after eating
  - fetor ex ore (halitosis)
  - borborygmi in the neck.

Examination

- Evidence of neurological and neuromuscular diseases causing dysphagia. However, the absence of neurological signs does not preclude the presence of significant pharyngeal neuromuscular dysfunction.
- The oral cavity and pharynx are carefully inspected for any mucosal lesions, masses and symmetry of soft palate.
- Examine neck for masses, e.g. goitre.
- Dysphagia due to underlying malignancy tends to lead to significant weight loss.
- Skin changes of connective tissue disorders, particularly scleroderma and CREST syndrome (calcinosis, Raynaud's phenomenon, (o)esophageal dysmotility, sclerodactyly and telangiectasia).
- Muscle weakness or wasting may suggest myositis (poly- or dermatomyositis).
- Signs of malnutrition, weight loss and pulmonary complications from aspiration.

Important causes of oesophageal and oropharyngeal dysphagia are given in Table 60.1.

Investigations

The majority of dysphagia requires early investigation, the main concern being risk of aspiration and possible malignancy.

Initial laboratory investigations should include:

- FBC
- urea and electrolytes (including creatinine)
- LFTs
- calcium
- magnesium
- phosphate
- coagulation.

Further tests are dictated by the clinical suspicion.

Gastroscopy provides both diagnostic and therapeutic benefits:

- biopsy of luminal lesions
- dilatation of benign strictures
- injection therapy for achalasia

- foreign bodies/food bolus removal.

Barium swallow study is useful in:

- detecting obstructive lesions (strictures, large hiatus hernia, achalasia)
- delineating postoperative anatomical relationship and intactness of anti-reflux repair.

Video-fluoroscopy is investigation of choice for:

- Evaluation of oropharyngeal dysphagia and tends to be performed by the speech and language therapist (SALT).
- A video-fluoroscopic swallowing study permits detailed examination of the swallow mechanism, including the opening characteristics of the upper oesophageal sphincter, which is often a blind spot at endoscopy or barium swallow examination because of lack of adequate distension.

CT scan of the neck:

- Can reveal rare structural causes such as cervical osteophytes or extraluminal malignancy.

CT chest/abdomen:

- Excludes pseudo-achalasia when extraluminal compression is suspected.

pH-oesophageal manometry:

- Is indicated if no structural abnormality is found.
- If available a high-resolution manometry (oesophageal pressure topography) study has greatest sensitivity in the diagnosis of achalasia and other motility disorders, and concurrent impedance-based assessment of oesophageal transit may provide additional information regarding the completeness of bolus transit in the oesophagus or non-acidic, non-erosive reflux, which can be missed with pH studies.

Management

- Assess risk of aspiration (see below), severity of dehydration and malnutrition.
- Correct fluid and electrolyte imbalance (watch out for magnesium and phosphate if malnourished) and make a detailed recording of intake in cases of severe dehydration and renal impairment.
- Keep '*nil-by-mouth*' if risk of aspiration and request full SALT assessment. The *water-swallow test* can be an initial screening to assess the risk of aspiration in conscious patients.
  - The patient is sat-up well.

- Give a teaspoonful of water.
- Observe the initiation of swallow and any occurrence of coughing or alteration in voice quality.
- If there are no adverse signs, the patient is given a larger quantity to drink from a glass.

- If water-swallow test is positive or equivocal, a full swallow screening should be carried out by the SALT team, which may include video-fluoroscopy as described above.
- The SALT team will advise on dietary modification using various thicknesses of diet for pharyngeal dysphagia and swallow therapy should be considered in order to minimize risk of aspiration. During swallow therapy, patients are taught postural manoeuvres and exercises to strengthen swallowing muscles to maintain oral feeding. Naso-enteral tube feeding may be necessary in some cases where adequate alimentation and hydration by mouth is not achieved. One has to consider risk of refeeding syndrome while commencing feeding in a patient at risk.
- For oesophageal dysphagia further assessment would be as shown in Figure 60.1.

Some important causes of dysphagia

Achalasia

Achalasia is defined by absent peristalsis and impaired deglutitive lower oesophageal sphincter (LOS) relaxation and diffuse oesophageal spasm by as evidenced by ≥20% of test swallows showing simultaneous or spastic contractions in the oesophagus. It is considered to be due to loss of ganglionic cells in the myenteric plexus of the oesophageal wall and impaired relaxation of LOS and can present in young adults.

Investigation

- Barium swallow shows oesophageal dilatation with a tapered 'bird beak' appearance at the gastro-oesophageal junction.
- Oesophageal manometry helps to confirm the diagnosis (lack of LOS relaxation on swallow).
- Endoscopy is required to exclude intraluminal lesions.
- CT scan of the chest/abdomen is sometimes considered to exclude an extraluminal lesion such as a tumour causing compression of the oesophagus (pseudo-achalasia).

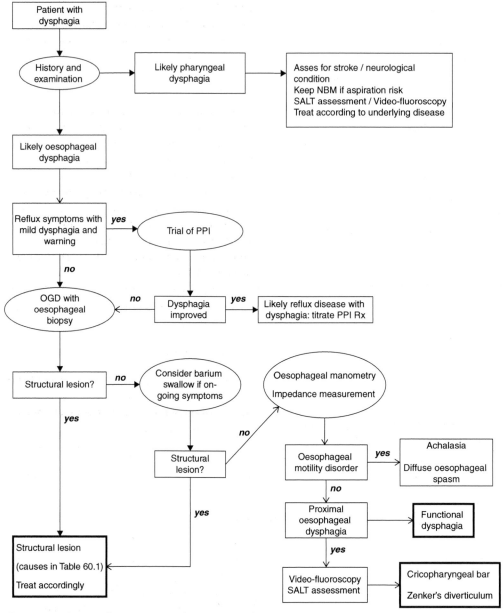

Figure 60.1 Algorithm for assessment and management of dysphagia.

Management

- *Dilatation of LOS*: balloon dilatation (3–4 cm diameter) has a success rate as high as 85% in the first year. Repeated dilatation is often required. The risk of oesophageal rupture of up to 5% is a significant concern.
- *Surgical myotomy* (Heller's myotomy) produces symptomatic relief in 90% of patients and is superior to pneumatic balloon dilatation in the surgically fit patient.
- *Botulinum toxin injection*: of the lower oesophageal sphincter (LOS) during endoscopy to cause paralysis of LOS and reduce pressure. Symptom improvement rates can be as high as 80%; however, repeat injections tend to be required, as the effect wears off with time (approx. 6 months). This is particularly helpful in elderly

patient where risk of complications of dilatation may be higher.

- *Medical treatment*: nitrate or calcium channel blocker such as nifedipine may only help in early achalasia, which tends however to progress over time.

Other oesophageal motility disorder

These usually cause chest pain and sometimes regurgitation and the dysphagia may be to both solids and liquids. This term includes [2]:

- diffuse oesophageal spasm
- nutcracker oesophagus
- rarely spasm of the lower oesophageal sphincter.

Investigation

- Confirmed by oesophageal manometry.

Management

- Is often difficult; it tends to include medication trials with calcium channel blocker or nitrate, and swallowing education (SALT).

Oesophageal stricture

Oesophageal strictures can be benign and malignant. Benign or peptic stricture is a complication of acid reflux; higher risk of malignancy is associated with older age, male gender and longer duration of reflux symptoms. Other conditions include:

- corrosive intake
- post-surgical resection for oesophageal or laryngeal cancer
- nasogastric tube placement
- infectious oesophagitis (such as caused by herpes zoster virus)
- radiation exposure.

Symptoms of peptic strictures are usually insidious but progressive, beginning with dysphagia to solids followed by dysphagia to liquids, heartburn and regurgitation.

Management

- Anti-acid medications (e.g. PPIs).
- Dietary modification for GORD such as no eating at bedtime, remaining upright after eating.
- Smoking cessation.

- Established cases with scarring may require oesophageal dilatation, which often needs repeating, normally up to a lumen diameter of 15 mm or bigger.

Oesophageal ring/web

- Oesophageal webs and rings are thin, fragile strictures that partially or completely compromise the oesophageal lumen causing intermittent dysphagia for solids, particularly when the ring diameter narrows to 13 mm or less.
- They can be solitary (often distal, probably linked to reflux) or multiple (e.g. due to NSAID intake).
- The sensation is usually short-lived, associated with chest discomfort, and relieved by regurgitating the food bolus, drinking liquids, or positional changes.
- Some patients present with acute dysphagia after swallowing a large piece of meat (termed the 'steak house' syndrome).

Eosinophilic oesophagitis

- Rare condition, usually affecting younger patients and causing intermittent dysphagia [3].
- Endoscopic findings are often subtle (furrows) or absent, and diagnosis is made on histology.
- Biopsies should be obtained from lower and mid-oesophagus at the time of endoscopy regardless of visual abnormalities in order to evaluate for eosinophilic oesophagitis.

Management

- Usually consists of topical steroids, e.g. beclometasone inhaler is advised to be swallowed 2–3 times a day [4].
- Dietary modification (e.g. six food elimination diet: milk, egg, wheat, soya, peanuts/tree nuts and seafood (fish/shellfish)) has shown success in children.

Oesophageal cancer

One of the common gastrointestinal malignancies, incidence is increasing (4/100 000 per year for squamous cell and 132/100 000 for adenocarcinoma worldwide) and carries a poor prognosis.

Risk factors include:

- smoking

Table 60.1 Causes of oesophageal and oropharyngeal dysphagia

Oesophageal dysphagia

Structural causes		Inflammatory causes	Motility causes	Anatomical causes	Systemic disease
Intramural	**Extramural**				
Primary cancer (squamous cell cancer, adenocarcinoma)	Mediastinal masses	Oesophagitis due to acid reflux disease	Idiopathic achalasia	Para-oesophageal hiatus hernia	Scleroderma
Secondary malignancy (metastasis from breast cancer, melanoma)	Bronchial cancer	Eosinophilic oesophagitis	Pseudo-achalasia	Oesophageal diverticulum	Lichen planus
GI stromal tumour	Oesophageal compression	Radiation oesophagitis	Diffuse oesophageal spasm	Schatzki's ring	Pemphigus and pemphigoid condition
Granular cell tumour		Pill-induced oesophagitis	Nutcracker oesophagus		
		Chemical oesophagitis	Chagas disease		

Oropharyngeal dysphagia

Central causes	Neuromuscular causes	Others
Stroke	Dermatomyositis	Zenker's diverticulum
Parkinson's disease	Poliomyelitis	
Brainstem disease	Muscular dystrophy	
Multiple sclerosis	Myasthenia gravis	
Motor neurone disease		
Head injury		
Drug such as phenothiazine		

- alcohol
- chronic stasis (e.g. chronic achalasia) for squamous cell cancer
- male sex, old age and chronic reflux and Barrett's oesophagus for adenocarcinoma.
  Symptoms include:
- dysphagia
- sometimes odynophagia
- eventually unintentional weight loss.

Investigation

- Diagnosis is made on endoscopy and histology.
- Staging is by means of CT chest/abdomen/pelvis.

- PET-CT scan and endoscopic ultrasound for loco-regional spread assessment for potential curative resection, *if* the patient is considered fit enough and *if* initial staging CT is negative.

Management

TNM classification is used to stage the disease (Table 60.2) and dictates treatment.

A multidisciplinary team approach is key to the successful management of patients with oesophageal cancer. A team consisting of gastroenterologist, radiologist, oncologist, palliative care, oncology nurse specialist and oesophago-gastric surgeon should review individual cases to decide the best treatment option for each patient.

Table 60.2 Staging and treatment options of oesophageal cancer

Disease extent	Stage	TNM classification	Treatment options
Confined to wall	0	TisN0M0	1. Photodynamic therapy 2. +/– EMR 3. Oesophagectomy
	I	T1 (intramucosal) N0M0	1. Photodynamic therapy 2. +/– EMR 3. Oesophagectomy
	I	T1 (submucosal) N0M0	Oesophagectomy
	IIA	T1–2N0M0	Oesophagectomy
Local lymph node involvement	IIB	T1–2 N1M0	Combined radiotherapy and chemotherapy
	III	T3 N1M0	
		T4 N0M0/T4N1M0	
Coeliac/supraclavicular lymph node involvement	IVA	Ta Na M1a	Combination chemotherapy and radiotherapy if in good health/palliative therapy
Distant metastasis	IVB	Ta Na M1b	Palliative therapy (e.g. oesophageal stent)

When to seek specialist advice for dysphagia

Where possible, multidisciplinary team involvement should be sought while managing patients with dysphagia who are suspected to have complex underlying aetiology or are on the verge of developing complications.

Oropharyngeal dysphagia

- The SALT team should be involved early to assess the swallowing in order to prevent the risk of aspiration.
- The stroke team should be involved in patients suspected of pharyngeal dysphagia due to stroke.
- ENT opinion is sought when oropharyngeal dysphagia is suspected.

Oesophageal dysphagia

A gastroenterologist should be involved early in:

- patients with complete oesophageal dysphagia
- those who are nutritionally compromised
- those at high risk of refeeding syndrome.

The oncology team should be involved where cause of dysphagia is found to be oesophageal cancer. Similarly palliative input should be requested in cases of advanced or metastatic malignancy where symptomatic treatment is the only practical option.

References

1. Lee BE, Kim GH. Globus pharyngeus; a review of its aetiology, diagnosis and treatment. *World J Gastroenterol* 2012; 18(20): 2462–2471.

2. Spechler SJ, Castell DO. Classification of oesophageal motility abnormalities. *Gut* 2001; 49: 145–151.

3. Prasad GA, Talley NJ, Romero Y, et al. Prevalence and predictive factors of eosinophilic esophagitis in patients presenting with dysphagia: a prospective study. *Am J Gastroenterol* 2007; 102: 2627.

4. Arora AS, Yamazaki K. Eosinophilic esophagitis: asthma of the oesophagus? *Clin Gastroenterol Hepatol* 2004; 2: 523–530.

Further reading

Cook IJ. Treatment of oropharyngeal dysphagia. *Curr Treat Options Gastroenterol* 2003; 6: 273–281.

Cook IJ. Diagnostic evaluation of dysphagia. *Nat Clin Pract* 2008; 7(5):1364–1370.

Kuo P, Holloway RH, Nguyen NQ. Current and future techniques in the evaluation of dysphagia. *J Gastroenterol Hepatol* 2012; 27: 873–881.

Lind CD. Dysphagia: evaluation and treatment. *Gastroenterol Clin North Am* 2003; 32(2): 553–575.

SIGN. Management of Patients with Stroke: Identification and Management of Dysphagia. SIGN Guideline 2010.

Syncope/collapse

Mark Dayer

(See also Chapter 24 'Fits and seizures' and Chapter 11 'Blackout/collapse: cardiac pacemakers')

Introduction

The terms 'blackout', 'syncope' and 'seizure' are used loosely and interchangeably in medicine.

A *blackout* is a temporary loss of memory or consciousness with complete recovery. The fact that it is transient is important to the definition. A blackout can have many causes (Figure 61.1). The three most common causes are:

- syncope
- epilepsy
- psychogenic attacks.

Syncope is defined as a transient deficiency of oxygen in the brain that results in a loss of consciousness, or a near loss of consciousness (*presyncope*). An *epileptic seizure* can also result in a loss of consciousness, but is defined as an episode of uncontrolled electrical activity of the brain. Psychogenic attacks presenting as transient loss of consciousness (TLoC) are referred to as *psychogenic pseudosyncope*.

TLoC is extremely common and will affect more than half of people during their lifetime. It accounts for 1–2% of emergency department visits. For most individuals it is a benign condition with no long-term adverse health consequences. However, it can be unsettling and worrying for patients and a proportion do have significant underlying disease. The accurate diagnosis of a blackout requires vigilance and a systematic approach. In this situation *the history is of paramount importance.*

This chapter will detail the principal cardiovascular causes of TLoC and detail the initial approach and management strategies for patients presenting in this way. It is extremely difficult to construct rules that are comprehensive enough to deal with every condition that may present with syncope and, to an extent,

experience and intuition are key. Neurological causes of transient loss of consciousness and differentiation from other causes of loss of consciousness are discussed in Chapter 24.

> **Scenario 61.1**
>
> *A 75-year-old man is referred by the ED. He 'collapsed' in the early hours of the morning in the bathroom. His wife recalls him getting out of bed to go to the toilet. She then heard a 'thud' and found him lying on the bathroom floor. She described him as 'pale and like he was asleep'. He came round after several seconds and initially after being a little disorientated he was soon 'back to normal' but unable to remember much of what happened. He has a past history of hypertension treated with bisoprolol 5 mg od and bendroflumethiazide 2.5 mg od. His ECG shows only a sinus bradycardia. He is keen to go home.*

Clinical approach

History

It is *imperative* to talk to both the person and any witnesses to obtain a detailed description of the event, including what happened both before and after. It is important to ascertain whether or not an episode of transient loss of consciousness has actually occurred. After obtaining a general description of the event, the following facts should be ascertained:

- posture prior to event – e.g. sitting or standing
- was the patient exerting themselves at the time of the event
- warning symptoms – e.g. feeling warm
- appearance – particularly the colour of the person during the event
- movement during the event

Acute Medicine, ed. Stephen Haydock, Duncan Whitehead and Zoë Fritz. Published by Cambridge University Press.
© Cambridge University Press 2015.

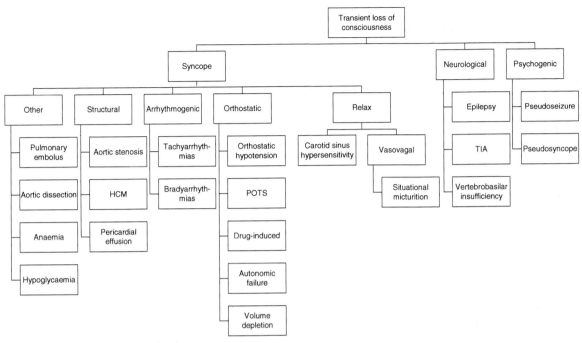

Figure 61.1 Causes of blackouts within three main groups.

- tongue biting
- other injuries sustained
- duration of the event
- whether the patient was confused whilst recovering
- presence of focal weakness.

It may transpire that the person has had a fall or has vertigo rather than a TLoC and therefore requires different management, beyond the scope of this chapter. If the history is not clear, however, it is safer to assume that they have had a TLoC, in which case:

- It is important to ascertain whether these events have happened before, how many times and when.
- A full past medical history should be obtained.
- Any family history of cardiac disease or sudden cardiac death is important to elicit.
- Medication, particularly diuretics and medications that lower blood pressure, should be recorded.

Examination

- Specific attention should be paid to the cardiovascular and neurological examination.
- Heart failure and murmurs may indicate significant underlying cardiac disease.

- Neurological signs, such as unilateral weakness, may indicate a neurological cause.
- Record vital signs including erect and supine blood pressure.
- The tongue should be carefully evaluated for tongue biting.
- Signs of bleeding, blood glucose, and response to carotid sinus massage may be useful depending on the clinical history (see later).

Initial investigations

A 12-lead ECG is imperative. NICE guidelines [1] recommend using a machine with automated interpretation, but it should be remembered that the interpretation may be inaccurate. Serious abnormalities that may require further evaluation include:

- inappropriate bradycardias, regardless of aetiology
- any sustained ventricular or supraventricular arrhythmia
- an abnormally short (QTc <350 ms) or long QT (QTc >450 ms) interval
- Brugada syndrome
- ventricular pre-excitation (Wolff–Parkinson–White syndrome)

- ventricular hypertrophy
- abnormal ST segments and T waves
- pathological Q waves
- left or right bundle branch block
- bifascicular and trifascicular block.

When the ECG is abnormal, other investigations, such as blood tests or a chest X-ray, may be indicated depending on the clinical scenario. When the ECG is abnormal, echocardiography should be undertaken. We have detailed many other conditions that may lead to syncope, which require specific investigations, but there will usually be other symptoms and signs.

Who needs admission and who needs specialist review?

One of the most difficult aspects of the management of a case of TLoC is deciding who needs admission, who needs specialist review and who can be safely reassured and not followed up. The decision to admit or discharge a patient will depend in part on local policies and how quickly outpatient assessment by an expert can be obtained. It is impossible to prescribe rules to cover all eventualities and experience and intuition are important.

Sometimes the decision is straightforward:

- A clear story of vasovagal syncope in the context of a normal examination and ECG can be safely reassured and discharged.
- Documented serious arrhythmias require specialist review prior to discharge.

It is the clinically stable patients where there is no clear cause that can be challenging to manage and clinical judgement is required. Generally speaking, higher risk patients will be older, may have abnormal ECGs or evidence of structural heart disease, they may have sustained an injury, and syncope will have occurred when sitting or lying. Lower risk patients will tend to have become syncopal whilst standing, they will be younger, and have a normal clinical examination and investigations.

To assist with such patients a number of syncope scoring systems have been developed, the most widely used and studied of which are the OESIL (Osservatorio Epidemiologico sulla Sincope nel Lazio) [2], and SFSR (San Francisco Syncope Rule) [3].

The OESIL score was derived from a study of 270 patients presenting with syncope. The study identified that four factors predicted an adverse outcome:

1. Age >65 years
2. A history of cardiovascular disease
3. Syncope without warning
4. An abnormal ECG.

The score ranged from 0 to 4 (an arithmetic sum of the number of risk factors) and mortality increased with the number of factors.

The SFSR was derived from a cohort of 684 patients. A rule that included five factors was found to be predictive of a serious outcome. These factors were:

1. Congestive heart failure
2. Haematocrit = less than 30%
3. Abnormal ECG
4. Shortness of breath
5. Systolic BP <90 mmHg at triage.

Both of these scoring systems performed well in the initial cohort of patients; however, both have fared less well when they have been validated by other studies. Therefore *neither of these scoring systems can be used to definitively answer the question, but may help clarify thinking.*

Current *NICE guidelines* recommend admission and review by a cardiologist within 24 hours for patients who have:

- any of the previously described ECG abnormalities
- cardiac failure
- transient loss of consciousness occurring on exertion
- a family history of sudden cardiac death in person aged <40 years and/or an inherited cardiac condition
- age over 65 years with no prodromal symptoms
- new or unexplained breathlessness
- a heart murmur.

A potential approach can be found in Figure 61.2. There are many, more complex approaches which have been suggested. Clearly these management suggestions are only that, and will not apply in all clinical situations. For example, it may be felt that an elderly patient with drug-induced postural hypotension requires admission to ensure that the situation has resolved.

Patients with any condition may require follow-up depending on the clinical context. For example, a single vasovagal event does not generally require follow-up, but if this is the third event in a week then the patient may well benefit from specialist management.

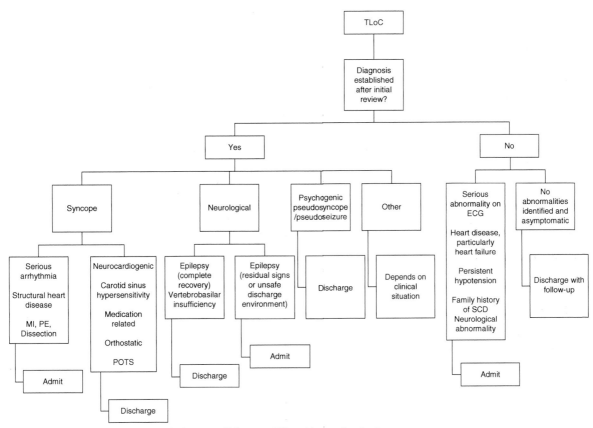

Figure 61.2 Deciding on admission, discharge and follow-up. SCD, sudden cardiac death.

When there is no clear diagnosis

After a thorough history, examination and basic investigations, there may be no clear diagnosis. NICE recommends subsequent referral of all patients for specialist cardiological opinion, except those in whom a firm diagnosis has been reached after initial assessment, or whose presentation is suspected to be due to a neurological cause, when onward referral to a neurologist is appropriate. You should make yourself aware of the local referral guidelines. NICE suggest that for all people with unexplained syncope an ambulatory ECG is appropriate, even if this is the first episode.

Driving restrictions

Although it is commonly overlooked, *all patients presenting with a loss of consciousness must be warned about the risks of driving*. There is detailed guidance on the DVLA website (www.dft.gov.uk/dvla/medical/aag. aspx) and reference should always be made to this site

as the advice changes frequently. Explaining to a patient that they cannot drive for a period of time is always difficult, but it is a crucial aspect of management.

Causes of syncope

Reflex syncope

Vasovagal syncope (VVS; also known as neurocardiogenic syncope)

Vasovagal syncope is the result of a reflex that results in vasodilation and bradycardia (occasionally tachycardia). It is the most common form of reflex syncope. Features that suggest a simple faint include:

- prolonged standing
- painful procedures, such as phlebotomy
- typical prodromal symptoms such as feeling hot immediately prior to an event.

If the history suggests that there has been a simple faint (vasovagal syncope) and it is a single episode then *no further action is required.* Patients with recurrent episodes, however, may have a significantly reduced quality of life and may benefit from seeing a cardiologist.

Typical patients are young and have no underlying medical problems, although older patients still suffer from VVS and it is still the most common cause of syncope in older patients. Typically, syncope is provoked by events such as venepuncture, although these may be difficult to identify in younger patients. Older individuals usually have more easy to identify triggers, for example micturition. The story of waking in the night to go to the toilet, followed by collapse, is particularly common in more elderly people; such patients can often sustain significant injuries.

Patients are typically aware that they may faint. They are usually sitting or standing. Lying flat typically restores consciousness within a short period, although feelings of malaise often persist for some time afterwards. Arrhythmias typically cause syncope that is more abrupt, whereas epilepsy causes syncope that is more prolonged. They may be aware when they come around that they are sweating. Witnesses may say that they looked pale and report that they were twitching and their eyes deviated to one side. A report of more prolonged tonic-clonic seizures is not typical for VVS. Tongue biting is unusual. Incontinence may occur.

The head-up tilt test produces a characteristic response that can be diagnostic, providing reasonable effort has been made to exclude other causes. Three responses are seen:

- The cardio-inhibitory response is characterized by sinus bradycardia and asystole.
- The vasodepressor response leads to hypotension.
- There is a mixed response with features of both. This is the most common, and characteristically hypotension precedes a fall in heart rate.

Management

Management of syncope may be *generally unsatisfactory.*

Lifestyle measures are the cornerstone of management:

- Education and reassurance as to the benign nature of the condition is key.
- Learning to recognize prodromal symptoms allows patients to change their posture (to a supine posture) or use physical counter pressure (e.g. hand grips) manoeuvres.

- Patients should be advised to avoid alcohol and remain well hydrated.
- Agents that lower blood pressure should be avoided.

Drug treatment is limited:

- Beta-blockers were thought to be helpful, but most trials have not supported their use.
- Fludrocortisone has not been shown to be effective in children and there are no trial data in adults.
- Midodrine, an alpha-agonist vasoconstrictor, may be effective, and is currently being trialled in POST IV [4].
- Serotonin reuptake inhibitors may also be helpful.
- Tilt-table training has not been shown to be helpful.
- Pacing may be helpful in patients with vasovagal syncope who have documented pauses associated with syncope of greater than 3 seconds or pauses of greater than 6 seconds without syncope; pacing has been shown to have a strong placebo effect.

Carotid sinus hypersensitivity

Carotid sinus hypersensitivity is an amplified response to stimulation of the carotid sinus baroreceptors. The resulting vagal activation/sympathetic inhibition leads to bradycardia and vasodilation, similar to vasovagal syncope. Patients may rarely report syncope on shaving or wearing a tight collar. It is a disease of older age and is rare below 40 years.

To make the diagnosis, carotid sinus massage should be performed:

- Massage for 10 seconds on each carotid body sequentially.
- Ensure full heart rate and blood pressure monitoring.
- It should not be performed if there has been a *stroke in the previous 3 months* or if there are *carotid bruits.*
- A fall in the blood pressure of greater than 50 mmHg or a pause of greater than 3 seconds is diagnostic.

Management

- General measures, as with vasovagal syncope, are recommended as first-line therapy.
- Drugs used to treat VVS may also be helpful although the data are more limited.

- Similarly, pacing may be helpful in those with a cardio-inhibitory response with induced pauses of greater than 3 seconds.

Orthostatic syncope

Orthostatic hypotension

Orthostatic hypotension has a typical history of syncope or presyncope shortly after standing. The diagnosis can be confirmed by measuring lying and standing blood pressure (over 3 minutes). Head-up tilt testing may be useful if the history is strongly suggestive, if lying and standing blood pressure measurements do not confirm the diagnosis. A fall of 20/10 mmHg or a decrease in the systolic blood pressure to less than 90 mmHg is considered positive.

Cardiovascular medications that lower blood pressure are a common cause. Diabetes, phaeochromocytoma, neurological conditions such as Parkinson's and conditions such as Ehlers–Danlos syndrome that affect collagen are also recognized.

Management

- General advice should be given to avoid hot environments/situations, including baths and saunas.
- Patients should be advised that suddenly getting up after lying down for a prolonged period is a behaviour that is particularly likely to bring on symptoms.
- Large meals may make the patient more vulnerable.
- Patients should be advised on waking to sit on their bed for a period of several minutes before standing.
- They should be taught physical counter manoeuvres.
- Elastic stockings may help.
- Patients should be advised not to restrict salt and to drink reasonable quantities of fluid (typically at least 2 L/day) unless other medical conditions prohibit.
- Specialist referral may be required to make a formal diagnosis, particularly if an underlying condition is suspected and sometimes to adjust medication.
- Medications such as fludrocortisone or the alpha-adrenoceptor agonist midodrine may be helpful [5].
- Pacing is not helpful.

Postural orthostatic tachycardia syndrome (POTS)

Postural orthostatic tachycardia syndrome [6] is a condition that tends to occur in younger adults. The diagnostic feature is a rapid rise in heart rate on standing associated with dizziness and light-headedness and sometimes syncope. Head-up tilt testing makes the diagnosis. A heart rate rise of greater than 30 beats per minute or an increase to 120 beats per minute within the first 10 minutes of tilt is diagnostic. Blood pressure does not fall excessively, but cerebral perfusion does.

Younger women are mainly affected. There may be a genetic element. The aetiology is uncertain and the disorder is probably heterogeneous. One intriguing hypothesis is that the heart is 'two sizes too small' and it has been postulated that it should be renamed The Grinch syndrome after the Dr Seuss character:

> The Grinch hated Christmas – the whole Christmas season … But I think that the most likely reason of all … may have been that his heart was two sizes too small.

There is usually evidence of hypovolaemia in addition.

Management

The best way to treat POTS remains uncertain.

- Volume expansion, with oral fluids, salt and possibly fludrocortisone may help.
- Physical exercise, particularly rowing, may also help.
- Some have used ivabradine successfully.
- A wide variety of other medications have been tried.

Arrhythmogenic syncope

Both tachycardias and bradycardias may cause syncope. In clinical experience, bradycardias are more common causes of syncope. Typically pauses of greater than 5 seconds may lead to syncope, although some people can tolerate much longer pauses. Both supraventricular (SVT) and ventricular tachycardias (VT) may cause syncope. Rates for sustained ventricular arrhythmias tend to have to be in excess of 180 bpm to lead to syncope, but rates as low as 140 bpm in severely diseased hearts may lead to syncope. Syncope is common in the context of SVTs too. In one study [7], almost 20% of patients with an SVT experienced syncope or presyncope. Surprisingly there was no difference in heart rates or the underlying mechanism of the arrhythmia between patients with and without syncope. The most common cause for syncope in the context of an SVT was, surprisingly, a vasovagal reaction.

Management

The management of arrhythmias is complex, and beyond the scope of this chapter.

- Device based therapy (see Chapter 11) is the mainstay of treatment for bradyarrhythmias and ventricular tachyarrhythmias.
- Ablation of the arrhythmic focus, particularly for supraventricular arrhythmias, is often performed.
- Generally, there is a low threshold to admit patients for monitoring who are thought to have been syncopal secondary to an arrhythmia. Patients who are admitted tend to be older, have injured themselves, and/or have a history of heart disease or an abnormal ECG; younger patients tend to be discharged.
- In patients in whom an arrhythmia is suspected (or cannot be excluded) who are deemed suitable for discharge or who are seen in the outpatient setting, prolonged ECG monitoring is recommended.
- A Holter monitor for as many days as is practical is recommended by NICE for patients with a single episode of unexplained syncope or with syncope several times per week.
- For patients with TLoC every 1–2 weeks an external event recorder is recommended.
- Those who are syncopal less often than once every 2 weeks should be offered an implantable loop recorder. This is a small device, around the size of a biro pen lid, but flatter, which can be implanted subcutaneously and will continuously monitor the ECG for around 3 years.

Note

There is always concern about patients with Wolff–Parkinson–White syndrome as there is a well-documented risk of sudden cardiac death. In one large study [8], patients presenting with a first episode of an AVRT who were followed up, had a rate of cardiac arrest that was approximately 0.8% per annum. The rate of syncope was considerably higher (approximately six times as high). Young men were at the highest risk of sudden cardiac death.

Structural heart disease can predispose to ventricular and supraventricular arrhythmias. Mitral valve disease is classically associated with atrial fibrillation.

Reduced left ventricular function of any aetiology predisposes to atrial fibrillation and, more importantly, ventricular arrhythmias. Arrhythmogenic right ventricular cardiomyopathy typically presents with ventricular arrhythmias. There are a number of 'channelopathies' (diseases which affect sodium and potassium channels in the heart) that also predispose to serious ventricular arrhythmias, including Brugada syndrome and long QT syndrome. Note that the characteristic ECG abnormalities may not be present at all times. A list of ECG abnormalities that should be looked for is given under 'Initial investigations' on pages 429–30.

Structural heart disease

Structural heart disease can cause syncope, particularly on exertion.

- Syncope is an established, although less common, symptom of severe aortic stenosis. The precise mechanism of syncope in patients with aortic stenosis remains unclear. Clinical examination should reveal the presence of significant aortic valve disease.
- Syncope can occur in patients with hypertrophic cardiomyopathy (HCM) either because of an arrhythmia (SVTs, VTs and asystole can occur) or secondary to haemodynamic disturbance – principally left ventricular outflow tract obstruction. Clinical examination and the ECG facilitate diagnosis; echocardiography and MRI are often required to confirm the diagnosis.
- Intracardiac tumours, for example left atrial myxomas, may present initially with syncope and presyncope.
- Pericardial effusions may also present with syncope and presyncope, particularly on exertion.

Other conditions

- Pulmonary embolism may present acutely with chest pain, shortness of breath and haemodynamic compromise. Syncope, particularly on exertion, is one well-recognized, but less common presentation, occurring in around 10% of patients with the condition.
- Aortic dissection is commonly misdiagnosed initially. Although the classic history is one of chest pain, radiating to the back, with haemodynamic compromise, it can present in

a variety of ways. A history of syncope is one recognized presenting feature. CT or MRI is the usual mode of imaging to confirm the diagnosis.

- It seems not uncommon for patients with syncope to be labelled as having had an episode of hypoglycaemia. This is unlikely, but not impossible. Syncope is a transient episode, whereas hypoglycaemia, unless treated, tends to progress and not reverse itself. There is one situation, however, in which transient hypoglycaemia can occur. Postprandial hypoglycaemia can cause a transient hypoglycaemia 1–2 hours after eating. It can occur after gastrectomy and bariatric surgery, but is commonly idiopathic. Modification of a patient's diet can ameliorate the condition.

- Anaemia when severe can lead to presyncope and syncope, particularly on exertion. Iron deficiency, interestingly, even in the absence of anaemia has been associated with vasovagal syncope. Erythropoietin is a successful treatment for syncope with a number of aetiologies.

References

1. Transient loss of consciousness ('blackouts') management in adults and young people. NICE clinical guideline 109. 2010.

2. Colivicchi F, Ammirati F, Melina D, Guido V, Imperoli G, Santini M. Development and prospective validation of a risk stratification system for patients with syncope in the emergency department: the OESIL risk score. *European Heart Journal* 2003; 24: 811–819.

3. Quinn JV, Stiell IG, McDermott DA, Sellers KL, Kohn MA, Wells GA. Derivation of the San Francisco Syncope Rule to predict patients with short-term serious outcomes. *Annals of Emergency Medicine* 2004; 43: 224–232.

4. Raj SR, Faris PD, McRae M, Sheldon RS. Rationale for the prevention of syncope trial IV: assessment of midodrine. *Clinical Autonomic Research* 2012; 22: 275–280.

5. Fu Q, Vangundy TB, Galbreath MM, et al. Cardiac origins of the postural orthostatic tachycardia syndrome. *Journal of the American College of Cardiology* 2010; 55: 2858–2868.

6. Frishman WH, Azer V, Sica D. Drug treatment of orthostatic hypotension and vasovagal syncope. *Heart Disease* 2003; 5: 49–64.

7. Brembilla-Perrot B, Beurrier D, Houriez P, Claudon O, Wertheimer J. Incidence and mechanism of presyncope and/or syncope associated with paroxysmal junctional tachycardia. *American Journal of Cardiology* 2001; 88: 134–138.

8. Pappone C, Vicedomini G, Manguso F, et al. Risk of malignant arrhythmias in initially symptomatic patients with Wolff-Parkinson-White syndrome: results of a prospective long-term electrophysiological follow-up study. *Circulation* 2012; 125: 661–668.

Further reading

Fitzpatrick AP, Cooper P. Diagnosis and management of patients with blackouts. *Heart* 2006; 92: 559–568.

Ventura R, Maas R, Ruppel R, et al. *Psychiatric conditions in patients with recurrent unexplained syncope. Europace: European Pacing, Arrhythmias, and Cardiac Electrophysiology* 2001; 3: 311–316.

Chapter 62

The unconscious patient

Christopher Westall and Kobus Preller

Introduction

Unconsciousness: a state of loss of awareness of self and environment from which the patient cannot be roused.

Coma: describes a state of unrousable unresponsiveness in which there is no coordinated response to external stimuli or inner need.

The difference between coma and unconsciousness is arbitrary; *coma implies a more prolonged duration and more profound unresponsiveness.*

The Glasgow Coma Scale (GCS) is the most widely used scale for describing the depth of unconsciousness (Table 62.1). A patient can be considered comatose at GCS scores of <8 (E2 V2 ≤M4).

- Always express GCS score in *absolute value and component score.*
- The motor element is the most sensitive predictor of severity and outcome.
- Presenting scores of 3–8 have a poorer prognosis than scores >8, but the *GCS is a poor predictor of outcome when the insult is not traumatic neurological injury* (original function of the scale).
- The GCS poorly reflects impairment of brainstem function.

The *Full Outline of UnResponsiveness (FOUR) score* (Table 62.2) is less commonly used but is a better descriptor of unconsciousness and a better prognostic indicator in non-trauma patients. The FOUR score does not include a verbal component and as such is more useful in dysphasic or intubated patients. A lower FOUR score describes a more profound unconsciousness.

Causes of unconsciousness

The causes of unconsciousness can be categorized in many ways. Generally they may be divided into primary neurological and systemic insults.

Table 62.1 The Glasgow Coma Scale

Eye opening (E)	Spontaneously	4
	To speech	3
	To pain	2
	No response	1
Verbal (V)	Normal speech	5
	Confused speech	4
	Inappropriate words	3
	Incomprehensible sounds	2
	No response	1
Motor (M)	Obeys commands	6
	Localizes to pain	5
	Withdraws from pain	4
	Inappropriate flexion to pain (decorticate posture)	3
	Inappropriate extension to pain (decerebrate) posture	2
	No response	1

1. Primary neurological insults

These may be associated with focal neurological deficits.

Traumatic head injury

Vascular

- Intracerebral haemorrhage: subdural, extradural or subarachnoid
- Cerebral infarction

Neoplastic

- Malignancy: primary or secondary with mass effect causing elevated ICP, obstructive hydrocephalus or haemorrhagic transformation
- Paraneoplastic syndrome
- Leptomeningitis
- Steroid psychosis

Acute Medicine, ed. Stephen Haydock, Duncan Whitehead and Zoë Fritz. Published by Cambridge University Press. © Cambridge University Press 2015.

Infective

- Meningitis: bacterial, fungal
- Encephalitis
- Cerebral malaria
- Cerebral abscess; either due to mass effect causing elevated ICP, obstructive hydrocephalus or haemorrhagic transformation

Inflammatory/autoimmune

- Cerebral vasculitis
- Autoimmune encephalitis: anti-voltage gated potassium channel or anti-NMDA receptor antibodies

Seizures

- Post-ictal
- Status epilepticus: convulsive and non-convulsive

Demyelination

- Central pontine myelinolysis
- Extra-pontine myelinolysis

Systemic insults

These are usually not associated with focal deficits.

Metabolic

- Hypoglycaemia
- Hepatic encephalopathy
- Uraemic encephalopathy
- Hypercapnia
- Hypothermia/hyperthermia
- Diabetic ketoacidosis/hyperglycaemic hyperosmolar state
- Hyponatraemia/hypernatraemia
- Hypercalcaemia/hypocalcaemia
- Hypomagnesaemia
- Wernicke's encephalopathy/B_{12} deficiency
- Hypothyroidism (myxoedema)
- Hypoadrenalism

Toxic

- Drugs: illicit and prescribed
- Benzodiazepines, opiates, antidepressants, neuroleptics, barbiturates, lithium
- Alcohols: ethanol, methanol
- Carbon monoxide
- Ethylene glycol
- Chemical weapons

Cardiovascular/reduced cerebral blood flow

- Shock (any cause)
- Arrhythmia
- Hypertensive encephalopathy

Psychiatric

- Catatonic state
- Severe depression

Scenario 62.1

A 25-year-old woman is admitted unconscious to the ED. She collapsed suddenly in front of friends on a night out in town. They were unable to rouse her and she was 'blue lighted' to the emergency department. Her friends are not aware of any medical problems and she had only a couple of drinks during the evening. Prior to the collapse she appeared entirely well. On arrival her GCS is 8 (E2 V2 M4).

You need to assess the patient and decide on immediate investigation and management.

Clinical assessment

Immediate assessment of the unconscious patient: the first 5 minutes

An unconscious patient is extremely vulnerable. Death will occur if asphyxiation secondary to airway obstruction occurs and neurological injury will be made worse if hypoxia, hypotension, hypoglycaemia and seizure activity are not immediately corrected. Assessment must be made rapidly with resuscitation in parallel; this should focus initially on airway, breathing and circulation. Always request help from nursing staff from the outset.

Cervical spine

- If there are signs of trauma or the presenting circumstances are unclear ensure that the cervical spine is immobilized and protected using a hard collar, blocks and tape or by manual in-line stabilization using an assistant.

Airway

- *Unconscious patients with a GCS <8* typically cannot maintain airway patency or protect their airway from aspiration and *usually require endotracheal intubation.* The clinical situation is the most important determinant when assessing whether a patient requires intubation. Patients

Table 62.2 The Full Outline of UnResponsiveness (FOUR) score

Eyes (E)			
	Eyes open and tracking/blink on command		4
	Eyes open, not tracking		3
	Eyes open only to speech		2
	Eyes open only to pain		1
	No eye opening		0
Motor (M)			
	Makes signs		4
	Localizes to pain		3
	Inappropriate flexion to pain (decorticate posture)		2
	Inappropriate extension to pain (decerebrate) posture		1
	No response or generalized myoclonus		0
Pupil reflexes	**Corneal reflexes**	**Cough**	
Present	Present	Present	4
One wide and fixed	Present	Present	3
Absent	Present	NA	2
Present	Absent	NA	2
Absent	Absent	Present	1
Absent	Absent	Absent	0
Respiration (R)			
Intubation	**Breathing**		
Not intubated	Regular		4
Not intubated	Cheyne–Stokes		3
Not intubated	Irregular		2
Not intubated	Apnoea		0
Intubated	Breathes above vent rate		1
Intubated	Breathes at vent rate		0

NA: not assessed.

with a GCS <8 due to a rapidly reversible or improving cause (e.g. hypoglycaemia or a post-ictal phase) may be managed with simple supportive measures. Conversely some patients presenting with a GCS ≥8 may benefit from early semi-elective intubation because it is anticipated that:

- they will deteriorate neurologically
- they will require transfer for investigation
- agitation is compromising treatment.

- In the absence of staff trained in rapid sequence intubation, airway patency should be maintained using airway manoeuvres and airway adjuncts such as an oropharyngeal, nasopharyngeal or supraglottic device as appropriate.
- *Airway adjuncts other than a cuffed endotracheal tube do not protect the patient against aspiration.* Aspiration is minimized by airway suctioning and

by nursing the patient head-down in the left lateral position.

Breathing

- Institute arterial oxygen saturation monitoring as soon as possible.
- Obtain an arterial blood gas early. This will provide useful information regarding oxygenation, adequacy of ventilation, usually a glucose level and a quick screen for metabolic disturbances. *Always look at the carboxyhaemoglobin level in an unconscious patient.*
- An unconscious patient may exhibit a disordered respiratory pattern. If this results in ineffective ventilation, the arterial $PaCO_2$ will rise, causing a respiratory acidaemia and further neurological depression. Hypercapnia and acidaemia are

harmful to cerebral blood flow and neurological function and should be avoided.

- Endotracheal intubation and mechanical ventilation may be required to maintain effective ventilation.
- Unconscious patients may present with coexistent lung injury by many mechanisms including aspiration of gastric contents and inhalation of smoke or water. Endotracheal intubation may be required to maintain arterial oxygen saturations.
- In the absence of staff trained in rapid sequence intubation, breathing should be supported by high-flow supplemental oxygen or manual ventilation using a self-inflating bag system.
- Some patients with known pulmonary disease are dependent on hypoxic respiratory drive. *Unless this is clearly the case, hypoxia should be corrected to achieve arterial oxygen saturations ≥94% until further history can be established.*

Circulation

- Institute cardiac monitoring as soon as possible. Obtain a 12-lead ECG.
- Obtain intravenous access as soon as possible; blood should be taken during venous cannulation for haematological, coagulation, biochemical and microbiological samples. Unnecessary samples can be discarded later.
- Mean arterial pressure should initially be maintained within the normal range (≥65 mmHg).
- The volume status of the patient should be carefully assessed and corrected. Hypotonic fluids such as glucose solutions should be avoided, as should large volume infusions unless clearly indicated, as both can promote cerebral oedema formation.
- Vasopressor support may be required early.

Disability

- The presenting GCS or FOUR score should be recorded as total score and breakdown; it may provide useful prognostic information at a later time. This is particularly important if the patient is subsequently anaesthetized for intubation.
- Is there evidence of seizure activity? Ongoing seizure activity may not always manifest as obvious tonic-clonic type activity, *subtle abnormal facial or localized limb movements should be*

actively searched out. Seizures should be treated promptly.

- Status epilepticus is defined as seizure activity lasting for more than 30 minutes or ongoing seizure activity without intervening recovery of consciousness. Persistence of seizure activity for >1 hour is associated with poorer neurological outcomes.

Exposure

If there is good evidence of an easily reversible cause for unconsciousness, this should be addressed as early as possible.

Glucose

- Measure capillary glucose as soon as possible.
- Hypoglycaemia <4 mmol/L should be treated with 50 mL of 50% glucose as an intravenous bolus.
- In suspected alcohol abuse or malnourishment, intravenous B-vitamins (thiamine 200 mg as Pabrinex, 1 pair of ampoules) should be given early and before glucose replacement. *Do not delay glucose therapy if severely hypoglycaemic.*

Secondary assessment of the unconscious patient

Once the patient is stabilized, a thorough assessment should be made to formulate a differential diagnosis, guide and prioritize investigation and identify key neurological features that may immediately alter management.

History

Ironically *there are few situations where a good history is as important.* Information should be gathered from every source available: friends and family, bystanders, emergency service personnel, ambulance call sheets and old medical records. The key aspects are:

- Where, how and by whom the patient was found.
- Time course of events. This will discriminate between a large number of potential causes.
- Prodromal features prior to unconsciousness. Epilepsy may be associated with a stereotyped, complex warning. Headache may point to subarachnoid haemorrhage. Chronic headache or (early morning) projectile vomiting suggests a space-occupying lesion.
- Past medical history.

- Medications. Ask specifically about opioids, anti-neuropathic analgesics, antidepressants and antipsychotics, thyroxine and long-term corticosteroids.
- Alcohol and illicit drug use.
- Foreign travel history.

General examination

The physical examination may provide useful clues in the absence of a corroborating history.

- *Look at how the patient is dressed.* Are they well groomed or unkempt? Is their dress incongruous to the time of day or weather?
- *Check the patient's pockets* and any items found with them. Is there evidence of illicit drug use, overdose or alcohol abuse? Are there any forms of identification or contact numbers for family and friends?
- *Does the patient have a characteristic smell* to suggest aetiology? Pay attention for ketotic breath (diabetic ketoacidosis), uraemic fetor or alcohol use.
- *Core temperature.* Pyrexia suggests infection or drug toxicity. Hypothermia suggests myxoedema or a prolonged lie (and can also be a manifestation of sepsis especially in the elderly).
- *The presence of pressure injuries* indicates immobility for a considerable time.
- *Are there signs of trauma* (CSF rhinorrhoea or otorrhoea, haemotympanum and bruising), rashes, needle marks to suggest IV drug use, finger-prick testing marks to suggest underlying diabetes, an AV fistula to suggest a dialysis patient, stigmata of chronic liver disease and the presence of a Medic Alert bracelet.
- *Psychogenic unconsciousness* can be extremely convincing but the neurological findings are usually inconsistent and cannot be explained by a neuroanatomical focus. There may be preserved self-protective reflexes. There will always be a preserved caloric reflex. Bell's phenomenon may be seen; the eyes deviate upwards and only sclerae are visible if the eyes are forcibly opened.

Assessment of key neurological features

1. Raised intracranial pressure

Cerebral perfusion pressure (CPP) = mean arterial pressure (MAP) – intracranial pressure (ICP):

$\sim$80 mmHg = $\sim$90 mmHg – <13 mmHg

The skull is a rigid container and hence the intracranial volume is fixed. An increase in intracranial blood, CSF or brain tissue volumes must be compensated by a change in the others. This concept is known as the Monro–Kellie doctrine. The brain can maintain a normal ICP for changes in volume up to 120 mL; beyond this, displacement of brain tissue through the skull outlet occurs. While herniation is the extreme consequence of raised ICP, cerebral perfusion is compromised long before this.

Causes of raised ICP

- Diffuse cerebral oedema; hypoxic brain injury, hepatic encephalopathy
- Mass effect; tumour, infarction with oedema, intracranial haemorrhage
- Venous outflow obstruction; venous sinus thrombosis, superior vena cava obstruction
- CSF flow obstruction; infection with high CSF protein, meningeal infiltrative disease

Recognized clinical syndromes

- *False localizing signs*: neurological examination findings that predict a neuroanatomical focus for pathology, when in fact the actual pathology is distant from this site. The most common false localizing sign is a sixth nerve palsy caused by mass effect from a cerebral tumour. The sixth nerve is particularly vulnerable as it can be stretched along its long intracranial course.
- *Central herniation*: there is downward displacement of the brainstem ultimately causing herniation through the foramen magnum. The clinical course is sequential midbrain, pons and medulla dysfunction. The Cushing response (bradycardia with marked hypertension) is only seen in the pre-terminal phase; it is a late sign and its absence does not indicate normal ICP.
- *Lateral herniation*: Mass effect exerted by a lesion in the temporal lobe may present with ipsilateral pupillary dilation (a 'blown' pupil), progressing to unilateral ptosis, ipsilateral third nerve palsy and central herniation.

2. Brainstem function

Brainstem dysfunction is an important prognostic feature and should always raise the possibility of raised

ICP. Dysfunction of the three components of the brain-stem can be separately assessed:

Midbrain

Cranial nerves III and IV

- Loss of the pupillary light reflex.
- Bilateral plantar extensor response.
- Decorticate posture (GCS M3).
- Cheyne–Stokes respiration: a cyclical progressive increase in the depth, and sometimes frequency, of inspiration before a peak then subsequent decrease in the depth of inspiration followed by a period of apnoea.

Pons

Cranial nerves V, VI, VII and VIII; pneumotaxic centre

- Loss of corneal reflex.
- Pupils fixed in mid-position.
- Loss of vestibulo-ocular reflexes as assessed by either the caloric or oculocephalic (doll's eyes) tests.
- Decerebrate posture (GCS M2).
- Apneustic respiration: a prolonged inspiratory phase followed by prolonged apnoea.
- Oculocephalic/doll's eyes reflex.
- Lateral rotation of head should result in slow conjugate deviation of both eyes in the direction opposite to head movement (i.e. the eyes appear to roll to continue looking up at the examiner). The reflex is absent if gaze is fixed (i.e. the patient always appears to be looking straight ahead).
- The caloric reflex.
- Injection of 50 mL of ice cold water into the external auditory meatus over one minute (provided that the meatus is not occluded by wax, foreign body or tumour) should cause deviation of the eyes to side of injection with fast nystagmus to the contralateral side. The reflex is absent if there is no deviation of the eyes.

Medulla

Cranial nerves IX, X, XII; respiratory centre; autonomic centres

- Fixed, dilated pupils.
- Loss of gag or cough reflex.
- Flaccid motor response (GCS M1).
- Ataxic/chaotic respiratory pattern, agonal breathing or apnoea.

3. Localizing neurology

The presence of neurological signs that localize pathology to a neuroanatomical focus suggests a:

- vascular aetiology
- space-occupying lesion.

The absence of localizing signs suggests a global cerebral insult such as:

- anoxic injury
- metabolic or endocrine disturbance
- drug- or toxin-induced coma
- post-ictal state
- hypothermia
- hypertensive encephalopathy.

4. Meningism

Neck stiffness is seen with meningeal irritation secondary to subarachnoid haemorrhage or meningitis.

Subsequent investigation

The clinical scenario will determine the plan of investigation. In some cases the cause of unconsciousness will be obvious and few investigations may be needed. In other cases a structured approach is necessary:

- *Brain imaging* should be obtained as soon as it is safe to do so, primarily to identify catastrophic intracerebral events or pathology amenable to urgent neurosurgical intervention. Non-enhanced CT is first line; if there is no evidence of haemorrhage on unenhanced imaging and there is a clinical suspicion of a space-occupying lesion, a contrast-enhanced scan can be performed immediately thereafter.
- *Lumbar puncture* should be performed if imaging is unremarkable.
- *EEG* should be requested early in the case of unexplained unconsciousness, particularly if there is a suspicion of seizure activity.
- *An urgent neurology opinion* should be sought if brain imaging is abnormal, but should not delay further investigation.
- Wider screens for metabolic disturbance and toxic insult should continue.

Laboratory analysis

Provided adequate samples are drawn at the time of venous cannulation, many tests can be subsequently requested, directed by the initial assessment. These may include:

Haematology and biochemistry

- Request standard samples: FBC, U&E, LFT, CRP and clotting.
- Serum ammonia levels are elevated in decompensated liver disease. An elevated level does not prove that hepatic encephalopathy is the cause of unconsciousness, but a normal level does exclude this. Very high levels should raise suspicion of significant cerebral oedema. The blood sample should usually be kept on ice.
- Endocrine assays, notably thyroid function, cortisol and the short Synacthen test.
- Serum vitamin B_1 and B_{12} levels.
- If unconsciousness is unexplained the osmolar gap should be calculated. A significant difference between the measured and calculated serum osmolality indicates the presence of an unmeasured osmotically active substance within the blood. This should raise the possibility of poisoning, usually with methanol or ethylene glycol. (Mannitol use will also result in a raised osmolar gap.)

Microbiology

- Blood cultures should be taken before administering antibiotics but should not delay first dose administration.
- Lumbar puncture for suspected meningitis (in the acute setting) *is never performed before antibiotics are given as it results in an unacceptable delay.*

Toxicology

- Serum drug levels can be measured for lithium, paracetamol and anticonvulsant medication among others.
- Most emergency departments use rapid assay urinalysis kits that detect common substances such as opioids, benzodiazepines and cannabinoids.
- Serum and urine can be sent for storage for retrospective analysis.

Imaging

Transfer of the unconscious patient to the radiology department can be extremely hazardous. Patient safety must always be prioritized and an unstable patient should only be transferred for imaging in exceptional circumstances; in these cases *urgent imaging must be expected to influence immediate treatment decisions.* A medical escort will always be required; the level and expertise of this escort is determined by clinical need.

Advantages of CT

- Widely available
- Quick to perform
- Easy to interpret
- Sensitive for acute haemorrhage

Disadvantages of CT

- Poor definition of posterior fossa (brainstem and cerebellum)
- Difficult to interpret subtle hyperacute and acute ischaemic changes or subacute changes during the 'isodense' phase
- May miss subtle cerebral pathology

Advantages of MRI

- Excellent resolution and superior to CT for acute ischaemia, space-occupying lesion and posterior fossa pathology

Disadvantages of MRI

- Limited availability, particularly out-of-hours
- Long set-up and acquisition times (up to 45minutes for full series)
- Requires specialist interpretation
- May be contraindicated in some patients with metallic implants
- Logistically challenging; requires MR-compatible ventilators and infusion pumps in ventilated patients

Cerebrospinal fluid examination

In an unconscious patient a lumbar puncture should only be performed if there is no evidence of raised ICP on imaging as clinical signs of raised ICP are less reliable in unconscious patients.
Indications for lumbar puncture:
- Suspected CNS infection
- Clinically suspected subarachnoid haemorrhage not proven by CT imaging
- All unconscious patients where the cause is unclear and brain imaging is unremarkable
- If coma remains unexplained, the LP should be repeated at 24 hours.

In every case:

- Record opening pressure.
- Describe the macroscopic appearance of the CSF.
- Send CSF for protein and glucose measurement.
- Send CSF for microscopy, cell count and Gram's stain.
- Assessment for xanthochromia/ spectrophotometry for bilirubin quantification.

Other CSF examinations are determined by the clinical situation and may include:

- viral PCR quantification
- specific microbiological tests: acid-fast bacilli, toxoplasma, listeria, India ink stain for fungi, meningococcal or pneumococcal PCR
- pathological CSF proteins including oligoclonal bands and 14-3-3 protein
- CSF antibodies for channelopathies and anti-neuronal antibodies
- S100B as a marker of CNS injury.

Electroencephalography

The EEG can provide useful information regarding the cause of coma:

- Different aetiologies show specific patterns of electrical activity, particularly in coma secondary to anoxic brain injury.
- May localize pathology to a neuroanatomical focus. The EEG may be used to support diagnosis of brainstem death or the locked-in syndrome.
- Only tool by which non-convulsive status epilepticus can be diagnosed. The risk of developing non-convulsive status is relatively high in coma, irrespective of cause.
- Repeated EEG assessment may be needed in prolonged coma to define evolving pathology, highlight new problems and guide prognosis.

General aspects of management

The management of the unconscious patient is two-fold: treatment of the underlying cause and protection of the patient from secondary injury.

Generic measures

Unconscious patients are particularly at risk of secondary injuries such as:

- stress ulceration of the gastrointestinal tract
- malnutrition
- constipation

- pressure injuries
- muscle contractures
- venous thromboembolism.

A comprehensive package of measures needs to be implemented to mitigate these risks.

Management of seizures

- *Secure the airway*: administer high-flow supplemental oxygen.
- *Secure intravenous access*: correct metabolic disturbances where possible, particularly hypoglycaemia.
- *Attempt to terminate seizure* with IV benzodiazepine; lorazepam is first choice at 0.1 mg/kg, approximately 2–4 mg. Rectal benzodiazepine can be given if IV access cannot be secured quickly.
- *If status epilepticus becomes established* IV phenytoin or fosphenytoin should be given as a loading bolus (15–18 mg/kg at a rate not greater than 50 mg/minute *for phenytoin*). Refractory status (duration of 60 minutes or longer) should be treated with general anaesthesia using propofol, midazolam or thiopental. *To avoid delay, anaesthetic or critical care staff should be informed early, usually at 30 minutes or if phenytoin has failed to terminate status* [1].
- In certain situations seizure activity may be secondary to drug overdose such as tricyclic antidepressants. In such cases specific guidance on the management of associated seizures may be available from the National Poisons Information Service (see Chapter 49) [2].
- Seizures secondary to hyponatraemia are extremely difficult to manage and ideally critical care colleagues should be involved. For profound hyponatraemia with seizures, 1–3 mL/kg boluses (typically 100 mL) of 3% sodium chloride should be administered at intervals of 10 minutes, to a maximum of three boluses, until seizure activity stops. Once seizures have stopped, the serum sodium should be corrected at a rate not greater than 12 mmol/day or 0.5 mmol/L per hour (see Chapter 50) [1].

When to involve neurosurgical centres (see also Chapter 22)

The following should *always* be discussed immediately with neurosurgical centres unless co-morbidity precludes aggressive medical intervention:

- subarachnoid haemorrhage
- extradural haemorrhage
- subdural haematoma
- head injury where there is persisting coma (GCS ≤8) after initial resuscitation, unexplained confusion for more than 4 hours, deterioration in GCS after admission, progressive focal neurological signs, seizure without full recovery, definite or suspected penetrating injury or CSF leak [3]
- evidence of raised ICP despite standard cerebroprotective measures where there is a confirmed space-occupying lesion
- evidence of raised ICP due to malignant middle-cerebral artery territory infarction (middle cerebral artery infarct associated with raised intracranial pressure due to cytotoxic oedema of a significant amount of cerebral tissue) as a decompressive craniectomy may be indicated.

Transfer of the neurosurgical patient

NICE have given clear guidance on the standards for transfer of neurosurgical patients, contained within the wider head injury guidelines; this includes:

- prioritizing resuscitation over transfer
- strict need for an appropriately trained medical escort (usually an anaesthetic registrar or above) [3].

Raised intracranial pressure

When raised ICP is suspected, critical care or *specialist neurocritical care involvement is an immediate priority*. Advanced neurophysiological monitoring may be indicated. In all cases cerebroprotective measures can be initiated while waiting for specialist input.

Standard cerebroprotective measures include:

- Endotracheal intubation with mechanical ventilation to achieve $PaCO_2$ of 4.5–5 kPa, maintain arterial oxygen saturations ≥97% or PaO_2 ≥11 kPa.
- Maintain cerebral perfusion pressure ≥70 mmHg by maintaining mean arterial pressure ≥90 mmHg with vasopressor support as necessary.
- Maintain a strictly neutral or slightly negative fluid balance to limit cerebral oedema formation.
- Maintain blood glucose 4–10 mmol/L using intravenous insulin or glucose infusion if necessary.
- Maintain normothermia (consider therapeutic hypothermia in special situations). Treat

hyperthermia with active cooling measures including paracetamol.
- Minimize obstruction to venous drainage; nurse the patient 30° head-up with the head in a neutral position, avoid tight endotracheal tube ties and avoid internal jugular central venous lines.
- Minimize acute rises in intracranial pressure due to agitation, cough or urinary retention through adequate use of sedative drugs, muscle relaxants and urinary catheterization.

Intracerebral tumours

- In the case of intracerebral tumours with significant vasogenic oedema and mass effect, start intravenous dexamethasone immediately (loading dose of 10 mg IV followed by 4 mg 6-hourly or 8 mg twice daily).

Mannitol

- Recommended when there are signs of raised ICP and is given before the institution of ICP monitoring or full cerebroprotective measures.
- An initial dose of 2 mL/kg 20% mannitol is infused over 20 minutes.
- Can be given through a peripheral IV cannula but the patient should have a urinary catheter.
- Reduction of ICP begins within a few minutes of infusion with benefit seen for up to 4 hours. Repeated doses should only be given under expert guidance.
- Some centres prefer to use hypertonic saline (1–2 mL/kg) as an alternative osmotic agent; however, it is only advisable to give hypertonic saline solutions of concentrations ≥3% via a central venous catheter; it is extremely irritant and can cause thrombophlebitis. Its clinical use is limited outside of the critical care environment [4].

Prognosis

Prognosis largely depends on the underlying aetiology, although poor prognostic markers include:

- more profound coma
- coma of longer duration
- persistent seizure activity.

Prognosis can often be uncertain, which creates a deeply unsatisfactory and difficult situation for the patient's relatives.

Brainstem death

There is no statutory definition of death in the UK. The Academy of Royal Colleges of the UK recommends a definition of death as:

> The irreversible loss of the capacity for consciousness combined with the irreversible loss of the capacity to breathe.

A comatose patient may be dead by these criteria without this being clinically obvious; in the era of modern intensive care medicine, ventilation can be artificially supported and sedative drugs are used to facilitate this. The capacity for consciousness and to breathe require intact integrative brainstem function; where brainstem function has been lost death will inevitably occur over a variable time-course with or without the withdrawal of life-sustaining therapy. The diagnosis of death by irreversible loss of brainstem function allows a doctor to relieve the burden of futile care on such patients [5].

Diagnosing brainstem death

1. Diagnosis must be made by two doctors of at least 5 years registration, one of whom must be a consultant, and both of whom must be competent in the procedure.
2. The testing doctors must not have any perceived or actual conflict of interest and neither doctor should be a member of a transplant team.
3. Testing must be performed by both doctors acting together.
4. Testing must be completed on two separate occasions. There need not be a long delay between the two sets of tests.

Preconditions necessary for the diagnosis of brainstem death

1. The patient has irreversible brain damage of a known aetiology

In cases where the aetiology is never fully established, despite extensive investigation, testing should be undertaken only if other reversible causes have been excluded.

2. Exclusion of potentially reversible causes of coma

1. Depressant drugs: the influence of depressant drugs must be excluded based on clinical judgement and drug-level measurement when possible.

2. Primary hypothermia: core temperature must be <34°C.
3. Potentially reversible circulatory, metabolic and endocrine disturbances:
- serum sodium <160 mmol/L but >115 mmol/L
- serum potassium >2 mmol/L
- serum glucose <20 mmol/L but >3.0 mmol/L
- serum magnesium and phosphate >0.5 mmol/L but <3.0 mmol/L
- PaO_2 >10 kPa
- $PaCO_2$ <6.0 kPa
- pH 7.35–7.45
- mean arterial pressure ≥60 mmHg
- endocrinopathies such as thyroid storm, myxoedema or hypoadrenal crisis must not be clinically suspected or have been excluded by hormonal assay.

3. Exclusion of potentially reversible causes of apnoea

1. The influence of neuromuscular blocking agents must be excluded by the presence of deep-tendon reflexes or by use of a nerve stimulator.
2. The influence of depressant drugs must be excluded.
3. Where coma follows a head injury, a cervical spine injury must be excluded.

Testing brainstem reflexes

1. The pupils are fixed and do not respond to light.
2. There is no corneal reflex.
3. The vestibulo-ocular (caloric) reflex is absent.
4. No motor response can be elicited within the cranial nerve or somatic distributions in response to supraorbital pressure.
5. There is no cough reflex response to bronchial stimulation by a suction catheter placed down the endotracheal tube to the carina or gag response to stimulation of the posterior pharynx with a spatula.
6. There is no spontaneous respiratory effort observed during a period of 5 minutes observation (the apnoea test). The patient's ventilation is adjusted such that the patient is subjected to a documented, objectively measured hypercarbic stimulus with mild respiratory acidaemia that would be expected to stimulate respiratory drive in that patient.

Organ donation

In the United Kingdom approximately 5500 organ transplants are performed each year; 70% of transplanted organs are taken from deceased donors, of which 60% are declared dead after brain death (DBD) [6].

The Human Tissue Act (2004) requires that consent be given for use of tissue for transplantation. Patients who are assessed for brainstem death inherently lack capacity to provide consent, so a *'best interests decision'* must be made on behalf of the patient in accordance with the Mental Capacity Act (2005) (see Chapter 59). A best interests decision must include an assessment of the patient's prior wishes and discussion with those with an appropriate relationship with the patient. While one adult cannot provide consent on behalf of another adult within the UK, assent or refusal for donation by the patient's representatives is usually respected. The counterpart legislation in Scotland, the Human Tissue Act (Scotland, 2006), uses the term 'authorize' rather than consent, a better reflection of the practical framework.

Arguably the best indicator of a patient's wishes is registration on the national donor registry. There are more than 19 million people on the UK register [1]. Authorization for donation is only obtained in about 60% of DBD patients on the register; the factors influencing family refusal to authorize donation include:

- entrenched religious and cultural belief
- uncertainty regarding the patient's wishes
- disagreements among the family group
- lack of understanding of brainstem death.

A previous discussion between donor and family concerning their wishes is a positive predictor for authorization.

Potential donors are identified by two clinical triggers: the diagnosis of a catastrophic brain injury and/or a decision to perform brainstem death tests or the intention to withdraw life-sustaining treatment which will result in circulatory death. The details of potential donors are passed to the Specialist Nurse for Organ Donation (SNOD), who may be resident in larger centres or on-call to cover a geographical region. The SNOD will then coordinate the clinical assessment of the patient, the approach to the patient's representatives for authorization and organ retrieval if authorization is granted [7].

References

1. National Institute for Health and Care Excellence. NICE clinical guideline 137. Epilepsy. www.nice.org.uk/nicemedia/live/13635/57779/57779.pdf. December 2012.

2. The Online database of the National Poisons Information Service. TOXBASE. www.toxbase.org.

3. National Institute for Health and Care Excellence. NICE clinical guideline 56. Triage, assessment, investigation and early management of head injury in infants, children and adults. www.nice.org.uk/cg56. September 2007.

4. Wakai A, Roberts IG, Schierhout G. Mannitol for acute traumatic brain injury. *Cochrane Database of Systematic Reviews* 2007, Issue 1. Art. No.: CD001049.

5. Academy of Royal Medical Colleges. A code of practice for the diagnosis and confirmation of death. www.aomrc.org.uk/publications/statements/doc_view/42-a-code-of-practice-for-the-diagnosis-and-confirmation-of-death.html. 2008.

6. NHS Blood and Transplant. Organ Donation and Transplant Activity Data: United Kingdom. Annual Data for financial years 2008/09 to 2011/12 and data for 2012/13. www.organdonation.nhs.uk/statistics/latest_statistics/. Published April 2013.

7. National Institute for Health and Care Excellence. NICE clinical guideline 135. Organ donation for transplantation: improving donor identification and consent rates for deceased organ donation. www.nice.org.uk/nicemedia/live/13628/57502/57502.pdf. December 2011.

Unsteadiness and balance disturbance

Edward Fathers

Introduction

Balance describes the ability to stand up and remain upright against the force of gravity. The ability to walk upright and remain balanced depends on a hierarchical system of muscles, nerves and interconnected pathways within the central nervous system. When assessing a person with the disorder of balance and gait it is very helpful to try and think about the problem anatomically.

Anatomy

The structures that control balance and movement are similar in all animals. The impulses are initiated in the cerebral cortex and then passed through the cerebral white matter tracts down towards the brainstem. There is input from the basal ganglia, thalamus, cerebellum and vestibular system. The pathways then continue down the spinal cord, then along peripheral nerves and eventually arrive at the muscles. Lesions in any of these anatomical structures can give rise to problems with balance and locomotion (Table 63.1).

> ### Scenario 63.1
>
> *A 63-year-old man with a past history of diabetes and hypertension presents with sudden onset of dizziness (vertigo), double vision and severe loss of balance. There have been several falls. There is numbness on the right side of the face. The symptoms began 4 days ago. He was unable to stand and walk for the first 3 days without holding on to someone else. He is now just able to walk unaided but is very unsteady. On examination he has normal speech, a slight drooping of the right eyelid and the right pupil is smaller than the left. His eye movements are abnormal; the left eye is slightly higher than the right, which gives rise to a vertical diplopia. He has nystagmus on horizontal gaze. He has reduced light touch sensation*

> *on the right lower face. He has normal tone and power in all four limbs but there is mild incoordination in the right arm and leg. His gait is unsteady and broad-based. The reflexes are generally brisk and plantar responses are equivocal.*

History

This is often difficult because the language used by patients who are trying to describe unsteadiness or abnormal movement and balance is frequently imprecise or misleading. You must spend time trying to understand exactly what the patient is trying to tell you. Avoid using leading questions where possible. Try to get a clear understanding of what they mean when they use specific words such as 'vertigo' or 'dizziness' as these often have different meanings to the non-specialist.

Dizziness

If the patient tells you that they feel dizzy then you must work out what they mean by this and document your interpretation in the notes. Most of the time patients are describing one of four different entities (see below). If you can classify the dizziness into one of these clinical phenotypes then it is often easier to identify the cause. As a neurologist with 15 years experience, I can confirm that this is actually a lot harder to do in practice!

- Try and let the patient describe how they feel without interrupting them or asking too many leading questions.
- If you don't feel you're getting anywhere, it can then be helpful to ask directly if there is a spinning sensation as if they had just got off a roundabout; this suggests vertigo.

Acute Medicine, ed. Stephen Haydock, Duncan Whitehead and Zoë Fritz. Published by Cambridge University Press.
© Cambridge University Press 2015.

Table 63.1 Correlation between site of lesion within nervous system and effect on balance and gait

Anatomical site of lesion	Impact on balance and gait
Cerebral cortex	May produce unilateral weakness, e.g. CVE
Basal ganglia	Often causes difficulty changing direction
Thalamus	Loss of proprioception
Cerebellum	Ataxia
Brainstem	Slurred speech, diplopia, facial numbness, vertigo
Vestibular system	Vertigo
Spinal cord	Sensory loss and weakness
Peripheral nerve	Weakness
Muscle	Proximal weakness

- Or do they feel like they are swaying as if they are on a ship at sea. This is not vertigo, and is often present in psychogenic dizziness.

When referring to 'dizziness' patients are often trying to describe one of the following:

- *Disequilibrium* is a state of altered balance, there is no symptom of vertigo. Patients will often complain that they feel unsteady and that other people have noticed that they lose balance. There may be a history of falls or tripping.
- *Vertigo* is an illusion of movement, which is usually rotatory but occasionally there is a sensation of tilting or complaint that the ground suddenly rushes upwards.
- *Presyncope* is a feeling of impending loss of consciousness often accompanied by sweating and nausea and a feeling of weakness.
- *Psychogenic dizziness* is often described as a general feeling of movement as if 'on a ship at sea'. There are no symptoms of vertigo, and the neurological examination is normal. There is no detectable abnormality of balance or gait. Symptoms are often exacerbated by anxiety and can be brought on by hyperventilation.

Assessment for each of the types of dizziness

Disequilibrium

History

Begin your assessment with careful history taking; the important points to cover are:

- *Onset and temporal pattern*: a long history in an older person is more likely to indicate a neurodegenerative disorder.
- *History of head trauma within the last 3 months*: a chronic subdural haematoma is very easy to miss.
- *Are the symptoms static, increasing or decreasing over time?* Disorders of the vestibular system typically improve over a few days. Posterior fossa space-occupying lesions typically worsen over days or weeks.
- *Have there been any falls?* Patients who fall over when changing direction are more likely to have an extrapyramidal disorder such as Parkinson's disease.
- *Enquire about medication*: many drugs can cause unsteadiness in the elderly, e.g. benzodiazepines, SSRIs, tricyclic antidepressants.
- *Sensory symptoms, can they feel where their feet are?* Could this be sensory ataxia due to loss of proprioception?

Examination

Perform a neurological examination of the head and limbs and then watch the patient walk.

Specific things to consider:

- Nystagmus may indicate a cerebellar or brainstem lesion.
- Reduced facial expression could suggest parkinsonism.
- Slurred speech is suggestive of a cerebellar lesion.
- Unilateral rest tremor in one hand combined with reduced finger-tapping speed on the same side is very suggestive of parkinsonism.
- Absent lower limb reflexes may indicate a peripheral neuropathy.
- Absent joint position sensation in the toes suggests a sensory ataxia.

Ask the patient to walk unaided for at least 10 metres:

- If they walk with the feet approximately 30 cm apart then they have an ataxic broad-based gait. Usually this is due to a cerebellar problem but can be due to loss of proprioception (sensory ataxia).
- Observe them changing direction (perform a 180° turn). Most people can do this with one or two steps; if it is more than this then that suggests either a cortical lesion or Parkinson's disease.

- If there is a slow and cautious gait, this can indicate a problem with the vestibular system.

  Perform Romberg's test. If they sway more with the eyes closed then this can suggest loss of proprioception or a vestibular lesion.

Vertigo

This is an illusion of movement, usually rotatory, due to an imbalance from tonic vestibular activity.

The cause may be:

- *Peripheral*: due to a problem in the semicircular canal or the vestibulocochlear nerve (vestibular neuritis).
- *Central*: due to a problem in the vestibular connections within the central nervous system.
- *Related to medication/toxicity*: there are a number of drugs that can cause vertigo: alcohol, benzodiazepines, barbiturates, phenothiazines, aminoglycoside antibiotics, anticonvulsants, aspirin, furosemide, chemotherapy agents.

History

What is the speed of onset?

Abrupt onset can indicate trauma, stroke, demyelination.

Subacute onset suggests vestibular neuronitis (often mistakenly referred to as viral labyrinthitis).

Chronic onset indicates drugs or a posterior fossa mass lesion.

Is the vertigo episodic or continuous?

- Benign paroxysmal positional vertigo is very common. Typically it causes brief episodes of vertigo lasting a few seconds to 1 minute in duration. Often they are triggered by a specific movement, for example turning over in bed or extending the neck to look up.
- In both *vestibular neuritis* and *stroke*, symptoms persist even with the head still. Patients who cannot stand at all are more likely to have had a stroke.

Are there any other accompanying symptoms?

- Unilateral tinnitus and deafness indicates a peripheral vestibular disorder probably within the middle ear.
- Look for other brainstem signs consistent with a central lesion (see below).

Examination tips

Patients with intermittent vertigo will often have a normal neurological examination. It is helpful then to perform a provocation test to try and induce the vertigo. *The Dix–Hallpike test* is performed on patients with episodic vertigo (Figure 63.1).

A positive result indicates a problem in the vestibular system. It is most frequently in the horizontal semicircular canals.

A word of *caution*: lesions within the brainstem can also result in a positive test; however, with central lesions the *nystagmus begins immediately*, it tends to *persist for much longer* and *does not tend to diminish with repeated tests*.

Central versus peripheral vestibular disorder causing vertigo

- Central lesions are usually much more disabling and cause more abnormal signs.

  - Usually cause much more unsteadiness. Often patients cannot walk unsupported.
  - Frequently cause severe symptoms that last many days.
  - There may be accompanying brainstem signs with a central lesion. Unilateral facial sensory disturbance, facial weakness or slurring of speech indicates a brainstem vascular lesion.
  - Look carefully for the presence of Horner's syndrome; this is associated with a lesion in the medulla (lower brainstem).

- Patients with a peripheral vestibular lesion tend not to have nystagmus unless it is induced by a provocation test such as the Dix–Hallpike manoeuvre.

  - Peripheral lesions usually start to improve within one day.

Presyncope (see Chapter 61)

It is usually fairly easy to differentiate the symptoms of presyncope from other types of dizziness.

History

- Patients usually describe an impending feeling that they are about to lose consciousness.
- They will often experience muffled hearing and dimming of the vision just prior to losing consciousness.

1. Position the patient on an examination couch so that they are sitting upright and staring straight ahead.

2. Request that the patient keep their eyes open throughout the test.

3. The patient's head is then turned to one side.

4. You then assist the patient in lying flat, this is to be done rapidly so that the head hangs over the end of the examination couch. I allow the head to fall back so that the neck extends, keep the head turned to the side.

5. You are looking to see if they develop nystagmus, which will accompany their symptom of vertigo. Typically a **positive test** will cause **nystagmus which has a rotatory and vertical component**. There is usually a delay of 10 seconds before it starts, it would usually last less than a minute.

6. If you repeat the test there is a smaller response with each repetition.

7. If there is no response when you perform the test then sit the patient back up, turn the head to the opposite side and repeat.

Figure 63.1 How to perform the Dix–Hallpike test. (If you have difficulty visualizing this description then there are excellent how-to-do-it videos on the internet.)

- There is often yawning, nausea, sweating and epigastric discomfort.
- Enquire regarding situations where the symptoms are likely to occur. If they occur when seated or lying down then consider cardiac arrhythmia as a possible cause.

Examination tips

- A cardiovascular examination must include a lying and standing blood pressure.
- Orthostatic hypotension is defined as a drop in systolic blood pressure of more than 20 mmHg or a fall in diastolic blood pressure of more than 10 mmHg within 3 minutes of standing up.
- It is a common mistake to measure the standing blood pressure within 30 seconds of the lying pressure; it is usually better to wait at least 2 minutes so that you do not miss clinically significant postural hypotension.

Variants of orthostatic hypotension are recognized:

1. Initial orthostatic hypotension is a transient drop in systolic blood pressure of at least 40 mmHg or in diastolic blood pressure of at least 20 mmHg within 15 seconds of standing.

2. Delayed orthostatic hypotension occurs after more than 3 minutes of standing.

Postural orthostatic tachycardia syndrome (POTS) is a syndrome of symptomatic orthostatic tachycardia in the absence of orthostatic hypotension. It mainly affects females aged between 15 years and 40 years.

It often causes dizziness (presyncope). The diagnostic criteria are:

- sustained heart rate increase of at least 30 beats per minute from supine to standing within 10 minutes of standing (or a heart rate that exceeds 120 bpm on standing)
- lack of orthostatic hypotension (systolic blood pressure does not fall by more than 20 mmHg and may increase with standing)
- symptoms of orthostatic intolerance (e.g. light-headedness, weakness, palpitations) develop with standing and resolve with lying down.

Psychogenic dizziness

History

- Is usually very long!
- Symptoms are often vague and descriptions such as 'giddiness' and 'muzziness' are common.
- Patients may feel that they are unsteady and cannot walk normally; however, there is no abnormality of gait visible to the onlooker.
- Symptoms tend to vary over time.
- There is often an illusion of movement as if 'on a ship at sea'. There is no history of vertigo, presyncope, weakness or falls.

Examination

- The neurological examination and assessment of the gait should all be normal.
- If you suspect that there may be a strong anxiety component then it can be instructive to request that the patient performs hyperventilation.
- Most normal individuals will feel a little strange after performing this for more than a minute or two.
- Patients with psychogenic dizziness will often start to feel off balance or dizzy within 20 seconds. If hyperventilation reproduces their symptoms in less than 30 seconds of starting then that can be very supportive evidence for a psychogenic disorder.

Investigations

The tests you need to perform depend on the likely anatomical site of the lesion causing the unsteadiness.

Peripheral vestibular lesion: audiogram, review medication and consider ENT referral.

Peripheral nerve lesion causing sensory ataxia: neuropathy screen, full blood count, urea and electrolytes, serum protein electrophoresis, serum B_{12}, thyroid function tests, fasting glucose.

Cerebellum: MRI brain, vitamin B_{12}, thyroid function tests, vitamin E, HIV, serum ACE.

Brainstem: MRI brain, ANA, serum ACE, ESR.

Cortex: MRI brain.

Scenario 63.1 continued

This man has developed severe disabling vertigo with brainstem symptoms and signs. The history is typical of a brainstem stroke (lateral medullary syndrome, giving rise to a right Horner's syndrome and right facial sensory loss combined with cerebellar signs and vertigo). The vertigo is caused by a lesion in the central vestibular pathways, which is why it is so disabling.

Further reading

Brandt T, Dieterich M, Strupp M. *Vertigo and Dizziness: Common Complaints*. London: Springer; 2013.

Visual disturbance

Kate R. Petheram and Chris Allen

Introduction

Disturbances of the visual system result from pathology in the:

- eye
- optic nerve
- optic tracts and visual pathways in the brain
- mechanisms that maintain binocular vision
- vestibular mechanisms maintaining ocular stability in the face of head movements
- occipito-parietal cerebral cortex.

As with all neurological symptoms, the management of these problems starts with a careful history, followed by a focused examination.

The nature of the visual disturbance is often dictated by the site of the anatomical pathology. Symptoms include:

- loss of acuity
  - acute
  - chronic
- visual field defects
- diplopia
- oscillopsia
- visual hallucinations.

> ### Scenario 64.1
>
> *A 76-year-old woman is referred by the emergency department. She gives a one-week history of unilateral headache. That evening whilst watching television, she developed sudden onset loss of vision in the left eye that was complete within 2–3 minutes. On examination the eyes are neither red nor painful. Vision is normal in the right eye but she is only able to recognize hand motion with the left eye. Eye movements are normal. Fundoscopy reveals a pallid swelling of the optic disc, the remainder of the fundus appears normal. You need to establish the diagnosis and institute appropriate management.*

History

Acute loss of acuity

Common causes of acute visual loss

- Central or branch retinal artery occlusion
- Central or branch retinal vein occlusion
- Acute retinal detachment
- Acute vitreous haemorrhage
- Optic neuritis
- Ischaemic optic neuropathy (associated headache)
- Acute angle closure glaucoma (associated headache)

If the visual loss is acute (coming on over seconds, minutes or hours) then ask more about:

Onset

- Very sudden onset suggests arterial pathology.
- If recurrent transient loss consider:
  - embolic episodes (amaurosis fugax)
  - migraine
  - ischaemic optic neuropathy
  - raised intracranial pressure (e.g. idiopathic intracranial hypertension).

Quality of visual loss

- Arterial occlusion causes profound loss of vision whereas other conditions, e.g. retinal vein occlusion, generally cause blurring and loss of colour saturation.
- Distortion of the visual image suggests macular disease.

Area of visual field affected

- Loss of central vision only suggests macular disease.

Acute Medicine, ed. Stephen Haydock, Duncan Whitehead and Zoë Fritz. Published by Cambridge University Press.
© Cambridge University Press 2015.

- Loss of left or right half or quarter field suggests homonymous hemianopia or quadrantanopia.
- Progression from periphery to centre suggests retinal detachment, retinal artery embolism or migraine.

Associated ocular symptoms/signs

- Pain and red eye suggests acute glaucoma.
- Headache, nausea, cracked glass effect (scintillating scotoma) suggests migraine.
- If there is pain on eye movements consider optic neuritis.
- Preceding floaters/flashing lights suggest retinal detachment and may go on to develop a vitreous haemorrhage.

General medical history

- Important to ask about vascular risk factors.
- If there is headache, jaw claudication and transient visual loss then giant cell arteritis must be excluded.
- Ask about previous or known neurological disease such as multiple sclerosis and migraine.

Chronic loss of acuity

Common causes of chronic visual loss

- Cataracts
- Macular degeneration
- Diabetic retinopathy
- Toxins
- Hereditary retinal disorders

  If the history is longer and goes back for days, weeks or months then the following questions are useful:

Past ocular history

- Cataract is a very common cause of reduced acuity and the majority are associated with normal age-related degenerative change but presenting in young or early middle age should prompt further investigation.
- *Ocular factors* to consider which cause cataract include trauma, high myopia, recurrent uveitis, ionizing radiation, excessive ultraviolet light exposure and infrared radiation.

General/past medical history

- Diabetes mellitus is a cause of cataract and retinopathy and a risk factor for non-arteritic ischaemic optic neuropathy.

- The following are risk factors for cataract: atopy, galactosaemia, hypocalcaemia, myotonic dystrophy.
- Toxins:
    - Steroid use, both topical and systemic, is a risk factor for cataract and glaucoma.
    - Drugs such as chloroquine and tamoxifen can cause toxic retinopathy.
    - Excessive alcohol use together with smoking and probably poor nutrition can cause an optic neuropathy known as tobacco-alcohol amblyopia.

Family history

- Especially useful in young patients.
- Examples of hereditary conditions affecting the ocular fundus include Leber's optic neuropathy and retinitis pigmentosa.

Visual field defect

Determining the area of visual field affected can be difficult from the history alone and patients can find these difficult to define. If the loss of vision was transient the patient may not know whether the defect was monocular or binocular. For example, a left-sided hemianopia is often misinterpreted as visual loss in the left eye.

Bitemporal hemianopia

- Patients may notice they bump into things.
- Caused by a lesion in the optic chiasm – classically by a pituitary adenoma but rarer causes include craniopharyngiomas, meningiomas and large internal carotid artery aneurysms.

Homonymous hemianopia

- If central vision is spared then the patient may only become aware of the defect by bumping into things on the affected side.
- If central vision is affected then the patient usually complains that he can only see half of what he is looking at.
- Caused by a lesion anywhere from the optic tract through to the visual cortex in the occipital lobe.
- The macular field is supplied by the middle cerebral artery so involvement suggests occlusion of that artery. This field is spared in posterior cerebral artery occlusion (macular sparing hemianopia).
- The more posterior the causative lesion, the more congruous or symmetrical the hemianopia.

- Common causes of homonymous hemianopia are vascular or neoplastic lesions in the contralateral hemisphere. Accompanying symptoms such as hemiplegia will help further localization. For example, a complete loss of motor and sensory function throughout the contralateral side of the body with a homonymous hemianopia suggests a lesion in the internal capsule supplied by small perforating branches of the middle and posterior cerebral arteries close to their origins.

Homonymous quadrantanopia

- Upper quadrantanopia caused by lesions in the temporal regions affecting lower parts of the optic radiation.
- Lower quadrantanopia caused by lesions in the parietal region.

Scotoma

- Defined as a *partial alteration in the visual field of one eye.*
- Can affect any area of the visual field and be any shape or size.
- It is caused by pathology in the *retina or the optic nerve.*
- A small scotoma that happens to affect the macular vision will have a major impact on vision whereas a relatively large scotoma affecting peripheral vision may go entirely unnoticed.

Diplopia

Diplopia is the *simultaneous perception of two images from one object* (double vision). It occurs when both eyes are functional but cannot converge on a target and is usually due to impairment of extraocular muscles or their innervation. In simple terms the two eyes are working but not moving in time with each other.

Check that diplopia is binocular

- Two clear images are present when both eyes are open, cured by covering either eye.
- Monocular 'diplopia' can be caused by cataract.

Position of images

- Horizontal, i.e. images side by side, usually caused by sixth nerve palsy
- Vertical or diagonal by any other cause

Intermittent diplopia

- Decompensating latent squint
- Myasthenia gravis or dysthyroid eye disease

History of head trauma

- Fourth nerve palsy
- Orbital fracture

General medical history

- Vascular history
- Symptoms of thyroid disease, raised intracranial pressure and myasthenia gravis

Oscillopsia

The term oscillopsia describes the illusion that stationary objects are moving.

It causes a reduction in visual acuity and is often associated with nausea. It most often results from abnormal eye movements or from an impaired vestibulo-ocular reflex. Patients with nystagmus may complain of this, although surprisingly infrequently.

Visual perception symptoms

Visual neglect or inattention

- Lesions near but not actually disrupting the fibres of the optic radiation may cause contralateral homonymous visual field neglect. Finger movement may be detected in all parts of the visual field during testing to confrontation but bilateral simultaneous visual stimulation reveals poor registration of stimuli from the affected hemi-field.
- It is most common following damage to the right hemisphere, usually parietal or temporo-parietal causing left-sided visual neglect. This is thought to reflect the right hemisphere's specialized function in spatial recognition and memory. If the left hemisphere is damaged the right can compensate for attention but not vice versa.

Visual hallucinations

A patient describes seeing something which is not there. The type of hallucination and situation in which it occurs can give a clue towards aetiology.

- *Simple elementary visual hallucinations* caused by irritation of the primary visual cortex, by a seizure for example, most often consist of brightly coloured geometric shapes that may move across the visual field and generally persist from a few seconds to a few minutes.

- *Complex visual hallucinations* are seen in Parkinson's disease, Lewy body dementia, delirium tremens, temporal lobe epilepsy and midbrain lesions.
- *Hypnogogic hallucinations* are very common and occur just before a person goes to sleep. Usually last for seconds to minutes. Can be associated with narcolepsy but are seen by 37% of the normal population.
- *Charles Bonnet syndrome*: these are usually non-threatening visions often of people or animals that occur in people with serious visual impairment. Usually occur in morning or evening but are not dependent on low light levels.

Examination

A focused examination should lead to a short list of differential diagnoses. For anatomical localization it may be helpful to approach the examination as to the cranial nerves involved. A short screening examination of the rest of the nervous system may reveal important signs unsuspected in the history and relevant to the diagnosis and consequent management.

Appearance of the eye

- Injection of the conjunctiva (red eye) suggests a primarily ocular condition and urgent ophthalmological care is often required.
- Proptosis can be detected best by looking at the patient from above; proptosis is suggested if the globe of the eye projects beyond the brow and suggests infiltration of the periorbital fat or ocular motor muscles as in thyroid eye disease (which may occur in a chemically euthyroid individual), a malignant neoplastic or infective disorder.
- Chemosis, oedema of the conjunctiva, suggests venous obstruction and if the proptosis is pulsatile, a carotico-cavernous fistula is present (almost always the result of head trauma).
- Look for ptosis which, if slight, may indicate Horner's syndrome (then accompanied by a smaller pupil on that side) or, if more significant, an oculomotor nerve lesion. It is always worth checking with the patient if they have always had a degree of eyelid drooping. However, do not forget myasthenia, which can present very

asymmetrically and mimic almost any eye movement abnormality. Fatiguability can be checked by asking the patient to close their eyes gently for about 30 seconds and then look upward for 30 seconds, during which one or both eyelids will be seen to droop.

Visual acuity (optic nerve – cranial nerve II)

- This is formally tested using a Snellen chart. Pinhole acuity suggests the best visual acuity achievable with the correct spectacles. Informally, asking a patient to read a piece of text with each eye in turn may be an adequate screen. *Colour vision* can be tested formally with the special plates but these are also available on a smartphone app or the patient can be asked if colour perception is normal with each eye.

Visual fields (cranial nerve II)

- Screening of fields to confrontation with both eyes open to finger movements is an adequate screen for homonymous visual field defects (of which a patient may not be aware), but can miss even quite major uniocular scotomas and bitemporal hemianopias.
- The former are likely to be noticed by the patient if he or she is tested with each eye in turn.
- The latter are very rare, happening in the context of substantial parasellar lesions and often require formal field-testing for confirmation.

Fundoscopy (cranial nerve II)

- This is essential primarily to exclude papilloedema.
- Cataracts that may be impairing vision can be seen during fundoscopy.
- Pallid retina with narrowed vessels of retinal artery occlusion, a cherry red spot may be seen at the fovea.
- Blood and thunder retina of retinal vein occlusion.
- Extreme disc pallor signifies optic atrophy that may follow optic neuritis; if this is unilateral a relative afferent pupillary defect will also be present.

Pupils (cranial nerves II and III and sympathetic nervous system)

- Look for pupils of different size.

- A very large pupil on one side suggests a third nerve palsy, if accompanied by ptosis.
- A pupil slightly smaller on one side with mild ptosis is seen in Horner's syndrome, signifying a lesion in the sympathetic outflow tract. Such a lesion may be in the dorsolateral brainstem (e.g. in a brainstem vascular event), in the region of the T1 spinal root (e.g. in an apical lung tumour, Pancoast syndrome) or in the wall of the carotid artery (e.g. in carotid dissection).
- Check with the patient that they are not known to have asymmetric pupils, as can happen in the entirely benign Holmes–Adie syndrome when the pupils are also very slow to react to light.
- An optic nerve lesion on one side will cause a relative afferent pupillary defect, where the commensal reaction to light on the other pupil will be stronger than the direct reaction.
- Loss of reaction to light with preserved accommodation (Argyll Robertson pupil) occurs from lesions in the midbrain tectum (classically in neurovascular syphilis) but more commonly can be seen in type 2 diabetes.

Eye movements (cranial nerves III, IV and VI)

- Look specifically for ptosis and obvious dysconjugate gaze (squint) and ask the patient if they have double vision as you test the conjugate movements of the eyes in all directions in an H shape.
- Diplopia will be maximal in the direction of action of the paretic muscle and the image carried by the paretic eye will be peripheral to the true image, so cover each eye in turn to see which muscle is paretic.
- A full third nerve palsy will produce complete ptosis and when the lid is raised, the eye will be directed down and out and the pupil will be dilated. A third nerve palsy without a dilated pupil is likely to be due to a microvascular lesion (diabetes or hypertension); compressive lesions of the third nerve (e.g. a posterior cerebral artery aneurysm) are more likely to involve the pupil because of the position of the pupillo-constrictor fibres on the periphery of the third nerve.
- A sixth nerve palsy will produce horizontal diplopia in the direction of gaze of that muscle as it fails to move out (abduct). The commonest cause of an isolated sixth nerve palsy is microvascular in the elderly and/or those with hypertension or diabetes. In a younger person an intrinsic brainstem lesion such as inflammatory demyelination is more likely. A sixth nerve palsy can be a false localizing sign of raised intracranial pressure, even when there is not displacement of intracranial contents such as in idiopathic intracranial hypertension.

- Trochlear (fourth) nerve palsies are very rare outside the context of a concussive head injury and cause diplopia on looking down, e.g. whilst going down stairs. The nerve is responsible for moving the already adducted eye downwards. In the presence of a third nerve lesion preventing adduction, the torsional effect of the superior oblique muscle can be seen to rotate the globe if the patient is asked to attempt to look at the end of his or her nose.
- During the examination of the eye movements it may be important to check that rapid goal-directed (saccadic) eye movements are intact to exclude the presence of the slowed or failed adduction which occurs in an internuclear palsy. This is a definite sign of an intrinsic brainstem (pontine) lesion, especially common in demyelinating disease.
- Nystagmus, when observed, is an important sign. In the absence of vertigo, nystagmus usually indicates brainstem disease (or disruption of brainstem mechanisms by drugs). This is due to disruption of the brainstem systems for maintaining gaze away from the straight-ahead position; the eyes drift back towards the midline only to be corrected with a saccade which jerks the eyes back to the desired direction of gaze. This fast corrective phase is thus always away from the centre in the commonest type of nystagmus, known as gaze-evoked nystagmus. Acutely, vestibular disturbances (such as labyrinthitis) may present with nystagmus but in this case it will be beating in a certain direction (and possibly rotatory), depending on which part of the vestibular apparatus is disturbed. Such peripheral vestibular nystagmus is always accompanied by vertigo and a lot of distress but is not sustained.

Investigations

A clear clinical differential will guide the necessary investigations. Images can be difficult to interpret in the absence of a clear history and the results of a relevant focused examination.

Blood tests

Necessary blood tests are usually suggested by the differential diagnosis.

- A significantly raised ESR may suggest in an elderly patient the presence of temporal arteritis which can also rarely present with sixth or third nerve lesions.
- If thyroid eye disease is suspected, thyroid autoantibodies should be requested in addition to thyroid function tests.

Imaging

- Magnetic resonance imaging of the head will reveal brain hemisphere lesions and also lesions in and behind the orbit and the cavernous sinus that might be causing loss of acuity or ocular motor signs and symptoms. If a recent vascular lesion is suspected diffusion-weighted imaging will be revealing.
- CT imaging will not visualize these areas with sufficient accuracy.

Visual evoked responses

- These are useful in detecting current or past optic nerve lesions even in the absence of any clear history or signs.

Lumbar puncture

- Seldom required in the acute stages of the investigation of visual symptoms; examination of the CSF may be required, once a mass lesion or hydrocephalus has been excluded, to identify the presence of inflammatory lesions in the nervous system (including the optic nerve).
- Examination of the CSF pressure will be a necessary part of the diagnosis and treatment of idiopathic intracranial hypertension.

Referral to specialties

Most conditions can wait until the next morning to be referred to ophthalmology or neurology. However, the following should be discussed urgently with ophthalmology:

1. Central retinal artery occlusion unless present for several days
2. Acute angle closure glaucoma
3. Acute ischaemic optic neuropathy suspected to be due to temporal arteritis
4. Acute loss of vision of less than 6 hours duration where the cause is uncertain.

Scenario 64.1 continued

It is extremely likely that this patient has acute ischaemia of the optic nerve due to temporal arteritis. Her ESR was raised at 100 mm/h. She was immediately started on high dose corticosteroids 60 mg od to protect vision in her right eye (50% chance of loss of vision in this eye if untreated). A temporal artery biopsy was performed 2 days later (needs to be performed within one week) confirming the diagnosis.

Further reading

Lueck CJ. Loss of vision. *Pract Neurol* 2010; 10: 315–325.

Chapter 65

Vomiting and nausea

Emma Greig

Introduction

Nausea and vomiting are common symptoms in both gastrointestinal (GI) and non-GI conditions. Nausea and vomiting are commonly acute but are considered chronic if present for longer than a month.

Definitions

Vomiting: the forceful expulsion of gastric contents through the mouth and may be involuntary or voluntary (derives from *vomere*, Latin for 'to discharge').

Nausea: the unpleasant sensations experienced prior to vomiting including autonomic features such as hypersalivation, sweating, tachycardia, altered respiration and pallor. Nausea can occur independently of vomiting (derives from *naus*, Greek for ship).

Retching: may precede *vomiting* and describes the involuntary effort to vomit against a closed glottis with no expulsion of gastric contents.

Vomiting should be distinguished from:

Regurgitation: undigested food contents are brought back in a less forceful way with no preceding nausea or somatic motor response.

Rumination: repetitive regurgitation of small amounts of food back into the mouth after swallowing.

Pathophysiology

Two areas within the medulla oblongata are responsible for coordination of vomiting:

The vomiting centre is situated within the lateral reticular formation in the nucleus tractus solitarius [1]:

- It is activated by vagal afferents as well as visceral nociceptors in the GI tract (reacting to irritants such as alcohol), peritoneum, mesentery, biliary tree, pharynx, vestibular apparatus and heart.
- It receives afferent inputs from higher centres in the central nervous system, which explains both functional (psychogenic) vomiting and vomiting precipitated by unpleasant smells, tastes and visual stimuli.

The chemoreceptor trigger zone (CTZ) is in the floor of the fourth ventricle within the area postrema:

- It is directly stimulated by drugs (e.g. opiates, cytotoxics and digoxin), metabolic causes (e.g. uraemia) and possibly radiation sickness and motion sickness.
- Once activated, the CTZ stimulates the vomiting centre with subsequent efferent impulses coordinating somatic muscle activity.
- Many neurotransmitters are involved, including acetylcholine (muscarinic receptors) and histamine (H_1 receptors) within the vestibular and vomiting centre and dopamine (D2 receptors) and 5-hydroxytryptamine ($5\text{-}HT_3$ receptors) in the CTZ and area postrema.
- Most antiemetics work by antagonizing these receptors.

Vomiting:

- Requires coordination of efferent impulses to somatic nerves in the pharynx, GI tract, abdominal muscles, diaphragm and respiratory muscles.
- Other autonomic pathways mediate the unpleasant sensations of nausea and vomiting

Acute Medicine, ed. Stephen Haydock, Duncan Whitehead and Zoë Fritz. Published by Cambridge University Press.
© Cambridge University Press 2015.

such as hypersalivation, altered respiration, tachycardia and sweating.

- Visceral vagal efferents produce the gastroduodenal motor response with reduced gastric antral motor activity and increased duodenal and jejunal reflux back into the stomach.
- Retching results from simultaneous contraction of the chest muscles, diaphragm and abdominal muscles against a closed glottis with vomit often reaching the lower oesophagus.
- Finally, a powerful and sustained contraction of the abdominal muscles, descent of the diaphragm, relaxation of the cardia and lower oesophageal sphincter, increased intra-abdominal pressure and an open glottis herald vomiting.

Scenario 65.1

A 36-year-old woman with type 1 diabetes is referred by the ED due to uncontrolled vomiting and epigastric pain. There is no diarrhoea. She describes similar but less severe episodes lasting a few days over the preceding 2–3 years with a number of brief emergency department attendances where she has been discharged with antiemetics and analgesia. She often knows when an attack is about to start and she then becomes extremely anxious. She has recently been referred by her GP to see the gastroenterology team in outpatients. On examination she is clearly distressed, with epigastric tenderness but no guarding or rebound. Initial investigations in the emergency department are unremarkable. A recent HbA$_{1c}$ level by her GP indicates that her diabetic control has not been good.

Approach to diagnosis and management

Most cases of nausea and vomiting result from minor infections such as viral gastroenteritis; however, vomiting also occurs in the early stages of a multiplicity of illnesses including life-threatening conditions and you will need to consider this variety of presentations when making a diagnosis (see Table 65.1).

- Quickly establish the severity of the patient's condition, which may require resuscitation using intravenous fluids and electrolytes as appropriate.
- Obtain a history, perform appropriate clinical examination and perform investigations to refine the differential diagnosis.
- Plan specific treatment as indicated by the diagnosis and consider the use of antiemetics and/or intravenous fluids as supportive therapy.

History

Features which should prompt clinical concern

- In prolonged or severe vomiting, significant fluid depletion may cause metabolic alkalosis and hypokalaemia; this should be identified and treated as an emergency.
- If abdominal pain is a major feature, then consider diagnoses such as bowel obstruction, perforation, pancreatitis, or acute cholecystitis and ask for early review by the surgical team as this could represent an acute surgical emergency.
- If there is evidence in the history of blood within vomit, melaena in the stool or on rectal examination, this is a potential medical emergency: treat as for haematemesis and melaena (see Chapter 26).
- While not a clinical emergency, a history of sudden onset vomiting (with or without diarrhoea) should prompt isolation of the patient with careful infection control measures to avoid dissemination to other patients, *irrespective of any exposure history*.

Relevant history helpful to make the diagnosis

- Ask about recent illnesses (such as gastroenteritis) in family members and other contacts.
- Has there been relevant travel abroad?
- Is diarrhoea present and, if so, does it contain mucus or traces of blood?
- Obtain a history of recent food consumption: e.g. out-of-date food, 'take-aways'.
- Consider a history of heartburn, as nausea may be the only symptom of gastro-oesophageal reflux.
- Is there blood in the vomit or bowel motion?
- Obtain an accurate and preferably corroborated alcohol history. Alcohol excess is a very common cause of acute nausea and vomiting, while chronic dependence is associated with early morning nausea and vomiting.
- Early morning vomiting is associated with pregnancy: consider in any female of childbearing age. If in doubt, perform a pregnancy test.
- Take a drug history including over-the-counter medication and recent changes in medication. A list of medications associated with nausea and vomiting is shown in Table 65.1.

Table 65.1 Causes and management of nausea and vomiting; the most common causes are shown in **bold** type

	Cause	Basic guide to management
Infection	**Viral infections:** **Norovirus** **Rotavirus** Hepatitis Herpesvirus (CMV, HSV, VZV) in immunocompromised **Bacterial infections:** secondary to pneumonia or urosepsis	Supportive management using fluids (intravenous or oral) and antiemetics such as prochlorperazine or metoclopramide Treat underlying bacterial infection with appropriate antibiotics and supportive management
Drugs	Prescribed: • Antibiotics (e.g. **metronidazole**, erythromycin, sulphonamides, aciclovir) • **Opiates** • NSAIDs • **Chemotherapeutic agents (e.g. cisplatin, methotrexate, tamoxifen)** • Digoxin (especially if toxicity) • Antiarrhythmics • Beta-blockers • Diuretics • Oral contraceptive pill • Oral hypoglycaemics • Azathioprine, sulfasalazine • Anti-Parkinson's medication, anticonvulsants Self-administered: • Alcohol	Stop likely culprit or swap for an alternative Antiemetic choice for cytotoxic-induced vomiting: 1. If chemotherapy regimen, consider 5-HT$_3$ receptor antagonist such as ondansetron 8 mg tds PO/IV. Add in dexamethasone 8 mg bd PO/IV to reduce/prevent vomiting post-chemotherapy 2. If opiate-related problem, then use oral or intramuscular cyclizine 50 mg tds PO/IM 3. Alternatives would be domperidone or metoclopramide using 10 mg tds PO Reduce/stop alcohol intake and offer support, e.g. Alcoholics Anonymous
Metabolic	Diabetic ketoacidosis Hypercalcaemia Hyponatraemia Uraemia Acute intermittent porphyria (AIP)	Supportive therapy Treat underlying cause and involve the appropriate specialist team early (diabetes and endocrinology), nephrology (uraemia) or gastroenterology (AIP)
Endocrine	**Pregnancy (especially first trimester)** Addison's disease Hyperthyroidism Hypo- and hyperparathyroidism	Pregnancy: mostly supportive for pregnancy. Antiemetics only for suspected hyperemesis gravidarum – try cyclizine 50 mg PO/IM Other conditions: treat underlying cause after input from the endocrinology team
Presentations with mechanical obstruction	Mechanical obstruction of small intestine: • Adhesions from previous surgery • Volvulus • Obstructed hernia • Tumour in small intestine or colon Mechanical obstruction of stomach: • Peptic ulcer disease (duodenal/pyloric channel) • Gastric/pyloric channel cancer • Crohn's disease causing stricturing • Pancreatic disease including pseudocyst formation or malignancy	Resuscitation with fluids, supportive therapy and early surgical opinion (within first 4 hours) Keep nil-by-mouth using intravenous fluids with placement of wide-bore NG tube to drain gastric contents For gastric outflow obstruction, early endoscopy +/– dilatation for non-malignant strictures with use of proton pump inhibitors (omeprazole 40 mg od) for peptic ulcer disease may prove invaluable (involve Gastroenterology next day)

	Cause	Basic guide to management
Other acute abdominal presentations	Acute pancreatitis Acute cholecystitis	Early surgical opinion with supportive therapy
Functional GI disorders	Functional obstruction of small intestine: • Postoperative ileus • Paralytic ileus • Chronic idiopathic intestinal pseudo-obstruction Functional obstruction of stomach: • Gastroparesis • Cyclical vomiting syndrome • Non-ulcer dyspepsia/irritable bowel syndrome • Psychogenic • Post-surgical • Idiopathic	Once you are sure that no acute surgical intervention is required, management is supportive (intravenous fluids and electrolytes) and an early gastroenterology opinion is necessary (next day). Supportive therapy includes enteral or parenteral nutrition as many of these conditions are chronic and worsen with malnutrition
Other significant non-gastrointestinal organic causes	Myocardial infarction Congestive cardiac failure	Treat as per hospital protocol. Involve a cardiologist as soon as possible
Central nervous system causes	Cerebral: • Migraine • Raised intracranial pressure • Brainstem lesions • Head injury • Tumours (especially near fourth ventricle) • Seizures Vestibular: • Labyrinthitis (usually viral) • Meniere's disease • Motion sickness	Migraine: supportive and domperidone 20 mg qds PO or 60 mg bd PR Raised intracranial pressure and tumours: involve Neurosurgery urgently (same day) Head injury: supportive Seizures: treat according to cause Antiemetics: try antihistamine with H_1 receptor antagonist properties such as cyclizine 50 mg tds PO/IM
Psychiatric	Anorexia nervosa Bulimia nervosa Psychogenic vomiting Depression	Ensure patient is clinically stable and not at risk of refeeding syndrome (see Chapter 67). Ask for early psychiatric input (next day)

- Consider immunocompromise by pre-existing illness or recent medication.
- Is there any associated abdominal pain?
- With recurrent symptoms of nausea and vomiting, consider the past medical history, including recent illness, but particularly past abdominal surgery causing bowel obstruction secondary to adhesions; prior gastric surgery (such as Billroth II gastrectomy) may cause bile staining within the vomit.
- Does the patient have diabetes mellitus? Acute vomiting may result from diabetic ketoacidosis while gastroparesis can cause chronic vomiting.
- Vomit which has a faeculent smell suggests small bowel obstruction, bacterial overgrowth or rarely gastrocolic fistula.

- Projectile vomiting is associated with pyloric stenosis.
- Associated vertigo, gait instability or nystagmus suggests labyrinthine disorders such as vestibular neuronitis.

In making a diagnosis for patients with chronic vomiting, the *pattern and type of vomiting* are important clues:

- Chronic vomiting occurring in the first hour after a meal is characteristic of a functional vomiting disorder and may suggest psychological causes and/or an eating disorder, particularly in the absence of abdominal symptoms such as pain.
- Large volumes of vomit containing partly digested food several hours after eating are indicative

of causes such as gastric outflow obstruction, gastroparesis or small bowel obstruction.

- The absence of retching implies regurgitation; the presence of undigested food implies rumination. Both these conditions are managed and investigated differently to nausea and vomiting and should be excluded with a careful history.

Examination

- It is essential to look for signs of dehydration: lethargy, reduced conscious level, dry mucous membranes, reduced skin turgor and delayed capillary refill. If appropriate, standing and lying blood pressures for postural hypotension will confirm the severity of vomiting and resultant dehydration.
- Examination of the abdomen is often normal, particularly if there is a non-GI cause; however, abdominal examination may reveal tenderness, guarding or rebound, implying an acute abdomen which will require surgical input. (Remember to examine the hernial orifices.)
- A gastric succussion splash (splashing sound heard over the left upper quadrant of the patient during sudden movement) suggests delayed gastric emptying.
- If gastroparesis is suspected, look for other evidence of autonomic neuropathy including orthostatic hypotension, orthostatic tachycardia, abnormal sweating and delayed bladder emptying.
- Loss of dental enamel may indicate recurrent vomiting due to bulimia or persistent reflux disease. If you suspect bulimia, then examine the knuckles for evidence of callus formation from self-inducing vomiting.
- Neurological causes are rare but should be considered: a full neurological examination with fundoscopy must be routine practice.
- Ideally inspect the vomit yourself to look for blood and bile.

Investigations to consider

Urine testing

- Dipstick urine for glucose.
- Dipstick urine for infection with lab analysis of mid-stream urine if positive as urosepsis is a common cause of vomiting, particularly in the

elderly who may have few other symptoms and signs.
- Consider a pregnancy test if there is any possibility of pregnancy.

Serology

- Full blood count, U&E, LFT, magnesium, phosphate, C-reactive protein: these basic investigations will determine the presence or absence of dehydration, infection, hypokalaemia and more rarely hypomagnesaemia and hypophosphataemia associated with persistent vomiting.
- Serum amylase (pancreatitis), random serum glucose (diabetic ketoacidosis), serum calcium (hypercalcaemia) and TFT (vomiting is also a feature of acute presentations of hypo- and hyperthyroidism).
- Consider investigation for corticosteroid deficiency (Addison's disease).
- In seriously ill patients, consider arterial blood gases to look for metabolic alkalosis with respiratory compensation (pH >7.44 and $PaCO_2$ >6.0 kPa).

Radiology

- Abdominal X-ray: if considering small or large bowel obstruction.
- Chest X-ray (erect): to exclude pneumonia or perforation.
- Ultrasound of the abdomen and biliary tree in suspected cholecystitis or pancreatitis.
- CT abdomen and pelvis will help to refine the differential diagnosis in the acute abdomen.
- CT head: if suspected raised intracranial pressure or cerebral lesion.
- Barium studies: barium meal or barium follow-through, useful in cases of chronic vomiting to confirm delayed gastric emptying.
- MRI: to investigate the small bowel in chronic nausea and vomiting.

Endoscopy

- Oesophagogastroduodenoscopy (OGD): to confirm or rule out peptic ulcer disease or inflammation and obtain histology if suspected malignancy.

- You will need to obtain consent for OGD and the risks to quote are: <1/1000 risk of perforation or haemorrhage with <1/200 risk of cardiorespiratory problems from sedation if used.

Motility studies

- Gastric scintigraphy using the tracer ^{99m}technetium to demonstrate gastric emptying using solid and liquid test meals.
- Scintigraphy cannot identify the specific cause, but may differentiate primary or secondary gastroparesis.

Management

Management is dependent on cause. Table 65.1 shows the causes of vomiting and nausea, with bold type indicating the most common causes. A basic guide to management for each cause is shown.

The mainstay of treatment is often supportive and this includes antiemetic treatment. Table 65.2 lists the classes of antiemetics, along with their mechanism of action and how to prescribe them safely. Be aware that:

- Most antiemetics antagonize neurotransmitter receptors involved in the pathophysiology of nausea and vomiting (see Introduction). Therefore it is important to understand their differing sites of action with your choice depending on the cause, preferred route of administration and safety.
- Some antiemetics (e.g. metoclopramide and domperidone) also exhibit prokinetic effects by speeding gastric emptying.
- The mechanism of action of glucocorticoids is unknown but they are effective and well tolerated in chemotherapy-induced vomiting; side effects include insomnia, hyperactivity, and mood disturbances. Dexamethasone (8 mg tds) is used as a single agent if mild symptoms are expected and with the addition of a 5-HT$_3$ receptor antagonist for more severe vomiting. Rarely, extreme vomiting due to chemotherapy may require co-therapy with dexamethasone, ondansetron and aprepitant.

Specific clinical situations

Gastrointestinal obstruction

- This is a surgical emergency which sometimes presents to MAU and requires prompt involvement of the surgical team.

- Keep nil-by-mouth and replace fluid and electrolyte deficiencies intravenously.
- As vomiting risks aspiration, place a wide-bore nasogastric tube to drain gastric/upper small bowel contents.
- Document fluid input and output carefully to allow accurate replacement and consider the electrolyte content of fluid losses in vomit or diarrhoea.
- Consider CT abdomen/pelvis to refine diagnosis and plan surgical intervention.
- Bowel obstruction for more than a few days may require nutritional support (probably parenteral) if clinically appropriate. Liaise with your hospital nutrition team.

Possible upper gastrointestinal malignancy

- All GI malignancies may present with vomiting, although it is more common in gastric and oesophageal cancer than tumours of the pancreas, biliary system or small bowel.
- History: alarm symptoms include dysphagia; dyspepsia; unintentional or progressive weight loss; persistent vomiting for over a month which is non-recurrent; painless jaundice (along with changes in colour of stool and urine); age >55 years; previous gastric surgery; family history of gastric cancer [3].
- The presence of alarm symptoms will most often prompt urgent outpatient referral using the 2-week wait pathway, although patients with severe vomiting, dehydration, or complete dysphagia may present directly to ED or MAU.
- Examination: look for anaemia, jaundice, objective evidence of weight loss, presence of an upper abdominal mass or hepatomegaly.
- Investigations: look for iron deficiency anaemia (for women, Hb <100 and ferritin <15 and for men Hb <110 and ferritin <30) and jaundice with a raised alkaline phosphatase suggestive of obstructive jaundice. If you suspect GI cancer of the oesophagus or stomach, then request OGD urgently (but not out-of-hours). If jaundice is present, then consider urgent (not out-of-hours) ultrasonography to establish whether biliary obstruction is present; if it is, then urgent endoscopic retrograde cholangio-pancreatography

Table 65.2 Antiemetics

Class	Receptor type(s)	Name of drug	Adult dose and route of administration	Uses	Comments and cautions
Anticholinergics	M_1 = muscarinic antagonist	Scopolamine	1.5 mg patch transdermal every 72 hours	Motion sickness	These are less sedative for managing travel sickness than antihistamines
		Hyoscine	10–20 mg PO 8-hourly		
Antihistamines	H_1 histamine antagonist	Cyclizine	50 mg PO or IM every 4–6 hours	Travel sickness and vestibular disorders. Cyclizine will counteract opiate-induced vomiting	Beware sedative effects
		Promethazine	12.5 to 25 mg PO/IM every 4 hours or 25 mg PR every 12 hours	First line in vomiting associated with pregnancy	
Phenothiazines	D_2 receptor (also some effect on M_1-muscarinic and H_1-histamine receptors) antagonists	Prochlorperazine	5–10 mg PO or IM 6–8-hourly, 2.5–10 mg IV 4-hourly, 25 mg PR 12-hourly, 3 mg buccal 12-hourly	Chemotherapy-induced vomiting or postoperative vomiting/nausea	Marked sedative effect, especially chlorpromazine. Risk of extrapyramidal side effects such as dystonia acutely and tardive dyskinesia in the longer term. Risk of hypotension in the elderly, especially using intravenous preparations
		Chlorpromazine	10–25 mg PO 4–6-hourly, 25 mg IV 3–4-hourly, 100 mg PR 6–8-hourly		
Benzamides	D2 receptors peripherally and centrally with weak 5-HT$_3$ receptor antagonist effect at high dose. Additional effect of stimulating cholinergic receptors on gastric smooth muscle cells and enhancing acetylcholine release at the neuromuscular junction	Metoclopramide	10 mg 8-hourly PO/IM/IV	Prokinetic (due to increased gastric emptying), therefore useful in gastrointestinal stasis. Higher doses can aid chemotherapy-induced emesis (due to 5-HT$_3$ activity) – especially cisplatin-induced symptoms. Migraine	Metoclopramide crosses the blood–brain barrier with risk of irreversible tardive dyskinesia in high doses prescribed long term. Risk of acute dystonic reactions including oculogyric crises, especially in young women and the elderly, and also causes akathisia and dystonia. Beneficial effect of speeding gastric emptying in and increasing tone of the lower oesophageal sphincter. Domperidone does not cross the blood–brain barrier, therefore lacks the neurological side effects of metoclopramide. Domperidone may be useful in Parkinson's disease to counter the nausea and vomiting induced by apomorphine and other dopaminergic drugs
		Domperidone	10 mg PO 8-hourly or 60 mg PR 12-hourly		

Class	Receptor type(s)	Name of drug	Adult dose and route of administration	Uses	Comments and cautions
Butyrophenones	D2 dopamine	Haloperidol	0.5–5 mg PO 8–12-hourly	Pre-anaesthetic agent or postoperative nausea and vomiting	Dose-dependent risk of prolonged QT syndrome and torsades de pointes
		Droperidol	0.625–2.5 mg IM		More rarely dystonia and hypotension
Serotonin receptor antagonists	5-HT$_3$ receptors centrally and peripherally	Ondansetron	8 mg PO 8-hourly or 8–16 mg IV single dose	Most useful for severe chemotherapy- and radiotherapy-induced vomiting	Asthenia and constipation (5–10%) Dizziness (10%; intravenous preparation only) ECG abnormalities noted with hypokalaemia/ hypomagnesaemia, heart failure including prolonged QT and torsades de pointes therefore monitor ECG
		Granisetron	2 mg PO 1 hour pre-chemotherapy then 1 mg 12 hours later or 1 mg before anaesthetic induction	Helpful for postoperative vomiting	Ondansetron should not be co-administered with apomorphine due to profound hypotension
Neurokinin receptor antagonists	NK1 receptors	Aprepitant	125 mg 1 hour pre-chemotherapy then 80 mg daily for the next 2 days	Chemotherapy-induced vomiting both acute and delayed and especially cisplatin-based regimens: give along with dexamethasone and a 5-HT$_3$ receptor antagonist for best effect	Use with caution in patients receiving drugs metabolized through the CYP3A4 pathway as these inhibit CYP3A4 metabolism

(ERCP) on the next ERCP list may be required to decompress the biliary tree. Refer the patient to gastroenterology.

- Management: as guided by results and if malignancy confirmed, then refer to the appropriate MDT. The specialist nurse is a useful resource for you, the patient and their family.

Palliative care management of nausea and vomiting

- Nausea and vomiting are common and distressing symptoms which need to be managed sensitively. Engage with palliative care services early as they will provide invaluable and specialist assistance for patients where further oncological or surgical treatment is not appropriate [4].
- Seek specialist advice from an oncologist to manage the direct complications of chemotherapy or radiotherapy.
- Treat any reversible causes: stop causative medication and treat constipation, hypercalcaemia, uraemia, infection, and gastric irritation (e.g. omeprazole 40 mg od).
- Manage according to the cause (see Table 65.1) and be aware that route of administration of antiemetics may need changing to intravenous, intramuscular or rectal preparations as gastrointestinal absorption may be limited.

Pregnancy

- 90% of pregnant women experience nausea and 50% experience vomiting in the first 9 weeks of pregnancy. Most symptoms resolve by 16 weeks of gestation [5].
- Prolonged vomiting and nausea (hyperemesis gravidarum) occurs in 3/1000 pregnancies with weight loss of 5% of pre-pregnancy weight, dehydration, electrolyte and nutritional deficiencies. This requires hospital admission for rehydration, antiemetics, thiamine (100 mg daily orally) and enteral or parenteral nutritional support to reduce risk to maternal and fetal health. On diagnosis of hyperemesis gravidarum, review pelvic ultrasound to diagnose multiple or molar pregnancy.
- Avoid drugs if possible. Anecdotal evidence suggests that ginger or wrist acupressure may help. All antiemetics are unlicensed in

pregnancy although several appear safe and are recommended in recent NICE guidance. Antihistamines such as oral promethazine (25 mg bd) or oral cyclizine (up to 50 mg tds) are first line, with prochlorperazine (10 mg tds orally or 3–6 mg buccally bd), ondansetron (8 mg bd) and metoclopramide (10 mg tds) used as second-line drugs.

- Recurrent vomiting may cause oesophagitis so consider using a proton pump inhibitor (omeprazole 20 mg od) or H_2-receptor antagonist (ranitidine 150 mg bd) to break this cycle.

Gastroparesis

- Gastroparesis is often secondary to diabetes mellitus so careful control of blood sugar is the mainstay of treatment, limiting further nerve damage and possibly reversing autonomic neuropathy [6].
- Nutrition must be considered and use of a percutaneous endoscopic gastrostomy (PEG) with a jejunal extension, a direct percutaneous endoscopic jejunostomy or placing a surgical jejunostomy allows predictable nutrition, and assists in glucose control.
- A trial of prokinetics may be beneficial (metoclopramide 10 mg tds or domperidone 10 mg tds) with some evidence for erythromycin (a motilin agonist) at up to 4 g daily.
- Gastric electrical stimulation (gastric pacing) is not routinely funded and remains experimental.

Functional disorders

Anorexia and bulimia nervosa

- Vomiting is a major feature of bulimia with 50% of patients exhibiting electrolyte disturbance with hypokalaemic, hypochloraemic metabolic alkalosis.
- Vomiting can occur in anorexia, possibly from delayed gastric emptying due to vagal nerve damage secondary to malnutrition.
- Treatment is supportive with intravenous fluids, antiemetics and psychiatric support.

Psychogenic vomiting

- This occurs in young women, during or shortly after meals. It is rarely preceded by nausea. It may be a manifestation of emotional disturbance but is rarely associated with psychiatric illness.

Cyclical vomiting

- Nausea and vomiting occurs in attacks lasting several days in association with headache, abdominal pain and fever.
- Patients are often well between episodes and frequently well informed about the appropriate medication to settle their vomiting (try ondansetron 8 mg tds).
- They may require brief admissions to maintain fluid input although nutrition is less of a problem if attacks are infrequent.
- Patients with frequent attacks may be helped by a range of medications including antidepressants, anticonvulsants and antimigraine preparations.

Scenario 65.1 continued

The symptoms of intermittent vomiting in a patient with poorly controlled diabetes should lead to the consideration of gastroparesis. This patient underwent gastric emptying studies that showed normal or slightly rapid emptying. Further investigations were also unremarkable. It was decided that her symptoms were in fact due to cyclical vomiting syndrome. She responded to a combination of lifestyle modifications (avoiding triggers, improved sleep patterns) and psychological support (associated anxiety symptoms).

References

1. Carpenter DP (1990) Neural mechanisms of emesis. *Can J Physiol Pharmacol* 68: 230.

2. British Medical Association and the Royal Pharmaceutical Society of Great Britain (2013) *British National Formulary*, 65th edn. BMJ Publishing Group.

3. NICE (2005) Referral guidelines for suspected cancer. National Institute for Health and Care Excellence. Clinical guideline 27. http://publications.nice.org.uk/referral-guidelines-for-suspected-cancer-cg27/guidance.

4. NICE (2012) Palliative cancer care – nausea and vomiting. National Institute for Health and Care Excellence. Clinical Knowledge Summaries. http://cks.nice.org.uk/palliative-cancer-care-nausea-vomiting.

5. NICE (2013) Nausea/vomiting in pregnancy. National Institute for Health and Care Excellence. Clinical Knowledge Summaries. http://cks.nice.org.uk/nauseavomiting-in-pregnancy.

6. Camilleri M, Parkman HP, Shafi MA, Abell TL, Gerson L; American College of Gastroenterology (2013) Clinical guideline: management of gastroparesis. *Am J Gastroenterol* 108: 18–37.

Weakness and paralysis

Kate R. Petheram, Chris Allen and Rob Whiting

(A) Assessment of the patient with motor weakness

Kate R. Petheram and Chris Allen

Scenario 66A.1

A 25-year-old man is referred urgently by his GP. He was fit and well until 2 days previously when he developed tingling and mild numbness in his fingers and toes. This morning his GP was called to see him because he was having difficulty walking. On examination he has significant lower limb weakness, especially proximally with hyporeflexia.

This chapter will help you develop an approach to reaching a differential diagnosis in the patient presenting with motor weakness.

Introduction

'Weakness' is a common presenting complaint to acute medical services. As well as referring to loss of muscle strength, patients may also use the term to describe fatigue, tiredness or lack of coordination. Initial management requires the formulation of a syndromal diagnosis from the history and a focused clinical examination to initiate appropriate investigations and start any necessary urgent treatment, whilst involving specialist teams as appropriate. For example, in a patient with lower motor neurone weakness due to Guillain–Barré syndrome (acute inflammatory demyelinating peripheral neuropathy, AIDP) the initial acute diagnosis is clinical and the tests that are urgently needed are those that will determine the acuity of treatment required (e.g. whether that patient needs intensive

care). On the other hand, in the patient with a rapidly evolving upper motor neurone lesion due a cord lesion, an MRI of the spinal cord (not the brain) will allow timely onward referral to neurosurgical services if a compressive lesion is found.

Weakness can be a symptom of pathology in any of the following anatomical domains:

- muscle
- neuromuscular junction
- peripheral nerve or nerve root
- pyramidal (spinal cord, brainstem, internal capsule)
- extrapyramidal (basal ganglia)
- motor cortex
- functional (behavioural).

The causative pathology of weakness can be suggested by:

- distribution of the weakness
- tempo of onset of the weakness
- accompanying symptoms
- site of the pathology suggested by the examination.

History

The history often suggests the anatomical location but is especially informative about the pathology of the lesion. Time spent in obtaining a clear history from the acutely weak patient is never wasted, even if this needs be partly second hand from accompanying relatives or obtained by phone from other witnesses. These are the important points upon which to focus:

- distribution of weakness
- tempo of onset
- accompanying symptoms and additional features in the history.

Acute Medicine, ed. Stephen Haydock, Duncan Whitehead and Zoë Fritz. Published by Cambridge University Press. © Cambridge University Press 2015.

Distribution of weakness

One arm or leg involved?

This is likely to be peripheral nerve or nerve root in origin. A pure monoparesis is unlikely to be spinal cord or above although occasionally can be cortical. However, remember Brown-Séquard syndrome (hemi-cord syndrome) where they are sensory signs (or symptoms) on the strong side.

One arm and one leg on the same side (hemiplegia/paresis)

This distribution suggests a cerebral hemisphere or brainstem lesion (or cervical hemi-cord lesion) but it is important to exclude significant motor signs (e.g. extensor plantar) on the other side. Brainstem lesions usually declare themselves by presenting with accompanying visual or cerebellar symptoms and signs.

Both legs (paraplegia/paresis)

This suggests a spinal cord lesion, especially if there is a sensory level on the trunk, unless there are lower motor neurone signs (absent reflexes, etc.) in which case multiple peripheral nerves may be involved (as in Guillain–Barré syndrome (AIDP)).

Weakness in all four limbs (quadriplegia/paresis)

This suggests a single lesion in the brainstem or high cervical cord or a diffuse pathology affecting peripheral nerves or muscles. Localizing the lesion causing a quadriparesis will require other clues from the history and examination. Here, again, determining by examination whether the weakness is upper or lower motor neurone or a mixture is fundamental.

Proximal, distal or global weakness?

Proximal weakness of all four limbs suggests a primary muscle disease, acute myositis or myopathy. This produces a waddling gait and/or difficulty rising from squatting or from deep armchairs as well as difficulty lifting objects with the arms. Proximal weakness of both lower limbs only can also occur in muscle disease but rarely can be a presentation of Guillain–Barré syndrome (AIDP).

Acute or subacute distal weakness usually suggests a more peripheral problem such as a peripheral neuropathy or spinal root disorder.

Facial involvement?

In the case of hemiplegia, facial involvement on the same side gives further support to a cerebral hemisphere lesion. If the facial involvement is contralateral then a brainstem lesion is probable. In a quadriparesis facial weakness could indicate either a brainstem lesion or peripheral nerve pathology. However, a brainstem lesion of sufficient size to give both a quadriparesis and bilateral facial weakness is very likely to also cause problems with other brainstem nuclei and tracts, including those mediating bulbar function and eye movements. Bilateral facial weakness without these features may be missed by observers if symmetrical but usually indicates myasthenia if ptosis also present and AIDP if it is not.

Bulbar or respiratory weakness?

A history of dysarthria or dysphagia should be sought to exclude a brainstem lesion or peripheral involvement of the bulbar muscles from myasthenia or AIDP (Guillain–Barré syndrome). Bulbar weakness may cause respiratory aspiration. Similarly a history of respiratory discomfort in the supine position may indicate weakness of the diaphragm in either AIDP or myasthenia.

Accompanying sensory symptoms?

A history of sensory symptoms may give a clue to the anatomical location of the problem. Sensory loss below a certain segmental level in the presence of a hemiparesis suggests a cord lesion at that level. Sensory symptoms in a root or peripheral nerve distribution (i.e. affecting parts of a limb rather than the whole) respectively suggest pathology there (see Chapter 4).

Tempo of onset

The rapidity of onset of weakness is often the best clue as to the pathological process.

Less than 5 minutes

Onset to peak deficit within seconds or minutes is highly suggestive of a vascular pathology (see part (B) of this chapter on the stroke patient). A stuttering onset with abrupt onset of weakness with recovery and then further decline may suggest rarer types of vascular lesions including dural venous sinus thrombosis (with venous haemorrhage) although lacunar stroke in the hemisphere or brainstem often presents in such a stuttering fashion. Rapid onset of a root lesion accompanied by pain indicates compression, usually from an intervertebral disc prolapse and rapid onset of a peripheral nerve lesion suggests vasculitis. If a person wakes from sleep with a deficit it may have been developing over some time; in the case of a peripheral nerve lesion this may be compressive such as a wrist drop due to radial nerve compression at the spiral groove of the humerus.

Minutes to hours

The weakness of hemiplegic migraine, usually accompanied or followed by a typical headache, evolves typically over 20–40 minutes and can last for several hours and sometimes days. Again vascular lesions can rarely present in a less dramatically sudden fashion. In this case the age and the presence or absence of stroke risk factors will help the diagnosis. A hemiparesis developing acutely after a lucid interval following even modest head trauma (especially to the temple) might suggest an extradural haematoma requiring prompt neurosurgical attention.

Days to a few weeks

Weakness evolving over days or a few weeks often suggests an inflammatory or autoimmune cause such as myasthenia, Guillain–Barré syndrome or central demyelination. For example, if a peripheral neuropathy comes on subacutely then Guillain–Barré syndrome (AIDP) has to be high on the list of likely diagnoses (see also Chapter 4). Central inflammatory demyelinating lesions (as occur in multiple sclerosis) will also come on over a few days but will have an upper rather than a lower motor pattern of weakness (i.e. with brisk tendon reflexes). Weakness from space-occupying lesions in the spine or cerebral hemispheres may appear to develop over days or a few weeks but there may a longer story of less dramatic symptoms obtainable with careful history taking. Myasthenia gravis can evolve over many weeks with fatiguable weakness of the face and eye muscles and then present more suddenly with bulbar failure.

Months

A more indolent picture with weakness coming on over a few months is more suggestive of a degenerative cause. Motor neurone disease is one example of this. Such conditions can present more acutely especially when, for example, the muscles of respiration are involved and there is intercurrent infection and ventilatory capacity appears to decompensate rapidly. In such a case a longer history of difficulty in walking or manual dexterity may be elicited or there may be a history of ventilatory discomfort in the supine position.

Years

Typically genetic conditions and some degenerative conditions present with problems going back many years although the patient may only just become aware of limitations imposed by their weakness. These are unlikely to present to the acute physician, again unless an intercurrent illness causes abrupt decompensation (for example with the heterogeneous group of mitochondrial disorders).

Accompanying symptoms and additional features in the history

Pain

Painful muscles with proximal limb weakness may suggest an inflammatory myositis or rhabdomyolysis. Patients with Guillain–Barré syndrome (AIDP) frequently have considerable pain in their back and limbs at presentation, often enough to raise suspicion of spinal root or spinal cord compression from an extrinsic lesion. Painful paraesthesia suggests peripheral neuropathy (most commonly occurring in alcoholic and diabetic neuropathy).

In a young person with no stroke risk factors, headache with hemiplegia may suggest hemiplegic migraine but this may warrant further investigation to exclude venous sinus thrombosis, a mass lesion or stroke pathologies. About one-third of patients with ischaemic stroke have a headache at presentation, whilst the rarer intracranial haemorrhages more frequently have an acute headache at presentation (see part (B) of this chapter on the stroke patient).

Fatiguability

Myasthenia gravis should be considered if weakness is better in the morning and reliably worse later in the day or improves with a relatively short rest, especially if associated with bulbar weakness (dysphagia getting worse towards the end of a meal or dysarthria towards the end of a conversation). Myasthenia gravis hardly ever presents with limb weakness unaccompanied by bulbar or eye muscle involvement (notably ptosis).

Patients with a subacute onset of an upper motor neurone paraparesis (usually due to inflammatory disease of the spinal cord) may report an apparent worsening after walking some distance but this is usually distinguishable from the more rapid fatiguability of myasthenia.

Sphincter disturbance

Bladder or bowel disturbance is more common in central rather than peripheral nervous system pathology and often suggests spinal cord pathology. Incontinence is a late feature of extrinsic spinal cord compression. The early appearance in the history of sphincter disturbance in a spinal cord (upper motor neurone) lesion, i.e. with only mild weakness, suggests intrinsic pathology (such as demyelination). However, bladder involvement from bilateral sacral root involvement at the cauda equina can occur with acute central lumbosacral disc protrusion when it is accompanied by bilateral sciatica and sacral sensory loss, which are usually more prominent than any weakness (although the ankle reflexes will be absent).

Visual disturbance

Diplopia suggests weakness of the extraocular muscles which can be either central from brainstem pathology, or peripheral affecting cranial nerves III, IV and VI outside the brainstem or the neuromuscular junction as in myasthenia (when it is always accompanied by ptosis, although this can be strikingly asymmetrical).

Nystagmus always suggests brainstem pathology and may not have been noticed by the patient. However, it should be remembered that myasthenia gravis can mimic almost any variety of eye movement abnormality.

Monocular visual loss may indicate inflammation of the optic nerve and hence, in the presence of weakness, more multifocal central nervous involvement (usually inflammatory).

A homonymous hemianopia suggests a cerebral hemisphere lesion. A transient hemianopia is a common feature of migraine but is usually accompanied by positive phenomena in the form of a scintillating scotoma or fortification spectra that move across the visual fields over minutes, leaving the hemianopic defect in their wake.

Speech and/or swallowing (bulbar) involvement

A history of dysphagia or dysarthria suggests weakness of bulbar muscles (cranial nerves IX, X and XII), termed a 'pseudobulbar palsy' when caused by an upper motor neurone lesion and a 'bulbar palsy' when from a lower motor neurone lesion. Where a disease affects both upper and lower motor neurones, as in motor neurone disease, these may coexist. If the problem is in the production of basic speech sounds (dysphonia), the problem is at the level of the larynx or its innervation.

A higher level language disturbance affecting speech content (i.e. dysphasia) and not just articulation is a result of a lesion in the left (usually) cerebral hemisphere.

Family history

A positive family history points towards a genetic diagnosis, or a genetic predisposition to more common diseases. Often patients' fears as to what might be the diagnosis will be conditioned by their family history. This may be misguided but if they are knowledgeable about a rare genetic condition present in their family (e.g. mitochondrial disease) it is worth considering this seriously, especially if the presenting syndrome seems to be unusual.

Examination

Having spent some time and trouble obtaining as clear a history as is possible, a short list of differential diagnoses should have been generated. Then there are two objectives in the neurological examination of a patient with weakness and both of these can be met without the expenditure of a lot of time.

- To differentiate between the possible diagnoses generated by the history with a focused examination.
- To screen for any accompanying neurological deficit not suspected from the history and provide a baseline for emergent problems.

Focused examination

- Is the weakness due to a motor innervation, neuromuscular junction or muscle lesion?
- If neural, is it an upper or lower motor neurone?
- Are there any accompanying sensory signs?
- Is there a single anatomical site of the lesion or is it multifocal or systematic?
- Is the weakness organic or functional?

Table 66A.1 demonstrates the main signs required to localize the site of the lesion in the motor system. With lower motor neurone lesions a basic knowledge of the myotomal distribution of the nerve roots and the motor innervation of the principal peripheral nerves (Tables 66A.2 and 66A.3) will allow one to distinguish peripheral nerve from nerve root (spinal roots or plexus). In the presence of an upper motor weakness

Table 66A.1 Differentiating the type of weakness on examination

	Functional	Extrapyramidal	Upper motor neurone	Lower motor neurone	Muscle	Neuromuscular junction (myasthenia)
Distribution of weakness	Not anatomical Hoover's sign	Asymmetric bradykinesia (fine motor control)	Arm extensors Leg flexors	Related to nerve/root	Usually proximal	Eye (including ptosis), bulbar, respiratory Face, neck
Reflexes	Normal	Normal	Brisk	Absent or reduced	Normal	Normal
Tone	Normal	Increased (lead pipe)	Increased (spastic)	Reduced or normal	Normal	Normal
Wasting	None	None	None	Present after interval	Not conspicuous	None
Fasciculation	None	None	None	Present (in established lesions)	None	None
Plantar reflex	Down (flexor)	Down (flexor)	Up (extensor)	Down (flexor) or mute	Down (flexor)	Down (flexor)
Gait	Bizarre Non-physiological	Festinant No arm swing	Spastic	Flapping	Waddling	Often not conspicuously abnormal

Table 66A.2 Upper limb motor innervation

Movement	Muscle(s)	Root	Reflex	Peripheral nerve
Shoulder abduction	Deltoid	C5		Axillary
Elbow flexion	Biceps Brachioradialis	C5/6 C6	Biceps Supinator	Musculocutaneous Radial
Elbow extension Finger extension	Triceps Extensor digitorum communis	C7	Triceps	Radial
Finger flexion	Flexor digitorum profundus Flexor pollicis longus	C8	Finger	Median (anterior interosseous branch) Ulnar
Finger abduction Thumb abduction	Dorsal interossei Abductor pollicis brevis	T1		Ulnar Median

of the limbs, the further localization of the lesion may require attention to the presence of eye movement abnormalities (see Chapter 64), especially nystagmus which indicates a brainstem lesion.

Alongside an assessment of the distribution of weakness, examination of the tendon reflexes is the most diagnostically useful part of the examination of a patient with weakness. Knowledge of the segmental innervation of the tendon reflexes is helpful in this context (Tables 66A.2 and 66A.3).

Wasting indicates the loss of motor neurones or axons at, or distal to, the anterior horns of the spinal cord grey matter but takes some time to develop and may not be conspicuous if the pathology is predominantly in the myelin (as in an inflammatory demyelinating neuropathy). Thus if the weakness is acute or subacute, wasting will not be present in lower motor lesions. Upper motor neurone lesions do not cause wasting (the increase in tone means there is no 'disuse') and the concept of wasting due to disuse is dubious and probably only happens in (rare) purely cortical lesions or in situations where movement is mechanically restricted (prolonged splinting, etc.) or inhibited by pain. However, the tendon reflex arc depends on intact

Table 66A.3 Lower limb motor innervation

Movement	Muscle	Root	Reflex	Peripheral nerve
Hip flexion	Iliopsoas	L1 and 2		Femoral and L1/2 spinal nerves
Knee extension	Quadriceps	L(3) 4	Knee	Femoral
Ankle dorsiflexion	Tibialis anterior	L4		Deep peroneal
Ankle inversion	Tibialis posterior	L4 (5)		Tibial nerve
Ankle eversion	Peronei	L5 (S1)		Superficial peroneal
Ankle plantar flexion	Soleus Gastrocnemius	S1	Ankle	Tibial
Hip extension	Gluteus maximus	L5 and S1		Sciatic
Knee flexion	Hamstrings	S1		Sciatic

afferent and efferent (motor) neurones and thus will be absent even early on in a lower motor neurone lesion.

If there is mixture of lower and upper motor neurone signs, for example, florid fasciculations and brisk reflexes, the presence or absence of sensory involvement is important. If sensation is normal with a mixture of lower and upper motor neurone it is highly suggestive of a motor system disease such as motor neurone disease.

If myasthenia is suspected, see if muscle power is fatiguable. Since ptosis and eye movement weakness are almost invariable in myasthenia, usually asymmetrically, ask the patient to look up at the ceiling (with the head in neutral position) and watch if the eyelid descends and ask him/her to look to follow a finger to one side with eyes only and see if diplopia occurs. If ptosis or diplopia is already present, ask the patient to gently close the eyes for a minute and then see if the ptosis or diplopia has improved briefly when the eyes are reopened. In the upper limb, check the patient's shoulder abduction power and see if this fatigues with repeated movement.

If functional weakness is suspected because the findings on examination do not make anatomical or physiological sense then test for Hoover's sign. Hold your hand under the apparently weak limb and ask the patient to flex their contralateral hip against resistance. If you feel pressure from the previously weak leg as it extends to synergistically counterbalance flexion of the other leg at the hip, Hoover's sign is present. However, extreme caution needs to exercised in making a diagnosis of entirely functional weakness since a person's emotional response to organic illness (especially in the presence of pain) often results in a functional component to a weakness that is principally organic in origin.

Investigations and management

A clinical differential diagnosis will enable the correct investigations to be performed with appropriate priority. In the acute situation the diagnoses for which urgent treatment is indicated should be ruled in or out first. When a lesion requiring urgent neurosurgical attention is in the differential (notably spinal cord compression), an image of the appropriate area should be sought as soon as the patient is confirmed to be safe from the cardiorespiratory aspect. If Guillain–Barré syndrome is suspected then assessment of respiratory function is more important than electrophysiological confirmation of the diagnosis. Any patient with bulbar symptoms or signs should be stabilized from a respiratory point of view before further diagnostic neurological investigations are performed.

Blood tests

All patients admitted should have routine *full blood count* and *electrolytes* measured. Other tests can be requested depending on the suspected diagnosis.

Creatine kinase may be raised in muscle disease.

Acetylcholine receptor antibodies are positive in approximately 80% of patients with generalized myasthenia gravis. Although these will not be available for days, the earlier the blood is sent the better.

Arterial blood gases are important especially if bulbar dysfunction and/or neurogenic hypoventilation are suspected.

ECG

In Guillain–Barré syndrome autonomic disturbance can lead to cardiac arrhythmias and a resting sinus tachycardia is frequently seen due to autonomic denervation of the heart. A baseline ECG and initial cardiac monitoring are therefore advised.

Neuroimaging

The modality of imaging required will depend on the suspected diagnosis and should be directed at the anatomical site suggested by the history and examination (scans should not be used as a substitute for clinical diagnosis). In the acute setting the emphasis should be on establishing diagnoses that need urgent treatment.

- For cerebral hemisphere lesions, CT brain imaging is quick and easily accessible. If a non-contrast scan is normal and the level of suspicion is high then a contrast scan should be requested. If venous sinus thrombosis is suspected then a CT venogram is indicated.
- For suspected acute spinal cord lesions MRI is the modality of choice (CT is of no value). The urgency again depends on the suspected diagnosis. If cord compression is suspected then same day imaging (*of the spinal cord*) for discussion with neurosurgeons is indicated. If a brainstem or cerebellar lesion is suspected then MRI will give more detailed information than CT.
- It is important to ensure cardiorespiratory stability before the patient attends the radiology department. Remember, for MRI the patient will be required to lie flat and still for at least 20 minutes.

Respiratory function tests

Forced vital capacity (FVC): this is a measure of the strength of the respiratory muscles. Peak flow is a measure of airway calibre and is *not* helpful in assessing neurogenic hypoventilation. FVC is especially useful in monitoring patients with suspected Guillain–Barré syndrome. A declining trend in FVC should prompt discussion with intensive care teams and closer observation on a high dependency or intensive care unit. A decline in FVC will precede blood gas changes in acute neurogenic hypoventilation unless bulbar dysfunction has led to aspiration.

Lumbar puncture

Lumbar puncture is most useful in patients whose weakness is suspected to be due to Guillain–Barré syndrome or central demyelination but is contraindicated if a mass lesion is suspected. In most cases of acute weakness it is not an investigation that is urgently indicated (as it is in suspected meningitis).

Neurophysiology

Nerve conduction studies and *electromyelography* look at nerve and muscle function but do not form part of the acute medical assessment of the weak patient and are best delegated to expert teams.

> **Scenario 66A.1 continued**
>
> *This young man's presentation is consistent with acute inflammatory demyelinating polyneuropathy (Guillain–Barré syndrome). The diagnosis was confirmed by nerve conduction studies. His FVC began to fall following admission and he was transferred urgently to the HDU for close monitoring.*
>
> (See also Chapter 4.)

Further reading

Ginsberg L. Neurology in practice: The bare essentials. Disorders of the spinal cord and roots. *Pract Neurol* 2011; 11: 259–267.

Overell JR. Peripheral neuropathy: pattern recognition for the pragmatist. *Pract Neurol* 2010; 10: 315–325.

Pritchard J. What's new in Guillain-Barré syndrome? *Pract Neurol* 2006; 6: 208–217.

(B) The stroke patient

Rob Whiting

Introduction

Stroke is the third commonest cause of death and the leading cause of adult disability worldwide. It affects approximately 15 million people each year, of whom 5 million will die and 5 million are left with a permanent deficit. In the UK it accounts for approximately 6% of all NHS and social care expenditure. A stroke is a syndrome characterized by:

- rapidly developing clinical symptoms/signs of focal loss of cerebral function (sometimes global, as in subarachnoid haemorrhage)
- no apparent cause other than that of vascular origin
- symptoms lasting more than 1 hour, and usually more than 24 hours (as compared to a transient ischaemic attack).

Prompt and accurate diagnosis of stroke is essential for:

- initiation of time-limited treatments
- identification of stroke aetiology
- timely management of vascular risk factors.

Arterial supply to the brain

The brain receives its blood supply by two routes. The two *vertebral arteries* arise as branches of the subclavian arteries and come together to form the *basilar artery* on the anterior surface of the pons. At the base of the brain they form the right and left posterior cerebral arteries. These constitute the posterior circulation. The two *internal carotid arteries* arise at the bifurcation of the common carotid arteries and at the base of the brain give rise to the *middle cerebral artery* and *anterior cerebral artery*. These constitute the anterior circulation. The vertebral and internal carotid arterial circulations communicate with each other through the small posterior communicating arteries that arise after the bifurcation of the vertebral artery. The two anterior cerebral arteries communicate via the *anterior communicating artery*. This arrangement results in an arterial loop (actually a heptagon) at the base of the brain called the *circle of Willis*. However, less than 50% of the population have a well-developed and symmetrical circle of Willis.

The anterior circulation supplies the forebrain including anterior cortex, basal ganglia, thalamus and internal capsule.

The posterior circulation supplies the posterior cortex, midbrain, cerebellum and brainstem.

Scenario 66B.1

You are called to the emergency department to receive a 76-year-old man who has been pre-alerted by the paramedics, who noted him to be FAST-positive with left-sided weakness and speech disturbance.

With the increasing use of thrombolytic therapy for acute ischaemic stroke, it is common for patients with focal neurological signs to be brought into hospital as an emergency. Many acute hospitals have a pre-alert system to prepare the on-call medical team to receive the patient as they arrive. This can mean that patients may arrive with the briefest of clinical information, and without any relevant past medical history.

History

Key points in the history which may point to a diagnosis of stroke include:

- rapid onset of deficit within minutes
- focal neurological symptoms which normally relate to a specific vascular territory
- predominantly negative neurological symptoms

- co-morbidities or medications which indicate an increased vascular risk.

Examination

Key objectives of the physical examination are to:

- determine the presence of focal neurological signs
- assess the severity and likely vascular territory of the stroke
- identify clues to the aetiology of the stroke.

Screening tools to facilitate detection of stroke

Screening tools such as the FAST (Face, Arm, Speech, Time) test have been developed to increase wider public awareness of stroke symptoms. Such basic screening tools will often overlook important signs, such as visual field loss and sensory inattention.

The ROSIER (Recognition of Stroke in the Emergency Room) tool is another validated assessment to facilitate early diagnosis of stroke and differentiation from common stroke mimics (Table 66B.1).

In many cases, the history and examination findings may make the diagnosis of stroke straightforward. However, non-vascular conditions may often manifest with a clinical picture very similar to an acute stroke syndrome (stroke mimics). Furthermore, strokes may sometimes present in atypical ways ('stroke chameleons'), leading to a delay in diagnosis and appropriate treatment.

Stroke mimics

Stroke mimics may account for 20–25% of suspected stroke presentations. Common mimics include:

Table 66B.1 The ROSIER tool to distinguish stroke from stroke mimics. Stroke is likely if total score is >0

Clinical features	Score for Yes	Score for No
Has there been loss of consciousness or syncope?	−1	0
Has there been seizure activity?	−1	0
Is there a new, acute onset:		
1. Asymmetric facial weakness?	+1	0
2. Asymmetric arm weakness?	+1	0
3. Asymmetric leg weakness?	+1	0
4. Speech disturbance?	+1	0
5. Visual field defect?	+1	0

- seizures
- sepsis
- toxic/metabolic disturbance
- syncope
- space-occupying lesion
- delirium
- peripheral vestibular disorder
- mononeuropathy
- functional disorder/medically unexplained symptoms
- migraine.

Non-classical presentations of stroke ('stroke chameleons')

These uncommon stroke presentations may imitate other diseases, often because the symptoms and signs may not correspond with a vascular territory, or the speed of onset is atypical.

Less common causes

Cervical artery dissection

- Clinical features include headache, neck or facial pain, Horner's syndrome, pulsatile tinnitus.
- There may be a history of mechanical trauma to head or neck, which may seem minor.
- Diagnosis is with MR angiography (particularly with fat-suppressed T1-weighted sequence), but can often be seen on CT angiogram.

Cerebral venous sinus thrombosis

- Headache is commonest symptom; focal neurological deficits can occur, depending on area of brain involved.
- Other manifestations include seizures, altered consciousness and papilloedema.
- A hypercoagulable risk factor is seen in 85% of cases (e.g. pregnancy and postpartum period, patients on oral contraceptive pill, malignancy, inherited thrombophilia, inflammatory disorders such as Behçet's, inflammatory bowel disease).
- Diagnosis is with MR/CT venography.

Reversible cerebral vasoconstriction syndrome

- Commonest clinical symptom is acute, severe headache (may be described as 'thunderclap')

- Other manifestations include motor seizures and visual disturbance (cortical blindness, flashing lights, scotomas). Confusion, apraxia, aphasia and ataxia may occur.
- Various associations, including pregnancy and puerperium (pre-eclampsia/eclampsia), hypercalcaemia, phaeochromocytoma, bronchial carcinoid, exposure to certain drugs (pseudoephedrine, SSRIs, sumatriptan, tacrolimus, cyclophosphamide, cocaine, ecstasy, LSD) and blood products (erythropoietin, IV immunoglobulin, red cell transfusion).

Atypical symptoms

Neuropsychiatric symptoms

- Strokes involving non-dominant frontal and parietal lobes may present with anosognosia, aprosodia, or disorders of diminished motivation (such as abulia or akinetic mutism). These symptoms may be mistaken for depression.

Delirium

- May be the presenting feature in a few patients; more common with haemorrhagic stroke. More commonly seen with strokes involving the right temporal gyrus, right inferior parietal lobe, or occipital lobe.

Altered consciousness

- A rapid drop in conscious level may accompany large strokes, especially intracerebral haemorrhages associated with a rapid rise in intracranial pressure.
- Patients with embolic occlusion of the distal basilar artery ('top-of-the-basilar' syndrome) may present with unconsciousness, quadriparesis, incontinence, pupillary abnormalities and oculomotor signs.
- Rarely, embolic occlusion of the artery of Percheron may cause bilateral infarction of the medial thalamus and rostral midbrain; this can manifest with coma and few other signs.

Peripheral nervous system symptoms

Acute vestibular syndrome

- A stroke is rarely the cause of dizziness. It accounts for only 3% of patients with dizziness and other symptoms, and only 1% of those presenting with vertigo in isolation without other symptoms and signs.

- In peripheral lesions, visual fixation on a stationary object may ameliorate symptoms, but not so much in central lesions. Ataxia is often more severe in patients with central lesions.
- The Dix–Hallpike manoeuvre and head impulse tests can differentiate central from peripheral causes of vertigo. (See Chapter 63.)

Monoparesis

- Isolated monoparesis is uncommon, accounting for approximately 5% of cases.
- Most commonly affects the arm (usually a middle cerebral artery territory lesion), but can also affect the leg (often an anterior cerebral artery territory lesion) or face (usually a subcortical event).
- Differential diagnosis can include spinal cord or root lesions, or peripheral nerve lesions.
- Assessment of cortical sensation (e.g. stereognosis, graphaesthesia and point localization) can aid correct diagnosis.

Assessing stroke severity and clinical classification

National Institutes of Health Stroke Scale (NIHSS)

This is a validated assessment used to measure the level of impairment caused by a stroke. There are 15 items, assessing conscious level, ocular gaze, visual fields, speech and language function, inattention, motor and sensory impairments, and ataxia.

The NIHSS is quick to perform and has good inter-observer reliability. It is thus a useful tool to monitor a patient's response to treatments such as thrombolytic therapy. There is a widely available online training programme to ensure that the assessment is standardized.

Bamford (Oxford Community Stroke Project; OCSP) classification of stroke

The OCSP classification [1] is a simple clinical scheme for subdividing patients with acute stroke into one of four subgroups, based on clinical criteria. The four main subgroups are shown in Table 66B.2.

Table 66B.2 The Bamford classification of stroke

Arterial territory	Clinical features
Total anterior circulation stroke (TACS)	All of: • Contralateral hemiplegia or severe hemiparesis +/– hemisensory loss • Contralateral hemianopia • New disturbance of higher cerebral function (e.g. dysphasia)
Partial anterior circulation stroke (PACS)	• Motor/sensory deficit and hemianopia • Motor/sensory deficit and new higher cerebral dysfunction • New higher cerebral dysfunction and hemianopia • Pure motor/sensory deficit less extensive than for lacunar syndromes (e.g. monoparesis) • New higher cerebral dysfunction alone (e.g. dysphasia)
Lacunar stroke (LACS)	Four main clinical syndromes: • Pure motor stroke (affecting at least 2 of 3 areas: face, arm, leg) • Pure sensory stroke (affecting at least 2 of 3 areas: face, arm, leg) • Ataxic hemiparesis (including dysarthria–clumsy hand syndrome and ipsilateral ataxia with lower limb paresis) • Sensorimotor stroke
Posterior circulation (POCS)	• Ipsilateral cranial nerve (III–XII) palsy with contralateral motor and/or sensory deficit • Bilateral motor and/or sensory deficit • Disorders of conjugate gaze (horizontal or vertical) • Cerebellar dysfunction without ipsilateral long tract deficit • Isolated hemianopia or cortical blindness

Table 66B.3 Outcome following stroke according to OCSP subtype

Outcome	OCSP subtype			
	TACI	PACI	LACI	POCI
30 days:				
Dead	39%	4%	2%	7%
Dependent*	56%	39%	36%	31%
Independent†	4%	56%	62%	62%
6 months:				
Dead	56%	10%	7%	14%
Dependent	39%	34%	26%	18%
Independent	4%	55%	66%	68%
1 year:				
Dead	60%	16%	11%	19%
Dependent	36%	29%	28%	19%
Independent	4%	55%	60%	62%

TACI: total anterior circulation infarct; PACI: partial anterior circulation infarct; LACI: lacunar infarct; POCS: posterior circulation infarct.

*Rankin score 3–5; †Rankin score 0–2.

Source: Bamford J, Sandercock P, Dennis M, Burn J, Warlow C. Classification and natural history of clinically identifiable subtypes of cerebral infarction. *Lancet* 1991; 337:1521–6.

The benefits of using this clinical classification are that:

- There is reasonable inter-observer reliability.
- It can be a useful predictor of infarct site and give an indication of likely underlying vascular pathology (and thus may guide appropriate investigation, e.g. carotid imaging, cardiac investigations, etc.).
- It is a useful predictor of infarct size, and can provide prognostic information in terms of mortality, long-term disability, and recurrence rates (Table 66B.3).

Investigation

Brain imaging

Timely brain imaging aids confirmation of diagnosis of stroke, identification of possible causes, and initiation of acute treatment. Royal College of Physicians guidelines (2012) recommend [2] that all stroke patients should receive brain imaging within 12 hours of arrival in hospital.

Indications for emergency brain imaging (next available slot, or at least within 1 hour) are as follows:

- symptom onset within 4½ hours (candidate for stroke thrombolysis)
- on anticoagulant treatment (warfarin, heparin, dabigatran, rivaroxaban, apixaban)

- depressed or deteriorating level of consciousness
- known bleeding tendency
- unexplained progressive or fluctuating symptoms
- papilloedema, neck stiffness or fever
- severe headache at onset of symptoms.

CT head

Pros

- Good for excluding acute brain haemorrhage and common mimics (e.g. subdural haematoma).
- Quick to perform, generally well tolerated and widely available.

Cons

- Has relatively low sensitivity (~26%) for detecting infarction in the first few hours.
- May be difficult to differentiate between infarction and haemorrhage a few days after onset.

MRI head

Pros

- Much more sensitive for detection of early ischaemia (~83%), especially using the diffusion-weighted imaging (DWI) and apparent diffusion coefficient map.

Cons

- May be less well tolerated by patients (e.g. if claustrophobic).
- Less widely available.

Other standard investigations

- *Blood tests*: FBC, ESR, U&E, LFT, cholesterol, glucose or HbA_{1c}.
- *12-lead ECG*: may indicate atrial fibrillation, LVH or ischaemic changes.
- *Carotid imaging*: patients with anterior circulation TIA or non-disabling ischaemic stroke.
- *Ambulatory ECG*: primarily to look for paroxysmal atrial fibrillation.
- *Echocardiogram*: if concerns about cardioembolic source; clues to this include abnormal ECG and recent cardiac symptoms, cerebral infarcts in multiple vascular territories, new murmur.

Management of acute ischaemic stroke

Stroke thrombolysis

Intravenous thrombolysis using alteplase (rt-Pa) should only be given in units with appropriately trained staff who know the contraindications to treatment and management of complications.

The major benefit is in *reducing the degree of long-term disability for stroke patients*. Its impact on survival is neutral: while there is an early (<7 days) risk of fatal and non-fatal intracerebral haemorrhage with thrombolysis, mortality at 6 months is not increased compared to patients who do not receive thrombolysis.

Benefits rapidly diminish with time; absolute benefits beyond 4½ hours are unproven. In a pooled meta-analysis of the major stroke thrombolysis trials [3], incorporating 3670 patients, the odds ratio (OR) for a favourable outcome with alteplase were as follows:

- rt-Pa at 0–90 minutes: 2.55 (95% CI 1.44–4.52)
- rt-Pa at 91–180 minutes: 1.64 (95% CI 1.06–1.68)
- rt-Pa at 181–270 minutes: 1.34 (95% CI 1.06–1.68)
- rt-Pa at 271–360 minutes: 1.22 (95% CI 0.92–1.61).

It is now licensed for use up to 4½ hours after stroke onset. While the licence is currently limited to patients aged between 18 and 80 years of age, the Third International Stroke Trial (IST-3) showed that patients over age 80 are as likely to benefit, especially when treated within 3 hours [4].

Recognized contraindications to stroke thrombolysis include:

- unknown time of onset
- known bleeding diathesis, or platelet count <100
- arterial puncture at a non-compressible site, or lumbar puncture, within 7 days
- on anticoagulation with warfarin (and INR >1.7), treatment-dose heparin, or newer oral anticoagulant
- major surgery within the last 14 days
- GI or urinary tract haemorrhage within the last 21 days
- any history of intracranial haemorrhage, brain tumour, intracranial arteriovenous malformation or aneurysm
- seizure at onset
- coma (GCS <8 or NIHSS item 1a score = 3)
- minor stroke symptoms (i.e. non-disabling)
- rapidly improving symptoms or signs (to the point of becoming non-disabling)
- clinical presentation suggestive of subarachnoid haemorrhage
- BP >185/110 in spite of attempts to lower blood pressure
- capillary glucose <2.7 mmol/L
- radiological signs of intracranial haemorrhage or diffuse swelling of cerebral hemisphere.

Potential complications of stroke thrombolysis

- Intracranial haemorrhage – occurs in approximately 4% of cases; may be fatal in up to 3%.
- Extracranial haemorrhage – occurs in approximately 1% of cases.
- Angio-oedema – occurs in approximately 1–2% of cases.

Aspirin

A large systematic review of antiplatelet use after ischaemic stroke showed that for every 1000 patients treated with aspirin there are 13 fewer deaths.

RCP guidelines [2] recommend aspirin 300 mg daily for the first 2 weeks, followed by secondary prevention depending on the aetiology of the stroke. If a patient is thrombolysed, aspirin should be withheld for the first 24 hours.

Surgical intervention

Carotid or middle cerebral artery (MCA) occlusion can result in a large area of infarction. This can lead to malignant swelling of the affected hemisphere (termed 'malignant MCA syndrome'). While it is uncommon, mortality is very high if left untreated.

Decompressive hemicraniectomy can reduce both mortality and disability in selected patients. A meta-analysis of three RCTs showed that it was associated with a number needed to treat (NNT) of 2 to reduce disability [5].

UK guidelines state that patients who meet the following criteria should be referred within 24 hours of stroke onset, and receive surgery within 48 hours:

- Aged ≤60 years
- Clinical deficits suggest infarction in the middle cerebral artery territory
- NIHSS score >15
- Decrease in conscious level to a score of 1 or more on item 1a of NIHSS
- CT signs of infarction of at least 50% of the cerebral hemisphere with or without additional infarction in the territory of the ipsilateral anterior or posterior cerebral artery (or infarct volume >145 cm^3 on DWI-MRI imaging).

Management of intracerebral haemorrhage (ICH)

Primary intracerebral haemorrhage accounts for approximately 10% of all strokes.

In patients on vitamin K antagonists (e.g. warfarin), clotting levels should be returned to normal using a combination of prothrombin complex concentrate and intravenous vitamin K. There is no antidote for the newer oral anticoagulants (e.g. dabigatran, rivaroxaban, apixaban), although they appear to be associated with a lower risk of intracerebral haemorrhage than warfarin.

Surgical intervention is occasionally indicated, especially in the following circumstances:

- small deep haemorrhages
- lobar haemorrhage without either hydrocephalus or rapid neurological deterioration
- a large haemorrhage and significant co-morbidities
- supratentorial haemorrhage with GCS <8, unless due to hydrocephalus.

Surgical intervention may be indicated in the context of hydrocephalus following ICH.

General management for all stroke patients

Stroke unit care

Organized, specialist care on a stroke unit is associated with significant benefit in terms of reduced disability and mortality when compared to standard care on a general medical ward.

The number needed to treat in a specialist stroke unit:

- to prevent one death is 22
- to prevent one patient losing their independence is 16.

In contrast to other interventions in stroke medicine, *this benefit can be offered to all patients.*

Physiological monitoring

There is evidence that implementation of multidisciplinary treatment protocols to manage fever, hyperglycaemia and dysphagia delivers significantly better outcomes in terms of death and dependency. Patients should have:

- regular neurological observations to enable early identification of a treatable complication, such as haemorrhage or hydrocephalus
- supplemental O_2 therapy only if O_2 saturations drop <95% and there is no contraindication
- treatment of hyperglycaemia to maintain blood glucose between 4 and 11 mmol/L.

The role of BP control in acute stroke remains uncertain; arterial hypertension in the acute setting is common, and associated with poor outcome.

- With respect to ischaemic stroke, the SCAST study [6] showed that BP lowering with candesartan had no benefit, and may cause harm.
- In hypertensive (BP >150/90 mmHg) patients with intracerebral haemorrhage, the INTERACT 2 trial [7] showed that early intensive BP lowering (to bring SBP <140 mmHg) is safe and may be associated with improved outcomes (mortality, disability and health-related quality of life).

Routine BP lowering is not recommended in UK guidelines, although these have not been updated since the publication of the INTERACT-2 study. The

RCP (2012) guidelines advise that BP should only be lowered if there is a hypertensive emergency or one or more of the following serious medical issues:

- hypertensive encephalopathy
- hypertensive nephropathy
- hypertensive cardiac failure/myocardial infarction
- aortic dissection
- pre-eclampsia/eclampsia
- intracerebral haemorrhage with systolic blood pressure >200 mmHg.

In patients who are candidates for stroke thrombolysis, BP should be reduced to below 185/110 mmHg. The most common parenteral agent that is used is labetalol.

Dysphagia assessment and management

Dysphagia after stroke is common, and can be associated with an increased risk of pulmonary complications and death. Early detection of dysphagia using a validated swallow screening tool can reduce these complications.

- All stroke patients should have their ability to swallow screened with such a tool (by an appropriately trained person) within 4 hours of hospital admission.
- Patients whose swallow is unsafe should be referred to the speech and language therapist for a more detailed dysphagia assessment. There should be a clear plan for provision of adequate nutrition and hydration. This might involve the use of thickened fluids or a modified-texture diet, or nasogastric tube feeding. The routine use of early gastrostomy tube feeding is not recommended.

Prophylaxis of venous thromboembolism (VTE)

VTE is a common complication of hemiplegic stroke: up to 50% of patients may have thrombus in the calf or thigh of the affected limb. Early mobilization and maintaining adequate hydration may play a role in reducing this risk.

Anticoagulation: prophylactic-dose low molecular weight (LMW) heparin may reduce the risk of VTE, but this benefit is offset by an increased risk of intracerebral haemorrhage. UK stroke guidelines state that anticoagulants should not be routinely used for VTE

prophylaxis. Where an individualized decision is made to use anticoagulants, LMW heparin is recommended over unfractionated heparin.

Mechanical compression: the CLOTS 1 and 2 trials showed no significant benefit from the use of knee- or thigh-length TED stockings. The CLOTS 3 study (published May 2013) showed that intermittent pneumatic compression devices applied to the paretic leg are associated with a significant reduction in both DVT risk and mortality at 6 months [8].

Secondary prevention

The risk of recurrent stroke is highest early after a TIA or stroke: it may be as high as 5% within the first week, and up to 20% within the first month. Therefore secondary prevention should start as soon as possible after the acute period, usually within 1 week of onset.

Antithrombotic treatment

Antiplatelet treatment is associated with a 22% reduction in the odds of a vascular event (MI, stroke or vascular death). The CAPRIE, ESPRIT and PROFESS trials showed that aspirin plus modified-release dipyridamole and clopidogrel monotherapy are equally effective in reducing the recurrent stroke risk. The PROFESS study showed that clopidogrel was better tolerated, with a trend to fewer bleeding events. Both options have been shown to be superior to aspirin monotherapy; in absolute terms this difference equates to one less vascular event per year per 100 patients.

RCP guidelines (2012) recommend [2] for patients with non-cardioembolic ischaemic stroke or TIA:

- Clopidogrel (75 mg daily, after a single loading dose of 300 mg) is recommended as first line.
- If clopidogrel is not tolerated, aspirin 75 mg od and dipyridamole (modified release) 200 mg bd should be used.

If clopidogrel and aspirin are not tolerated, dipyridamole monotherapy may be used.

Atrial fibrillation

Patients with a TIA or stroke who are found to be in atrial fibrillation are at a higher risk of cardioembolic stroke. Risk calculators such as the $CHADS_2$ or CHA_2DS_2VASc score may help stratify this risk.

- Studies show that anticoagulation with warfarin can reduce the recurrent stroke risk by about 68%. Aspirin is poor at reducing this risk; thus anticoagulation is recommended as the standard of treatment. It should not be commenced until brain imaging has excluded haemorrhage, or where the BP is uncontrolled.

- In patients with disabling stroke anticoagulation should usually be deferred for at least 14 days. It should be started immediately after TIA using either LMW heparin or a newer oral anticoagulant. The HAS-BLED tool is a useful aid to determining contraindications to anticoagulation.

Carotid stenosis

Carotid endarterectomy (CEA) is of proven benefit for patients with at least moderate stenosis of the internal carotid artery ipsilateral to the stroke.

- For patients with a severe (>70% by North American Symptomatic Carotid End arterectomy Trial (NASCET) criteria) stenosis, CEA is associated with at least a 15.6% absolute risk reduction in ipsilateral stroke over 5 years. For those with a moderate (50–69% by NASCET criteria) stenosis, the absolute risk reduction is 4.5%.

RCP guidelines [2] state that, for patients with non-disabling stroke or TIA, CEA should be performed within 1 week of symptom onset.

Blood pressure

BP reduction after TIA or stroke prevents further vascular events.

- The PROGRESS study showed that the use of two antihypertensive agents reduced BP by 12/5 mmHg, and resulted in a 42% reduction in recurrent stroke, and a 35% reduction in major coronary events.
- RCP guidelines recommend a target clinic BP <130/80 mmHg, except in patients with severe bilateral carotid stenosis, where the target systolic BP should be 130–150 mmHg.

For patients aged <55 years or African/Caribbean patients of any age:

- Start treatment with a long-acting calcium-channel blocker or thiazide-like diuretic.
- If target BP is not achieved, add an ACE inhibitor or angiotensin-II receptor blocker.

For patients aged >55 years and not of African/Caribbean origin:

- Start treatment with an ACE inhibitor or angiotensin-II receptor blocker.

Lipid-lowering treatment

The SPARCL trial [9] showed that statin treatment in patients with TIA or stroke is associated with a relative risk reduction of 15% for recurrent stroke, and 35% for major coronary events.

UK guidelines recommend:

- Offer statin (e.g. simvastatin 40 mg nocte) to all patients with TIA or ischaemic stroke unless contraindicated; aim for total cholesterol <4 mmol/L and LDL-cholesterol <2 mmol/L.
- Avoid statin therapy in patients with recent intracerebral haemorrhage, or use with caution if it is required for other indications.

References

1. Bamford J, Sandercock P, Dennis M, Burn J, Warlow C. Classification and natural history of clinically identifiable subtypes of cerebral infarction. *Lancet* 1991; 337: 1521–1526.

2. National Clinical Guidelines for Stroke, 4th edn. Royal College of Physicians; 2012.

3. Lees KR, Bluhmki E, von Kummer R et al. Time to treatment with intravenous alteplase and outcome in stroke: an updated pooled analysis of ECASS, ATLANTIS, NINDS, and EPITHET trials. *Lancet* 2010; 375: 1695–1703.

4. The IST-3 Collaborative Group. The benefits and harms of intravenous thrombolysis with recombinant tissue plasminogen activator within 6 hours of acute ischaemic stroke (the third international stroke trial [IST-3]): a randomised controlled trial. *Lancet* 2012; 379: 2352–2363.

5. Vahedi K, Hofmeijer J, Juettler E, et al. Early decompressive surgery in malignant infarction of the middle cerebral artery: a pooled analysis of three randomised controlled trials. *Lancet Neurol* 2007; 6: 215–222.

6. Sandset EC, Bath PM, Boysen G, et al., SCAST Study Group. The angiotensin-receptor blocker candesartan for treatment of acute stroke (SCAST): a randomised, placebo-controlled, double-blind trial. *Lancet* 2011; 377: 741–750.

7. Anderson CS, Heeley E, Huang Y, et al. Rapid blood-pressure lowering in patients with acute intracerebral haemorrhage. *N Engl J Med* 2013; 368: 2355–2365.

8. CLOTS Trials Collaboration. Effectiveness of intermittent pneumatic compression in reduction of risk of deep vein thrombosis in patients who have had a stroke (CLOTS 3): a multicentre randomised controlled trial. *Lancet* 2013; 382(9891):516–24.

9. The Stroke Prevention by Aggressive Reduction in Cholesterol Levels (SPARCL) Investigators. High-dose atorvastatin after stroke or transient ischemic attack. *N Engl J Med* 2006; 355: 549–559.

Further reading

Edlow JA, Selim MH. Atypical presentations of acute cerebrovascular syndromes. *Lancet Neurol* 2011; 10: 550–560.

McArthur KS, Quinn TJ, Dawson J, Walters MR. Diagnosis and management of transient ischaemic attack and ischaemic stroke in the acute phase. *BMJ* 2011; 342: d1938.

McArthur KS, Quinn TJ, Higgins P, Langhorne P. Post-acute care and secondary prevention after ischaemic stroke. *BMJ* 2011; 342: d2038.

Nor AM, Davis J, Sen B, Shipsey D, Louw SJ, Dyker AG, Davis M, Ford GA. The Recognition of Stroke in the Emergency Room (ROSIER) scale: development and validation of a stroke recognition instrument. *Lancet Neurol* 2005; 4: 727–734.

Warlow C, et al. *Stroke – Practical Management*, 3rd edn. Blackwell Publishing; 2008.

Weight loss

Emma Greig

Introduction and background

The basic mechanism of weight loss is simple: *reduced energy absorption or increased energy expenditure.* Weight loss may be voluntary, including a deliberate weight-reducing diet or increase in exercise, or involuntary, with progressive involuntary weight loss indicating a potentially serious medical or psychosocial problem.

Scenario 67.1

An 80-year-old woman is admitted from the community at the request of her GP. She has been visited by her niece who lives in another part of the country. This niece was horrified by her aunt's appearance as she has lost several stones in weight since her husband's funeral. While there is very little food in the house, it is unclear whether there are other reasons for her weight loss. You need to urgently assess the patient regarding the causes of weight loss, make a plan for investigation and management and assess nutritional status to include a safe feeding regime.

Clinical assessment

While weight loss is seldom the primary reason for admission, it is clinically important if 5% of body weight has been lost over 6 months and must be investigated if loss is >10%. An involuntary loss of >20% is frequently associated with nutritional deficiencies, protein-energy malnutrition and multi-organ dysfunction. However, weight loss is a crude measurement with no distinction between reduction in fat and lean muscle tissue. Sarcopenia is age-related loss of muscle mass, which contributes significantly to reduced mobility and independence in the elderly [1]. This contrasts with loss of body fat, which often improves clinical outcomes in e.g. diabetes mellitus.

How to assess for malnutrition

- Assessment of malnutrition risk should be carried out within 24 hours of arrival in hospital by nursing staff. The Malnutrition Universal Screening Tool (MUST) is a five-step validated assessment tool for adults encompassing:
  - percentage weight loss
  - acute disease effect (illness and factors which may temporarily prevent oral intake)
  - body mass index (which requires a height and weight).

The output is a score which reflects malnutrition risk and creates a management plan [2].

- Significant weight loss or MUST >2 prompts timely interventions including fortified foods, dietetics review, sip supplements or, for more intractable problems, consideration of enteral or parenteral feeding.
- Always consider and prevent refeeding syndrome when planning nutritional intervention.
- There are no serological markers of malnutrition: *low serum albumin invariably reflects acute phase responses* including sepsis or surgery rather than malnutrition.

History

- *Is weight loss intentional or unintentional?* Intentional weight loss in a non-obese patient may indicate anorexia nervosa so sensitive questions should be asked.
- *Has there been a change in calorie intake?*
- *Are they avoiding certain foods?* Avoidance of wheat/gluten may indicate coeliac disease; avoidance of fibre may suggests stricturing disease

---

Acute Medicine, ed. Stephen Haydock, Duncan Whitehead and Zoë Fritz. Published by Cambridge University Press. © Cambridge University Press 2015.

in small bowel (Crohn's disease or gastrointestinal malignancy) while avoiding solid food boluses (bread and meat) may indicate oesophageal strictures.

- *Has their appetite changed?* A decrease in appetite is common and short-lived in many infections but also occurs in upper gastrointestinal (GI) conditions including malignancy and peptic ulceration.
- *Is there increased appetite with weight loss?* Consider hyperthyroidism, uncontrolled diabetes mellitus, malabsorption (usually associated with diarrhoea).
- *What is the actual weight loss?* Corroborative evidence of the usual weight from previous clinical contacts is helpful; ask about looser fit of clothes/jewellery.
- *Is weight loss progressive or has it stabilized?*
- *Are there associated symptoms* of vomiting, diarrhoea or abdominal pain indicating a primary GI cause?
- *Is dysphagia (difficulty in swallowing) present?* Distinguish from odynophagia (pain on swallowing).
- *Is there evidence of dementia?* Think about a mini-mental test score.
- *Is there evidence of anxiety or depression?* Be aware that anxiety or phobia about a potential diagnosis of cancer may itself lead to weight loss.
- Obtain an accurate drug history and include over-the-counter and herbal preparations: many medications may temporarily affect weight (see Table 67.1).
- For elderly patients and those with physical or mental frailties, it is important to ask about recent changes in family circumstances. The ability to perform activities of daily living including shopping, food preparation and eating may be temporarily or permanently disrupted by the death of a spouse or incapacity of others who have undertaken these roles.
- Remember dentition: are there difficulties with chewing? In elderly patients, poor fitting or lost dentures limit the number and type of calories consumed.
- If the cause of weight loss remains elusive, a thorough review of systems helps determine any organic pathology as disease processes leading to weight loss can involve all body systems (see Table 67.1).

Examination

There are many physical causes of unexplained weight loss. Look for primary organic disease but also physical findings associated with nutritional deficiency (see Table 67.2).

- Perform a thorough examination looking for signs of malignancy. The probability of abnormal physical findings is >55% for those with malignancy, but 3% for those with a psychiatric disorder [3].
- Measure height and weight to establish body mass index (BMI). For patients who cannot stand, ulnar length, knee height and demispan estimate height while mid-upper arm circumference estimates weight using a conversion chart [2].
- Presence or absence of oedema may alter dry weight by 2–5 kg.
- Examine teeth for signs of dental enamel erosion from persistent vomiting (bulimia or part of disease process).

Investigations to consider

Blood tests

- Initial tests: FBC, U&E, creatinine, glucose, LFT, TSH, C-reactive protein, ESR, calcium. Further investigations are dictated by the results from this initial screen.
- If the patient is at risk of malnutrition, *baseline bloods for refeeding syndrome are essential*: magnesium, phosphate and potassium.
- A nutritional screen is helpful before enteral or parenteral feeding starts: zinc, selenium, ferritin, B_{12}, red cell folate, vitamins A, D, E and INR (a functional assay for vitamin K status).
- If anaemia (iron deficiency +/– folate deficiency) with or without GI symptoms, consider coeliac antibody testing using anti-tissue transglutaminase antibodies (tTG). If tTG levels are raised or if tTG levels are normal and IgA low, then consider requesting duodenal biopsies to make a formal diagnosis of coeliac disease.

Urine

- Dipstick urine and culture (if evidence of infection).

Table 67.1 Causes of weight loss

	Involuntary weight loss	Voluntary weight loss
Drugs	Alcohol Opiates Amphetamines/cocaine Drug withdrawal (psychotropic medication/cannabis) Adverse effects of prescription drugs: topiramate, SSRIs, levodopa, digoxin, metformin, exenatide, liraglutide, NSAIDs, cytotoxics, antiretrovirals Herbal and non-prescription drugs: caffeine, dandelion, herbal diuretics, nicotine, St John's wort, guarana, 5-hydroxytryptophan, aloe	Prescription drugs for treating obesity: orlistat, sibutramine, metformin Drugs abused in weight loss: amphetamines, thyroxine, caffeine, dandelion, herbal diuretics, nicotine, St John's wort, guarana, 5-hydroxytryptophan, aloe
Medical disorders	Malignancy (GI, lung, lymphoma, renal, prostate, breast) GI diseases: peptic ulcers, Crohn's disease, coeliac disease, gastroparesis, ulcerative colitis, dysphagia (any cause) Endocrine diseases: hyperthyroidism, diabetes mellitus, adrenal insufficiency Infectious diseases: HIV, viral hepatitis, TB, lung abscess End-stage cardiac disease causing cardiac cachexia Severe lung disease: obstructive or restrictive Renal disease: nephrotic syndrome, chronic glomerulonephritis, renal failure Neurological conditions such as stroke, dementia, Parkinson's disease, motor neurone disease Chronic inflammatory conditions, e.g. severe rheumatoid arthritis	
Psychiatric disorders	Food-related delusions as part of any psychiatric disorder Depression Generalized anxiety disorder Bipolar disorder Dementia	Anorexia nervosa Bulimia nervosa
Lifestyle	Especially elderly: Social isolation (reduces calories eaten) Financial limitations Problems with teeth/chewing	Dieting Chronic vigorous exercise (often with dieting), e.g. distance runners, gymnasts

Radiology

- *Chest radiograph*: useful to diagnose primary or secondary malignancy, TB, chest sepsis, lymphadenopathy.
- *Abdominal ultrasound scan*: useful for primary and secondary malignancy in liver, pancreatic disease, significant lymphadenopathy.
- *CT scan* (chest, abdomen and pelvis) should be reserved for the most significant weight loss (>10%) or for those where physical examination suggests a malignant cause.

Management

- Whatever the cause, supportive therapy using additional calories is essential alongside investigation and management of underlying organic or psychosocial causes.

- *If the gut works, you should use it!* Oral intake should be first line with enteral tube feeding next, then parenteral (intravenous) feeding only if the gut has failed.
- Involve a dietitian at an early stage to determine individual nutritional requirements, which are the same whichever route is chosen to supplement calories. Use a food chart to measure the volume and type of food consumed.
- Remember to determine individual refeeding risk as this establishes how quickly artificial feeding can proceed.

Refeeding syndrome

- Potentially life-threatening shifts in fluid and electrolytes occur when a patient with malnutrition is given artificial feeding.

Table 67.2 Physical signs in micronutrient and macronutrient deficiency

Tissue	Sign	Suspected or possible deficiency
Hair	Corkscrew and coiled hairs which have not emerged from a keratinized follicle	Vitamin C deficiency (scurvy)
	Flag sign – depigmentation of hair in a linear stripe corresponding to times of nutritional stress	Protein-calorie malnutrition (mainly protein)
	Hair pluckability (easy pluckability of >3 hairs painlessly from the crown)	Protein-calorie malnutrition (mainly protein)
Mouth	Angular stomatitis/cheilitis (sores at the side of the mouth and inflammation of the lips, respectively)	Iron deficiency and/or pyridoxine, riboflavin or niacin deficiency
Tongue	Glossitis (absence of papillae)	Iron, B_{12} or folate deficiency
Eyes	Xerophthalmia	Vitamin A deficiency
Teeth	Gingivitis with swollen, retracted and bleeding gums	Vitamin C deficiency (scurvy)
Skin	Perifollicular petechiae	Vitamin C deficiency
	Purpura and bruising	Vitamin C and/or vitamin K deficiency
	Scaly dermatitis	Vitamin A deficiency or excess, zinc deficiency and essential fatty acid deficiency
	Dermatitis with hypo- and hyper-pigmentation	Niacin deficiency (pellagra)
	Pitting oedema	Possible protein-calorie malnutrition (mainly protein)
	Pressure ulcer	Protein calorie malnutrition (mainly protein)

Adapted from: Morgan SL (1996) Nutritional assessment of patients. In: *A Diagnostic Guide to Clinical Gastroenterology.* Eds. Kumar D, Christensen J. Churchill Livingstone, New York.

- Hallmark feature is hypophosphataemia, but hypomagnesaemia, hypokalaemia, alterations in sodium and fluid balance and disordered glucose, protein and fat metabolism may occur [4].
- In starvation, the body switches from carbohydrate to protein and fat metabolism so reintroducing carbohydrate increases insulin and decreases glucagon. This stimulates glycogen, fat and protein synthesis requiring phosphate and other co-factors. Insulin stimulates transporters moving potassium, magnesium and phosphate into cells, lowering serum levels which may precipitate cardiac dysfunction and arrhythmias.
- Particularly high risk of refeeding syndrome with one or more of:
  - BMI <16 kg/m^2
  - involuntary weight loss of >15% in 3–6 months
  - little or no nutritional intake for >10 days
  - low baseline potassium, phosphate and magnesium.
- Moderate risk of refeeding if any two of:
  - BMI <18.5 kg/m^2
  - involuntary weight loss >10% in 3–6 months

- little or no nutritional intake for 5 days
- history of alcohol misuse or medications including insulin, antacids, chemotherapy or diuretics.

Treatment/avoidance

- Start feeding at 5–10 kcal/kg body weight/24 hours with careful rehydration and individually tailored increases to full feeding over 4–7 days depending on daily blood results (potassium, magnesium, phosphate).
- Consider cardiac monitoring in light of the arrhythmia risk, especially if electrolyte levels are particularly low.
- Replace electrolytes orally, enterally or parenterally depending on serum levels, local guidelines and their likely absorption. Use 2–4 mmol/kg per day for potassium, 0.3–0.6 mmol/kg per day for phosphate and 0.2 mmol/kg per day for intravenous magnesium and 0.4 mmol/kg per day for oral magnesium with daily blood tests to assess and monitor.
- Do not delay feeding to correct electrolytes first; do this alongside starting nutrition.

Table 67.3 How to place a nasogastric (NG) tube

1. Explain the procedure to the patient – obtain verbal consent
2. Mark the tube at a distance from xiphisternum to nose via the tip of the earlobe (this is usually 50–60 cm)
3. Lubricate the tube by dipping the end into water, and check that the guidewire moves easily within the tube
4. Ask the patient if either nostril is blocked or if they have a preference
5. Sit the patient upright with the head level and pass the tube into the preferred nostril directly backwards to about 10–15 cm
6. If able to swallow safely, ask them to take a sip of water then swallow when you say so, advancing the tube as they swallow
7. If there are no problems, continue to advance the tube to the mark made earlier
8. Stop advancing and withdraw the tube at any stage if the patient is distressed, cyanosed or coughing as this suggests that the tube is in the bronchial tree
9. If there is difficulty with swallowing the tube, the patient could tip their head forward at the critical moment
10. Once in place, remove the guidewire and test a gastric aspirate using pH paper
11. Document tube placement in the notes including pH of the aspirate, the depth of insertion in cm and also the length of tube outside the patient
12. If you need to check an X-ray due to problems with not obtaining an aspirate or getting an aspirate where pH >5, then ensure you have received specific training in X-ray interpretation. There is a helpful online module [7]

- Vitamins/minerals: before feeding, give at least the first dose of either oral thiamine 200–300 mg/daily or intravenous thiamine (Pabrinex vials 1 and 2 tds for 72 hrs) along with vitamin B compound-strong 1–2 tablets daily and a multivitamin and trace element preparation. Continue all vitamins/minerals for at least 10 days [5].

Oral intake

- Dietitians' advice may include supplemented foods using calorie-dense products including cheese, custard and biscuits. The next line is sip supplements using cartons which are high in calories and protein (such as Fortisips or Ensure) or small volume supplements including Calogen and Procal.

Enteral feeding

- Enteral tube feeding, using nasogastric (NG) or percutaneous endoscopic gastrostomy (PEG) tube, is a medical treatment by law so starting, stopping or withholding feeding is a medical decision. The wishes of a competent patient must be taken into account but in cases where the patient is not competent to decide, consult family, carers, their GP to make a decision in the patient's best interests [6].
- In cases where it is unclear that the patient will benefit from feeding, then consider a limited 2-week trial of feeding, taking care to explain the parameters to relatives and carers.
- A dietitian should supervise all enteral feeding with an individually tailored plan to support calorie intake.

- Indications include:
  - swallowing disorders (post-stroke, multiple sclerosis, Parkinson's disease, motor neurone disease)
  - unconscious patients (post-head injury or ventilated patients)
  - upper GI obstruction (oesophageal strictures)
  - partial intestinal failure (postoperative ileus, inflammatory bowel disease, short bowel syndrome)
  - increased nutritional requirements (cirrhotic liver disease, cystic fibrosis, renal disease)
  - psychological problems (depression or anorexia nervosa).
- NG feeding is most appropriate in the short term. See Table 67.3 for advice on placement. Feeding using a misplaced nasogastric tube is considered a '*never event*', so extreme care must be taken to check the position of an NG tube before feed or drug administration [8]. Beware timing of acid-suppressing medications such as proton pump inhibitors and H_2-receptor antagonists as these will affect pH.
- Consider PEG placement if tube feeding will be required for >4–6 weeks. Ethical issues are even more important and patients must be reviewed by a nutrition support team ideally led by a consultant gastroenterologist.
- Aspiration of gastric contents can occur despite correctly placed NG and PEG tubes so the patient should lie at >30° angle during feeding and for 30 minutes afterwards. Consider a prokinetic

(metoclopramide or domperidone) if gastric emptying appears impaired.

- Other complications of enteral feeding include diarrhoea, bloating and nausea.
- Nasojejunal feeding tubes and surgically placed jejunostomies are useful for post-pyloric feeding in cases of gastric outlet obstruction (peptic ulceration or malignancy) and delayed gastric emptying (gastroparesis). Involve a gastroenterologist or GI surgeon if needed.

Parenteral nutrition (PN)

- PN is used to manage patients with intestinal failure resulting from intestinal resection or disease-associated malabsorption characterized by the inability to maintain protein-energy, fluid, electrolyte or micronutrient balance.
- Short-term hospital PN indications include postoperative ileus or small bowel fistulas while indications for longer-term home PN include surgical complications such as short bowel syndrome or vascular insufficiency and disorders of gut motility [9].

Complications of PN

- Infection: particularly line sepsis as PN is administered centrally and requires scrupulous asepsis. If line sepsis is suspected, *paired central and peripheral blood cultures are essential and the line should not be used until infection is ruled out.*
- Liver disease: especially in patients with a short gut who may develop liver failure.
- Gallstones.
- Catheter occlusion.
- Central venous thrombosis.
- Nephrolithiasis.

References

1. Cruz-Jentoft AJ, Baeyens JP, Bauer JM, et al. (2010) Sarcopenia: European consensus on definition and diagnosis. Report of the European Working Group on Sarcopenia in Older People. *Age Ageing* 39: 412–423.

2. Malnutrition Advisory Group as subgroup of British Association of Parenteral and Enteral Nutrition (2004) Malnutrition Universal Screening Tool. www.bapen. org.uk/pdfs/must/must_full.pdf.

3. Metalidis C, Knockaret DC, Bobbaers H, Vanderschueren S (2008) Involuntary weight loss. Does a negative baseline evaluation provide adequate reassurance? *Eur J Int Med* 19: 345.

4. Mehanna HM, Moledina J, Travis J (2008) Refeeding syndrome: what is it and how to prevent and treat it. *Br Med J* 336: 1495–1498.

5. National Institute for Health and Care Excellence (2006) Nutrition support in adults. Clinical guideline CG32. nice.org.uk/page.aspx?o=cg032.

6. Stroud M, Duncan H, Nightingale J (2003) Guidelines for enteral feeding in adult hospital patients. *Gut* 52(Suppl VII): vii1–vii12.

7. Law R, Bennett J (2011) Reducing the risk of feeding through a misplaced nasogastric tube. PowerPoint presentation with a multiple choice questionnaire to test knowledge. www.trainingngt.co.uk/site/home.aspx.

8. National Patients Safety Agency. Patient Safety Alert NPSA/2011/PSA002: Reducing the harm caused by misplaced nasogastric feeding tubes in adults, children and infants. March 2011. www.npsa.nhs.uk/corporate/news/reducing-the-harm-caused-by-misplaced-nasogastric-feeding-tubes-in-adults-children-and-infants/.

9. Lal S, Teubner A, Shaffer J (2006) Review article: intestinal failure. *Aliment Pharmacol Ther* 24: 19–31.

Index

Note: page numbers in *italics* refer to figures and tables, those in **bold** refer to boxes